Introduction to Ultrasound

William J. Zwiebel, M.D.
Professor of Radiology
University of Utah School of Medicine
Chief, Imaging Service
Department of Veterans Affairs
Medical Center
Salt Lake City, Utah

Roya Sohaey, M.D.
Assistant Professor of Radiology
University of Utah School of Medicine
Salt Lake City, Utah
Co-Director, Women's Imaging
Grand Valley Radiology
Holland, Michigan

W.B. SAUNDERS COMPANY
A Division of Harcourt Brace & Company
Philadelphia   London   Toronto   Montreal   Sydney   Tokyo

W.B. SAUNDERS COMPANY
A Division of Harcourt Brace & Company

The Curtis Center
Independence Square West
Philadelphia, Pennsylvania 19106

Library of Congress Cataloging-in-Publication Data

Introduction to Ultrasound / William J. Zwiebel, Roya Sohaey.

p.   cm.

ISBN 0–7216–6947–6

1. Diagnosis, Ultrasonic.   I. Sohaey, Roya.   II. Title.
   [DNLM: 1. Ultrasonography—methods. WN 208Z98i 1998]

RC78.7.U4Z95   1998

616.07′543—dc20

DNLM/DLC   96-18778

INTRODUCTION TO ULTRASOUND   ISBN 0–7216–6947–6

Printed in the United States of America.

Last digit is the print number: 9   8   7   6   5   4   3   2   1

To my wife, Margaret Batson, M.S., C.N.M., who endured years of this project while mothering our young children, Colin and Aaron, with great love and expertise.

W.J.Z.

To my husband, David Boston, M.D., for taking unsurpassed care of everything else (especially Brett and Haley) while I took care of this book; and to my father, Manutchehr Sohaey, M.D., whose pursuit of education led him thousands of miles from home and provided me with unlimited opportunities.

R.S.

Preface

A monumental epic; more than ten years in the making! You might think we are talking about a Cecil B. De Mille classic film, but in fact we are talking about this book. In 1986, I (W.J.Z.) started working on a general ultrasound textbook with a colleague at the University of Utah. At that time, encyclopedic ultrasound tomes and bare-bones primers were in print, but there was nothing in between. A textbook was needed that had reasonable depth, yet could be read in the course of a one- or two-month training rotation. So work was begun on the "ideal" ultrasound textbook, and it was assumed that the project could be completed in one year. This timeframe, needless to say, grossly underestimated the size of the task! To begin with, the ultrasound literature proved to be far more vast than the authors had ever imagined. Then there was the not-so-simple task of condensing all of that information into a concise package. Finally, there was the reality of locating, photographing, and labeling thousands of illustrations. The one-year deadline quickly slipped away and then faded from memory. Subsequently, the textbook project was shelved because Dr. Zwiebel acquired an oppressive clinical load and his coauthor entered a community radiology practice, reluctantly giving up the project. The book was revived in 1992, with Roya Sohaey as coauthor. The timeframe for completing the text, once again, was wildly optimistic. (Some people never learn!) But at long last, the ultrasound textbook was finished in 1997.

We are very happy with the product, and we hope you will be happy with it as well. We have remained true to our objective of producing a relatively brief, readable text, packed with as much information as possible. To accomplish this goal, we have focused on clinically relevant material, and we have presented this material with concise syntax that goes directly "to the point." Instead of composing reams of text, we have frequently let illustrations "tell the whole story." Similarly, we have used lists and tables widely to condense factual details and to summarize key points.

Because of our efforts to be concise, certain subjects are noticeably abbreviated. For instance, we do not dwell on the "deeper" aspects of ultrasound physics. Basic physical principles are included that are essential for operating an ultrasound machine, but these principles are presented in a clinically relevant, non-mathematical format. We also do not dwell on ultrasound scanning techniques, feeling that ultrasound scanning is learned through practice and not by reading a book. The essential components of specific ultrasound examinations *are* presented, however, in tabular form.

In addition to being concise and factual, we have written this text in language that is suitable for technologists in training as well as for physicians. Technical, anatomic, and pathologic terms are extensively defined and illustrated throughout the text, and the writing, overall, is at a fairly basic level. To further the goal of making this text accessible to technologists, we have asked the publishers to keep the price reasonable. This objective has necessitated grouping the color illustrations in a "well." We realize that this arrangement is inconvenient, but publishing color illustrations throughout the text would at least double the price of the book, possibly making it too expensive for trainees.

Writing a medical textbook is an arduous and seemingly interminable task. The readers are the primary beneficiaries of this effort, but the authors also benefit educationally to a degree unappreciated by most readers! As any instructor knows, "digesting" teaching material is an excellent way to assimilate knowledge. Stated differently, you have to know something pretty well before you can teach it. Although the original coauthor of this text gave up this project with sadness, he did not regret the effort expended, considering how much he had learned in the process. We understand his feelings. Although writing this textbook has been a long and sometimes painful task, the effort has greatly expanded our clinical capabilities. We hope that the readers benefit proportionally from our efforts.

William J. Zwiebel, M.D.
Roya Sohaey, M.D.

Acknowledgments

Many individuals helped with this project, but I am particularly grateful to the following: Don Cubberly, M.D., radiologist with Inland Imaging, Spokane, Washington, the original coauthor of this text; Susan Cole, R.V.T., Vascular Laboratory Technical Director, Bristol Royal Infirmary, Bristol, England, who kindly shared her office with me in 1992; Peter N. T. Wells, Ph.D., Professor and Chairman, Department of Medical Physics and Bioengineering, University of Bristol (England), who hosted the sabbatical that got this project restarted; Janet Carne, of the same department, for speedy and accurate transcription; Dixie Zumwalt, Imaging Service, Salt Lake City Veterans Affairs Medical Center, for transcription, correspondence, and for handling the myriad details associated with writing a textbook; and, finally, the excellent medical illustrators, Julian Maack, Medical Illustrations Service, University of Utah Medical Center, and Alex James, freelance illustrator, Bristol, England.

W.J.Z.

I am most grateful to my radiology partner, Paula Woodward, M.D., for her support and encouragement throughout this long project. She was generous with her time and enthusiasm, and I couldn't have done it without her. I am especially appreciative of our excellent sonographers at the University of Utah Medical Center, Becky Weintraub, Catherine Townsend, Ruth Zollinger, Lezlie Morrison, Diane Engelby, and Jillyn Myers, for their image contributions and patience. I profusely thank Renate Hulen for her secretarial magic. Finally, I wish to acknowledge the outstanding artistic skills of Julian Maack, Director, Medical Illustrations Service, University of Utah Medical Center.

R.S.

Contents

Section 1
Basics

INTRODUCTION

One begins, of course, with the basics. In the field of diagnostic ultrasound, the basics are physics, instrumentation, and safety, and all three of these subjects are addressed in this section. Practitioners of diagnostic sonography, by and large, have limited backgrounds in physics and engineering, and for this reason the two chapters that make up this section are *really* basic. The goal here is to convey fundamental concepts about diagnostic ultrasound in such a way that they can be understood by virtually anyone, including the authors. More sophisticated readers may be disappointed in the content of these chapters, but these individuals will be pleased to know that numerous highly technical sources exist from which they can obtain additional information.

Chapter 1

Basic Ultrasound Physics and Instrumentation

William J. Zwiebel

Ultrasound physics and instrumentation[1-5] are reviewed briefly in this chapter, principally in the format of captioned illustrations. This is an unusual approach for teaching ultrasound physics, but I feel that this method conveys the concepts of ultrasound physics well and is relatively painless.

Physicists or engineers reading this chapter may be horrified to find that only a few mathematical formulas are presented! I have avoided the use of mathematical formulas because the majority of medical personnel have not been trained to think in mathematical terms. A mathematical format, therefore, can make ultrasound physics seem more complicated than necessary.

DEFINITIONS

A few definitions are in order at the outset. Please review these briefly now and return to them as needed as you proceed through this and the following chapter.

B-mode—Abbreviation for "brightness modulation mode," which is the basis for all ultrasound images. Echoes are converted into bright dots that vary in intensity (are modulated) according to the strength of the echo.

Farfield—The portion of the ultrasound image distant from the transducer.*

Frame rate—The rate at which the image on an ultrasound display screen (television monitor) is renewed. The frame rate must exceed 20 frames per second to avoid image "flickering."

Frequency—The number of ultrasound waves per second (Fig. 1–1).

Gray scale—The display of various levels of echo brightness in shades of gray; as opposed to a "bistable" display in which only black and white are shown.

Nearfield—The portion of the ultrasound image near the transducer.*

Pulse echo sonography—Ultrasound technique using a single transducer to send short bursts (or pulses) of ultrasound into the body and alternately "listen" for echoes.

Pulse repetition frequency—The number of ultrasound pulses sent into the body per second.

RADAR—Abbreviation for "radio detection and ranging."

Range—Technical synonym for "distance."

Real time—Abbreviated term meaning "in real time"; that is, movement is depicted on the display screen as it occurs, without an appreciable delay.

Scanhead—The composite of the ultrasound crystal, its electrical attachments, and its housing. In short, the entire ultrasound sending and receiving device that comes into contact with the patient.

Scanner—The entire ultrasound instrument, including the scanhead.

SONAR—Abbreviation for "sound navigation and ranging."

Sonography—The process of generating images with ultrasound (analogous to the term "photography").

Transducer—A device that converts one form of energy into another. The ultrasound crystal is the heart of the transducer. It converts electrical energy to ultrasound (mechanical energy) and vice versa.

---

*These terms are defined here in a general sense. Nearfield and farfield actually refer to specific portions of an ultrasound beam, which is beyond the scope of this chapter.

Two-dimensional image—An image that has width and height. Photographs and television images are two-dimensional.

Ultrasound—Sound that exceeds a frequency level of 2000 cycles per second (2 kilohertz).[1] For medical diagnosis, ultrasound frequencies of 2.5 to 10 million cycles per second (2–10 megahertz) are used commonly.

Wavelength—The distance encompassed by each ultrasound wave (Fig. 1–1).

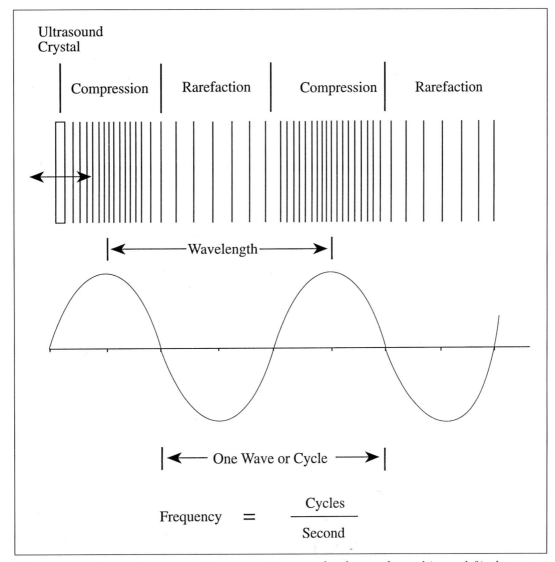

Figure 1-1—Illustration of an Ultrasound Wave. As the ultrasound crystal (upper left) vibrates, it sends an ultrasound *wave* into the body that consists of alternating *compression* and *rarefaction* zones (that is, the tissues are alternately compressed and stretched as the wave passes through).

The ultrasound wave can be illustrated as a graph, as seen in the midportion of this figure. Each complete "wave" or cycle contains one compression and one rarefaction zone, and each wave is represented on the graph as one peak and one valley. The *wavelength* is the distance between consecutive peaks (as shown here), consecutive valleys, or consecutive crossings of the baseline.

The *frequency* is the number of waves (or cycles) per second. The term *hertz*° is commonly used when referring to frequency. One cycle per second equals 1 hertz (Hz); therefore, 1000 cycles per second equals a kilohertz (KHz) and 1,000,000 cycles per second equals a megahertz (MHz). When we say that a certain ultrasound transducer operates at 5 megahertz, we are using shorthand meaning that it operates at 5 million cycles per second.

°This term honors a famous German physicist named Hertz (not the car rental company).

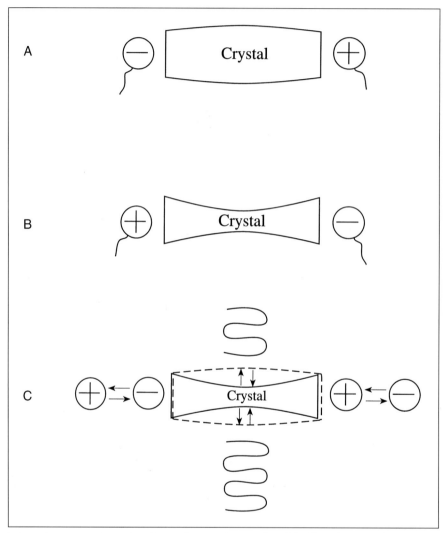

Figure 1-2—Ultrasound Production. Ultrasound is produced by the vibration of a synthetic crystal that possesses *piezoelectric* properties. When an electrical potential is applied to a piezoelectric crystal, it either expands (**A**) or contracts (**B**), depending on the polarity of the electrical connections. Ultrasound is generated when a rapidly alternating electrical potential causes the crystal to vibrate (**C**).

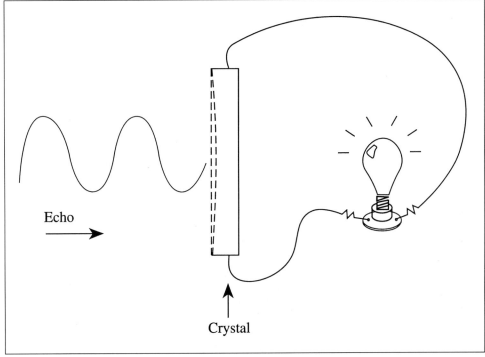

Figure 1-3—Ultrasound Reception. Ultrasound "echoes" reflected from objects within the body are detected by the same piezoelectric crystal that produced the ultrasound waves. The returning waves deform the crystal, generating a minute electrical potential that is sensed by the instrument and recorded electronically. This electrical potential is exceedingly weak and could not possibly light a light bulb, as facetiously shown here.

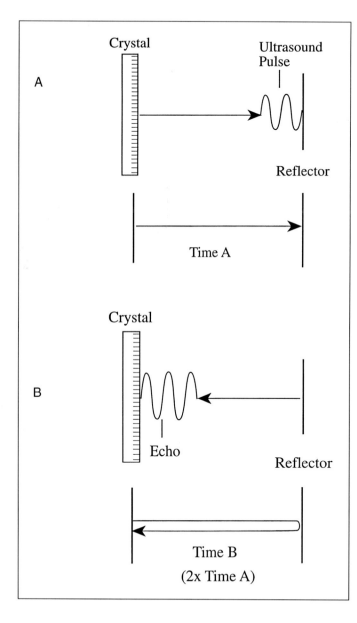

Figure 1-4—Pulse-Echo Sonography. For most medical applications, the piezoelectric crystal is stimulated electrically for only very short periods and produces, therefore, brief "pulses" of ultrasound (**A**). The ultrasound crystal then "listens" for echoes from structures within the body (**B**). Ultrasound pulses are very short; and the listening period is about 1000 times longer than the sending period.

For a businessperson, time is money, but for an ultrasound instrument, time is distance; that is to say, distance is measured as the *transit time* of the ultrasound pulse—from the ultrasound crystal to a reflector and then back to the crystal (Time B in part **B**). The *longer* the transit time, the *greater* the distance from the crystal to the reflector. To calculate distance, the instrument assumes that ultrasound travels through soft tissues at a uniform velocity of 1540 meters per second.[2] Transmission velocity actually is not uniform for all soft tissues, but image distortion resulting from velocity variation usually is insignificant.

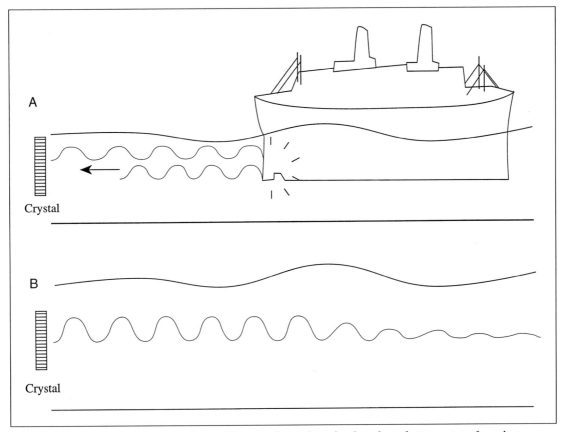

Figure 1-5—Reflecting Interfaces. Ultrasound is reflected only at boundaries, or *interfaces*, between two materials that have *different* acoustic properties. **(A)** Ultrasound pulses transmitted throughout the ocean are reflected when they strike a ship, since the steel from which the ship is made has vastly different acoustic properties than the adjacent water. **(B)** If ultrasound pulses traveling through the ocean do not encounter a ship, or anything other than water, they will travel outward until they fade from existence (from frictional forces), and they never will return to the transducer.

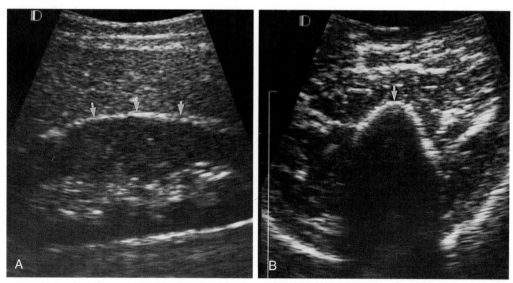

Figure 1-6—Echo Strength, Factor 1. A major factor affecting echo strength is the *degree* to which the acoustic properties differ for materials making up a reflecting interface (or boundary). This difference is called the *acoustic impedance mismatch.* The greater the mismatch, the greater the reflection, and the less ultrasound penetrates the interface. For instance, as shown in **(A)**, strong echoes are generated at the boundary between the liver and perinephric fat (arrows) because the acoustic properties of these tissues are different. The acoustic impedance mismatch is not so great as to block ultrasound transmission entirely, however, and deeper structures are clearly visible. **(B)** In contrast, virtually all the ultrasound energy is reflected at a bone/soft tissue boundary (arrow) because the acoustic mismatch between bone and soft tissue is very great. An "acoustic shadow" occurs distal (deep) to the bone since virtually all the ultrasound is reflected.

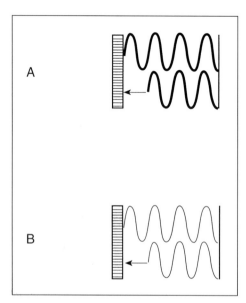

Figure 1-7—Echo Strength, Factor 2. The strength of an ultrasound echo also is governed by the inherent *strength of the ultrasound beam.* A powerful ultrasound pulse **(A)** generates stronger reflections than a weak pulse **(B).** It might seem that the strongest possible ultrasound beam should be used to enhance image quality, but three factors necessitate the restriction of beam strength: (1) if echoes are too strong they will "overwhelm" the ultrasound receiver, causing "white out"; (2) excessive beam strength (ultrasound power) can cause tissue damage; and (3) excessive beam strength could generate heat perceptible by the patient.

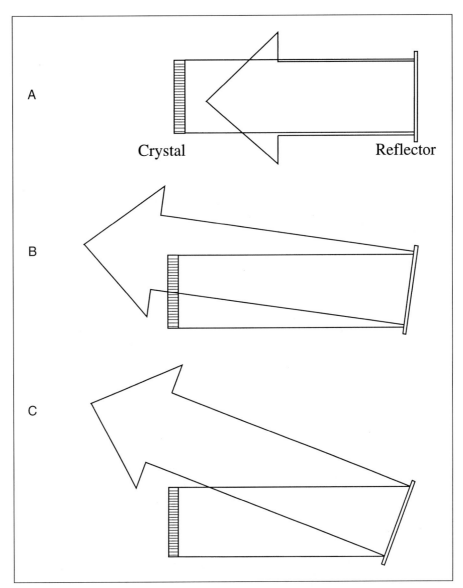

Figure 1-8—Echo Strength, Factor 3. The strength of a reflection also is affected by the angle at which the ultrasound beam strikes a reflecting interface. In technical jargon, this angle is called the *angle of incidence.* As is the case with light, the angle of incidence of an ultrasound beam equals the angle of reflection. **(A)** Maximum reflection back to the transducer, hence the strongest echo, occurs when the angle of incidence is 90°; that is, when the reflector is perpendicular to the ultrasound beam. **(B)** The strength of the echo wanes as the angle of incidence decreases. **(C)** At some point, the ultrasound beam is deflected away from the crystal and no echo is recorded.

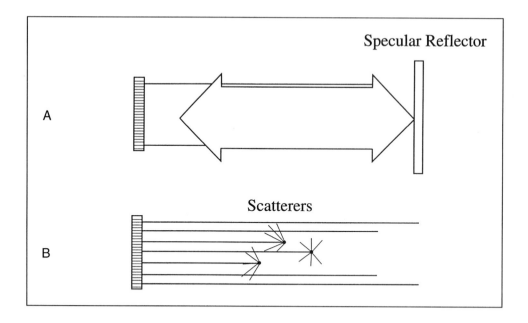

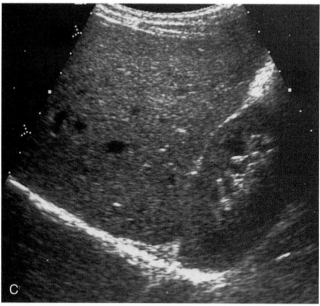

Figure 1-9—Echo Strength, Factor 4. The size of the reflector significantly affects the strength of an ultrasound reflection. Reflecting interfaces fall into two classes: (**A**) *specular reflectors,* which are large compared with the ultrasound beam and produce high-intensity, unidirectional reflections, and (**B**) *scatterers,* or tiny, punctate reflectors that scatter a small portion of the ultrasound beam in virtually all directions. (A chip in an automobile windshield acts as a scatterer when struck by the beam of an oncoming headlight.) (**C**) Specular reflectors provide the broad outlines of organs, whereas scatterers provide the "sonographic texture" within the organs. This texture actually arises from a phenomenon called speckle, as discussed in Chapter 9. Early ultrasound instruments could display only strong specular reflections; therefore, they could display only the outlines of large anatomic structures.

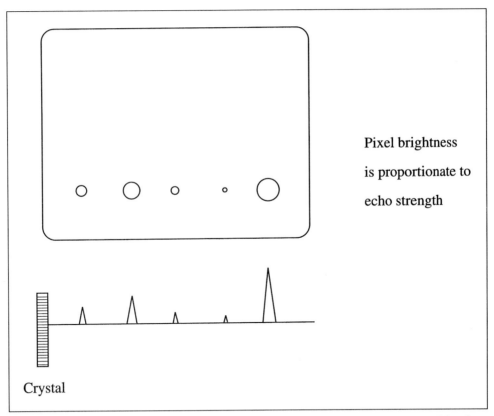

Pixel brightness

is proportionate to

echo strength

Crystal

Figure 1-10—The B-Mode Display. All standard ultrasound images are brightness modulated, or "B-mode" images. Bright dots or *pixels* (short for picture elements) make up the picture, and the brightness of each pixel (illustrated here by the size of the circle) is modulated (adjusted) in proportion to the strength of each echo (illustrated by the height of the spikes).

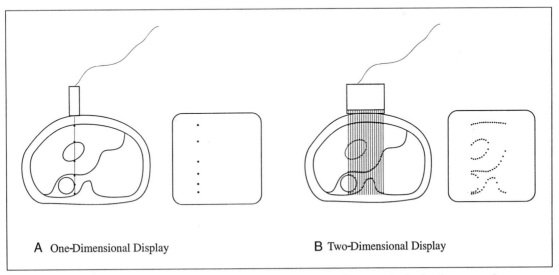

A One-Dimensional Display   B Two-Dimensional Display

Figure 1-11—One- and Two-Dimensional Displays. (A) The B-mode display from a single ultrasound crystal is a one-dimensional series of bright dots. This is the ultimate "ice-pick" or "searchlight" view of the world. **(B)** Multiple "ice-pick" views are assembled to form a two-dimensional (width and height) image, as illustrated here with a linear array transducer. With linear array devices, multiple "ice-pick" views are lined up side-by-side, like the teeth of a comb.

An array transducer contains multiple elements that can be fired singly or in groups. The elements of a linear array are fired beginning at one end and proceeding to the other. The result is a series of "echo lines" that collectively are called a frame. When the frame is complete, it is displayed on a television screen, and the process of accumulating a new set of echo "lines" begins all over.

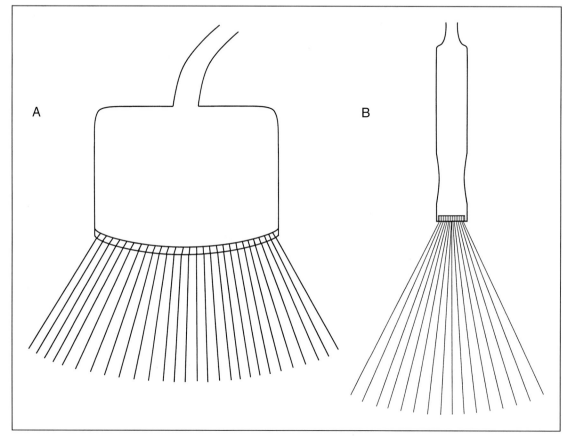

Figure 1-12—Sector Images. Pie-shaped images resembling a *sector* of a circle are used commonly in medical sonography. These images are produced in two ways: **(A)** A curved array may be used. Such arrays operate in the same way as linear arrays, but the transducer elements are oriented on a curved surface. **(B)** A second technique for creating a sector image involves a mini-linear array in which the elements are fired in a certain way to generate a series of radially oriented ultrasound beams (see subsequent figures). With either system, multiple one-dimensional lines of echo information are obtained and stored for subsequent assembly as a two-dimensional image.

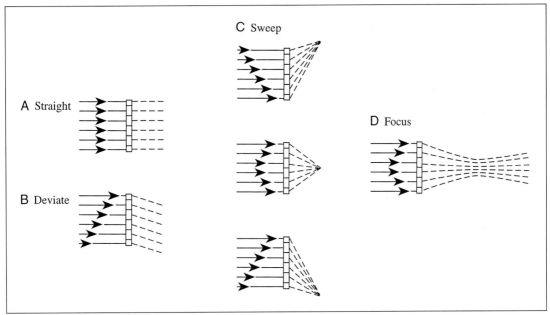

Figure 1-13—Electronic Beam Formation, Steering, and Focusing. Many ultrasound instruments utilize a "phased array" ultrasound crystal to create, steer, and focus the ultrasound beam. Each crystal element produces a "wavelet," or little ultrasound wave. The wavelets merge at a short distance from the crystal to form a unified *"wavefront."* **(A)** If all the array elements are fired simultaneously, the resultant wavefront moves straight outward from the crystal. **(B)** If each succeeding crystal element is fired a little later than the next, then each wavelet is out of phase with the adjacent wavelet (i.e., the peaks and valleys do not line up). This lack of synchronization causes the wavefront to deviate from a straight path. By changing the element firing delay, the wavefront may be made to deviate a little or a lot. **(C)** For sector image formation (as shown in Figure 1–12*B*), the firing delay is altered sequentially, causing the ultrasound beam to sweep through a sector of a circle. As the beam sweeps through its arc, multiple pulses of ultrasound are sent out along different lines of sight and ultrasound echoes are acquired for each of these lines. These echo lines are stored for display as a two-dimensional image. **(D)** The firing delay mechanism also may be used to focus the beam. This feature is operator controlled, permitting the focal zone to be placed in areas of interest. An analogous method is used to "return focus," or to enhance crystal sensitivity for echoes that arise from specified depths within the body.

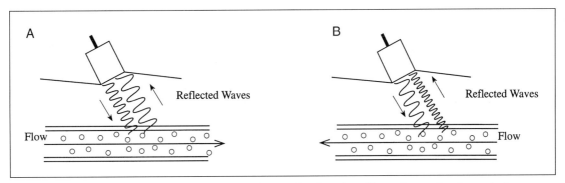

Figure 1-14—Doppler Ultrasound Principles. The Doppler effect refers to the *change* in frequency that occurs when ultrasound is reflected from moving objects. **(A)** If the objects (e.g., red blood cells) are moving *away* (relatively) from the transducer, then the reflected (returning) waves have a *longer* wavelength and a *lower* frequency than the incident (outgoing) waves. **(B)** If the reflecting objects are moving *toward* the transducer, then the reflected waves have a *shorter* wavelength and a *higher* frequency than the incident waves. The frequency difference between the incident and reflected wave is called the *Doppler shift*. The size of the Doppler shift is directly proportionate to the *velocity* of the reflectors. *In essence, Doppler ultrasound provides two pieces of information: (1) the direction of the Doppler shift (increase or decrease) indicates the direction of blood flow; and (2) the size of the shift indicates the velocity of blood flow.*

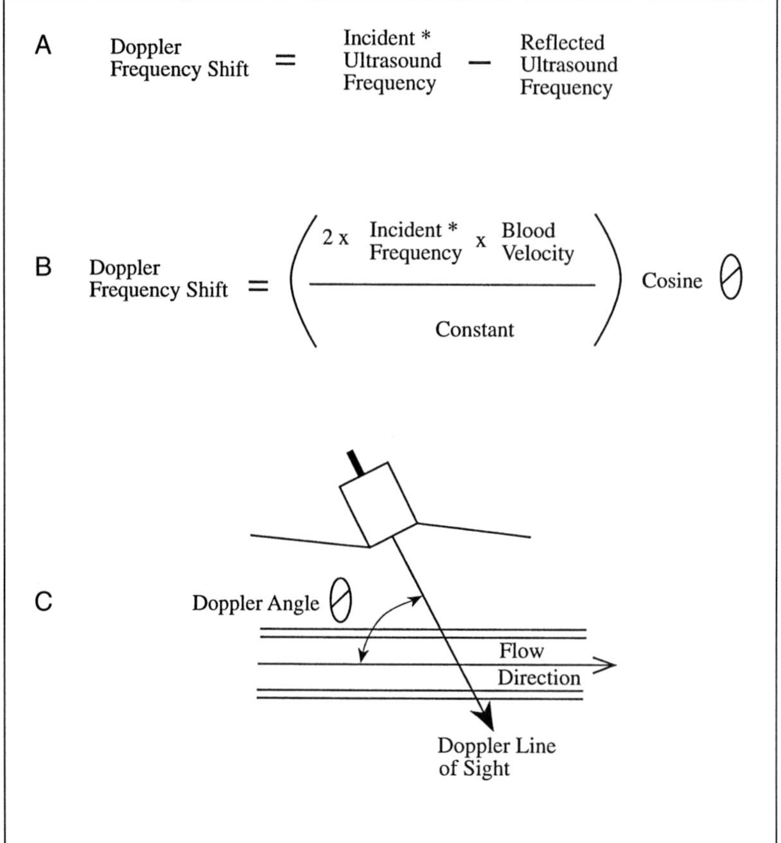

A   Doppler Frequency Shift   =   Incident * Ultrasound Frequency   —   Reflected Ultrasound Frequency

B   Doppler Frequency Shift   = $\left(\dfrac{2 \times \text{Incident * Frequency} \times \text{Blood Velocity}}{\text{Constant}}\right)$ Cosine θ

C

Doppler Angle θ

Flow Direction

Doppler Line of Sight

* The incident frequency refers to the ultrasound beam sent into the body.

Figure 1-15—The Doppler Formula. **(A)** The Doppler frequency shift is the frequency difference between the incident (outgoing) ultrasound beam and the returning echoes. **(B)** The Doppler frequency shift may be predicted using the *Doppler formula,* which is illustrated here. Since the incident frequency and the constant are known, the Doppler frequency shift is proportionate to two unknown variables: the velocity of the reflector (blood), and the Doppler angle. **(C)** *The Doppler angle* is illustrated with the Greek letter theta (θ). The Doppler angle can be determined with modern ultrasound instruments, permitting the Doppler equation to be solved (electronically) for the only remaining variable, the reflector velocity (the velocity of blood flow).

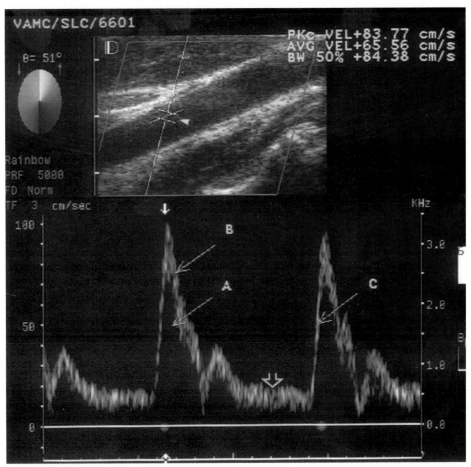

Figure 1-16—Duplex Sonography. The term *duplex sonography* refers to the simultaneous display of an ultrasound image and Doppler information. The display screen typically shows the following information:

B-mode image—A two-dimensional, B-mode image of the area of interest is shown at the top of the display.

Sample volume—The region where Doppler information is obtained is called the sample volume. This is shown by parallel lines on the B-mode image (arrowhead).

Doppler angle—the Doppler angle (see Figure 1–15C) is visible on the B-mode image and also is displayed numerically (θ = 51 degrees, upper left corner of display).

Flow direction—Flow away from the transducer is shown above the spectrum baseline, and flow toward the transducer is shown below the baseline. (In this case, all flow is away from the transducer; i.e., above the baseline.)

Velocity distribution—the z axis, or the brightness of the spectral display elements, and the width of the spectrum, correlate with the distribution of velocities (frequency shifts) in the sample volume. To better understand the z axis, imagine that the spectrum display is made up of tiny pixels, or picture elements, with each corresponding to a specific moment in time and a specific velocity (frequency shift). At the moment in time indicated by arrow A, the picture elements corresponding to 50 cm/sec are black, indicating that no blood cells are moving at 50 cm/sec. At the same moment, pixels corresponding to 75 cm/sec (arrow B) are gray, indicating that a moderate number of blood cells are moving at that velocity. Picture elements corresponding to arrow C are white, indicating that a large proportion of blood cells are moving at about 50 cm/sec at that moment in time. Note also that the spectrum is very narrow (just a thin line) at C, indicating that at that moment in time most of the blood is moving at the same velocity. In contrast, the spectrum is much thicker (broader) at B, indicating that the range of velocities is much wider at moment B. Note also that a wide range of velocities is present throughout diastole, as indicated by a broad diastolic spectrum (open arrow).

Moment-by-moment velocity data—The vertical arrow at the bottom of the spectrum display represents a moment in time. The numbers at the top right of the display show the maximum velocity (PKc VEL), the average velocity (AVG VEL), and velocity range (BW 50%) within the sample volume at the moment indicated by the vertical arrows.

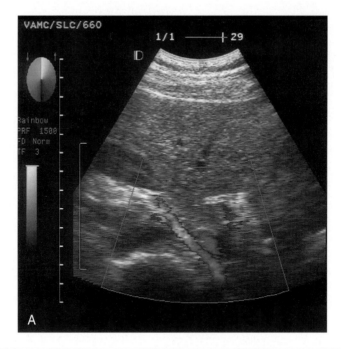

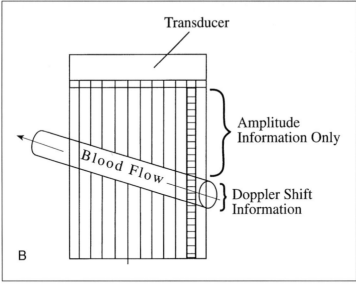

Figure 1-17—Principles of color Doppler sonography. (**A**) Color Doppler sonography refers to the representation of blood flow in color on a two-dimensional ultrasound image, as shown here. See this figure in the Color Plates. (**B**) Color Doppler images are produced as follows: Stationary reflectors generate echo amplitude information but do not generate a Doppler shift. Stationary reflectors, therefore, are shown in shades of gray. Flowing blood generates a Doppler shift *in addition* to amplitude information, and all Doppler-shifted echoes are shown in color. The direction of flow is shown by the color hue. For instance, red may represent flow in one direction (relative to the transducer), and blue may represent flow in the opposite direction. The velocity of blood flow is represented by the shade of color. For instance, lower velocities might be dark red, and higher velocities pink. Note the color wheel in the left upper corner of part **A.** This wheel indicates the coding for flow direction and velocity. (See Color Figure 1–17A following page 108.)

REFERENCES

1. Curry TS, Dowdey JE, Murry RC: Christensen's Physics of Diagnostic Radiology, 4th ed. London, Lea and Febinger, 1990, pp 323–371.
2. Kremkau FW: Diagnostic Ultrasound; Principles, Instrumentation, and Exercises, 2nd ed. Philadelphia, Grune and Stratton, 1984, pp 5–153.
3. Fish P: Physics and Instrumentation of Diagnostic Medical Ultrasound. New York, John Wiley and Sons, 1990, pp 7–179.
4. Kremkau FW: Doppler Ultrasound; Principles and Instruments. Philadelphia, WB Saunders, 1990, pp 73–182.
5. Zagzebski JA: Physics and instrumentation in Doppler and B-mode ultrasonography. *In* Zwiebel WJ: Introduction to Vascular Ultrasonography, 3rd ed. Philadelphia, WB Saunders, 1992, pp 19–44.

Chapter 2

Image Optimization, Ultrasound Artifacts, and Safety Considerations

William J. Zwiebel

This chapter provides instruction on how to adjust an ultrasound instrument to produce the clearest and most informative ultrasound images. It also provides information on commonly encountered ultrasound artifacts that can be beneficial or problematic diagnostically. Finally, this chapter considers the bioeffects of ultrasound and ultrasound safety. Many of the terms used in this chapter are defined in the preceding chapter, and the reader should refer to these definitions as needed.

IMAGE OPTIMIZATION

Computerized automation has made it relatively easy to adjust ultrasound instruments; nonetheless, sonographers must be familiar with basic principles of ultrasound physics and instrumentation to optimize the function of diagnostic ultrasound devices. Many instruments now are equipped with preset power, gain, and echo-processing parameters that are tailored to specific applications, such as obstetric or abdominal diagnosis. In spite of these conveniences, it remains necessary to "fine tune" the image repeatedly in the course of most sonographic examinations.[1–3]

Six steps are suggested for image optimization:

1. Select a *scanhead* (see definition in preceding chapter) with an ultrasound frequency appropriate to the depth of operation.
2. Choose the appropriate *preprogrammed instrument setup* (e.g., abdomen, pelvis, superficial structures).
3. Adjust the *field of view* to encompass the area of interest.
4. Adjust the *focal depth.*
5. Adjust the *gain and power* settings to provide a uniform level of echoes throughout the image.
6. Select *pre- and postprocessing* settings as needed, to enhance specific image features.

For convenient reference, these six steps are listed in Table 2–1. Each of the six steps will be considered in turn.

Scanhead Selection

Each scanhead contains a piezoelectric crystal that produces a range of ultrasound frequencies, but this range is limited. Different scanheads are required, therefore, for different ultrasound tasks. For example, a 7.5- or 10-MHZ scanhead is ideal for examining the thyroid gland, but these scanheads would be useless for examining the liver or kidneys. At most, a scanhead may be designed to function at three frequencies (e.g., 2.5, 3.5, and 5 MHz); therefore, the need to switch from one scanhead to another is inevitable. Image resolution with higher ultrasound frequencies, such as 5 to 10 MHz, generally is superior to resolution with lower frequencies (2 to 4 MHz), but high-frequency ultrasound cannot penetrate deeply into the body since the ultrasound beam is attenuated (weakened) more

Table 2-1. Ultrasound Instrument Adjustment Protocol

1. Scanhead
   Select a scanhead with a frequency appropriate to the depth of examination.
2. Programmed Setup
   Select the appropriate preprogrammed instrument setup.
3. Field of View
   Adjust the field of view such that the display screen is filled with useful information.
4. Focal Depth
   Place the focal region in the area of maximum interest.
5. Time-compensated Gain (TCG) and Output Power
   First adjust the TCG, and then adjust the output power to produce a uniformly bright image and optimal echo strength.
6. Pre- and Postprocessing
   Select the pre- and postprocessing settings to enhance areas of interest.

readily than a low-frequency beam. In choosing a scanhead, therefore, a compromise must always be struck between resolution and attenuation. Generally, 7.5- to 10-MHz scanheads are used for very superficial structures, such as the thyroid gland or breast; 5.0-MHz scanheads are used for intermediate depths; and 3.0-MHz scanheads are used for deeper structures, such as the abdominal contents. In some cases, even lower frequencies (2 to 2.5 MHz) are useful for abdominal examination in large patients, particularly when Doppler information is desired.

The shape of the ultrasound image also must be considered in scanhead selection. Sector scanheads with a small "footprint," or area of skin contact, are desirable for working in close confines, such as between the ribs. In contrast, a broad nearfield, as provided by a linear or curved array, is advantageous for examining superficial structures such as the thyroid.

The final factor to be considered in scanhead selection is the inherent resolution of a particular scanhead design. In general, linear array scanheads offer better resolution than curved arrays, and curved arrays offer better resolution than sector scanheads. When high resolution is desired (e.g., obstetric imaging), the sonographer should take advantage of the superior resolution of linear arrays wherever possible.

Programmed Settings

The instrument settings that are optimal for different ultrasound examinations vary widely. For example, fetal echocardiography requires the following: (1) a high pulse repetition frequency and frame rate, needed for visualizing rapidly moving structures; (2) a high-contrast, "edge-enhanced" gray scale image to visualize minute cardiovascular structures; and (3) a color Doppler velocity range appropriate for intracardiac flow. These instrument settings are vastly different from those that optimize abdominal images; namely: (1) a relatively low pulse repetition frequency and frame rate (abdominal viscera do not move fast); and (2) a broad gray scale image that enhances "tissue texture" resolution.

Because it can be quite difficult to arrive at the right combination of instrument settings for a given examination, ultrasound instruments are preprogrammed for specific applications, such as abdominal sonography, peripheral vascular examination, and obstetric sonography. The sonographer can pick and choose among these applications as needed. It is important to use the proper preset adjustment package for the examination at hand, or else image quality may suffer greatly. If the preset programs do not fit the needs of a given ultrasound department, then they can be modified as needed, or entirely new programs can be created for specific applications. The manufacturer can provide assistance and recommendation for such program modifications.

Field of View

The image size should always be adjusted so that the display screen is filled with useful information, as illustrated in Figure 2–1. Do not be a "postage stamper," who scrunches a tiny image into the corner of the display! Conversely, do not magnify the image so greatly that orientation is impossible.

Focus

The term "focus" is used broadly, since ultrasound "focusing" involves electronic techniques that may be quite different from optical focusing. Nevertheless, two important points must be made concerning ultrasound focusing: First, maximum resolution occurs in the focal zone, and resolution may decrease significantly at a distance from the focal zone—therefore, the focal zone should always correspond to the area of maximum diagnostic interest (Fig. 2–2). Second, if a broad field of resolution is desirable, multiple focal areas should be used rather than a single focal zone; the trade-off, however, is a reduction of frame rate.

Time-Compensated Gain

As an ultrasound beam travels through the body, two processes diminish the strength or "intensity" of the beam: (1) the beam is attenuated, meaning that mechanical energy (vibration) is converted to heat; and (2) the beam becomes dispersed or spread out as it is reflected and refracted at acoustic interfaces. Because of attenuation and dispersion, distant ultrasound echoes are *much* weaker than near echoes; therefore, distant echoes must be amplified much more than near echoes to produce an image that is uniformly bright from the nearfield to the farfield (from top to bottom) (Fig. 2–3). The term "time-compensated gain" describes the process of amplifying distant echoes more than near echoes. Stated literally, the *gain* (amplification) is increased to *compensate* for the effects of transit *time*. Since distance equals time in ultrasound parlance, we also could say that gain is increased to compensate for distance from the scanhead.

Ultrasound attenuation varies markedly as the scanhead is moved from one position to another in the course of an ultrasound examination, and

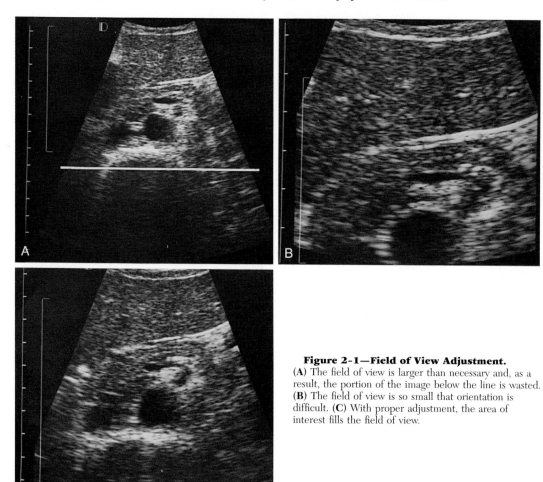

Figure 2-1—Field of View Adjustment.
(A) The field of view is larger than necessary and, as a result, the portion of the image below the line is wasted.
(B) The field of view is so small that orientation is difficult. (C) With proper adjustment, the area of interest fills the field of view.

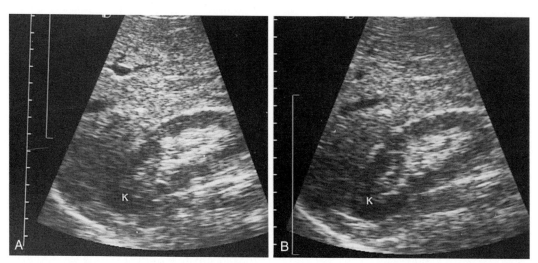

Figure 2-2—Effects of Focal Zone Adjustment. (A) The focal zone (bracket at left of image) is too high, and as a result the superior pole of the kidney (K) is indistinct. (B) With the focal zone properly positioned, the upper pole of the kidney (K) is clearly seen.

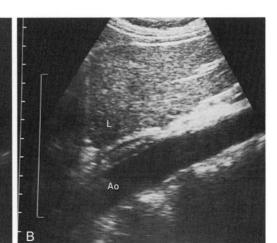

Figure 2-3—Time-Compensated Gain. (A) In this image, the TCG is improperly set, resulting in poor visualization of the posterior portion of the liver (L) and the aorta (Ao). **(B)** With proper TCG adjustment, the liver (L) and the aorta (Ao) are seen clearly.

time-compensated gain (TCG°) must therefore be adjusted *repeatedly* to maintain uniform image intensity. Proper TCG adjustment is particularly important in the pelvis to insure clear visualization of the female reproductive organs through the distended bladder.

Power

The strength, or power, of the ultrasound beam sent into the patient may be adjusted by the sonographer. The power of the beam is measured in absolute terms as watts per square centimeter. Ultrasound power also is measured with a relative term called the decibel (dB), and this term is particularly important since it typically is used for instrument power settings. The decibel is a logarithmic expression that *compares* the power of two ultrasound beams. If two beams differ in intensity by 1 dB, then the power difference is tenfold; that is, one beam is ten times more powerful than the other. Thus, 2 dB equates to a 100-fold difference in power, and 3 dB equates to a 1000-fold difference, and so on. Output power controls on ultrasound instruments frequently are calibrated in dB, *relative to the maximum or minimum output of the instrument and scanhead in use.* The term "relative" is crucial; the power output settings of one instrument do not equate to those of another instrument, and the output of one scanhead does not equate to that of another scanhead. The *actual* power output may vary greatly from one instrument or scanhead to another. Many instruments are programmed to prohibit output power levels

above certain limits, per the requirements of the United States Food and Drug Administration.

Image quality is affected significantly by output power, but it is not necessarily true that more power equates to superior image quality. Output power must be tailored to match the scanhead and the echo processing components. It is best, therefore, to begin with the power setting that is preprogrammed for a specific diagnostic application. If visualization of deep structures is limited even though TGC is maximized, then it may be advisable to increase the output power (Fig. 2–4). If an increase in output power merely fills the image with noise, then no benefit is derived, and it may be preferable to switch to a lower frequency scanhead to reduce ultrasound beam attenuation.

Preprocessing and Postprocessing

The echo information that returns from the patient is processed in two ways before the image is assembled on the display screen. First, the "raw" echo signal from the transducer is "preprocessed," prior to storage of the echo information; second, the stored echo information is "postprocessed," prior to display on the image screen.

Preprocessing principally determines which echoes are saved and which are discarded, on the basis of echo strength. For example, with one preprocessing program, high-intensity echoes are stored and low-intensity echoes are discarded. With another program, only the low-intensity echoes are saved, and with yet another program, echoes are retained over a wide range of intensities.

°The abbreviations TCG, for time-compensated gain, and TGC, for time gain compensation, are equivalent and may be used interchangeably.

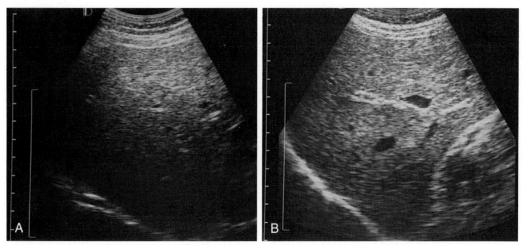

Figure 2-4—Effects of Output Power Adjustment. (A) The TGC has been maximized in this example, yet the posterior aspect of the liver and the diaphragm are poorly seen because output power is low. (B) With increased output power, and readjustment of the TGC, the posterior aspect of the liver is seen clearly.

Postprocessing concerns the selection of stored echoes for display on the image monitor. This selection process is based on echo amplitude or gray scale level. To understand postprocessing, consider that a television monitor may display 32 shades of gray but that a much broader range of echo intensities exists in storage. A decision must be made as to which echoes are shown on the display and which are not. One option might be to show the entire range of echoes but to compress them into 32 gray shades. The resultant image would have wide latitude, but subtle gray scale differences would be lost. Another option might be to show primarily the low-level echoes. This approach would enhance subtle tissue "texture" differences, but the image might be "noisy" and indistinct. Finally, high-intensity echoes might be displayed while the low-intensity echoes are ignored. The latter approach would emphasize structural borders, such as the edges of blood vessels, but gray scale "texture" might be lost. The potential effects of postprocessing are illustrated in Figure 2–5.

From a practical perspective, it is best to begin pre- and postprocessing adjustments with the programmed settings provided by the manufacturer. Preprocessing generally is left at the programmed setting, and only postprocessing is adjusted to enhance specific components of the image. Postprocessing is particularly useful since frozen images can be postprocessed "after the fact" to emphasize areas of interest.

IMPORTANT ULTRASOUND ARTIFACTS

As noted earlier, several commonly occurring ultrasound artifacts affect ultrasound interpreta-

tion, either positively or negatively. There is a vast array of ultrasound artifacts, but we will consider only the most important ones; namely, enhanced through-transmission, acoustic shadowing, lateral edge shadows, reverberation artifacts, slice thickness artifacts, and "side lobe" artifacts.[1–11]

Enhanced Through-Transmission

Earlier in this chapter, we considered the need to adjust the time-compensated gain (TCG) so that weaker echoes from deeper structures are amplified more than stronger echoes from near structures. The TCG adjustment assumes that ultrasound attenuation is relatively uniform throughout the tissues imaged, but attenuation actually varies considerably from one point to another in most clinical applications. If the ultrasound beam passes through an area of unexpectedly low attenuation, deeper structures receive stronger ultrasound pulses and produce stronger echoes than the gain settings anticipate. As a consequence, echoes from the deeper structures are overamplified and are much brighter than other echoes at a similar depth (Fig. 2–6). The resultant artifact is called "enhanced through-transmission," since ultrasound transmission is enhanced in the low-attenuation area.[1–6]

Enhanced through-transmission is a crucial diagnostic feature of fluid-filled structures such as cysts and abscesses. A mass should be regarded as fluid-filled only if enhanced through-transmission is evident. A low-attenuation mass that does *not* show enhancement may be a homogeneous

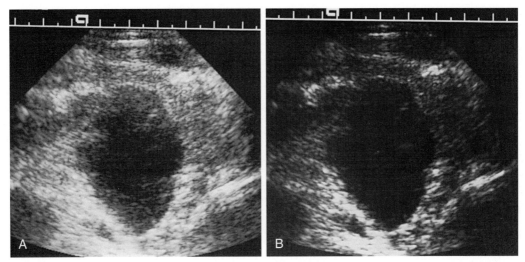

Figure 2-5—Effects of Postprocessing. (Subject: pelvic cyst.) **(A)** Postprocessing is adjusted to display a wide range of echo intensities that makes the image somewhat cluttered. **(B)** Postprocessing is adjusted to display only high-level echoes, which produces a sharper, "edge-enhanced" image, but low-level echoes are lost.

solid mass (e.g., lymphoma), rather than a fluid-filled structure.

Acoustic Shadowing

The converse of enhanced through-transmission is acoustic shadowing.[1–5, 7] In this case, a highly reflective or highly attenuating area blocks transmission of the ultrasound beam, leading to weak or absent distal echoes (Fig. 2–7). The result is a hypoechoic or echo-free area, called an acoustic shadow, distal to the highly reflective or highly attenuating structure. Acoustic shadows can hinder visualization of important structures, but they also can be of great diagnostic value, as is the case with gallstones. They are an essential diagnostic feature of gallstones, and an object in the biliary tree should not be regarded as a gallstone if it does not produce an acoustic shadow.

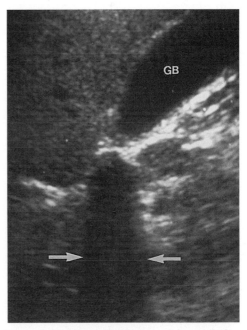

Figure 2-6—Enhanced Through-Transmission. A band of high-intensity echoes (arrows) is present distal to a renal cyst (C). The intensity of these echoes is greater than that of other echoes at similar depths because the ultrasound beam is attenuated very little as it traverses the homogeneous cyst fluid.

Figure 2-7—Acoustic Shadow. A distinct shadow (arrows) is seen distal to a gallstone impacted in the gallbladder (GB) neck. The shadow is caused by virtually complete deflection of the ultrasound beam by the gallstone.

Lateral Edge Shadows

Acoustic shadows may occur distal to the walls of well-encapsulated lesions, as a result of reflection and refraction of the ultrasound beam in the lesion wall (Fig. 2–8). These shadows, which are called lateral edge shadows,[1–5, 7] are a useful diagnostic feature of cysts but are seen only when high-frequency, high-resolution instruments are used. Lateral edge shadows are not specific for cysts, for such shadows also occur with well-encapsulated solid lesions.

Reverberation Artifacts

Reverberations are common and annoying artifacts that occur in the form of parallel lines oriented perpendicular (more or less) to the ultrasound beam[1–5] (Fig. 2–9). They are generated when an ultrasound beam bounces back and forth between strong specular reflectors, or between a specular reflector and the transducer. The net result is an increase in the time required for the ultrasound beam to get back to the transducer (remember, time is distance in ultrasound). Several features serve to identify reverberation artifacts: (1) they usually are multiple; (2) they are parallel and repeat at regular intervals; (3) one or more strong specular reflectors often can be identified as the source of the artifact; and (4) succeeding reverberations become weaker, since the beam is attenuated as it bounces back and forth between the reflectors.

Comet Tail Artifacts

Reverberations also may occur *within* small, very dense objects, such as small metal fragments or cholesterol crystals, as illustrated in Figure 2–10. A characteristic "comet tail" artifact results from these internal reverberations. This artifact consists of short parallel lines that taper and "fade out" distal to the object.[1–5, 8, 9]

Slice Thickness Artifacts

An ultrasound image is shown on a television monitor as if it has only two dimensions, width and height. The ultrasound slice actually has three dimensions, width, height, and thickness, but slice thickness is not shown. As illustrated in Figure 2–11, the compression of three dimensions into two may superimpose objects and cause diagnostic ambiguity.[1–5, 10] Slice thickness artifacts include cysts that appear echogenic and spurious thickening of the gallbladder wall.

Off-Axis Ultrasound Beams

We typically assume that an ultrasound transducer produces a single ultrasound beam that propagates straight outward from the crystal, but

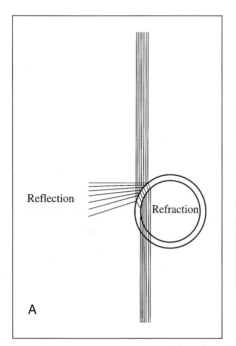

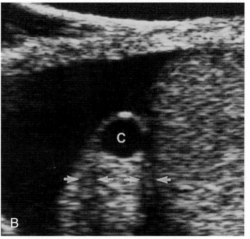

Figure 2-8—Lateral Edge Shadows. **(A)** Reflection occurs at the surface of a sharply marginated object, and refraction occurs within the wall of the object. These phenomena generate an edge shadow. **(B)** In this clinical example, lateral edge shadows (arrows) are seen distal to the wall of an epididymal cyst (C).

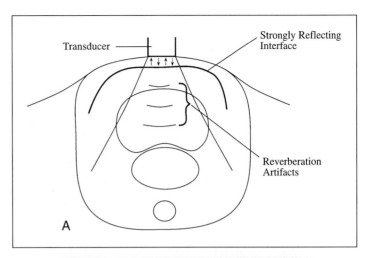

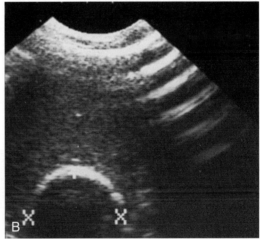

Figure 2-9—Reverberation Artifacts. **(A)** Reverberation occurs when the ultrasound beam bounces back and forth between strongly reflecting surfaces. In this diagram, the sound beam bounces (arrows) between the transducer face and a strongly reflecting superficial interface. Reverberation artifacts are produced that are superimposed on deeper structures as uniformly spaced parallel lines. Note that the distance between these lines is twice the distance between the reflectors. **(B)** In this clinical example, prominent reverberation artifacts are seen along the right side of the image. These were produced by reverberation between the transducer and a rib.

this is not really the case. In addition to the main beam, all ultrasound transducers produce off-axis beams that are known by names such as side lobes or grating lobes[1-5, 11] (Fig. 2–12A). These off-axis ultrasound beams are significantly weaker than the main beam; nevertheless, they may generate echoes that are mistakenly placed in the midst of the "real" echoes from the main beam. Two different types of artifacts may result from off-axis ultrasound beams. First, and most commonly, the image may be "peppered" with a haze of spurious echoes that reduces detail (Fig. 2–12B). Second, spurious structures are superimposed on real structures (Fig. 2–12C).

Mirror Image Artifacts

An object in the ultrasound image is represented twice in the mirror image artifact, once in its correct location and a second time in an artifactual "mirror image" location. Mirror image artifacts are most commonly seen adjacent to

the diaphragm, where an "extra" diaphragm may appear in the image (Fig. 2–12C), or an echoic liver lesion may be shown twice: once in the liver where it belongs and a second time in the lung, where it does not belong (or vice versa).

Mirror image artifacts are caused by two basic fallacies in the way ultrasound machines think.[2, 4, 5] First, the ultrasound machine assumes that all echoes that return to the transducer arise from structures along the beam axis. This is not true, because off-axis ultrasound beams occur, as illustrated in Figure 2–12. The second fallacy is that the ultrasound beam always travels in a straight line to and from a reflector. This also is not the case, for reflection and refraction may divert the beam. These two fallacies of "ultrasound machine thinking" cause ambiguity in ultrasound distance measurements (range ambiguity). Ambiguous distance measurements lead to misplacement of objects in the ultrasound image. Two additional examples of mirror image artifacts are shown in Figure 2–13.

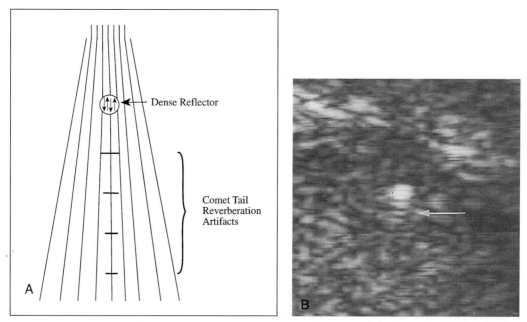

Figure 2-10—Comet Tail Artifacts. (**A**) Reverberation of the ultrasound beam (arrows) within a dense object produces comet tail artifacts seen distal to the object. (**B**) In this clinical example, a distinct comet tail (arrow) is seen deep to a dense object (possibly crystalline cholesterol) within the gallbladder.

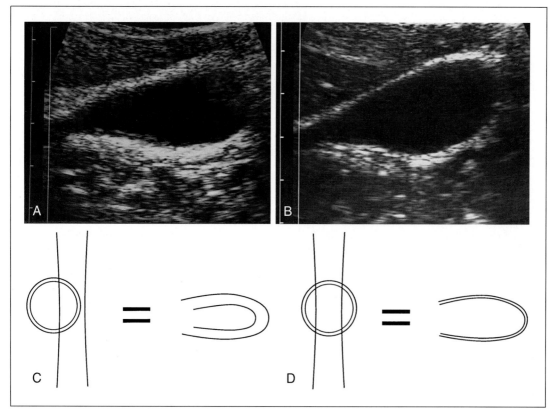

Figure 2-11—Slice Thickness Artifact. (**A**) The gallbladder wall appears thick in this clinical example, but this thickening is artifactual. (**B**) With proper position of the scan plane, the gallbladder wall is thin and sharply defined. (**C**) Artifactual wall thickening in this example occurred when the slice thickness fell partially within the gallbladder lumen and partially outside the lumen. (**D**) The gallbladder wall was correctly shown when the beam axis passes through the diameter of the gallbladder lumen, minimizing the effect of slice thickness.

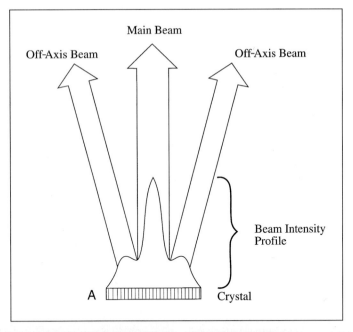

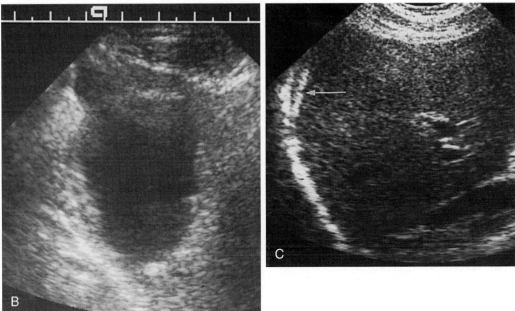

Figure 2-12—Artifacts Due to Off-Axis Ultrasound Beams. (A) Ultrasound transducers produce off-axis, secondary ultrasound beams in addition to the main central beam. (B) The diffuse punctate echoes within this pelvic cyst probably are caused by off-axis ultrasound beams striking reflectors outside the cyst. (C) A mirror image of the diaphragm (arrow) is generated by an off-axis beam that strikes a part of the diaphragm that is not in the image plane.

ULTRASOUND POWER MEASUREMENT

It was noted previously that the power of an ultrasound beam may be quantified with a unit of measure called the decibel. Measurements in decibels are useful for describing the *relative* power output of a device, but the decibel does not have an absolute value, and the *actual* power cannot be described with this term. Decibel calibration is like saying that a vehicle is running at a certain percent of its maximum power; for one vehicle, a given percentage might be 50 horsepower and for another vehicle the same percentage might be 150 horsepower.

The watt is a commonly used *absolute* value

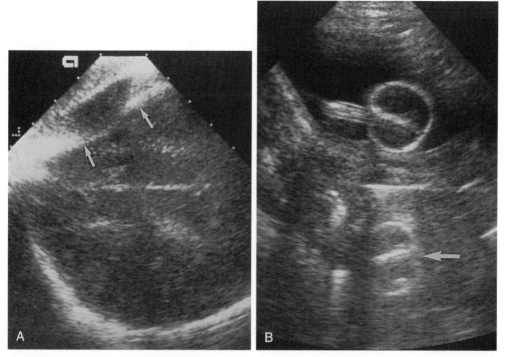

Figure 2-13—Mirror Image Artifacts. (A) A mirror image artifact of the skull (arrows) of this premature infant was mistaken for the margin of an extra-axial fluid collection. No fluid was present on a computed tomogram performed in response to this finding. **(B)** A mirror image of a Foley catheter (arrow) is seen distal to the real image within the bladder.

for measuring acoustic power, and a number of methods are available for accurately measuring ultrasound power in watts.[3, 12–15] The measurement process is complicated, however, by two factors: (1) power intensity varies markedly from moment to moment in pulsed ultrasound applications, since the ultrasound pulses are interspersed with long "listening" periods; and (2) ultrasound power varies markedly from one point to another within the beam due to the effects of attenuation and focusing. The existence of these factors creates three potential choices for describing pulsed ultrasound power: (1) as a temporal peak or temporal average; (2) as a pulse peak or pulse average; and (3) as a spatial peak or spatial average. The most commonly used measures are spatial peak temporal average (SPTA), reported in milliwatts per square centimeter (mW/cm^2); and spatial peak pulse average (SPPA), reported in watts per square centimeter (W/cm^2).

In the United States, the Food and Drug Administration has authority to regulate diagnostic ultrasound instruments and requires extensive verification of output power for all devices used for medical purposes. A standardized system for displaying output power has not been adopted by manufacturers of ultrasound instruments, but it is likely that such a system will be adopted or required in the future.

It is noteworthy that output power varies markedly among presently available diagnostic ultrasound instruments; furthermore, for a given instrument, output also may vary markedly from one application to another.[12, 14–16] Output power generally is quite low for applications involving linear array transducers. Sector scanners generally require slightly higher power than linear arrays, and spectral Doppler applications require the greatest power output of all. The output power of modern pulsed ultrasound instruments varies from 0.02 mW/cm^2 SPTA for some linear array applications to 4000 mW/cm^2 SPTA for some Doppler applications (note: the high end is 4 $watts/cm^2$!).[12, 15] The power output of diagnostic ultrasound instruments has risen steadily over the history of medical sonography and has taken a particularly great jump in recent years.[12, 15, 16] This recent increase in power has raised additional concern with respect to the safety of ultrasound diagnosis.

ULTRASOUND SAFETY

The safety of ultrasound is of elementary importance and has been the subject of extensive investigation since ultrasound was first used for diagnostic purposes early in the 1950s. Four physical effects of ultrasound are of principal concern: (1) tissue heating resulting from frictional resistance to wave transmission; (2) streaming of suspended particulate matter or cell structures; (3) direct vibratory effects on membranes and other cell structures; and (4) cavitation phenomena.[12–15] The greatest concern has centered on tissue heating and cavitation.

Tissue heating in response to ultrasound is directly proportionate to beam intensity and the duration of exposure. Furthermore, a 1-degree centigrade (C) elevation of tissue temperature is an accepted threshold for tissue damage (i.e., tissue damage is thought not to occur if the temperature rise is under 1 degree C).[13, 14] It is generally accepted that tissue heating occurs in humans during diagnostic ultrasound exposure, but it is not known whether heating ever is sufficient to cause biologic damage.[13]

Cavitation refers to the formation and/or expansion of microbubbles within a liquid medium in response to the rapid pressure oscillations induced by the ultrasound wave.[12–14] During the rarefaction (pressure reduction) phase of an ultrasound beam, microbubbles form and/or expand, creating cavities. These cavities decrease in size or collapse during the compression phase. As the ultrasound waves pass through tissue, massive and rapid alteration of cavity size may occur, potentially causing violent movement or actual streaming of cell contents, as well as other direct physical damage. In the worst case, violent expansion and collapse of cavities causes tremendous shock waves, local heating, and the formation of "sonochemicals," including free radicals.[14]

Cavitation, unlike tissue heating, is not precisely related to beam intensity or exposure time and can occur at quite low ultrasound output levels. No threshold is thought to exist, therefore, for cavitation damage. The generation of cavitation with ultrasound appears to depend on the attainment of very precise conditions, and it is not known whether cavitation occurs in humans during diagnostic ultrasound exposure.[12–14]

Safety Experiments

Concerns about ultrasound safety have been focused on biologic damage that might injure or kill an organism directly, and teratogenic effects that might injure or kill the offspring of an organism. These concerns have generated bioeffects studies that fall into several general categories: (1) mechanistic experiments that address the nature of ultrasound damage (e.g., heat production and cavitation); (2) outcome experiments that

address the effects of ultrasound exposure on mammalian and nonmammalian tissues (e.g., insonation of cultured cells, mice, or rats in an attempt to detect adverse effects on the individuals or their offspring); and (3) epidemiologic studies of humans exposed to ultrasound.[12–15] The results of such experiments can be summarized as follows:

1. Potentially damaging physical effects of ultrasound, such as heating and cavitation, have been demonstrated convincingly in vitro. Although these phenomena potentially could occur in humans at current diagnostic ultrasound exposure levels, it has not been demonstrated that these effects in fact do occur, and no potential adverse effects of these phenomena have been revealed by epidemiologic studies.[12–14]

2. Potentially adverse effects of ultrasound at diagnostic levels have been shown in certain tissue culture and laboratory animal studies, but independently verified adverse effects have not been demonstrated at output power levels of 100 mW/cm^2 or less for unfocused beams and 1000 mW/cm^2 or less for focused beams. The American Institute of Ultrasound in Medicine suggests, therefore, that these output power levels are safe for diagnostic purposes. It is postulated, furthermore, that significantly higher output power would be required to produce adverse effects in humans.[13]

3. Epidemiologic studies in humans have not documented any adverse effects of ultrasound exposure, including exposure to fetuses.[13]

4. No adverse effects of diagnostic ultrasound on patients or ultrasound operators have become apparent empirically during more than 40 years of clinical use.[13]

Is Ultrasound Safe?

What about the bottom line: is ultrasound safe? After 40 years of diagnostic ultrasound experience, we can say that we *think* ultrasound is safe, even though we know that ultrasound can cause cellular damage in an in vitro setting at currently used output levels. It is likely that we will never be able to prove conclusively that ultrasound is safe. The increase in output power that has occurred in recent years is noteworthy.[16] Some diagnostic instruments clearly operate above the recognized safe limit of 1000 mW/cm^2. Although it is likely that the upper limit of safe operation exceeds 1000 mW/cm^2,[13] we would do well to be cautious, especially during Doppler examination of fetuses. Output power is apt to be maximum during spectral Doppler examination, and the risk of biologic effects, at least empirically, is at its greatest in the early stages of fetal development. Therefore, in my opinion, fetal ultrasound exposure should be kept as low as possible during the first trimester, and it should particularly be minimized during the period of embryogenesis (the first 9 weeks of pregnancy). In keeping with this philosophy, I feel that fetal Doppler examination should be conducted only when absolutely necessary during the first trimester of pregnancy.

REFERENCES

1. Curry TS, Dowdey JE, Murry RC: Christensen's Physics of Diagnostic Radiology, 4th ed. London, Lea and Febinger, 1990, pp 323–371.
2. Kremkau FW: Diagnostic Ultrasound; Principles, Instrumentation, and Exercises, 2nd ed. Philadelphia, Grune and Stratton, 1984, pp 5–153.
3. Fish P: Physics and Instrumentation of Diagnostic Medical Ultrasound. Chichester, John Wiley and Sons, 1990, pp 7–179.
4. Laing FC: Commonly encountered artifacts in clinical ultrasound. Semin Ultrasound 4:27–43, 1983.
5. Kremkau FW: Artifacts in ultrasound imaging. J Ultrasound Med 5:227–237, 1986.
6. Filly RA, Sommer FG, Minton MJ: Characterization of biological fluids by ultrasound and computed tomography. Radiology 134:167–171, 1980.
7. Robinson DE, Wilson LS, Kossoff GP: Shadowing and enhancement in ultrasound echograms by reflection and refraction. J Clin Ultrasound 9:181–188, 1981.
8. Ziskin MC, Thickman DI, Jacobs Goldenberg N, Lapayowker MS, Becker JM: The comet tail artifact. J Ultrasound Med 1:1–7, 1982.
9. Thickman DI, Ziskin MC, Jacobs Goldenberg N, Linder BE: Clinical manifestations of the comet tail artifact. J Ultrasound Med 2:225–230, 1983.
10. Goldstein A, Madrazo BL: Slice-thickness artifacts in gray-scale ultrasound. J Clin Ultrasound 9:365–375, 1981.
11. Laing FC, Kurtz AB: The importance of ultrasonic side-lobe artifacts. Radiology 145:763–768, 1982.
12. Fish P: Physics and Instrumentation of Diagnostic Medical Ultrasound. Chichester, John Wiley and Sons, 1990, pp 201–220.
13. Lizzi F, Mortimer A, Miller M, et al: Bioeffect considerations for the safety of diagnostic ultrasound. J Ultrasound Med 7:9(suppl):1–38, 1988.
14. Miller DL: Update on safety of diagnostic ultrasonography. J Clin Ultrasound 19:531–540, 1991.
15. Kremkau FW: Doppler Ultrasound; Principles and Instrumentation. Philadelphia, WB Saunders, 1990, pp 173–181.
16. Henderson J, Wilson JR, Jago JA, Whittingham TA: A survey of the acoustic outputs of diagnostic ultrasound equipment in current clinical use. Ultrasound Med Biol 21:699–705, 1995.

The Pancreas

INTRODUCTION

The development of gray scale ultrasound in the mid-1970s added a significant new dimension to pancreatic diagnosis. For the first time, the pancreas could be visualized effectively with an imaging procedure. For a short period, sonography reigned as the premier pancreatic imaging technique, but this reign was short indeed! In the early 1980s, computed tomography (CT) came into widespread use and proved to be more effective than ultrasound, in certain respects, for pancreatic diagnosis. The pancreas, nonetheless, is commonly a direct or indirect subject of sonographic examination. Furthermore, the pancreas and its surrounding vessels are important orienting landmarks for ultrasound assessment of other upper abdominal viscera. Sonographers and sonologists° alike must be familiar, therefore, with the normal and pathologic appearance of the pancreas.

The principal limitation of pancreatic sonography is inconsistent visualization of the gland due to overlying bowel gas and other factors discussed in Chapter 3. Visualization of the pancreatic tail is particularly limited.[1-11] CT more consistently and precisely defines pancreatic anatomy. CT, therefore, is more sensitive than sonography for detecting pancreatic abnormality, and CT permits more confident diagnosis of pancreatic disorders.[3, 12-16] Magnetic resonance imaging (MRI) has emerged as a promising method for pancreatic diagnosis,[15-18] principally because this technique offers better soft tissue differentiation than does CT. MRI may be of particular value for the detection of small intrapancreatic neoplasms, but this technique is not likely to displace CT as the primary modality for pancreatic diagnosis.

If CT is the predominant method for pancreatic imaging, what then is the role of ultrasound? First, sonography remains useful as the initial study in jaundiced patients. Bile duct dilatation is more accurately diagnosed with ultrasound than with CT (Chapter 15). Furthermore, pancreatic masses causing ductal obstructions generally are large and easily detected with ultrasound. Second, the pancreas is visualized well in at least two thirds of upper abdominal sonograms,[1-11] and important pancreatic disorders (suspected or unsuspected) are commonly detected with ultrasound. Finally, sonography is an especially effective diagnostic tool in pediatric patients, in whom pancreatic visualization is more successful than in adults. Ultrasound, therefore, is the primary mode of pancreatic diagnosis in children.

Sonography is not recommended as a primary imaging procedure when occult pancreatic carcinoma or islet cell tumor is a primary diagnostic consideration. Ultrasound also is not recommended for assessment of complications of pancreatitis, or for the diagnosis of chronic pancreatitis. CT is the imaging procedure of choice in these circumstances.

REFERENCES

1. Arger PH, Mulhern CB, Bonavita JA, Stauffer DM, Hale J: An analysis of pancreatic sonography in suspected pancreatic disease. J Clin Ultrasound 7:91–97, 1979.

°Sonographer = person who creates an ultrasound image; analogous to a radiographer. Sonologist = person who interprets an ultrasound image; analogous to a radiologist.

2. Levitt RG, Geisse GG, Sagel SS, Stanley RJ, Evens RG, Koehler RE, Jost RG: Complementary use of ultrasound and computed tomography in studies of the pancreas and kidney. Radiology 126:149–152, 1978.
3. Hessel SJ, Siegelman SS, McNeil BJ, Sanders R, Adams DF, Alderson PO, Finberg HJ, Abrams HL: A prospective evaluation of computed tomography and ultrasound of the pancreas. Radiology 143:129–133, 1982.
4. McCain AH, Berkman WA, Bernardino ME:

Pancreatic sonography: Past and present. J Clin Ultrasound 12:325–332, 1984.

5. Filly RA, London SS: The normal pancreas: Acoustic characteristics and frequency of imaging. J Clin Ultrasound 7:121–124, 1979.

6. Taylor KJW, Buchin PJ, Viscomi GN, Rosenfield AT: Ultrasonographic scanning of the pancreas. Prospective study of clinical results. Radiology 138:211–213, 1981.

7. Doust BD, Pearce JD: Gray-scale ultrasonic properties of the normal and inflamed pancreas. Radiology 120:653–657, 1976.

8. Weill A, Schraub A, Eisenscher A, et al: Ultrasonography of the normal pancreas. Radiology 123:417, 1977.

9. Laval-Jeantet P, Gardeur D, Taboury J, et al: Anatomie echographieque du pancreas normal. J Radiol Electrol 57:149, 1976.

10. Haber K, Freimanis AK, Asher WM: Demonstration and dimensional analysis of the normal pancreas with gray scale echography. AJR Am J Roentgenol 126:624, 1976.

11. Coleman BG, Arger PH, Rosenberg HK, et al: Gray-scale sonographic assessment of pancreatitis in children. Radiology 146:145–150, 1983.

12. Haaga JR, Alfidi RJ, Havrilla TR, Tubbs R, Gonzalez L, Meaney TF, Corsi MA: Definitive role of CT scanning of the pancreas. Radiology 124:723–730, 1977.

13. Husband JE, Meire HB, Kreel L: Comparison of ultrasound and computer-assisted tomography in pancreatic diagnosis. Br J Radiol 50:855–862, 1977.

14. Stanley RJ, Sagel SS, Levitt RG: Computed tomographic evaluation of the pancreas. Radiology 124:715–722, 1977.

15. Stainer E, Stark DD, Hahn PF, Saini S, Simeone JF, Mueller PR, Wittenberg J, Ferrucci JT: Imaging of pancreatic neoplasms: Comparison of MR and CT. AJR Am J Roentgenol 152:487–491, 1989.

16. Semelka RC, Kroeker MA, Shoenut JP, Kroeker R, Yaffe CS, Micflikier AB: Pancreatic disease: Prospective comparison of CT, ERCP, and 1.5-T MR imaging with dynamic gadolinium enhancement and fat suppression. Radiology 181:785–791, 1991.

17. Vallet AD, Romano W, Bach DB, Passi RB, Taves DH, Munk PL: Adenocarcinoma of the pancreatic ducts: Comparative evaluation with CT and MR imaging at 1.5 T. Radiology 183:87–95, 1991.

18. Reimer P, Saini S, Hahn PF, Mueller PR, Brady TJ, Cohen MS: Techniques for high-resolution echo-planar MR imaging of the pancreas. Radiology 182:175–179, 1992.

Chapter 3

The Pancreas: Sonographic Technique and Anatomy

William J. Zwiebel

VASCULAR LANDMARKS

The pancreas lies adjacent to a number of major vessels that serve as orienting landmarks for sonographic examination.[1-4] Our discussion of the pancreas therefore includes the nearby vessels with which the reader should become intimately familiar. The correct identification of these vascular landmarks is the foundation for virtually all ultrasound studies of the upper abdomen. When "lost" in the upper abdomen, the experienced sonographer immediately seeks out the peripancreatic vessels in an attempt to become oriented.

STEP-BY-STEP SURVEY OF PANCREATIC ANATOMY

The pancreas (Fig. 3–1) is divided into five portions: the head, neck, body, tail, and uncinate process. These anatomic divisions are largely descriptive, since well-defined landmarks do not separate one portion of the pancreas from another. In this section, we will present the anatomic features of each pancreatic segment and at the same time describe the technique for visualizing that segment. The usual order of sonographic examination will be followed, beginning with the pancreatic body and then proceeding to the tail, neck, head, and uncinate process.

The Body

Pancreatic examination usually begins with the body, for this portion of the gland is most easily identified with ultrasound. To find the body, first identify the superior mesenteric artery (SMA) and the superior mesenteric vein (SMV) on transverse images (Fig. 3–2A). The SMA is distinctive because it is surrounded by a highly echogenic triangle of fat. With the SMA and SMV in view, move the image plane cephalad slightly, until the splenic vein and pancreatic body come into view (Fig. 3–2B). The identity of the splenic vein should be confirmed by demonstrating its confluence with the SMV, forming the portal vein. The body of the pancreas lies ante-

rior to the splenic vein; therefore, this vein is an excellent landmark for locating the pancreas. The point of contact between the pancreas and the splenic vein is variable, however, as seen in Figure 3–3. Because of this variability, the splenic vein may not be visible when the body of the pancreas is *optimally* seen, and vice versa.

The Tail

The tail of the pancreas follows the course of the splenic vein and "points" to the hilum of the spleen (Figs. 3–1 and 3–4). The tail usually angles obliquely toward the left upper quadrant. Less commonly, the pancreatic tail is transversely oriented or is angled obliquely downward. Regardless of its orientation, the tail usually is identified by following the plane of the splenic vein toward the splenic hilum. The pancreatic tail

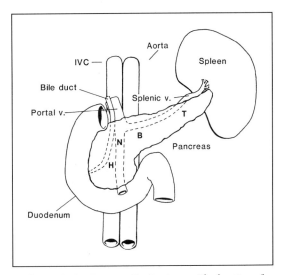

Figure 3-1—Pancreatic Anatomy. The location of head (H), neck (N), body (B), and tail (T) of the pancreas is shown. (The uncinate process is illustrated elsewhere.) Note the following anatomic features: (1) The head of the pancreas overlies the inferior vena cava (IVC) and extends inferior from the body. (2) The tail of the pancreas follows the splenic vein toward the splenic hilum. (3) The bile duct curves laterally through the pancreatic head. (4) The duodenum "caresses" the pancreatic head.

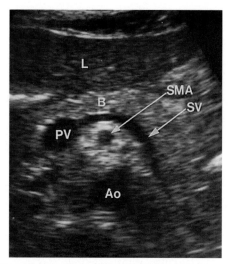

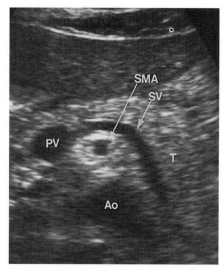

Figure 3-2—Transverse Sonogram of the Pancreatic Body (B). Note that the pancreas is more echogenic than the liver (L) and lies anterior to the splenic vein (SV) and the superior mesenteric artery (SMA). Note the echogenic fat around the SMA, and the distinctive relationship among the SMA, the splenic vein, the portal vein (PV), and the aorta (Ao). *This constellation of vessels is the primary orienting landmark for upper abdominal scanning.*

Figure 3-4—Transverse Sonogram of the Pancreatic Tail (T). Note that the tail dips posteriorly and parallels the course of the splenic vein (SV). PV = portal vein; SMA = superior mesenteric artery; Ao = aorta.

always dips posteriorly into the pericolic gutters, as shown in Figure 3–4.

In most cases, the pancreatic tail has a tapered configuration, but in some instances the diameter of the tail may be greater than that of the body. This bulbous shape is more common in children than in adults. It should not be assumed, therefore, that a bulbous pancreatic tail necessarily represents a mass lesion.

The Neck

After examining the pancreatic tail, the sonographer should return to the body of the gland (still in the transverse plane) and then proceed toward the right, to locate the pancreatic neck and head. The neck is a thin segment, located anterior to the portosplenic confluence, that connects the body and head (Figs. 3–1 and 3–5). The neck may be seen best in oblique image planes, as described in the next section.

The Head

The pancreatic head is longitudinally oriented and is best seen, therefore, on longitudinal sections. In most individuals, the pancreatic head lies anterior to the inferior vena cava (IVC), more or less, and for that reason it often is seen optimally when the IVC is clearly in view. The head also lies immediately caudal to the portal vein

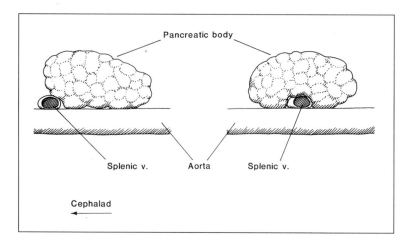

Figure 3-3—Relationship of the Pancreatic Body and the Splenic Vein. In the left figure, the splenic vein lies at the superior edge of the pancreatic body, and in this case, the pancreas is seen most clearly on transverse images slightly *below* the splenic vein. In the right figure, the splenic vein is more centrally located over the pancreas, and the pancreatic body is seen best on images *through* the splenic vein.

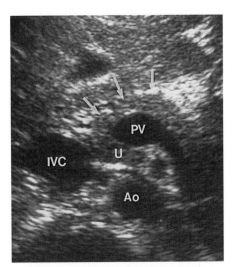

Figure 3-5—Transverse Sonogram of the Pancreatic Neck. The neck (arrows) is the relatively thin bridge of tissue that passes anterior to the portal vein (PV). The uncinate process (U) is seen posterior to the portal vein. IVC = inferior vena cava; Ao = aorta.

(Figs. 3–1 and 3–6). The pancreatic head also may be seen well on oblique scans angled from the left upper to right lower quadrant. *Neophyte sonographers commonly fail to examine the bulk of the pancreatic head,* because they do not realize how far the head extends inferior to the pancreatic body. In this scenario, the neophyte visualizes the pancreatic body on transverse scans, as shown in Figure 3–2, and perhaps sees part of the head but, in failing to use oblique or longitudinal views, does not see the bulk of the head.

KEY ANATOMIC RELATIONSHIPS OF THE HEAD

Several important anatomic relationships of the pancreatic head are illustrated in Figures 3–7 through 3–10. Please review these figures before proceeding, as their contents are not repeated in the text.

The Uncinate Process

The uncinate process is a small, triangular portion of the pancreas that projects medially from the pancreatic head, between the SMV and the IVC. As seen on transverse images (Figs. 3–6A and 3–10), the uncinate process resembles a medially pointed arrowhead. This arrowhead should be sharply pointed. A bulbous uncinate configuration suggests inflammation or neoplasia.

TECHNICAL PROTOCOL

A technical protocol for pancreatic sonography is presented in Table 3–1. In most instances, the pancreas is examined in conjunction with other upper abdominal structures, such as the liver, biliary tree, and kidney. Protocols for examining these areas are listed elsewhere in this text.

TECHNICAL CAVEATS
Dealing with Gas

Pancreas-obscuring gas often is present within the stomach or duodenum, and numerous techniques have been devised to displace gas from

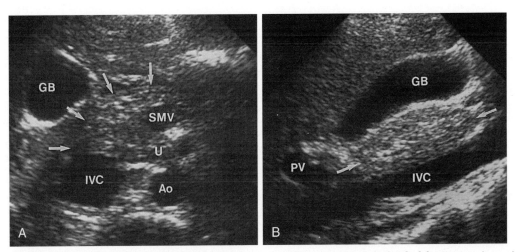

Figure 3-6—Sonograms of the Pancreatic Head. (A) An oblique view shows the head of the pancreas (arrows). The uncinate process is indicated by the letter U. SMV = superior mesenteric vein; Ao = aorta. IVC = inferior vena cava; GB = gallbladder. **(B)** A longitudinal view along the inferior vena cava (IVC) shows the full cephalocaudad extent of the pancreatic head (arrows). Note that the pancreatic head lies *inferior* to the portal vein (PV) and *adjacent* to the IVC. GB = gallbladder.

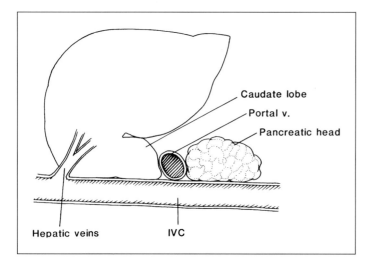

Figure 3-7—Relationship of Structures along the IVC. Proceeding inferiorly from the diaphragm, the following structures lie anterior to the IVC: the hepatic veins, the caudate lobe of the liver, the portal vein, and the pancreatic head. Note that the pancreatic head lies *inferior* to the portal vein, and the caudate lobe lies *superior* to the portal vein.

Figure 3-8—Anatomic Relationships of the Pancreatic Head. The common bile duct dives *posteriorly* into the pancreatic head, whereas the gastroduodenal artery rises up *anterior* to the head. The latter vessel defines the anterior margin of the gland. The pancreatic head lies adjacent to the inferior vena cava and may actually indent the cava slightly.

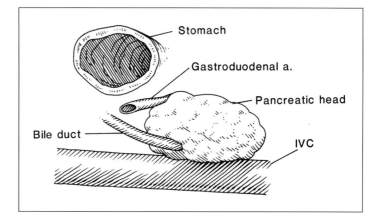

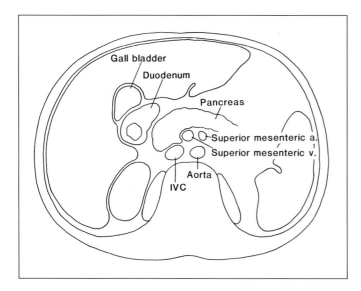

Figure 3-9—Relationship of the Pancreatic Head, the Duodenum, and the Gallbladder. The duodenum intervenes between the gallbladder and the pancreatic head. Fluid in the duodenum or gallbladder must not be mistaken for pathology, such as a pseudocyst or abscess.

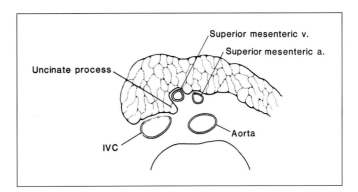

Figure 3-10—The Uncinate Process, as seen on transverse images.

these viscera.[5–12] Ingestion of a large volume of fluid has been advocated most commonly as a gas-displacing method (everything from water to oatmeal has been tried). I occasionally use water ingestion to define the pancreatic head, but in my experience, fluid ingestion does not improve pancreatic visualization in many patients, and I do not use this method routinely. Possibly the best aid for pancreatic visualization is to use effectively the acoustic window provided by the liver. The "liver window" is most effective in deep inspiration and, in some cases, with the patient standing.[9, 10, 13]

Mesenteric Fat

Excessive parapancreatic and mesenteric fat also may limit sonographic visualization of the pancreas.[14–18] Two factors contribute to the fat problem. First, fat scatters and attenuates the ultrasound beam. Second, fat interspersed among the pancreatic lobules (Fig. 3–11) may

Table 3-1. Pancreatic Sonography Protocol

Vascular Landmarks
With transverse images, identify the aorta, inferior vena cava (IVC), superior mesenteric artery, superior mesenteric vein, splenic vein, and portal vein.

Body, Tail, and Neck
Examine the body, tail, and neck of the pancreas with transverse images. Note the size of the body and tail, echogenicity, and the appearance of the pancreatic duct. Document normal and abnormal features with hard copy images.

Head
Examine the head, first with oblique images (left upper to right lower quadrant), and then with longitudinal images (usually along the course of the IVC). Note the size of the head, echogenicity, and the appearance of the uncinate process. Document normal and abnormal features with hard copy images.

Other Structures
Examine the rest of the upper abdomen, using protocols listed elsewhere in this text.

cause the pancreas to "blend in" with the surrounding retroperitoneal fat. This problem may be compounded by senescent pancreatic atrophy. In some elderly patients, only a small amount of pancreatic tissue is present, and the pancreatic bed contains mostly fat. I know of no technical "tricks" for overcoming fat-related pancreas visualization problems.

The Posterolateral Approach

A technique has been described for scanning the pancreatic tail through the left kidney from a posterolateral approach,[13] but only in rare instances have I been able to identify the *normal* pancreatic tail with this method. The posterolateral approach appears to be valuable, however, for visualization of pancreatic masses. Furthermore, the posterolateral approach is very useful for surveying the upper lesser sac for fluid collections such as abscesses or pseudocysts.

PANCREATIC ECHOGENICITY AND TEXTURE

Pancreatic echogenicity either *equals* or *exceeds* hepatic echogenicity in normal adults.[1, 3, 4,]

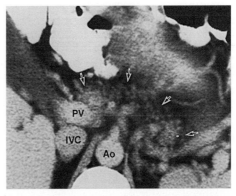

Figure 3-11—Computed Tomogram of a Fat-Replaced Pancreas (arrows). Note the dark fat intervening among the rounded pancreatic lobules. PV = portal vein; IVC = inferior vena cava; Ao = aorta.

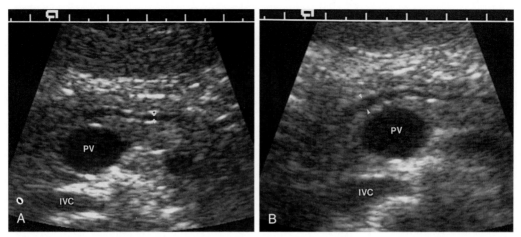

Figure 3-12—The Pancreatic Duct. (A) Sonogram of the duct (cursors) as seen on a transverse scan of the pancreatic body. PV = portal vein; IVC = inferior vena cava. (B) Note that the size of the duct (arrowheads) increases as it passes through the pancreatic head. PV = portal vein; IVC = inferior vena cava.

[13, 16, 17, 19] This is a very important sonographic observation, since most pathologic processes diminish pancreatic echogenicity, making the gland less echogenic than the liver. Pancreatic echogenicity also equals or exceeds hepatic echogenicity in about 90% of children. In the remaining 10% of children, the normal pancreas is *less* echogenic than the liver. Thus, a hypoechoic pancreas does not always signify pathology in a child.

The "texture" of the normal pancreas is slightly coarser than that of the liver, in both adults and children. Pancreatic texture varies from one individual to another, however, perhaps in relation to the quantity of fat interposed among the pancreatic lobules.

PANCREATIC DIMENSIONS

The normal dimensions of the pancreas have been defined by a large number of studies.[3, 4, 19–23] In adults, the pancreatic head is 2.5 cm or less in its maximum anteroposterior (AP) dimension. The body and tail in adults normally do not exceed 2 cm AP. Caution must be used in applying these measurements when the pancreatic head or tail "droops" prominently to the right or left of the spine. Such a configuration exaggerates the AP measurement. Caution also must be exercised in interpreting pancreatic size in young adults, since the pancreas is larger in young individuals than it is later in life. A diagnosis of enlargement should be made cautiously in a young patient, therefore, when measurements approximate the upper limit of normal.

Childhood pancreatic dimensions, as correlated with age, are listed in Table 3–2.[21] As noted previously, the pancreatic tail in children may have a bulbous appearance.

THE PANCREATIC DUCT

The main pancreatic duct* (hereafter called the "duct")[24–28] traverses the gland as shown in Figure 3–1. The duct is largest in the pancreatic head and tapers smoothly throughout the body and tail. The most commonly visualized portions lie within the body and tail. These portions are more or less perpendicular to the ultrasound beam, facilitating their visualization. If imaging conditions are good, the duct lumen is seen as a sonolucent zone bounded by the echogenic duct wall (Fig. 3–12). With less optimal imaging conditions, the lumen is not resolved, and the wall is seen as an echogenic line. The wall, when seen, should be smooth and should appear as parallel lines. A wavy or irregular duct wall is highly suggestive of chronic pancreatitis.[26]

The normal pancreatic duct lumen is 2 mm or less in diameter (inner-to-inner), as seen in the pancreatic body.[24, 26, 28–30] A dimension greater

---

*The main duct also is called Wirsung's duct. The secondary pancreatic duct (the duct of Santorini) traverses the pancreatic head but seldom is seen with ultrasound.

Table 3-2. Pancreatic Dimensions in Children

	Maximum Anteroposterior Dimensions (cm ± 1 standard deviation)		
Age	*Head*	*Body*	*Tail*
1 mo–1 yr	1.5 ± 0.5	0.8 ± 0.3	1.2 ± 0.4
1–5 yr	1.7 ± 0.3	1.0 ± 0.2	1.8 ± 0.4
5–10 yr	1.6 ± 0.4	1.0 ± 0.3	1.8 ± 0.4
10–19 yr	2.0 ± 0.5	1.1 ± 0.3	2.0 ± 0.4

From Siegel MJ, Martin KW, Worthington JL: Normal and abnormal pancreas in children; US studies. Radiology 165:15–18, 1987.

than 2 mm in the body is highly specific for ductal obstruction or chronic pancreatitis, as discussed in the next chapter. The duct diameter in the pancreatic head is variable and may normally be as large as 5 mm adjacent to the duodenum.[25, 28] Ductal measurements in the head, therefore, have less diagnostic value than measurements made in the body or tail.

REFERENCES

1. Filly RA, London SS: The normal pancreas: Acoustic characteristics and frequency of imaging. J Clin Ultrasound 7:121–124, 1979.
2. Doust BD, Pearce JD: Gray-scale ultrasonic properties of the normal and inflamed pancreas. Radiology 120:653–657, 1976.
3. Sample WF: Techniques for improved delineation of normal anatomy of the upper abdomen and high retroperitoneum with gray-scale ultrasound. Radiology 124:197–202, 1977.
4. Filly RA, Carlsen EN: Newer ultrasonographic anatomy in the upper abdomen: II. The major systemic veins and arteries with a special note on localization of the pancreas. J Clin Ultrasound 4:91–96, 1975.
5. den Orth JOO: Sonography of the pancreatic head aided by water and glucagon. Radiographics 7:85–100, 1987.
6. duCret RP, Jackson VP, Rees C, Lowe R, Davison NE: Pancreatic sonography: Enhancement by metoclopramide. AJR Am J Roentgenol 146:341–343, 1986.
7. Bowie JD, MacMahon H: Improved techniques in pancreatic sonography. Semin Ultrasound 1:170–177, 1980.
8. Crade M, Taylor KJW, Rosenfeld AT: Water distention of the gut in the evaluation of the pancreas by ultrasound. AJR Am J Roentgenol 131:348–349, 1978.
9. Jacobson P, Crade M, Taylor KJW: The upright position while giving water for the evaluation of the pancreas. J Clin Ultrasound 6:353–354, 1979.
10. MacMahon H, Bowie JD, Breezhold C: Erect scanning of the pancreas using a gastric window. AJR Am J Roentgenol 132:587–591.
11. Warren PS, Garrett WJ, Kossoff G: The liquid-filled stomach—an ultrasonic window to the upper abdomen. J Clin Ultrasound 6:315–320, 1978.
12. Weighall SK, Wolfman NT, Watson N: The fluid-filled stomach; A new sonic window. J Clin Ultrasound 7:353–356, 1979.
13. Taylor KJW, Buchin PJ, Viscomi GN, Rosenfield AT: Ultrasonographic scanning of the pancreas. Radiology 138:211–213, 1981.
14. den Orth JOO: Prepancreatic fat deposition: A possible pitfall in pancreatic sonography. AJR Am J Roentgenol 146:1017–1018, 1986.
15. Bree RL, Schwab RE: Contribution of mesenteric fat to unsatisfactory abdominal and pelvic ultrasonography. Radiology 140:773–776, 1981.
16. Marks WM, Filly RA, Callen PW: Ultrasonic evaluation of normal pancreatic echogenicity and its relationship to fat deposition. Radiology 137:475–479, 1980.
17. Worthen NJ, Beabeau D: Normal pancreatic echogenicity: Relation to age and body fat. AJR Am J Roentgenol 139:1095–1098, 1982.
18. So CB, Cooperberg PL, Gibney RG, Bogoch A: Sonographic findings in pancreatic lipomatosis. AJR Am J Roentgenol 149:67–68, 1987.
19. Arger PH, Mulhern CB, Bonavita JA, Stauffer DM, Hale J: An analysis of pancreatic sonography in suspected pancreatic disease. J Clin Ultrasound 7:91–97, 1979.
20. Coleman BG, Arger PH, Rosenberg HK, et al: Gray-scale sonographic assessment of pancreatitis in children. Radiology 146:145–150, 1983.
21. Siegel MJ, Martin KW, Worthington JL: Normal and abnormal pancreas in children: US studies. Radiology 165:15–18, 1987.
22. McCain AH, Berkman WA, Bernardino ME: Pancreatic sonography: Past and present. J Clin Ultrasound 12:325–332, 1984.
23. DeGraaff CS, Taylor KJW, Simonds BD, et al: Gray scale echography of the pancreas. Radiology 128:157–161, 1978.
24. Ohto M, Saotome N, Saisho H, Tsuchiya Y, Ono T, Okuda K, Karasawa E: Real-time sonography of the pancreatic duct: Application to percutaneous pancreatic ductography. AJR Am J Roentgenol 134:647–652, 1980.
25. Berland LL, Lawson TL, Foley WD, Geenen JE, Stewart ET: Computed tomography of the normal and abnormal pancreatic duct: Correlation with pancreatic ductography. Radiology 141:715–724, 1981.
26. Lawson TL, Berland LL, Foley WD, Stewart ET, Geenen JE, Hogan WJ: Ultrasonic visualization of the pancreatic duct. Radiology 144:865–871, 1982.
27. Hadidi A: Pancreatic duct diameter: Sonographic measurement in normal subjects. J Clin Ultrasound 11:17–22, 1983.
28. Cornud SBF, Benacerraf ASR: Etude du canal de Wirsung normal en échographie temps réel. Radiology 65:35–39, 1984.
29. Mack E: Clinical aspects of pancreatitis. Semin Ultrasound I/3:166–169, 1980.
30. Levitt RG, Geisse GG, Sagel SS, Stanley RJ, Evens RG, Koehler RE, Jost RG: Complementary use of ultrasound and computed tomography in studies of the pancreas and kidney. Radiology 126:149–152, 1978.

Chapter 4

Pancreatitis

William J. Zwiebel

ACUTE PANCREATITIS

Etiology

The most common cause of acute pancreatitis in the United States is impaction of a calculus in the distal common *bile* duct.[1-4] The impacted calculus blocks the pancreatic duct where it joins the duodenum and usually blocks the bile duct as well. The resultant back pressure in the pancreatic ductal system causes acute pancreatitis. Calculi may be present *within* the pancreatic duct in patients with chronic or recurrent pancreatitis, but such calculi seldom obstruct the duct and seldom cause acute pancreatitis. Pancreatic neoplasms also may obstruct the pancreatic duct and cause acute pancreatitis, but this presentation is uncommon.[1]

The second most common cause of acute pancreatitis in the United States is chemical injury from excessive alcohol consumption.[1-4] This injury can present as an episode of acute pancreatitis, or it may be clinically silent and relentless, as discussed later. Pancreatic injury can result from other chemical agents, but such injury occurs only rarely.

Trauma is an additional common cause of acute pancreatitis in adults and is the most commonly recognized cause in children.[5] Two mechanisms are recognized: (1) direct, violent or surgical injury, and (2) indirect injury induced by nearby surgical manipulation.

Pancreatic carcinoma with ductal obstruction may present with acute pancreatitis, but this is a relatively uncommon occurrence.

Pathology

The pathology of acute pancreatitis,[1-37] once initiated, proceeds along a common pathway, regardless of cause. If the inflammatory process is relatively mild and massive cellular disruption does not occur, then pancreatitis is self-limiting and resolution may be expected. If extensive cellular breakdown occurs, however, the intercellular fluid becomes laden with digestive enzymes, which cause parenchymal autolysis. If the lytic process disrupts the pancreatic ductal system, pancreatic secretions may extravasate widely into the pancreatic bed, the anterior perinephric

space, and the mesentery. Occlusion or rupture of blood vessels invariably accompanies severe pancreatitis.

Together, the autolytic process and vascular injury may cause a variety of complications, including the following: (1) necrosis of small or large portions of the gland; (2) massive inflammation in the pancreatic bed, contiguous retroperitoneal structures, and contiguous portions of the mesentery; (3) retroperitoneal hemorrhage (hemorrhagic pancreatitis); (4) fluid collections within or extrinsic to the pancreas (including pseudocysts); (5) abscess formation; and (6) fistulas between the bowel and the pancreatic bed, or between the bowel and pseudocysts.*

The Roles of Imaging Procedures in Acute Pancreatitis

The primary roles of imaging procedures in acute pancreatitis are to identify significant complications, to follow their course, and to help determine when intervention is needed for management of complications. Imaging procedures generally should not be used to diagnose acute pancreatitis, except perhaps in children with unexplained abdominal pain.[2, 34] Acute pancreatitis, in most instances, is diagnosed clinically and with laboratory tests.[1-4, 6, 7]

Profound intestinal ileus in acute pancreatitis often limits the value of sonography, since gas in aperistaltic bowel obscures the pancreatic bed. Ileus does not interfere significantly with computed tomographic (CT) examination, and for this and other reasons, CT is the imaging procedure of choice in acute pancreatitis.[7-9, 18] The diagnostic superiority of CT should not dissuade sonographers and sonologists from learning about acute pancreatitis, however. In some cases, abnormalities related to acute pancreatitis may be noted incidentally on examinations performed for other reasons; furthermore, sonography is the primary method for diagnosis of acute pancreatitis in children. Magnetic resonance imaging also

---

*The term "phlegmonous pancreatitis" is sometimes applied when the inflammatory process is massive, but "phlegmon" implies infection, which, in fact, is uncommon in acute pancreatitis.

may be used to detect and evaluate acute pancreatitis,[9, 10] but as of this writing, the value of this technique appears limited.

Uncomplicated Acute Pancreatitis

Acute but uncomplicated pancreatitis is identified sonographically by pancreatic enlargement and *decreased pancreatic echogenicity*[2, 7, 8, 17, 18] (Fig. 4–1). These inflammatory changes may make the pancreas unusually visible, and in some cases the enlarged pancreas may resemble a large, sonolucent sausage. Sonographic detection of these pancreatitis-related abnormalities is especially important when pancreatitis is not suspected clinically (e.g., in a patient with epigastric pain attributed to peptic disease or cholecystitis). In such instances sonographic diagnosis may greatly expedite the diagnostic process.

Unfortunately, altered pancreatic echogenicity is not always an accurate predictor of pancreatitis, for several reasons. First, pancreatic echogenicity may remain normal in acute pancreatitis, even when the severity of the process causes clinical symptoms and biochemical findings. Normal pancreatic echogenicity, therefore, does not

exclude the diagnosis of acute pancreatitis. Second, in rare instances, echogenicity may be *increased* in acute pancreatitis, apparently because of hemorrhage or the accumulation of proteinaceous debris within the parenchyma.[7] Third, a false-positive diagnosis of pancreatitis may occur if the liver is abnormally echogenic due to hepatocellular disease, making the pancreas appear *relatively* lucent. Finally, the normal pancreas may be less echogenic than the liver in children, as discussed later.

Fluid Collections

A variety of ambiguous and overlapping terms have been used to describe fluid collections associated with pancreatitis.[7, 8, 11, 13, 14, 19–21, 27, 29] In an effort to clarify this matter, a clinically based classification system has been devised that defines four types of pancreatitis-related fluid collections: (1) acute fluid collections; (2) pseudocysts; (3) pancreatic necrosis; and (4) abscesses.[2] It is worthwhile to note the definitions of these entities.

Acute fluid collections include any pancreatitis-related fluid collections that appear within 4 weeks of the onset of pancreatitis. These vary in

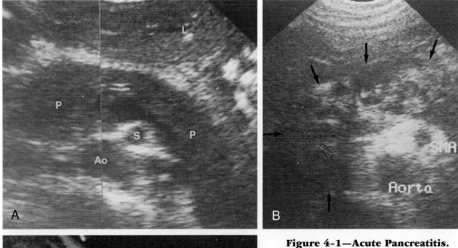

Figure 4-1—Acute Pancreatitis.
(A) A composite view of the pancreas (P) demonstrates enlargement of the gland (the head measures 3.5 cm AP) and reduced echogenicity as compared with the liver (L). S = superior mesenteric artery; Ao = aorta. **(B)** Gross pancreatic bed edema is represented by mottled echogenicity (arrows) on this transverse view. The pancreas per se is not visible. SMA = superior mesenteric artery. **(C)** Longitudinal view of a dilated extrahepatic bile duct (BD) and a markedly edematous (hypoechoic) pancreatic bed (arrows).

composition and may be located in, near, or distant from the pancreas. They are not encapsulated and often resolve spontaneously. Bacteria may be present, but the contents are not grossly purulent.

Pseudocysts, in contrast to acute fluid collections, *persist for more than 4 weeks after the onset of pancreatitis* and generally are well defined and rounded. These fluid collections are rich in pancreatic juices and are encapsulated by a well-defined wall of granulation or fibrous tissue. This wall generally is not visible, however, on imaging studies. Bacteria may be present, but the contents of pseudocysts are not grossly purulent. The crucial feature that defines a pseudocyst is its age. Collections less than 4 weeks old should not be called pseudocysts. The prefix "pseudo" refers to the fact that these collections are void of an epithelial lining and therefore are not true cysts.

Pancreatic necrosis refers to devitalization of a portion of the pancreas (necrosis of the entire gland is uncommon), typically leading to liquefaction and formation of a fluid collection. The collection may be sterile or infected, and in the latter case it is called *infected necrosis.* Pancreatic necrosis is important, for it portends a high incidence of morbidity and mortality, particularly when infected (discussed later).

Abscess refers to a grossly purulent, pancreatitis-related fluid collection of any age. Thus, the term "infected pseudocyst" should not be used! A distinction should be made, however, between infected necrosis and pancreatitis-related abscess in the general sense, for infected necrosis carries a particularly bad prognosis.

Sonographic Findings. Pancreatitis-related fluid collections tend to form along the usual routes that the acute inflammatory process follows.[2, 7, 11-13, 19] Thus, they occur most commonly within the pancreatic substance, in the pancreatic bed, or in the lesser peritoneal space. Other common locations are the anterior pararenal space, adjacent to the pancreatic tail, and within the transverse mesocolon.° Pancreatitis-related fluid collections are notorious, however, for presentation in unusual and distant locations, such as the pelvis, mediastinum, and pleural space. The explanation for this phenomenon lies in the ability of enzyme-laden pancreatic fluid to digest/dissect along tissue planes.

Acute pancreatitis-related fluid collections or pseudocysts classically present as well-circumscribed, rounded masses with typical cyst features, including anechoic contents, and enhanced through-transmission of ultrasound (Fig. 4–2). It should be noted, however, that the ultrasound features of these fluid collections may vary widely from the classic appearance. The fluid collections may contain debris from tissue necrosis, inflammation, infection, or hemorrhage; consequently, the fluid contents may exhibit varying levels of echogenicity (Fig. 4–3), from faintly echogenic to markedly echogenic.[7, 11, 20, 29] Echogenic material may be dispersed throughout the contents or may form a dependent layer.

The shape of these collections also is variable.[7, 19] The fluid that extravasates from the pancreas tends to dissect between tissue planes in

---

°The anatomy of the lesser peritoneal space is presented in Chapter 24. Perinephric space anatomy is presented in Chapter 16.

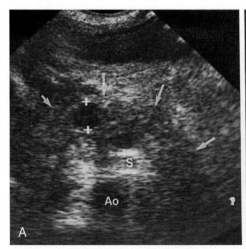 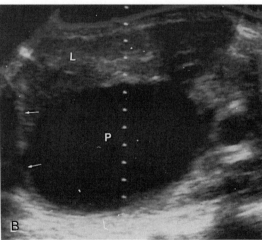

Figure 4-2—Classic Pseudocyst Appearance. (A) A transverse sonogram shows a 1.5-cm pseudocyst (cursors) in the pancreatic head. It is anechoic and exhibits enhanced through-transmission. Arrows = pancreas; S = superior mesenteric artery; Ao = aorta. **(B)** A longitudinal sonogram through the left upper quadrant of the abdomen demonstrates an 11-cm pseudocyst (P) in the lesser sac. The pseudocyst is sharply marginated and anechoic, and exhibits enhanced through-transmission. Arrows = diaphragm; L = liver.

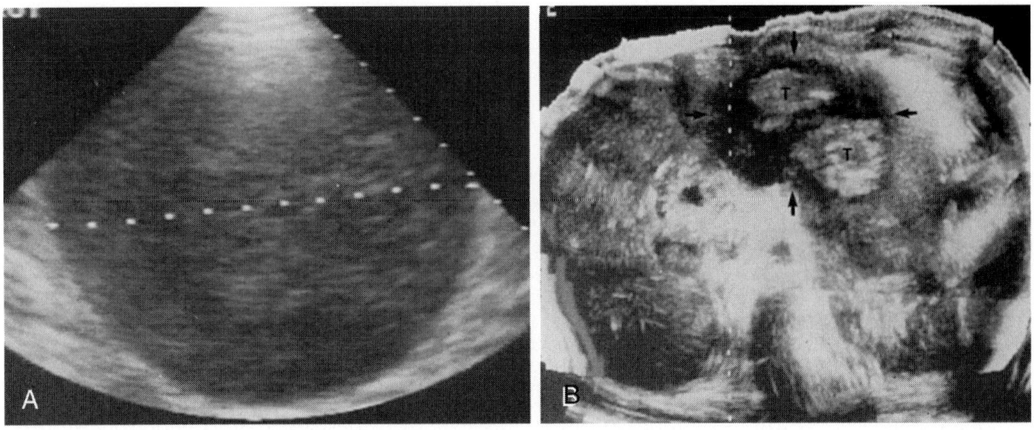

Figure 4-3—Variation in Pseudocyst Appearance. (A) Longitudinal image of an 11-cm pseudocyst with moderately echogenic contents. (B) Transverse image of a pancreatic bed pseudocyst (arrows) containing strongly echogenic, retracted thrombus (T).

acute pancreatitis; therefore, such collections may have an irregular shape. With resorption or spontaneous decompression (into the bowel or peritoneal space), pseudocysts may lose turgor. As a result, the usual rounded shape may give way to an irregular configuration. Irregular, collapsed pseudocysts may have a bizarre appearance and may resemble solid masses.

Ultrasound cannot generally differentiate between pseudocysts and other fluid collections.[7, 11, 19, 20] The wall of a pseudocyst generally is too thin for sonographic visualization. Rarely, very chronic pseudocysts may have visible wall or even a strongly echogenic, calcified rim.

Sonographic Detection. Sonography performs reasonably well for the detection of large, pancreatitis-related fluid collections (96% sensi-

tivity for cysts larger than 3 cm), but ultrasound identifies only about 75% of the fluid collections seen with computed tomography, since many of these collections are smaller than 3 cm[19] (Fig. 4–4). Because even small fluid collections or pseudocysts (under 3 cm) may be symptomatic or may be associated with significant complications, the detection of all collections is desirable. Computed tomography, therefore, is the imaging procedure of choice for imaging fluid collections arising from acute pancreatitis.

Differential Diagnosis. A host of cystic and solid masses may mimic the appearance of a pancreatitis-related fluid collection. These include pancreatic carcinoma (5% to 10% have cystic components), cystic pancreatic neoplasms (e.g., cystadenoma), hematomas, splanchnic arte-

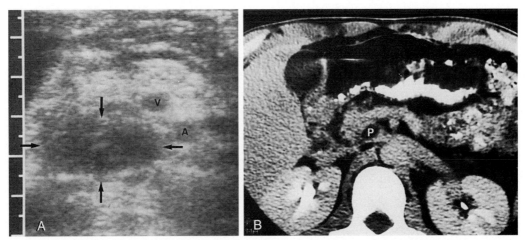

Figure 4-4—Superior CT Visualization of a Pseudocyst. (A) A transverse sonogram demonstrates an edematous region (arrows) in the pancreatic head. A pseudocyst was not identified. V = superior mesenteric vein; A = superior mesenteric artery. (B) A transaxial CT scan on the same date as the sonogram clearly demonstrates a small pseudocyst (P) in the uncinate process.

rial aneurysms, abscesses, and "simple" cysts (which are rare).[20–26, 30, 32, 34]

Pseudocyst Follow-up. The widespread use of ultrasound and CT in pancreatitis has taught us a great deal about the natural history of pancreatitis-related fluid collections.[7, 13, 17–19, 27, 35, 36] We have learned that fluid collections are much more common in pancreatitis than previously suspected, and that about 20% to 40% resolve spontaneously, with a mean disappearance time of 4 to 6 weeks. Persistent fluid collections (more than 4 weeks), defined as pseudocysts, may communicate with the pancreatic duct, in which case they may predispose the patient to recurrence of acute pancreatitis.* Persistent pseudocysts also may cause pain and are subject to superinfection, spontaneous rupture (into the peritoneum or into the bowel), and erosion into blood vessels. Pseudocyst rupture is said to carry a 50% mortality rate, regardless of the route of decompression.[7, 19]

Because significant complications may accompany a persistent pseudocyst, intervention is recommended for pseudocysts larger than 5 cm in diameter that do not show evidence of regression or resolve completely within 6 weeks of an episode of acute pancreatitis.[20]

The time-honored solution for a chronic pseudocyst is surgical marsupialization to the bowel. Percutaneous catheter drainage has been advocated as a safe and less morbid means of pseudocyst drainage, but this technique is not appropriate in all cases.[28]

Pancreatic Necrosis

Pancreatic necrosis (see earlier definition)[1, 2, 14–16, 18] usually is diagnosed with CT, by lack of

---

*Ductal communication is identified via endoscopic retrograde pancreatography.

enhancement of the affected portion of the gland. If large areas of liquefaction occur, however, pancreatic necrosis may be recognized sonographically, since a characteristic fluid collection develops in the pancreatic bed.[14–16] This fluid collection is tubular and has the same general configuration as the pancreas, as shown in Figure 4–5. Echogenicity of the contained fluid varies with the amount of macroscopic debris.

Pancreatic Abscess

A pancreatitis-related abscess occurs when a fluid collection becomes secondarily infected.[2, 7, 11, 13, 27–33] Abscesses are difficult to differentiate from noninfected fluid collections. The only finding that suggests abscess formation is the presence of gas within the collection, as revealed by strong ultrasound reflections and acoustic shadows (Fig. 4–6). Since gas is the only distinctive finding, imaging studies can detect *only* abscesses caused by gas-forming organisms. In the absence of accumulated gas, infected and noninfected collections have no definitive sonographic or CT characteristics. The track record of CT for abscess detection is superior to that of ultrasound (50% versus 31% sensitivity),[30] but neither of these results is worth raving about. Furthermore, chemical processes or fistulous communication with the bowel may cause gas to accumulate in pancreatitis-related fluid collections, mimicking the appearance of abscess.[30, 31, 33] Needle aspiration is an effective means for abscess diagnosis, but caution is recommended, as needle aspiration may introduce bacteria to a sterile fluid collection, with serious adverse consequences.

As noted previously, clinical differentiation between infected pancreatic necrosis and run-of-

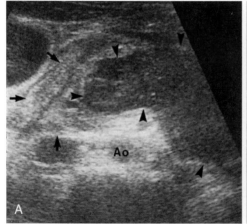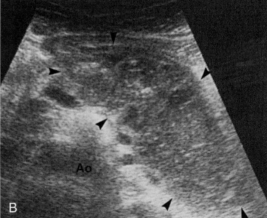

Figure 4-5—Pancreatic Necrosis. (A) A transverse sonogram demonstrates residual pancreatic tissue (arrows) in the head of the pancreas, which partially surrounds a large necrotic area (arrowhead). Ao = aorta. **(B)** A transverse sonogram slightly to the left of **A** demonstrates replacement of the pancreatic body and tail by an encapsulated collection of moderately echogenic, necrotic debris (arrowheads). Ao = aorta.

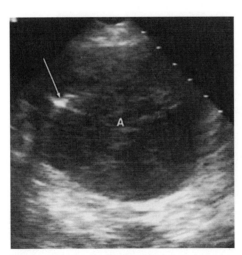

Figure 4-6—Pancreatitis-Related Abscess. A transverse sonogram through a lesser sac abscess (A) demonstrates low-level, heterogeneous echoes and a bright focus (arrow). The latter is an infection-related gas bubble.

the-mill pancreatitis-related abscess is of vital importance since infected pancreatic necrosis carries a poor prognosis.[2, 16, 18]

Acute Pancreatitis in Childhood

Etiology. Blunt abdominal trauma is a primary cause of acute pancreatitis in children (about 50% of cases), and child abuse is the etiology of such trauma in most instances.[33, 34, 36] Other identifiable causes include infection (mumps and other viral illnesses), biliary or pancreatic ductal obstruction, and systemic disorders, such as cystic fibrosis, hypercholesterolemia, and uremia.[36] In at least 30% of cases, the cause of childhood acute pancreatitis cannot be identified.[33, 36]

The Role of Sonography. The diagnosis of acute pancreatitis may be difficult to confirm clinically in pediatric patients, and in such instances sonography may be a useful tool. The sensitivity of ultrasound for acute pancreatitis in children is low (about 70%), but the specificity and positive predictive values exceed 90%.[33] Thus, positive sonographic findings may be quite valuable in difficult-to-diagnose cases. Sonography is recommended, therefore, as a *primary* modality for diagnosis of acute pancreatitis in children, whereas sonography is not recommended as a primary diagnostic tool in adults.

Ultrasound Findings. The most important sonographic sign of acute pancreatitis in children is focal or diffuse pancreatic enlargement.[33, 35] A valuable parameter for defining pancreatic enlargement in children is a ratio of the largest AP

dimension of the body or tail to the transverse dimension of a nearby vertebral body. A ratio greater than 0.3, coupled with a hypoechoic appearance, is highly suggestive of acute pancreatitis.[33] Hypoechogenicity (compared with the liver) is not as specific a sign of pancreatitis in children as in adults, since about 10% of normal glands are hypoechoic in children.[37–39] Pancreatic duct and common bile duct dilatation are other important signs of acute pancreatitis in children.

Ultrasound is more successful for the identification and follow-up of pancreatitis-related fluid collections in children than in adults because children generally are lean and relatively easy to examine.[35, 36] The sonographic features of acute fluid collections and pseudocysts in children are the same as those described previously.

CHRONIC PANCREATITIS

The term "chronic pancreatitis" refers to chronic pancreatic inflammation, which leads ultimately to parenchymal destruction, pancreatic atrophy, scar formation, and the accretion of intraductal calculi.[29, 40–56] Chronic pancreatitis may have multiple causes, including the obstructive effects of biliary calculi, but in Western nations the toxic effect of alcohol is the most common cause. The precise mechanism of alcohol injury is not known, and the susceptibility of some individuals to alcohol-related pancreatitis is unexplained. Although alcohol can cause damaging episodes of acute pancreatitis, the principal destructive effects of alcohol seem to be slowly progressive and insidious.

Chronic pancreatitis usually causes epigastric pain and/or symptoms of malabsorption (from loss of exocrine function). In some patients with chronic pancreatitis, however, symptoms are absent.[44]

Pancreatic calcification is a significant feature of chronic pancreatitis. The calculi generally are small (up to a few millimeters in diameter) and are thought to form as proteinaceous plugs in the side branches of the pancreatic duct.[41] These deposits accrete calcium salts and subsequently become visible radiographically or sonographically. The calculi typically "line up" parallel to the main pancreatic duct, since they form in the branches of this duct,[40] but this pattern is lost in advanced cases owing to architectural distortion and diffuse calculus formation. Pancreatic ductal dilatation is a common feature of chronic pancreatitis, but calculus-related obstruction generally is *not* the cause of such dilatation.[48] Ductal dilatation is caused initially by spasm and edema[44] and later by scarring. With progressive ductal dilatation, calculi that form in the branch ducts

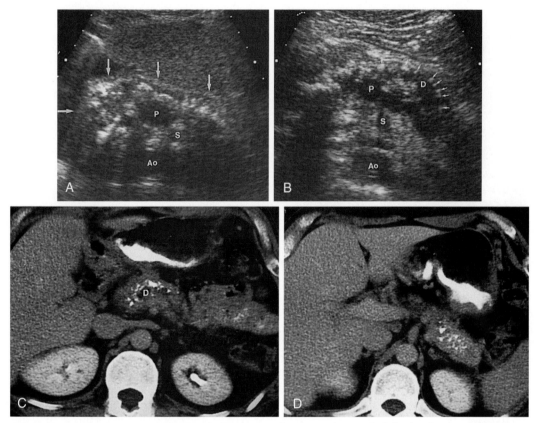

Figure 4-7—Chronic Pancreatitis. (A, B) The pancreas (large arrows) is poorly defined and contains multiple strongly echogenic calcifications, as seen on these transverse images. Note in **B** that the calcifications (small arrows) line up adjacent to a dilated segment of the pancreatic duct (D). P = portosplenic confluence; S = superior mesenteric artery; Ao = aorta. **(C, D)** Computed tomograms of the same patient demonstrate the periductal location of the calculi. D = dilated pancreatic duct.

"fall into" the main pancreatic duct, but they do not obstruct the duct primarily.

The Role of Sonography and Computed Tomography

Ultrasound and computed tomography (CT) serve to document the diagnosis of chronic pancreatitis in patients with obscure abdominal pain or pancreatic insufficiency, to exclude pancreatic carcinoma as a cause of abdominal pain, and to identify pseudocysts complicating chronic pancreatitis.[7, 29, 35, 40, 43, 45–53, 57–61] Endoscopic retrograde pancreatography is used to document and evaluate ductal obstruction, which is a common finding in chronic pancreatitis.

Ultrasound is particularly valuable for identifying chronic pancreatitis in children.[7, 29, 45, 47, 53, 58–61] In adults, however, CT is the diagnostic procedure of choice, because pancreatic morphology is better seen with CT, and because chronic pancreatitis is more easily differentiated from other pancreatic disorders, such as carcinoma or senescent atrophy.[7, 46–48, 52]

Sonographic Findings

Pancreatic abnormalities may be found sonographically in about 85% of patients with chronic pancreatitis.[45] In the remaining cases, the gland is normal in appearance. The most common ultrasound findings (Fig. 4–7) are nonhomogeneity (57%), generalized increased echogenicity (53%), and focal strong echoes, with or without acoustic shadows (40%).[45] The latter findings are caused by large calculi that are resolved as discrete structures. The pancreatic margins frequently are poorly defined in severe chronic pancreatitis. In such instances, only a vaguely outlined area of increased echogenicity is seen in the usual location of the pancreas (Figs. 4–7 and 4–8).

Pancreatic ductal abnormalities are frequently visible sonographically, consisting of dilatation, irregularity, and intraductal calculi[29, 43, 45, 47, 51] (Figs. 4–8 and 4–9). An irregular or beaded duct configuration is typical of chronic pancreatitis, whereas a smooth duct margin is typical of neoplastic dilatation. The configuration of the duct, however, does not reliably indicate benign or neoplastic obstruction.[29, 43, 46, 51]

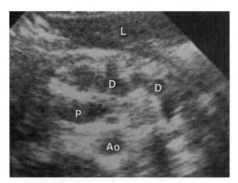

Figure 4-8—Varicose Pancreatic Duct in Chronic Pancreatitis. The pancreatic duct (D) is dilated (5 to 8 mm) and markedly tortuous (varicose). The borders of the pancreas are ill-defined, and the scarred pancreatic tissue is much more echogenic than the adjacent liver (L). P = portosplenic confluence; Ao = aorta.

Bile duct dilatation (usually slight) is present in about 30% of patients with chronic pancreatitis.[46] Biliary dilatation almost always is a *secondary* finding, rather than the cause of chronic pancreatitis.[46, 47] This is an important differential point between acute and chronic pancreatitis.

The Problem of the Inflammatory Mass

Destruction of the pancreatic tissue in chronic pancreatitis generally results in shrinkage of the gland, but in some cases, focal or diffuse pancreatic enlargement may occur. Focal enlargement (seen in 7% to 30% of patients) is a particularly thorny diagnostic problem, since differentiation from pancreatic carcinoma may be difficult. To make matters worse, calcifications may be seen both in chronic pancreatitis and pancreatic carcinoma. In some cases, focal enlargement is caused by a chronic pseudocyst, but in others it is caused by a fibrotic inflammatory mass.[45, 46, 48] Such

masses generally occur in the pancreatic head or body.

Three features appear to be valuable for identifying inflammatory pancreatic masses: (1) hyperechogenicity (as compared with normal pancreatic echogenicity); (2) extensive, diffusely scattered small (ductal) calculi within the mass; and (3) dilated side branches distributed throughout the mass. These features, as seen with CT or ultrasound, are reported successfully to identify 67% to 77% of inflammatory pancreatic masses.[45, 46, 49] In cases *without* these features, the inflammatory mass is hypoechoic (relative to the normal pancreas) and may be somewhat heterogeneous. These findings are identical to those of pancreatic carcinoma, as considered in the following chapter.

The most accurate means for differentiating between inflammatory and neoplastic pancreatic masses appears to be percutaneous needle aspiration, which provides a definitive diagnosis in up to 94% of cases.[49]

Chronic Pancreatitis Associated with Cystic Fibrosis

Cystic fibrosis affects all exocrine glands, including the pancreas. In this condition, abnormally viscid pancreatic secretions form concretions in the small pancreatic ducts, leading to glandular atresia, fibrosis, and fatty degeneration.[57]

The predominant sonographic finding in cystic fibrosis[58-63] is increased echogenicity of the pancreas, which has not been found to correlate with the severity of exocrine dysfunction. Massive fatty replacement has been noted in some cases,[59] and in rare instances, 1- to 2-cm cysts are scattered throughout the gland. Pancreatic ductal dilatation, calcification, and pseudocysts

Figure 4-9—Intraductal Calculi in Chronic Pancreatitis. Two calculi (arrows) are visible in a dilated pancreatic duct (cursors = 7.6 mm) on this transverse image. S = superior mesenteric artery; SV = splenic vein.

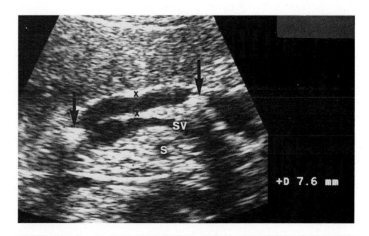

are encountered *rarely* in patients with cystic fibrosis. The absence of these findings emphasizes the pathogenetic differences between this and other forms of chronic pancreatitis. Bile duct dilatation also occurs in cystic fibrosis patients with chronic pancreatitis, but the incidence is unknown.[62]

REFERENCES

1. Stenberg W, Tenner S: Acute pancreatitis. N Engl J Med 330:1198–1210, 1994.
2. Bradley EL III: A clinically based classification system for acute pancreatitis. Arch Surg 128:586–590, 1993.
3. Arger PH, Mulhern CB, Bonavita JA, Stauffer DM, Hale J: An analysis of pancreatic sonography in suspected pancreatic disease. J Clin Ultrasound 7:91–97, 1979.
4. Police AM, Waxman K, Smolin M, Tominga G, Landau S, Mason GR: Development of gallstone pancreatitis: The role of the common channel. Arch Surg 119:1299–1300, 1984.
5. Roy CL, Silverman A, Cozzetto FJ: Pediatric Clinical Gastroenterology, 2nd ed. St Louis, CV Mosby, 1975, pp 648–650.
6. Moossa AR: Current concepts: Diagnostic tests and procedures in acute pancreatitis. N Engl J Med 311:639–643, 1984.
7. Federle MP, Burke VD: Pancreatitis and its complications: Computed tomography and sonography. Semin Ultrasound 5:414–427, 1984.
8. Silverstein W, Isikoff MB, Hill MC, Barkin J: Diagnostic imaging of acute pancreatitis: Prospective study using CT and sonography. AJR Am J Roentgenol 137:497–502, 1981.
9. Semelka RC, Kroeker MA, Shoenut JP, Kroeker R, Yaffe CS, Micflikier AB: Pancreatic disease: Prospective comparison of CT, ERCP, and 1.5-T MR imaging with dynamic gadolinium enhancement and fat suppression. Radiology 181:785–791, 1991.
10. Reimer P, Saini S, Hahn PF, Mueller PR, Brady TJ, Cohen MS: Techniques for high-resolution echo-planar MR imaging of the pancreas. Radiology 182:175–179, 1992.
11. Jeffrey RB, Laing FC, Wing VW: Extrapancreatic spread of acute pancreatitis: New observations with real-time US. Radiology 159:707–711, 1986.
12. Jeffrey RB, Federle MP, Laing FC: Computed tomography of mesenteric involvement in fulminant pancreatitis. Radiology 147:185–188, 1983.
13. Siegelman S, Copeland BE, Saba GP, Cameron JL, Sanders RC, Zerhouni EA: CT of fluid collections associated with pancreatitis. AJR Am J Roentgenol 134:1121–1132, 1980.
14. Burrell M, Gold JA, Simeone J, Taylor K, Dobbins J: Liquefactive necrosis of the pancreas. Radiology 135:157–160, 1980.
15. White EM, Wittenberg J, Mueller PR, Simeone JF, Butch RJ, Warshaw AL, Neff CC, Nardi GL, Ferrucci JT: Pancreatic necrosis: CT manifestations. Radiology 153:343–346, 1986.
16. Johnson CD, Stephens DH, Sarr MG: CT of acute pancreatitis: Correlation between lack of contrast enhancement and pancreatic necrosis. AJR Am J Roentgenol 156:93–95, 1991.
17. Hill MC, Barkin J, Isikoff MB, Silverstein W, Kalser M: Acute pancreatitis: Clinical vs. CT findings. AJR Am J Roentgenol 139:263–269, 1982.
18. Balthazar EJ, Robinson DL, Megibow AJ, Ranson JHC: Acute pancreatitis: Value of CT in establishing prognosis. Radiology 174:331–336, 1990.
19. Williford ME, Foster WL, Halvorsen RA, Thompson WM: Pancreatic pseudocyst: Comparative evaluation by sonography and computed tomography. AJR Am J Roentgenol 140:53–57, 1983.
20. Laing FC, Gooding GAW, Brown T, Leopold GR: Atypical pseudocysts of the pancreas: An ultrasonographic evaluation. J Clin Ultrasound 7:27–33, 1979.
21. Hashimoto BE, Laing FC, Jeffrey RB, Federle MP: Hemorrhagic pancreatic fluid collections examined by ultrasound. Radiology 150:803–808, 1984.
22. Thurber LA, Cooperberg PL, Clement JG, Lyone EA, Gramiak R, Cunningham J: Echogenic fluid: A pitfall in the ultrasonographic diagnosis of cystic lesions. J Clin Ultrasound 7:273–278, 1979.
23. Dennis JW, Aranha GV, Greenlee HB, Hoffman JP, Prinz RA: Carcinoma masquerading as a pancreatic pseudocyst on ultrasound. Am Surg 50:334–339, 1984.
24. Haney PJ, Whitley NO: CT of benign cystic abdominal masses in children. AJR Am J Roentgenol 142:1279–1281, 1984.
25. Gooding GAW: Ultrasound of a superior mesenteric artery aneurysm secondary to pancreatitis: A plea for real-time ultrasound of sonolucent masses in pancreatitis. J Clin Ultrasound 9:255–256, 1981.
26. Shultz S, Druy EM, Friedman AC: Common hepatic artery aneurysm: Pseudopseudocyst of the pancreas. AJR Am J Roentgenol 144:1287–1288, 1985.
27. Agha FP: Spontaneous resolution of acute pancreatic pseudocysts. Surg Gynecol Obstet 158:22–26, 1984.
28. vanSonnenberg E, Wittich GR, Casola G, Brannigan TC, Karnel F, Stabile BE, Varney RR, Christensen RR: Percutaneous drainage of infected and noninfected pancreatic pseudocysts: Experience in 101 cases. Radiology 170:757–761, 1989.
29. Cotton PB, Lees WR, Vallon AG, Cottone M, Croker JR, Chapman M: Gray-scale ultrasonography and endoscopic pancreatography in pancreatic diagnosis. Radiology 134:453–459, 1980.
30. Woodard S, Kelvin FM, Rice RP, Thompson WM: Pancreatic abscess: Importance of conventional radiology. AJR Am J Roentgenol 136:871–878, 1981.
31. Alexander ES, Clark RA, Federle MP: Pancreatic gas: Indication of pancreatic fistula. AJR Am J Roentgenol 139:1089–1093, 1982.
32. Vernacchia FS, Jeffrey RB, Federle MP, Grendell JH, Laing FC, Wing VW, Wall SD: Pancreatic abscess: Predictive value of early abdominal CT. Radiology 162:435–438, 1987.
33. Torres WE, Clements JL, Sones PJ, Knopf DR: Gas in the pancreatic bed without abscess. AJR Am J Roentgenol 137:1131–1133, 1981.
34. Fleischer AC, Parker P, Kirchner SG, James AE: Sonographic findings of pancreatitis in children. Radiology 146:151–155, 1983.
35. Coleman BG, Arger PH, Rosenberg HK, Mulhern CB, Ortega W, Stauffer D: Gray-scale sonographic assessment of pancreatitis in children. Radiology 146:145–150, 1983.
36. Slovis TL, Von Berg VJ, Mikelic V: Sonography in the diagnosis and management of pancreatic pseudocysts and effusions in childhood. Radiology 135:153–155, 1980.
37. Garel L, Brunelle F, Lallemand D, Sauvegrain J:

Pseudocysts of the pancreas in children: Which cases require surgery? Pediatr Radiol 13:120–124, 1983.

38. Coleman BG, Arger PH, Rosenberg HK, et al: Gray-scale sonographic assessment of pancreatitis in children. Radiology 146:145–150, 1983.

39. Siegel MJ, Martin KW, Worthington JL: Normal and abnormal pancreas in children: US studies. Radiology 165:15–18, 1987.

40. Weinstein BJ, Weinstein DP, Brodmerkel GJ: Ultrasonography of pancreatic lithiasis. Radiology 134:185–189, 1980.

41. Sarles H, Sarles JC, Camatte R, et al: Observations on 205 confirmed cases of acute pancreatitis, recurring pancreatitis, and chronic pancreatitis. Gut 6:545–559, 1965.

42. Paulino-Netto A, Dreiling DA, Baronofsky ID: The relationship between pancreatic calcification and cancer of the pancreas. Ann Surg 151:530–537, 1960.

43. Gosink BB, Leopold GR: The dilated pancreatic duct: Ultrasonic evaluation. Radiology 126:475, 1978.

44. Kissaine JM, Lacy PE: Pancreatitis and diabetes mellitus. *In* Kissaine JM (ed): Anderson's Pathology, 8th ed. St Louis, CV Mosby, 1985, pp 1238–1239.

45. Alpern MB, Sandler MA, Kellman GM, Madrazo BL: Chronic pancreatitis: Ultrasonic features. Radiology 155:215–219, 1985.

46. Luetmer PH, Stephens DH, Ward EM: Chronic pancreatitis: Reassessment with current CT. Radiology 171:353–357, 1989.

47. Huntington DK, Hill MB, Steinberg W: Biliary tract siltation in chronic pancreatitis: CT and sonographic findings. Radiology 172:48–50, 1989.

48. Karasawa E, Goldberg HI, Moss AA, Federle MP, London SS: CT pancreatogram in carcinoma of the pancreas and chronic pancreatitis. Radiology 148:489–493, 1983.

49. DelMaschio A, Vanzulli A, Sironi S, Castrucci M, Mellone R, Staudacher C, Carlucci M, Zerbi A, Parolini D, Faravelli A, Cantaboni A, Garancini P, Di Carlo V: Pancreatic cancer versus chronic pancreatitis: Diagnosis with CA 19-9 assessment, US, CT, and CT-guided fine-needle biopsy. Radiology 178:95–99, 1991.

50. Isikoff MB, Hill MC: Ultrasonic demonstration of intraductal pancreatic calculi: A report of two cases. J Clin Ultrasound 8:449–452, 1980.

51. Kuligowska E, Miller K, Birkett D, Burakoff R: Cystic dilatation of the pancreatic duct simulating pseudocysts on sonography. AJR Am J Roentgenol 136:409–410, 1981.

52. Shuman WP, Carter SJ, Montana MA, Mack LA, Moss AA: Pancreatic insufficiency: Role of CT evaluation. Radiology 158:625–627, 1986.

53. Lees WR, Vallon AG, Denyer ME, et al: Prospective study of ultrasonography in chronic pancreatic disease. Br Med J 1:162–164, 1979.

54. Lawson TL, Berland LL, Foley WD, Stewart ET, Geenan JE, Hogan WJ: Ultrasonic visualization of the pancreatic duct. Radiology 144:865–871, 1982.

55. Berland LL, Lawson TL, Foley WD, Geenen JE, Stewart ET: Computed tomography of the normal and abnormal pancreatic duct: Correlation with pancreatic ductography. Radiology 141:715–724, 1981.

56. Blangy S, Cornud F, Sibert A, Benacerraf R: Etude du canal de Wirsung normal en échographie temps réel. Radiology 65:35–39, 1984.

57. Oppenheimer EM, Esterly JR: Pathology of cystic fibrosis: Review of the literature and comparison with 146 autopsied cases. Perspect Pediatr Pathol 2:241, 1975.

58. Phillips HE, Cox KL, Reid MH, McGahan JP: Pancreatic sonography in cystic fibrosis. AJR Am J Roentgenol 137:69–72, 1981.

59. Daneman A, Gaskin K, Martin DJ, Cutz E: Pancreatic changes in cystic fibrosis: CT and sonographic appearances. AJR Am J Roentgenol 141:653–655, 1983.

60. Shawker TH, Linzer M, Hubbard VS: Chronic pancreatitis: The diagnostic significance of pancreatic size and echo amplitude. J Ultrasound Med 3:267–272, 1984.

61. Swobodnik W, Wolf A, Wechsler JG, Kleihauer E, Ditschuneit H: Ultrasound characteristics of the pancreas in children with cystic fibrosis. J Clin Ultrasound 13:469–474, 1985.

62. Gaskin KJ, Donna LM, Waters RN, Howman-Giles R, De Silva M, Earl JW, Martin HCO, Kan AE, Brown JM, Dorney SFA: Liver disease and common-bile-duct stenosis in cystic fibrosis. N Engl J Med 318:340–346, 1988.

63. Hernanz-Schulman M, Teele RL, Perez-Atayde A, Zollars L, Levine J, Black P, Kuligowska E: Pancreatic cystosis in cystic fibrosis. Radiology 158:629–631, 1986.

Chapter 5

Pancreatic Neoplasms

William J. Zwiebel

From a sonographer's perspective, pancreatic neoplasms fall into two groups: solid and cystic lesions (Table 5–1). Each group will be considered in turn, but emphasis will be on solid lesions because they are by far the most common. Among solid pancreatic tumors, carcinoma is of greatest importance, as this lesion accounts for 75% of all pancreatic tumors.

PANCREATIC CARCINOMA

Pancreatic ductal carcinoma (hereafter called pancreatic carcinoma)[1–3] is a deadly malignancy that originates in the ductal epithelium. Approximately two thirds of pancreatic carcinomas occur in patients 60 years of age or older. This neoplasm is rare under the age of 40 years, and a lesion other than carcinoma should be considered when a solid pancreatic tumor is detected in younger individuals. In such cases, an inflammatory mass, a neuroendocrine tumor, or a papillary epithelial neoplasm is a consideration. The latter tumor is particularly suspect when a solid pancreatic tumor is discovered in a young woman.[1, 3]

The reported 5-year survival for pancreatic carcinoma ranges from 1% to 12%. These low survival statistics are principally due to the insidious development and aggressive nature of the tumor. Metastasis is to regional lymph nodes, the liver, the lungs, and the peritoneum.

The prospects for survival are better with an "ampullary carcinoma," localized to the ampulla of Vater. Tumors that originate here are better differentiated than other pancreatic carcinomas and attract clinical attention early because of bile duct obstruction.[1, 2]

The Role of Ultrasound

Sonography is reported to be 56% to 94% sensitive for pancreatic carcinoma.[4–13] A reasonable sensitivity figure probably is around 70%, if patient selection bias is excluded. Most carcinomas are detected in the setting of painless jaundice or a palpable mass. In these cases, sonography is the procedure of choice for confirming that a pancreatic mass is present and is causing biliary obstruction. Computed tomography (CT) is the procedure of choice for staging a pancreatic carcinoma, because CT is more sensitive than sonography for metastasis detection, and CT more clearly defines local tumor extent. Magnetic resonance imaging (MRI) ultimately may find a role in pancreatic carcinoma staging, but its value is not currently well defined.

Ultrasound is *not* the primary modality with which to search for an *occult* pancreatic carcinoma in a *nonjaundiced* patient. Computed tomography is the procedure of choice for occult lesions.

Sonographic Findings

The size of pancreatic carcinomas ranges widely at the time of sonographic diagnosis, from under 2 cm to more than 10 cm. The typical tumor is about 4 cm in diameter[2, 9, 10, 16–20] and therefore grossly distorts the pancreatic contours. Approximately 75% of pancreatic carcinomas are located in the head and neck of the gland (to the right of the superior mesenteric vein), and the remainder are located in the body and tail.[9, 16] Carcinomas that obstruct the common bile duct generally are smaller at presentation than tumors originating elsewhere in the gland. On rare occa-

Table 5-1. Differential Considerations for Pancreatic and Peripancreatic Masses

Solid-Appearing Masses

Pancreatic carcinoma
Inflammatory mass
Complicated pseudocyst
Peripancreatic adenopathy
Neuroendocrine tumor
Aneurysm
Papillary neoplasm of the pancreas
Benign microcystic neoplasm

Cystic Masses

Benign epithelium-lined cyst
Pseudocyst (or other pancreatitis-related collection)
Abscess
Aneurysm
Pancreatic bed metastasis°
Papillary neoplasm
Microcystic neoplasm
Macrocystic neoplasm

°Especially sarcoma metastases.

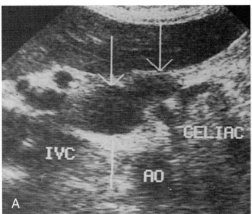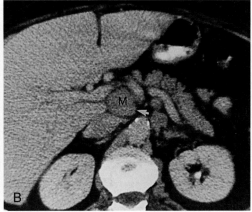

Figure 5-1—Small Pancreatic Carcinoma. (A) An oblique sonogram demonstrates a homogeneous, hypoechoic neoplasm (arrows) replacing the pancreatic head and body. The head is slightly enlarged (3 cm anteroposterior). This pancreatic carcinoma appears similar to focal acute pancreatitis (see Figure 4–4A). IVC = inferior vena cava; AO = aorta; celiac = celiac artery. **(B)** A CT scan at a corresponding level demonstrates the mass (M) in the pancreatic head. Note that the uncinate process (arrow) is rounded rather than pointed (its normal configuration).

sions, carcinoma infiltrates the gland diffusely, producing enlargement and irregularity without a focal mass. This appearance may mimic acute pancreatitis.

Pancreatic carcinoma is not encapsulated; hence the junction of the tumor with the normal pancreas is not sharply defined in most instances. A rounded tumor configuration with a smooth or slightly irregular border is the rule. Pancreatic carcinoma generally is less echogenic overall than the normal pancreas (Fig. 5–1), but a degree of heterogeneity is the rule and coarse, strong reflections commonly are interspersed in the hypoechoic tumor background (Fig. 5–2). Small cystic spaces are present in approximately 10% of tumors, and these can be mistaken for pancreatitis-related pseudocysts. Calcification is

identified occasionally in pancreatic carcinoma (through typical strong focal reflections and acoustic shadows), and it should be noted, therefore, that calcification is not specific for chronic pancreatitis. Pancreatic duct and common bile duct dilatation (Fig. 5–3) occurs in about 40% and 70% of cases, respectively.[9, 19] The "double duct sign" of pancreatic carcinoma refers to simultaneous dilatation of both the pancreatic and bile ducts.

Pancreatic carcinoma metastasizes most commonly to peripancreatic tissues, peripancreatic nodes, porta hepatis nodes, and the liver.[9, 21] It is essential to search these areas carefully during sonographic examination. Look in particular for thickening of tissues around the celiac artery or the root of the superior mesenteric artery, as these are early findings of metastasis. Nodal metastases are round-to-ovoid, 10 to 15 mm in size, homogeneous in texture, and moderately echogenic.[9, 21] Hepatic metastases are relatively small (1 to 3 cm), spherical and hypoechoic, and typically are numerous.[9]

NEUROENDOCRINE TUMORS

Neuroendocrine tumors are relatively uncommon, yet they are the second most important pancreatic tumors after pancreatic carcinoma.[1, 2, 22–34] These tumors have traditionally been called "islet cell tumors" because they were thought to originate in the islets of Langerhans, which are "nests" of endocrine tissue scattered throughout the pancreatic parenchyma. More recently, however, it has been determined that these tumors actually arise from pluripotential ductal cells,[30] rather than the islets of Langerhans. The term

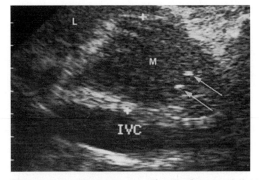

Figure 5-2—Large Pancreatic Carcinoma. A 4 × 6-cm mass (M) arising from the pancreatic head is seen on this longitudinal image along the inferior vena cava (IVC). Note that the mass is slightly heterogenous and about equal in echogenicity to the liver (L). Bright echoes due to calcification (arrows) are visible in the inferior portion of the mass.

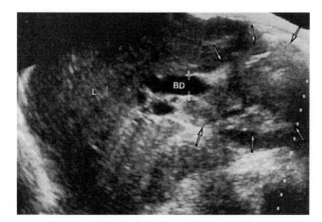

Figure 5-3—Massive Bile Duct Dilatation in Pancreatic Carcinoma. A longitudinal sonogram demonstrates marked dilatation (15-mm diameter) of the extrahepatic bile duct (BD) caused by a large pancreatic carcinoma (arrows) situated in the head of the pancreas. L = liver.

"islet cell tumor" has been replaced, therefore, with "neuroendocrine tumor," which describes the functional class to which these tumors belong. Neuroendocrine tumors may arise from a number of tissues located throughout the body, including the pancreas, stomach, and other abdominal viscera. They may be benign or malignant, and the malignant potential varies according to cell type.

Gastrointestinal neuroendocrine tumors are commonly named with respect to the enzyme secreted—e.g., insulinoma, gastrinoma, glucagonoma, and so on. Approximately two thirds of these tumors produce enzymes in sufficient quantity for clinical detection.[24] In such cases, the endocrine effects are the presenting clinical feature, and the tumor may be small and difficult to identify. Nonfunctioning neuroendocrine tumors, in contrast, tend to grow unnoticed and often are very large (10 to 20 cm) at the time of diagnosis.[2, 31] Nonfunctioning tumors generally are detected as palpable masses or are detected because of the compressive effects of the tumor (e.g., pain or visceral obstruction).

The most important neuroendocrine tumors, by far, are insulinomas and gastrinomas. Insulinomas are very frequently located in the pancreas. They usually are solitary and usually are benign. Because of these features, an experienced surgeon can palpate 80% to 90% of these tumors at operation without any imaging localization.[30] Gastrinomas are much more likely than insulinomas to be multiple, extrapancreatic, and malignant; therefore, preoperative localization has greater potential value for gastrinomas than for insulinomas. It should be noted that *about 90% of extrahepatic gastrinomas are located in the "gastrinoma triangle,"* the corners of which are (1) the junction of the cystic and common bile ducts; (2) the second and third portions of the duodenum; and (3) the neck and body of the pancreas.

Gastrinomas may be associated with the multiple endocrine neoplasia (MEN) syndrome, defined as hyperplasia or neoplasia occurring simultaneously in two or more endocrine tissues. When gastrinomas occur in the MEN syndrome, they usually are multiple in location and may be dispersed throughout the pancreas.

Imaging Objectives

The role of imaging procedures in the diagnosis of gastrointestinal neuroendocrine tumors is subject to debate, and it is clear that the cost of an extensive imaging evaluation must be weighed against the clinical effectiveness of imaging assessment.[30] For insulinomas, preoperative ultrasound and CT are recommended, supplemented by intraoperative sonography to detect nonpalpable pancreatic tumors. For gastrinomas, a more detailed preoperative evaluation may be desirable, and ultrasound, CT, and MRI all may be applicable. In MEN patients, imaging localization of gastrinomas is difficult or impossible. This limitation has prompted the suggestion that MEN-gastrinoma patients should be treated medically with H_2 blockers, and that surgical resection should be restricted to large tumors detected with a limited imaging examination.[30] Scintigraphy is recommended for neuroendocrine tumor imaging principally in patients with signs or symptoms of postoperative recurrence.

The Role of Ultrasound

Ultrasound sensitivity for extrahepatic neuroendocrine tumors is poor overall (20% to 60%),[22–24, 27, 30, 32, 33] but sonographic detectability varies with cell type and level of function. Excellent sonographic results are reported for nonfunctioning tumors because of their large size, whereas poor results are reported for functioning insulinomas and gastronomas because these tumors usually are small.[24] Ultrasound continues to have a role in the diagnosis of gastrointestinal neuroendocrine tumors for three reasons: (1) about 60% of insulinomas can be detected with transabdominal sonography;[30] (2) virtually all insulinomas can be detected with intraoperative ultrasound[30, 34]; and (3) no single imaging modality performs very well, and the combined sensitivity for all imaging modalities (85%)[32] exceeds that of any individual methods. Pancreatic neuroendocrine tumors, in particular, may be seen with ultrasound when they cannot be identified with other imaging techniques.[30, 33]

Sonographic Findings

The great majority of gastrointestinal neuroendocrine tumors (Fig. 5–4) are spherical or ovoid, hypoechoic (relative to normal pancreas), and homogeneous.[22, 28–33] They are well defined but not encapsulated, and the texture of the tumor is "finer" than that of the surrounding parenchyma. Less common ultrasound appearances include echogenicity equaling or exceeding that of the normal pancreas, and a "halo" appearance. Large, nonfunctioning tumors tend to have a heterogeneous ultrasound "texture" caused by liquefaction necrosis and calcification. Malignant neuroendocrine tumors frequently metastasize to the liver,[35] and a careful search for hepatic metastases is advisable, as these usually are detected more easily than are primary tumors. The metastatic lesions do not have specific ultrasound features.

PERIPANCREATIC ADENOPATHY

The head and body of the pancreas are surrounded by several lymph node chains that are commonly enlarged by metastasis or inflammation.[21, 36–38] Normal lymph nodes are not seen sonographically, but enlarged metastatic or inflamed modes may be visualized. Metastatic nodes have a characteristic appearance, regardless of the tumor of origin: they are round or ovoid, homogeneous, discretely margined, and hypoechoic relative to other solid abdominal tissues. Multiple adjacent metastatic nodes may coalesce and form a large mass. In the early stages of coalescence, the boundaries between nodes remain visible, producing a pseudoseptated appearance. In later stages, the boundaries between nodes are obliterated.[21]

To differentiate between peripancreatic nodes and a primary pancreatic tumor, the sonographer must note that the pancreas is displaced by enlarged lymph nodes but appears normal otherwise[37] (Fig. 5–5). A helpful ancillary finding is absence of pancreatic or common bile duct dilatation, which is a common feature of primary pancreatic neoplasms.[21, 37]

BENIGN CYSTS

Benign, epithelium-lined cysts of the pancreas occur rarely and are analogous in structure to benign cysts of the liver and kidney. Such cysts are usually seen in patients with polycystic kidney disease. The sonographic findings are the same as those described for hepatic cysts (Chapter 7).

CYSTIC PANCREATIC NEOPLASMS

Three types of pancreatic neoplasms are cyst-like on sonographic examination: papillary neo-

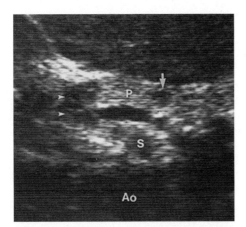

Figure 5-4—Malignant Neuroendocrine Tumor (Gastrinoma). A 1-cm hypoechoic mass (arrow) is present in the body of the pancreas, as seen on this transverse image. The patient had recurrent gastritis and evidence of gastric hypersecretion. The hypoechoic area in the pancreatic head (arrowheads) is an artifact caused by duodenal gas (acoustic shadow). S = SMA; Ao = aorta.

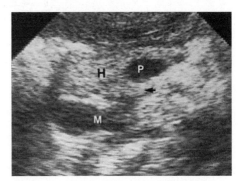

Figure 5-5—Extrapancreatic Nodal Mass. A transverse scan through the pancreatic head (H) and uncinate process (arrow) demonstrates a portion of a nodal mass (M) posterior to the pancreas. Note that the configuration of the pancreas is normal. P = portosplenic confluence.

plasms, benign microcystic neoplasms, and macrocystic neoplasms.[1, 2, 39–50] Because these tumors are rare, they will be discussed only briefly.

Papillary Neoplasm of the Pancreas

The papillary neoplasm is a rare tumor of exocrine origin that most commonly occurs in young women. The malignant potential of this neoplasm is low, and resection may be curative. Pancreatic carcinoma rarely occurs under the age of 40 years; therefore, a papillary neoplasm is a particularly worthy consideration in a young woman with a pancreatic mass.

Large areas of hemorrhagic necrosis are a typical feature of this tumor and impart a cystlike sonographic appearance. The liquefied areas are surrounded by thick, shaggy walls.[1, 40, 45–47] In some cases, however, papillary neoplasms are solid appearing, and such tumors are indistinguishable from pancreatic carcinoma.

Benign Microcystic Adenoma

Benign microcystic adenoma of the pancreas[1, 39, 41–43, 48] is called "serous cystadenoma" in the older medical literature. This tumor, which originates from the endocrine pancreas, has no malignant potential. As implied by the name "microcystic," the tumor consists of innumerable small, epithelium-lined cysts that generally range from less than 1 mm to 2 cm in size. Larger cysts are present occasionally, and focal calcification is a common feature.

Microcystic adenomas occur most commonly in the pancreatic head. The sonographic appearance varies with the size of the cysts.[39, 42, 43, 48] If all the cysts are very small, the tumor appears solid, and echogenicity ranges from hypoechoic to hyperechoic relative to the normal pancreas. In some cases, larger cysts (usually not exceeding 2 cm in diameter) may be embedded in the tumor mass. If these larger cysts are numerous, a distinct multicystic appearance may be seen.

Macrocystic Tumors

Macrocystic adenoma and macrocystic adenocarcinoma[1, 2, 39, 41–44, 49, 50] are relatively new pathologic terms that replace the older names: "mucinous cystadenoma" and "mucinous cystadenocarcinoma" of the pancreas. The new terms are recommended to differentiate between the potentially malignant macrocystic neoplasms (macrocystic adenocarcinoma) and the uniformly benign microcystic pancreatic tumors.

Macrocystic neoplasms arise from exocrine tissue and present clinically as large masses (typically 15 to 20 cm in diameter). The tumor consists of either a single, epithelium-lined cyst or multiple cysts with relatively sparse solid elements. In contradistinction to microcystic adenoma, the cysts exceed 2 cm in diameter, and the tumor usually is located in the pancreatic tail. Focal cyst wall calcification is common.

The sonographic appearance of macrocystic tumors[18, 41–44, 50] (Fig. 5–6) varies with the number and size of the cysts and the amount of solid tissue in the cyst walls. The range of findings is similar to that seen with cystadenoma and cystadenocarcinoma of the ovary, as discussed in Chapter 31. Sonographic differentiation between benign and malignant macrocystic tumors is not possible.

PANCREATIC MASS DIFFERENTIAL

When a mass is identified in the pancreatic bed, one should not immediately spring to the diagnosis of pancreatic carcinoma but should consider other diagnostic possibilities, as outlined in Table 5–1. Most of the lesions listed in this table are discussed in this or the preceding chapter. Epigastric aneurysm is included in Chapter 26.

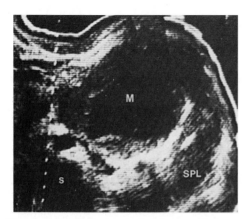

Figure 5-6—Macrocystic Carcinoma of the Pancreatic Tail. A transverse sonogram demonstrates an 8.5 × 10-cm cystic mass (M) with thick, irregular walls, located in the usual position of the pancreatic tail. Macrocystic carcinoma of the pancreas was diagnosed at surgery. SPL = spleen; S = spine.

REFERENCES

1. Kissaine JM, Lacy PE: Pancreas and diabetes mellitus. *In* Kissaine JM, ed. Anderson's Pathology, 8th ed. St Louis, CV Mosby, 1985, pp 1238–1239.
2. White M, Wittenberg H: Pancreatic neoplasia. Semin Ultrasound CT MR 5:401–413, 1984.
3. Balthazar EJ, Subramanyam BR, Lefleur RS,

Barone CM: Solid and papillary neoplasm of the pancreas. Radiology 150:39–40, 1984.

4. Arger PH, Mulhern CB, Bonavita JA, Stauffer DM, Hale J: An analysis of pancreatic sonography in suspected pancreatic disease. J Clin Ultrasound 7:91–97, 1979.

5. Essel SJ, Siegelman SS, McNeil BJ, Sanders R, Adams DG, Alderson PO, Finberg HJ, Abrams HL: A prospective evaluation of computed tomography and ultrasound of the pancreas. Radiology 143:129–133, 1982.

6. Taylor KJW, Buchin PJ, Viscomi GN, Rosenfield AT: Ultrasonographic scanning of the pancreas. Radiology 138:211–213, 1981.

7. Haaga JR, Alfidi RJ, Havrilla TR, Tubbs R, Gonzalez L, Meaney TF, Corsi MA: Definitive role of CT scanning of the pancreas. Radiology 124:723–730, 1977.

8. Karasawa E, Goldberg HI, Moss AA, Federle MP, London SS: CT pancreatogram in carcinoma of the pancreas and chronic pancreatitis. Radiology 148:489–493, 1983.

9. Shawker TH, Garra BS, Hill MC, Doppman JL, Sindelar WF: The spectrum of sonographic findings in pancreatic carcinoma. J Ultrasound Med 5:169–177, 1986.

10. Cohen MM, Switzer PJ, Cooperberg PL: Sensitivity of ultrasonography in the diagnosis of pancreatic cancer. Can Med Assoc J 120:453–455, 1979.

11. Taylor KJW, Buchin PJ, Viscomi GN, et al: Ultrasonographic scanning of the pancreas. Radiology 138:211, 1981.

12. Pollack D, Taylor KJW: Ultrasound scanning in patients with clinical suspicion of pancreatic cancer: A retrospective study. Cancer 47:1662, 1981.

13. Hessel SJ, Siegelman SS, McNeil BJ, et al: A prospective evaluation of computed tomography and ultrasound of the pancreas. Radiology 143:129, 1982.

14. Steiner E, Stark DD, Hahn PF, Saini S, Simeone JF, Mueller PR, Wittenberg J, Ferrucci JT: Imaging of pancreatic neoplasms: Comparison of MR and CT. AJR Am J Roentgenol 152:487–491, 1989.

15. Vellet AD, Romano W, Bach DB, Passi RB, Taves DH, Munk PL: Adenocarcinoma of the pancreatic ducts: Comparative evaluation with CT and MR imaging at 1.5 T. Radiology 183:87–95, 1992.

16. Neumann CH, Hessel SJ: CT of the pancreatic tail. AJR Am J Roentgenol 135:741–745, 1980.

17. Weinstein DP, Wolfman NT, Weinstein BJ: Ultrasonic characteristics of pancreatic tumors. Gastrointest Radiol 4:245–251, 1979.

18. Itai Y, Araki T, Tasaka A, Maruyama M: Computed tomographic appearance of resectable pancreatic carcinoma. Radiology 143:719–726, 1982.

19. Wittenberg J, Simeone JF, Ferrucci JT, Mueller PR, vanSonnenberg E, Neff CC: Non-focal enlargement in pancreatic carcinoma. Radiology 144:131–135, 1982.

20. La Seta F, Cottone M, Marceno MP, Maringhini A, Sciarrino E, Pagliaro L: L'ecografia nei pazienti con sospetto clinico di carcinoma pancreatico: Analisi di une studio prospettico. Radiol Med 69:538–540, 1983.

21. Zeman RK, Schiebler M, Clark LR, Jaffe MH, Paushter DM, Grant EG, Choyke PL: The clinical and imaging spectrum of pancreaticoduodenal lymph node enlargement. AJR Am J Roentgenol 144:1223–1227, 1985.

22. Günther RW, Klose KK, Rückert K, Kuhn F-P, Beyer J, Klotter H-J, Cordes U: Islet-cell tumors: Detection of small lesions with computed tomography and ultrasound. Radiology 148:485–488, 1983.

23. Günther RW: Ultrasound and CT in the assessment of suspected islet cell tumors of the pancreas. Semin Ultrasound CT MR 6:261–275, 1985.

24. Shawker TH, Doppman JL, Dunnick NR, McCarthy DM: Ultrasonic investigation of pancreatic islet cell tumors. J Ultrasound Med 1:193–200, 1982.

25. Raghavendra BN, Glickstein ML: Sonography of islet cell tumor of the pancreas: Report of two cases. J Clin Ultrasound 9:331–333, 1981.

26. Rifkin MD, Weiss SM: Intraoperative sonographic identification of nonpalpable pancreatic masses. J Ultrasound Med 3:409–411, 1984.

27. Gorman B, Charboneau JW, James EM, Reading CC, Galiber AK, Grant CS, van Heerden JA, Telander RL, Service FJ: Benign pancreatic insulinoma: Preoperative and intraoperative sonographic localization. AJR Am J Roentgenol 147:929–934, 1986.

28. Dunnick NR, Long JA, Krudy A, Shawker TH, Doppman JL: Localizing insulinomas with combined radiographic methods. AJR Am J Roentgenol 135:747–752, 1980.

29. Krudy AG, Doppman JL, Jensen RT, Norton JA, Collen MJ, Shawker TH, Gardner JD, McArthur K, Gorden P: Localization of islet cell tumors by dynamic CT: Comparison with plain CT, arteriography, sonography, and venous sampling. AJR Am J Roentgenol 143:585–589, 1984.

30. Gorman B, Reading CC: Imaging of gastrointestinal neuroendocrine tumors. Semin Ultrasound CT MR 16:68–75, 1996.

31. Eelkema EA, Stephens DH, Ward EM, Sheedy PF: CT features of nonfunctioning islet cell carcinoma. AJR Am J Roentgenol 143:943–948, 1984.

32. Frucht H, Doppman JL, Norton JA, Miller DL, Dwyer AJ, Frank JA, Vinayek R, Maton PN, Jensen RT: Gastrinomas: Comparison of MR imaging with CT, angiography, and US. Radiology 171:713–717, 1989.

33. London JF, Shawker TH, Doppman JL, Frucht HH, Vinayek R, Start HA, Miller LS, Miller DL, Norton JA, Jensen RT, Gardner JD, Maton PN: Zollinger-Ellison syndrome: Prospective assessment of abdominal US in the localization of gastrinomas. Radiology 178:763–767, 1991.

34. Clyne CAC, Greene WJ, Paisey RB: Intra-operative ultrasound localization of an insulinoma undetected pre-operatively. J Clin Ultrasound 19:419–420, 1991.

35. Willis RA: The spread of tumors in the human body. New York, Butterworths, 1975, p 216.

36. Wernecke K, Peters PE, Galanski M: Pancreatic metastases: US evaluation. Radiology 160:399–402, 1986.

37. Schnur MJ, Hoffman JC, Koenigsberg M: Gray-scale ultrasonic demonstration of peripancreatic adenopathy. J Ultrasound Med 1:139–143, 1982.

38. Swartz TR, Ritchie WGM: Bile duct obstruction secondary to lymphomatous involvement of the pancreas. J Clin Ultrasound 11:391–394, 1983.

39. Friedman AC, Lichtenstein JE, Dachman AH: Cystic neoplasms of the pancreas. Radiology 149:45–50, 1983.

40. Radin DR, Colletti PM, Forrester DM, Tang WW: Pancreatic acinar cell carcinoma with subcutaneous and intraosseous fat necrosis. Radiology 158:67–68, 1986.

41. Lloyd TV, Antonmattei S, Freimanis AT: Gray scale

sonography of cystadenoma of the pancreas: Report of two cases. J Clin Ultrasound 7:149–151, 1979.

42. Wolfman NT, Ramquist NA, Karstaedt N, Hopkins MB: Cystic neoplasms of the pancreas: CT and sonography. AJR Am J Roentgenol 138:37–41, 1982.

43. Fond A, Bret PM, Bretagnolle M, Thiesse P, Marion D, Dubreuil A, Labadie M: Ultrasound and percutaneous fine needle biopsy of cystic tumors of the pancreas. J Belge Radiol 67:277–284, 1984.

44. Itai Y, Ohhashi K, Nagai H, Murakami Y, Kokubo T, Makita K, Ohtomo K: "Ductectatic" mucinous cystadenoma and cystadenocarcinoma of the pancreas. Radiology 161:697–700, 1986.

45. Yandow D: Case of the fall session: Acinar cell carcinoma. Semin Ultrasound 1:153–155, 1980.

46. Friedman AC, Lichtenstein JE, Fishman EK, Oertel JE, Dachman AH, Siegelman SS: Solid and papillary epithelial neoplasm of the pancreas. Radiology 154:333–337, 1985.

47. Lin J-T, Wang T-H, Wei T-C, Sheu J-C, Sung J-L, How S-W, Su C-T: Sonographic features of solid and papillary neoplasm of the pancreas. J Clin Ultrasound 13:339–342, 1985.

48. Buck JL, Hayes WS: Microcystic adenoma of the pancreas. RadioGraphics 10:313–322, 1990.

49. Itoh S, Ishiguchi T, Ishigaki T, Sakuma S, Maruyama K, Senda K: Mucin-producing pancreatic tumor: CT findings and histopathologic correlation. Radiology 183:81–86, 1992.

50. Itai Y, Kokubo T, Atomi Y, Kuroda A, Haraguchi Y, Terano A: Mucin-hypersecreting carcinoma of the pancreas. Radiology 165:51–55, 1987.

The Liver and Spleen

INTRODUCTION

The liver is readily accessible to ultrasonic examination because it is a large solid organ with a broad area of contact with the abdominal wall. Due to its accessibility, the liver is visualized during virtually all sonographic examinations of the upper abdomen, either as the primary subject of investigation or as a "window" to other organs. The liver is covered in greater detail in this text than some other subjects, for it is an especially important organ from a sonographic perspective.

The spleen also is readily visualized sonographically and is examined regularly in the course of sonographic studies. The spleen is not often the primary subject of sonographic study, but splenomegaly and other important pathologic findings may be noted sonographically. The spleen, furthermore, is an important "window" to the lesser peritoneal space (lesser sac) and the left subphrenic and pleural spaces.

This section includes material on anatomy, sonographic technique, and important pathologic findings in the liver and spleen.

Chapter 6

The Liver: Sonographic Technique and Anatomy

William J. Zwiebel

SONOGRAPHIC TECHNIQUE

An established examination protocol should be followed during examination of the liver, to ensure that all pertinent areas are studied. The recommended protocol is outlined in Table 6–1, and selected sonographic views from this protocol are illustrated in Figures 6–1 and 6–2. Both the liver and biliary tree are included in Table 6–1, since these areas typically are examined as a unit, but the technical aspects of biliary tract scanning are not included in detail. This subject is presented in Chapter 12.

The image planes listed in the hepatobiliary protocol (Table 6–1) were chosen to optimize anatomic orientation. To this end, transverse and longitudinal image planes are emphasized, but the use of oblique images is inevitable in the course of hepatobiliary imaging. When oblique images are used, the sonographer should include orienting landmarks whenever possible. For example, an image showing a liver mass might include the right kidney and the inferior vena cava for orientation.

HEPATIC ANATOMY

General Features

The liver parenchyma produces a uniform pattern of medium-level echoes[1-3] (Figs. 6–1 and 6–2). In adults (and older children), the overall "brightness," or echogenicity, of the liver *equals or exceeds* the brightness of the renal cortex, but the liver is *less* bright than the pancreas or abdominal fat. In normal infants and young children, the liver may be less bright than the renal cortex. This difference between adults and young children has nothing to do with the liver. It is due instead to a relatively high level of kidney echogenicity in young children (Chapter 16).

The sonographic "texture" of the liver (Figs. 6–1 and 6–2) is neither extremely fine grained nor coarse. Both a fine-grained and a coarse

texture suggest hepatocellular disease (Chapter 9). Normal hepatic parenchyma transmits ultrasound quite well. Diseased parenchyma, on the other hand, may attenuate the sound beam.

The liver is encompassed by a well-defined capsule, but this capsule is not visible sonographically. The surface of the liver should be smooth. A nodular surface suggests cirrhosis, as discussed in Chapter 9.

Portal and Hepatic Veins

Portions of the portal and hepatic veins[3-8] are seen in all normal livers, and differentiation between these vessels generally is quite simple. The portal veins are oriented more or less transversely and converge at the porta hepatis, whereas hepatic veins are oriented longitudinally and converge on the inferior vena cava (IVC) at the diaphragm (Fig. 6–3A). Portal veins have highly echogenic walls, due to a thick investment of collagenous tissue (Fig. 6–3B). In contrast, the hepatic veins exhibit well-defined but echo-poor margins. Blood flow in the portal veins is *into* the liver, whereas blood flow in the hepatic veins is *out of* the liver (toward the IVC).

The portal vein is seen in about 97% of normal patients, and failure to visualize the portal vein, therefore, portends pathology such as venous thrombosis.[6] The portal vein splits at the porta hepatis into right and left branches (Fig. 6–4A) that supply the right and left hepatic lobes. The right branch is prominently seen on longitudinal sections, as shown in Figure 6–3B. The left branch is prominently seen on transverse images, as shown in Fig. 6–2A. A large, anteriorly directed branch arises from the left portal vein (Fig. 6–4B). This so-called "ascending" branch is an important anatomic landmark, as discussed later. *The junction of the ascending and left portal branches may easily be mistaken for the junction of the right and left portal veins, and care must be taken to avoid this error.*

Hepatic vein anatomy is a little more variable than portal vein anatomy, but the "standard" pat-

Table 6-1. Technical Protocol for Hepatobiliary Sonography

Liver Examination

A. Supine, longitudinal survey of the liver
   1. Sweep from left to right through the liver with longitudinal sections. *Do not miss the dome of the liver, high under the diaphragm.*
   2. Note the hepatic texture, look for masses and biliary dilatation, note the shape and surface features (if visible) of the liver, and confirm that the inferior vena cava and portal vein are patent.
   3. Record representative images:
      a. Far left lobe (Fig. 6–1*A*)
      b. Through the aorta (Fig. 6–1*B*)
      c. Through the inferior vena cava (Fig. 6–1*C*)
      d. Through the right lobe (Fig. 6–1*D*)
      e. Views of pathologic findings
B. Supine, transverse survey of the liver
   1. From a subcostal approach, sweep through the left lobe from superior to inferior. Repeat this process for the midregion and the right lobe. *Do not overlook the right lateral aspect of the liver, near the abdominal wall.*
   2. Note the normal features cited in A2 above. Confirm patency of the major hepatic veins at the diaphragm (see Figure 6–5) and the left and right portal veins.
   3. Record representative images:
      a. Through the left portal vein (Fig. 6–2*A*)
      b. High, mid, and low through the middle and right portions of the liver (Fig. 6–2*C*)
      c. Views of pathologic findings
C. Supine or left decubitus intercostal views
   1. Supplement the above survey, if needed, with additional oblique views obtained between the right ribs. These views may help you visualize the dome of the liver, the diaphragm, the portal vein, and the right hepatic vein.
   2. Record representative images.

Gallbladder Examination

A. Supine, long axis views° of the gallbladder
   1. Survey the gallbladder, including the neck, body, and fundus.

   2. Note the size, shape, and overall appearance of the gallbladder. Examine the gallbladder wall for thickening, irregularity, polyps, and other abnormalities. Look for gallstones and other abnormal intraluminal material.
   3. Record representative normal and pathological findings.
B. Supine, short axis views† of the gallbladder
   1. Repeat the gallbladder survey from the short axis perspective.
   2. Record representative normal and pathologic findings.
C. Decubitus, prone, and/or upright long axis views of the gallbladder
   1. Confirm mobility of calculi and search carefully for calculi that might not be visible on supine views.
   2. Record representative normal and pathologic findings.

Biliary Examination

A. Intrahepatic ducts
   1. During the liver examination, search for evidence of intrahepatic bile duct dilatation. Use color Doppler imaging to differentiate between ducts and blood vessels.
   2. Record representative normal and pathologic findings.
B. Extrahepatic ducts
   1. Survey the extrahepatic bile duct with the patient supine or in the left decubitus position. Obtain both "Mickey Mouse" and "sandwich" (long axis) views (chapter 12). Use color Doppler to differentiate between duct and vessels. *Be sure to look at both the proximal and distal portions of the duct.*
   2. Measure the extrahepatic duct proximally and distally. Look for wall irregularity, calculi, or masses. Look for pancreatic masses or pancreatic duct dilatation.
   3. Record representative images:
      a. Mickey Mouse view at porta hepatis
      b. Transverse or oblique image of the distal duct in the pancreatic head
      c. Longitudinal views of the extrahepatic duct (proximal and distal)
      d. Representative pathologic findings

°"Long axis" means along the length of the gallbladder.
†"Short axis" means perpendicular to the long axis plane.

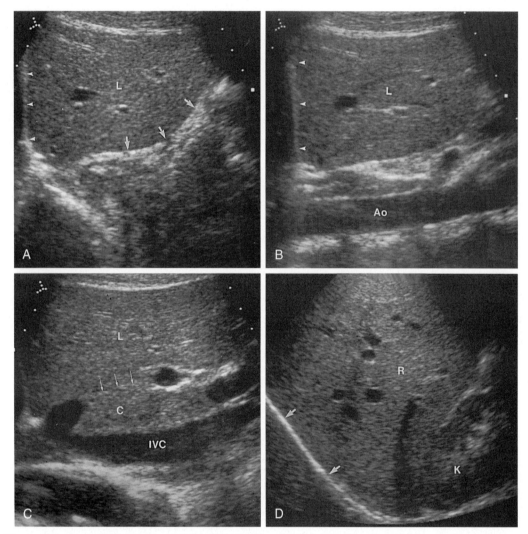

Figure 6-1—Longitudinal Views of the Normal Liver. (A) Left lobe (L) and upper lesser sac (arrows). Arrowheads = diaphragm. **(B)** Left lobe (L) in the plane of the aorta (Ao). Arrowheads = diaphragm. **(C)** Left (L) and caudate (C) lobes in the plane of the inferior vena cava (IVC). The fissure for the ligamentum venosum (arrows), which separates the left and caudate lobes, is barely visible in this asthenic individual. **(D)** Right lobe (R) and right kidney (K). Note that the kidney is slightly less echogenic than the liver. Arrows = diaphragm.

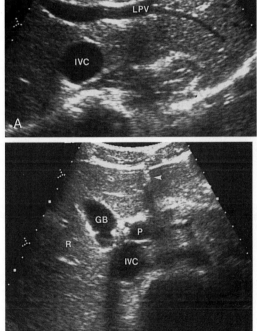

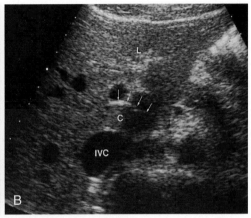

Figure 6-2—Transverse Views of the Normal Liver. (A) Left lobe of the liver in the plane of the left portal vein (LPV). Note the ascending portion of the left portal view (arrow). IVC = inferior vena cava. **(B)** The left (L) and caudate (C) lobes are separated by the fissure for the ligamentum venosum (arrows). The plane of this image is slightly inferior to **A**. IVC = inferior vena cava. **(C)** Right lobe (R) at the level of the gallbladder fossa (GB). IVC = inferior vena cava; P = portal vein; arrowhead = falciform ligament.

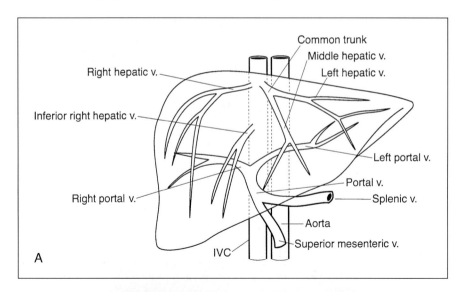

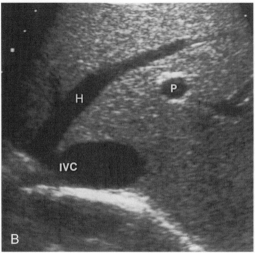

Figure 6-3—Portal and Hepatic Veins. (A) The right and left portal veins are transversely oriented and converge at the porta hepatis. The hepatic veins are more longitudinally oriented and converge with the inferior vena cava at the diaphragm. (B) Hepatic veins (H) have "naked" margins. The portal veins (P) are surrounded by echogenic fat. Note that hepatic veins increase in size as they near the confluence with the inferior vena cava (IVC).

tern, shown in Figure 6–5, is present in about 90% of adults: three main hepatic veins (right, middle, and left) drain the liver, and the middle and left veins merge just before they enter the IVC.[8] (See Figure 6–5, following page 108.)

Variations of hepatic vein anatomy include absence of the right hepatic vein, duplication of major trunks, and the existence of multiple small veins rather than the three large trunks. Accessory hepatic veins drain the right lobe directly into the IVC in about 10% of individuals, and these may be seen occasionally with ultrasound.[7]

Hepatic Arteries

The proper hepatic artery and its right and left branches are commonly visualized at the porta

hepatis. Arterial branches generally are not seen deep within the liver owing to their small size.

Doppler Flow Signatures

The portal veins, the hepatic veins, and the hepatic artery branches can be readily identified by their Doppler ultrasound flow characteristics[9] (Fig. 6–6). Portal veins exhibit low velocity flow that undulates slightly in response to respiration. The audible portal vein signals have a "windstorm" sound. Flow in the hepatic veins is pulsatile and is characterized by alternate forward and reverse flow components. This pattern is caused by fluctuations in right atrial pressure during the cardiac cycle. The hepatic artery and its tributar-

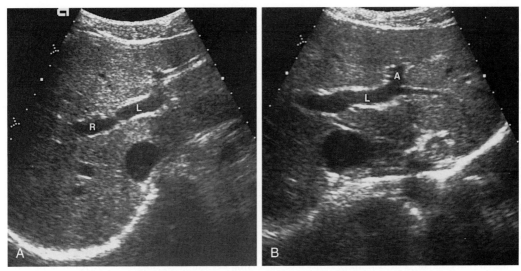

Figure 6-4—Portal Vein Anatomy. (A) Transverse scan showing the bifurcation of the portal vein into right (R) and left (L) branches. (B) The "ascending" branch (A) extends anteriorly from the left portal vein (L).

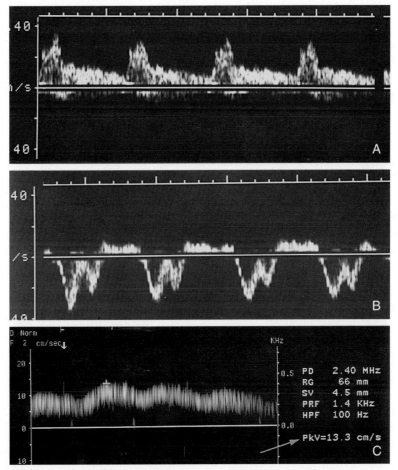

Figure 6-6—Normal Vascular Signatures. (A) Hepatic artery flow is characterized by a low-resistance arterial flow pattern (wide systolic peaks and continuous forward flow in diastole). (B) Hepatic vein flow exhibits a distinctive, pulsatile, to-and-fro pattern. (C) Portal vein flow undulates slightly with cardiac activity and respiration and always is hepatopedal (toward the liver). Cursor and arrow = normal peak velocity of 13.3 cm/sec.

ies produce "low resistance" arterial signals (broad systolic peaks and a large amount of forward flow in diastole). These arterial signals are readily distinguished from portal and hepatic vein signals.

LOBES AND SEGMENTS

The liver is divided, albeit incompletely, into lobes and segments.[2-4, 10-13] The boundaries of these lobes and segments are defined using a system known as the functional anatomy of the liver.[10-12] This system describes lobar anatomy in relation to blood supply, biliary drainage, and hepatic venous drainage. In essence, functional anatomy describes potential surgical resection planes and may be used, therefore, to predict the resectability of hepatic tumors. Knowledge of functional liver anatomy is essential as this system is in standard use.

The functional anatomic system is outlined in Table 6–2 and in Figures 6–7 and 6–8. The latter figure, showing the "H" concept, is particularly helpful for visualizing hepatic lobar anatomy. The contents of Table 6–2 and Figures 6–7 and 6–8 are not repeated in the text; therefore, this material should be reviewed carefully.

The Maverick Caudate

The caudate lobe (Table 6–2, Fig. 6–2*B*) is the maverick of functional lobar anatomy because of its circulatory peculiarities. Unlike the other lobes, the caudate is supplied with blood by both the right and left portal vein branches and the right and left hepatic artery divisions. Venous drainage, furthermore, is via small veins that enter the IVC directly, independent of the main hepatic vein trunks. It appears that these circulatory peculiarities account for the relative sparing of the caudate lobe in some cases of cirrhosis.[13] Direct venous drainage into the IVC, furthermore, may have protective value in cases of hepatic vein thrombosis and may be of great importance following lobar hepatic resection.

Anatomic Variance

The size of the individual hepatic lobes varies greatly in normal individuals,[14-17] and the resultant shifts of lobar/segmental boundaries may be dramatic. The most common anatomic variant is a small left lobe, and in such cases the right lobe is compensatorily enlarged. Rarely, either the left or the right lobe is absent (lobar agenesis). Anomalies of lobar size may be recognized sonographically by two potential findings: (1) little or no hepatic tissue may be present either to the

left or right of the gallbladder; and (2) the gallbladder may be displaced markedly—to the left if the left lobe is small, and to the right if the right lobe is small. In extreme cases, the gallbladder may lie to the left of midline, or far posterior on the right.

A "Riedel's lobe" is a common morphologic variant that may be mistaken for a right upper quadrant mass. Riedel's lobe is not really a lobe; rather, it is a tongue-like projection that extends caudally from the inferior margin of the right lobe.

ASSESSMENT OF LIVER SIZE

Sonographic evaluation of liver size is somewhat difficult because the liver is irregularly shaped and the size of individual lobes varies. Marked enlargement or shrinkage may be appreciated with gestalt assessment, but more precise evaluation of liver size is desirable. Various hepatic measurement schemes have been devised,[17-19] but the simplest appears to be the best—midclavicular line (MCL) measurement of the greatest longitudinal dimension of the right hepatic lobe (Fig. 6–9). In adults, a 13-cm MCL measurement is a highly reliable cut-off for normal livers, and an MCL measurement that equals or exceeds 16 cm suggests hepatomegaly. The likelihood of hepatomegaly increases in direct proportion to the MCL measurement. For example, in cadaver studies, about 75% of livers measuring 15.5 cm (MCL) actually are enlarged (by weight or volume). In contrast, virtually all 20-cm (MCL) livers actually are enlarged.[17]

THE DIAPHRAGM

The dome of the diaphragm[20-22] is readily visualized sonographically as a strongly echogenic, curvilinear structure located adjacent to the liver (Fig. 6–1) and spleen. The strong diaphragmatic echoes emanate from the pleural and peritoneal surfaces.[20]

Because the diaphragm is readily visualized, it serves well to differentiate between pleural and peritoneal space abnormalities. In some instances, the distinction between pleural and peritoneal processes can be made more easily with ultrasound than with computed tomography.

PERIHEPATIC SPACES

Peritoneal reflections, ligaments, and other structures divide the peritoneal space around the liver into numerous compartments called the perihepatic spaces.[22] These spaces, as shown in Figure 6–10, are common sites for the accumula-

Text continued on page 69

Table 6-2. Hepatic Lobes and Segments

Division	Definition	Vasculature
Right lobe	All tissue to the right of a plane through the gallbladder fossa, IVC, and middle hepatic vein	Right portal vein, hepatic artery, right and middle hepatic veins
Anterior segment, right lobe	Portion of right lobe anterior to the right hepatic vein	Same
Posterior segment, right lobe	Portion of right lobe posterior to the right hepatic vein	Same
Left lobe	All tissue to the left of a plane through the gallbladder fossa, IVC, and middle hepatic vein (excluding the caudate lobe)	Left portal vein, left hepatic artery, middle and left hepatic veins
Medial segment, left lobe	Portion of left lobe medial to the falciform ligament and the ascending portion of the left portal vein	Same
Lateral segment, left lobe	Portion of left lobe lateral to the falciform ligament and the ascending portion of the left portal vein	Same
Caudate lobe	Tissue posterior to the fissure for the ligamentum venosum, left of the IVC, and superior to the portal-splenic junction	Variable: Left or right portal vein and hepatic artery; middle or left hepatic veins; direct venous communication with the IVC

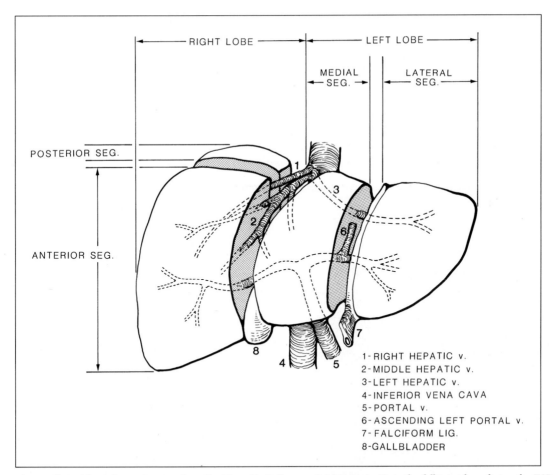

Figure 6-7—The Planes Separating the Hepatic Lobes and Segments. Note the following boundaries: the IVC (4), gallbladder (8), and middle hepatic vein (2) separate the right and left lobes; the falciform ligament (7) and ascending portal branch (6) separate the medial and lateral segments of the left lobe.

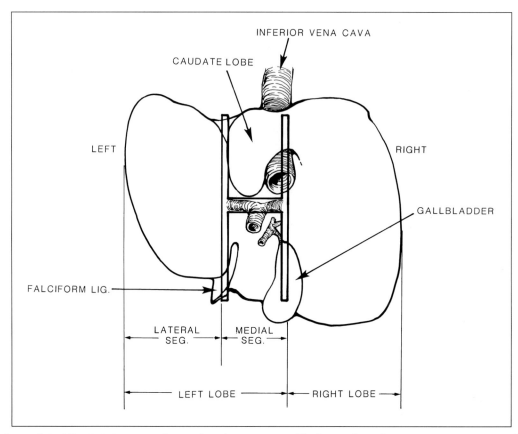

Figure 6-8—The "H" Concept of Hepatic Lobar Anatomy. The liver is shown from a posterior perspective. The upright on the patient's right separates the right and left lobes (it passes through the gallbladder fossa, the IVC, and the middle hepatic vein [not shown]). The upright on the patient's left separates the lateral and medial segments of the left lobe and marks the lateral border of the caudate lobe (it passes through the falciform ligament, the ascending portion of the left portal vein (not shown), and the left hepatic vein (not shown). The crossbar of the H is the bifurcation of the portal vein into right and left branches. It marks the inferior border of the caudate lobe.

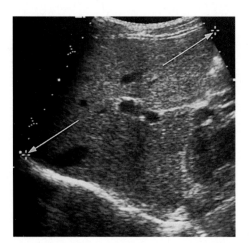

Figure 6-9—Midclavicular Line Measurement of the Normal Liver. Arrows = 14 cm.

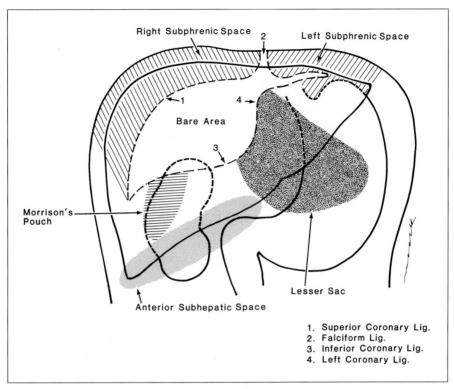

Figure 6-10—The Major Perihepatic Spaces.

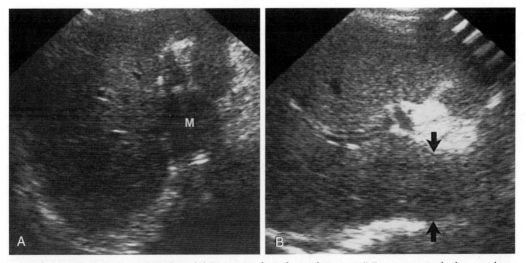

Figure 6-11—Shadow Pseudolesion. (A) It appears that a hypoechoic mass (M) is present in the liver on this transverse image. This is a pseudolesion caused by attenuation of the ultrasound beam by overlying echogenic structures. **(B)** A view of the same area (arrows) from a different perspective reveals no abnormality. Shadow pseudolesions are caused by acoustic shadows from the costal cartilage, the portal veins, hepatic fissures, and hepatic ligaments. Misdiagnosis may be avoided by scanning the apparent mass in more than one plane. If a mass disappears when viewed from a different projection, then a pseudomass is likely.

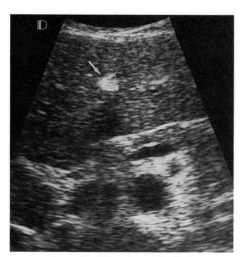

Figure 6-12—Ligamentum Teres Pseudolesion.
On transverse scans, the echogenic fat (arrow) surrounding
the ligamentum teres should not be mistaken for a mass.
Avoid this error by showing continuity between the fat and
the falciform ligament, and by visualizing the hypoechoic
ligamentum teres or a vessel in the center of the
pseudomass (neither are seen here).

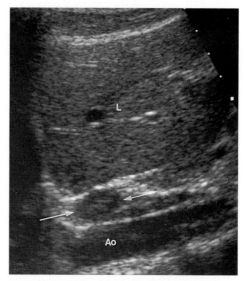

**Figure 6-13—Gastroesophageal Junction
Pseudolesion.** The gastroesophageal (GE) junction
(arrows) may be visible on longitudinal images (as shown
here) or on transverse images (not shown). It lies posterior
to the left lobe of the liver (L) and adjacent to the aorta
(Ao) or the spine. The GE junction frequently has a
rounded, masslike shape that may be mistaken for a
neoplastic mass by a neophyte sonographer. Familiarity with
the normal appearance prevents this error, as does
swallowing—when the patient swallows, a brightly
echogenic stream of bubbles passes through the
pseudolesion.

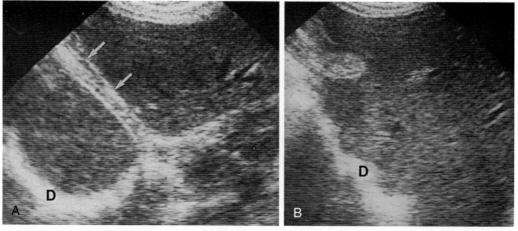

Figure 6-14—A Diaphragmatic Fold (also called an accessory diaphragmatic fissure)[25, 26] is a cleft in the hepatic
parenchyma that contains fat and, in some cases, a fold of the diaphragm. **(A)** On longitudinal section, this cleft has a
characteristic "tram track" appearance (arrows). D = diaphragm. **(B)** On transverse images, a diaphragmatic fold has a "bull's
eye" appearance. D = diaphragm. Misdiagnoses can be avoided through familiarity with the unique appearance of a
diaphragmatic fold.

tion of pus and other pathologic fluids. The right and left subphrenic spaces, Morrison's pouch, and the lesser peritoneal sac are particularly noteworthy as sites where fluid may collect.

NORMAL STRUCTURES THAT MIMIC PATHOLOGY

Several normal hepatic structures can generate sonographic findings that may be mistaken for liver disease.[23–26] These pseudomasses have several sources: (1) acoustic shadows, (2) the ligamentum teres, (3) accessory fissures, and (4) the gastroesophageal junction. Hepatic pseudolesions are illustrated and discussed in Figures 6–11 through 6–14.

REFERENCES

1. Platt JF, Rubin JM, Bowerman RA, Marn CS: The inability to detect disease on the basis of renal echogenicity. AJR Am J Roentgenol 151:317–319, 1988.
2. Kane RA: Sonographic anatomy of the liver. Semin Ultrasound 2:190–197, 1981.
3. Marks WM, Filly RA, Callen PW: Ultrasonic anatomy of the liver: A review with new applications. J Clin Ultrasound 7:137–146, 1979.
4. Sexton CC, Zeman RK: Correlation of computed tomography, sonography, and gross anatomy of the liver. AJR Am J Roentgenol 141:711–718, 1983.
5. Chafetz J, Filly RA: Portal and hepatic veins: Accuracy of margin echoes for distinguishing intrahepatic vessels. Radiology 130:725–728, 1979.
6. Merritt CBR: Ultrasonographic demonstration of portal vein thrombosis. Radiology 133:425–427, 1979.
7. Makuuchi M, Hasegawa G, Yamazaki S, et al: The inferior right hepatic vein: Ultrasonic demonstration. Radiology 148:213–217, 1983.
8. Cosgrove DO, Arger PH, Coleman BG: Ultrasonic anatomy of hepatic veins. J Clin Ultrasound 15:231–235, 1987.
9. Taylor KJW, Burns PN, Woodcock JP, et al: Blood flow in deep abdominal and pelvic vessels: Ultrasonic pulsed Doppler analysis. Radiology 154:487–493, 1985.
10. Pagani JJ: Intrahepatic vascular territories shown by computed tomography (CT). Radiology 147:173–178, 1983.
11. Mukai JK, Stack CM, Turner DA, Gould RJ, Petasnick JP, Matalon TAS, Doolas AM, Murakami M: Imaging of surgically relevant hepatic vascular

and segmental anatomy. Part 1. Normal anatomy. AJR Am J Roentgenol 149:287–292, 1987.
12. Lafortune M, Madore F, Patriquin H, Breton G: Segmental anatomy of the liver: A sonographic approach to the Couinaud nomenclature. Radiology 181:443–448, 1991.
13. Dodds WJ, Erickson SJ, Taylor AJ, Lawson TL, Stewart ET: Caudate lobe of the liver: Anatomy, embryology, and pathology. AJR Am J Roentgenol 154:87–93, 1990.
14. Pietri H, Boscaini M, Berthezene P, Durbec JP, Cros R, Sarles H: Hepatic morphotypes. Their statistical individualization using ultrasonography. J Ultrasound Med 7:189–196, 1988.
15. Belton R, VanZandt TF: Congenital absence of the left lobe of the liver: A radiologic diagnosis. Radiology 147:184, 1983.
16. Radin DR, Colletti PM, Ralls PW, Boswell WD, Halls JM: Agenesis of the right lobe of the liver. Radiology 164:639–642, 1987.
17. Gosink BB, Leymaster CE: Ultrasonic determination of hepatomegaly. J Clin Ultrasound 9:37–41, 1981.
18. Niederau C, Sonnenberg A, Mueller JE: Sonographic measurements of the normal liver, spleen, pancreas, and portal vein. Radiology 149:537–540, 1983.
19. Niederau C, Sonnenberg A: Liver size evaluated by ultrasound: ROC curves for hepatitis and alcoholism. Radiology 153:503–505, 1984.
20. Fried AM, Cosgrove DO, Nassiri DK, et al: The diaphragmatic echo complex: An in vitro study. Invest Radiol 20:62–67, 1985.
21. Callen PW, Filly RA, Sarti DA: Ultrasonography of the diaphragmatic crura. Radiology 130:721–724, 1979.
22. Rubenstein WA, Auh YH, Wahlen JP, et al: The perihepatic spaces: Computed tomographic and ultrasound imaging. Radiology 149:231–239, 1983.
23. B'onhoff AJ, Linhart P: A pseudolesion of the liver caused by rib cartilage in B-mode ultrasonography. J Ultrasound Med 4:135–137, 1985.
24. Mitchell SE, Gross BH, Spitz HB: The hypoechoic caudate lobe: An ultrasonic pseudolesion. Radiology 144:569–572, 1982.
25. Auh YH, Rubenstein WA, Zirinski K, et al: Accessory fissures of the liver: CT and sonographic appearance. AJR Am J Roentgenol 143:565–572, 1984.
26. Arenson AM, McKee JD: Hypertrophied muscular bands in the region of the foramen of Bochdalek as a cause for an accessory fissure within the liver. Ultrasound Med Biol 11:461–465, 1985.
27. Prando A, Goldstein HM, Bernadino ME, Green B: Ultrasonic pseudotumors of the liver. Radiology 130:403–407, 1979.
28. Berland LL: Focal areas of decreased echogenicity in the liver at the porta hepatis. J Ultrasound Med 5:157–159, 1986.

Chapter 7

Cysts and Cystlike Hepatic Lesions

William J. Zwiebel

This chapter considers hepatic lesions that typically have a fluid-containing or cystlike sonographic appearance. Solid-appearing lesions, including benign and malignant neoplasms, will be discussed in the chapter that follows. The cystic/solid approach to hepatic masses may seem a little odd at first glance, but this approach represents a real-life perspective of hepatic masses, in which the sonographer first assesses the appearance of a mass and attempts to determine whether it is a cyst, a cystlike lesion, or a solid mass.

DIFFERENTIAL DIAGNOSIS

With rare exceptions, sonographic findings do not specifically indicate the etiology of cystlike hepatic masses, and in most cases, therefore, a differential diagnosis is indicated. Table 7-1 is a checklist of differential considerations for "cystic" hepatic masses. In many instances this list may be shorted by considering the patient's history, symptoms, and signs, as well as the results of other diagnostic studies. Note that some of the cystlike lesions inclued in Table 7-1 are actually solid masses that merely appear cystic on ultrasound examination.

TRAUMATIC FLUID COLLECTIONS

General Concepts

Computed tomography is the primary method for evaluating liver trauma, but occasionally trau-

Table 7-1. Differential Diagnosis of Fluid-Containing Hepatic Masses

---

Hematoma
Biloma
Benign cyst
Pyogenic abscess
Amebic abscess
Echinococcal cyst
Caroli disease
Necrotic metastasis
Primary cystic neoplasm
Sonolucent solid neoplasm

---

matic lesions are the subject of sonographic examination, either as an incidental finding or as the primary point of concern. In evaluating hepatic trauma, the sonographer should attempt to determine the following: (1) the location and extent of injury; (2) the size of the resulting hematoma; (3) whether the liver capsule is intact; and (4) whether a hematoma is intra- or extrahepatic.[21]

Hematoma

The most common manifestation of liver trauma is hematoma formation (Fig. 7-1). The appearance of a hepatic hematoma is governed in part by its location and the extent of hepatic injury.[1-3] Subcapsular hematomas (Fig. 7-1B) tend to be lens-shaped, because the extravasated blood is confined by the adherent liver capsule. Deep intrahepatic hematomas (Fig. 7-1C) generally reflect the configuration of the underlying liver laceration and may be linear, spherical, ovoid, irregular, or even branching in shape. Blood extravasated from the liver may collect in the perihepatic spaces or may become dispersed within the peritoneal cavity. Noncoagulated, peritoneal-space blood may be indistinguishable from ascites and other peritoneal fluid collections.

The sonographic appearance of a hematoma in the liver, or at any other location in the body, is governed by its age and by a variety of hematologic and technical factors; hence, there is some variability from case to case.[1-8] Nevertheless, a general pattern of sonographic findings unfolds as a hematoma is formed and ages (Fig. 7-1). Recently coagulated blood is moderately echogenic and homogeneous in texture. Echogenicity fades rapidly, however, over a period of hours, as thrombus forms and then retracts. With retraction, a matrix of echogenic fibrinoid material appears that is surrounded by anechoic expressed serum. After 24 hours, most hematomas contain clumps and strands of echogenic material surrounded by anechoic fluid. The proportion of echogenic components decreases over a period

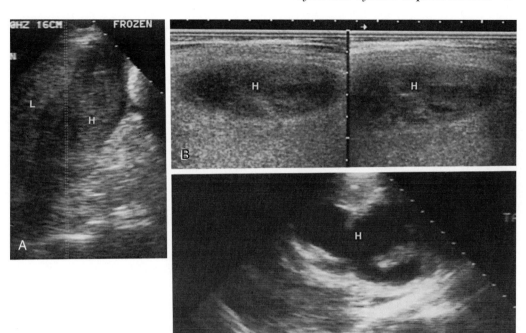

Figure 7-1—Variable Sonographic Appearances of Hematomas. (A) Four hours after percutaneous liver biopsy, a hematoma (H) with uniform, low-level echogenicity is seen adjacent to the right lobe of the liver (L). **(B)** About 3 days after liver biopsy, a slightly heterogeneous hepatic hematoma (H) is seen in a subcapsular location (different patient from *A*). Note the lens shape that is characteristic of a subcapsular hematoma. **(C)** Three weeks after blunt liver trauma, an intrahepatic hematoma (H) is virtually anechoic. The stellate shape of this collection reflects the configuration of the liver laceration.

of days to weeks, as the clot is lysed by naturally occurring processes. Within a month after formation, most hematomas are entirely anechoic.

Hematomas in the liver, or elsewhere in the abdomen, gradually diminish in size over a period of months, assuming that hemorrhage does not recur. Transient *enlargement* of hematomas older than 1 month may occur, apparently due to the imbibition of fluid.[1] In general, however, delayed enlargement suggests secondary infection and must be viewed with concern. Large hepatic hematomas may persist for months but eventually resolve, leaving no trace of abnormality.[3]

Biloma

In addition to causing hemorrhage and hematoma formation, trauma may disrupt the biliary system and cause intra- or extrahepatic leakage of bile. Abrupt and massive leakage causes peritonitis that is sufficiently severe to be recognized clinically. With smaller or slowly occurring leaks, however, the inflammatory response may be quite mild, and such leaks may be insidious. The inflammatory response to extravasated bile generates a pseudocapsule that encloses the collection, forming a biloma. These encapsulated

collections tend to be quite large (5 to 15 cm) at the time of clinical diagnosis.[9–11]

On ultrasound examination,[9–11] bilomas are well defined, anechoic intra- or extrahepatic masses without a visible capsule. Small bilomas are rounded in configuration, whereas larger collections conform in shape to adjacent anatomic boundaries. Dependent echogenic debris is occasionally present. Ultrasound features do not distinguish between bilomas and other fluid collections.

BENIGN CYSTS

Pathology and Clinical Features

Benign hepatic cysts[12–23] are thought to originate from remnants of the original, blind bile duct system of the embryo, which is replaced by a secondary, permanent system.[12, 13] The cysts (Fig. 7–2) are lined with epithelium identical to that of normal bile ducts and are filled with clear fluid thought to be secreted by the cyst lining. Cysts are uncommon in infants and children but frequently are present in middle-aged or elderly adults.[20] It is assumed, therefore, that cysts en-

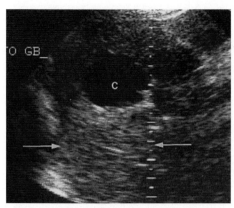

Figure 7-2—Cardinal Features of a Liver Cyst.
(1) The cyst (C) contents are anechoic; (2) the wall is invisible and smooth (although slightly undulant due to pressure from surrounding structures); and (3) enhanced through-transmission is evident (arrows).

Table 7-2. Sonographic Features of Benign Hepatic Cysts

Anechoic
Invisible wall
Smooth inner surface
No or minimal loculation
Enhanced through-transmission
Lateral edge shadows

cysts, an additional abnormality probably exists.[12, 16, 22]

Sonographic Findings

Benign hepatic cysts, whether solitary or multiple, have characteristic sonographic findings, as listed in Table 7–2 and illustrated in Figure 7–2. Before a lesion is deemed a benign cyst, four cardinal cyst characteristics must be demonstrated: (1) anechoic contents; (2) enhanced through-transmission of ultrasound (see Chapter 2); (3) an invisible wall; and (4) a relatively smooth interior border.[17] These features deserve emphasis, for they are applicable to benign cysts at any location, including the kidneys.

First, benign cysts remain anechoic even at high-gain settings because the cyst fluid does not contain crystals or other suspended material. This fluid impedes ultrasound transmission very little, leading to enhanced echogenicity of structures distal to the cyst, as discussed in Chapter 2. Homogeneous, solid tumors, such as lymphoma, may appear anechoic in some circumstances, but the degree of distal enhancement is not as great as with cysts of equivalent size.

Second, the wall of a benign cyst is invisible sonographically, and the inner surface of the cyst is smooth. A thick or irregular wall suggests a lesion other than a benign cyst.

Third, benign cysts may be slightly irregular

large slowly and become more conspicuous with time.

The great majority of hepatic cysts are asymptomatic, but pressure from very large cysts may cause pain, biliary obstruction, or compressive dysfunction of surrounding viscera.[14–16, 20–22] Intracyst hemorrhage and cyst infection also may cause symptoms. Percutaneous drainage may be warranted in symptomatic cases. A sclerosing agent, such as alcohol, may be used in such cases to prevent reaccumulation of cyst fluid.[14, 15, 19]

Multiple hepatic cysts (Fig. 7–3) are present in about 30% to 50% of patients with dominant (adult) polycystic kidney disease (DPKD).[12, 16, 21, 22] Conversely, about 50% of patients with *multiple* hepatic cysts have DPKD. Multiple hepatic cysts also may occur in children or adults with a congenital disorder termed "fibropolycystic disease."[12] Hepatic dysfunction rarely results from multiple cysts; therefore, *when liver dysfunction occurs in a patient with multiple hepatic*

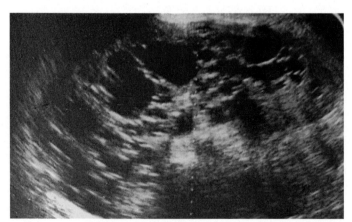

Figure 7-3—Multiple Hepatic Cysts.
A transverse sonogram demonstrates multiple hepatic cysts of varying size in a patient with autosomal dominant polycystic kidney disease.

in shape, because of pressure from surrounding structures, and minimal septation also may occur. Grossly irregular shape or a multilocular appearance is not a feature of benign cysts, however.

Fourth, localized crescentic calcification occurs rarely in the walls of benign liver or renal cysts, but such calcification is also a feature of hepatic echinococcus cysts, as discussed later.[22] Coarse and extensive calcification suggests other conditions, such as a chronic hematoma or a degenerated echinococcus cyst.

Finally, high-resolution images of benign cysts may demonstrate lateral edge shadows, which result from refraction and reflection at the cyst wall (Chapter 2). Although these shadows support the diagnosis of benign cyst, they are not specific and may occur distal to any well-encapsulated mass, whether fluid-filled or solid.

Diagnostic Accuracy and Differential Diagnosis

Sonographic diagnosis of benign hepatic cysts appears to be extremely accurate, but this impression is not confirmed by a body of data such as that which exists for renal cysts (see Chapter 21). It is well recognized, however, that other pathologic lesions may mimic exactly the sonographic appearance of benign hepatic cysts, including bilomas, hematomas, abscesses, necrotic neoplasms, and parasitic cysts (especially echinococcus).[17, 22, 23] Hence, when clinical circumstances require absolute accuracy, percutaneous cyst aspiration should be performed.

PYOGENIC HEPATIC ABSCESS

Hepatic abscesses are common cystlike lesions of the liver. These abscesses may result from bacterial, fungal, or parasitic infection. We will first consider pyogenic (bacterial) abscesses, which generally are caused by gram-negative organisms. Bacteria may gain access to the liver via hematogenous (usually portal) and cholangitic routes, by direct extension from adjacent infection sites, and by penetrating injury.[24–27]

Clinical Features

In most instances, pyogenic hepatic abscesses are highly symptomatic and represent a serious, life-threatening condition. Hepatic abscesses also may occur, however, in much less dire circumstances, and the signs and symptoms of these insidious infections may be deceptively mild. Blood cultures are positive in only about 50% of patients with hepatic abscesses, and clinical diagnosis, therefore, may be difficult.[24–29]

Sonographic/Pathologic Correlation

The classic sonographic appearance of a pyogenic hepatic abscess is a spherical or ovoid lesion that (1) is well defined but not distinctly encapsulated, (2) has an irregular border, (3) is hypoechoic or anechoic, (4) has a fine-grained to coarse echo texture, and (5) exhibits enhanced through-transmission of ultrasound.[22, 28–33] *A cluster of fluid collections with these features* (Fig. 7–4) *is particularly suggestive of hepatic ab-*

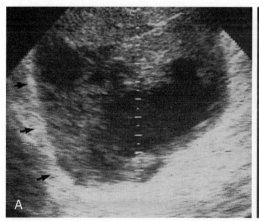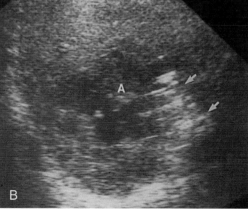

Figure 7-4—Pyogenic Liver Abscesses. (A) A longitudinal scan through the left lobe of the liver demonstrates a cluster of interconnected fluid collections with irregular borders. This clustered appearance is highly suggestive of pyogenic liver abscess. The patient was 2 months postcholedochojejunostomy. Arrows = diaphragm. (B) A longitudinal scan through the right hepatic lobe demonstrates a poorly marginated, lobulated, heterogeneous abscess (A) that contains gas (bright reflections marked by arrows). The patient was an emaciated, homeless alcoholic who presented with abdominal pain and sepsis.

scess.[22] In spite of these "typical" features of hepatic abscesses, the sonographic appearance is quite variable. In large measure, this variability relates to the pathologic stage at which the abscess is examined. An abscess begins as an accumulation of neutrophils in an area of parenchymal infection. At this stage, the liver is likely to appear normal sonographically. Liquefactive necrosis ensues and causes the abscess cavity to form. With highly suppurative infection, the abscess contents are apt to be watery and are either anechoic or sonolucent. Alternatively, if liquefaction is less complete, the contents are apt to be debris-ladened and echogenic. In some cases abscesses may be more echogenic than normal hepatic parenchyma.[30-32]

About 20% of abscesses contain gas,[22, 34] which causes strong reflections and prominent acoustic shadows (Figs. 7–4B, 7–5). Occasionally the supernatant, echogenic gas may obscure the remainder of the abscess. In most cases, however, the bright reflections are not a problem, for they serve as a "beacon" that identifies the pathologic area.

Sonographic Accuracy

The sensitivity of ultrasound for pyogenic hepatic abscesses is reported as 75% to 90%.[28-33] Abscesses that are overlooked sonographically most often are located high under the diaphragm and far lateral in the right lobe. These locations are notorious hiding places for hepatic mass lesions of any kind and always deserve close scrutiny.

INTRAHEPATIC GAS

The discussion of pyogenic hepatic abscess provides a good opportunity to review the differential diagnosis of intrahepatic gas.[22, 35-42] Sonographic detection of gas within the liver portends serious abnormality and is an indication, therefore, for thorough investigation.

Sonography is very sensitive for intrahepatic gas, even when present in small quantities, because the vast acoustic impedance mismatch at a gas/liver boundary produces very strong reflections. Larger gas collections may generate acoustic shadows, but tiny gas bubbles do not block enough of the ultrasound beam to cause a shadow. In some cases, gas bubbles may produce comet tail artifacts,[40] which are described in Chapter 2.

Causes

Intrahepatic gas may be located in the parenchyma, the bile ducts, or the portal veins. Parenchyma gas may be introduced by violent or surgical trauma but more typically is due to hepatic abscess. Gas may accumulate in the biliary tract as a result of serious and even life-threatening conditions, such as ascending cholangitis, gallbladder empyema, and communication of the biliary tree with an abscess cavity. More commonly, however, gas in the biliary tree has an innocuous cause, such as cholecystojejunostomy, sphincterotomy (Oddi), or percutaneous biliary drainage. Portal vein gas generally is regarded as an ominous finding related to ischemic bowel

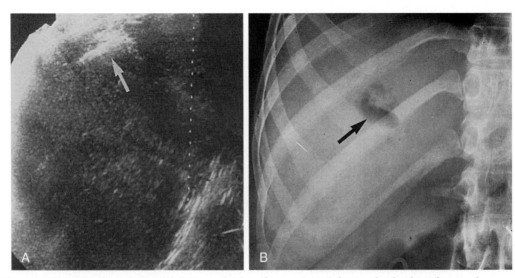

Figure 7-5—Parenchymal Gas. (A) Stationary bright reflections (arrow) due to a localized intrahepatic abscess were the only hepatic abnormalities detected with ultrasound. **(B)** A radiograph exposed shortly after the sonogram confirmed the existence of intrahepatic gas. The patient was status post gastric bypass (for obesity) complicated by peritoneal space abscess.

necrosis or a severe suppurative process involving the bowel. These conditions should always come to mind when portal vein gas is encountered, but it is noteworthy that gas may be present in the portal venous system in far less dire circumstances, including uncomplicated gastric distention.[35–42]

Localization

The mere sonographic detection of intrahepatic gas is of limited diagnostic value. The accurate localization of gas to the parenchyma, the biliary system, or the venous system is essential for determining its significance.[35, 37–42] Intraparenchymal gas (Fig. 7–5) is easiest to localize, since it remains stationary in spite of respiratory motion or changes in patient position.

Gas within the major portal veins (Fig. 7–6) also is easily localized, since the portal veins are readily visualized with ultrasound in most patients. Portal vein gas produces tiny but strong reflections that are *transitory* and move rapidly toward the periphery of the liver. Gas may be seen concomitantly in the superior mesenteric vein, the splenic vein, or less commonly in the hepatic veins.

Biliary tract gas may be more difficult to localize than portal vein gas, since intrahepatic bile ducts, for the most part, are not visualized with ultrasound. Proper localization is facilitated, however, by a tendency for biliary tract gas to coalesce *centrally* within the liver as coarse bubbles or linear collections. In many cases, biliary

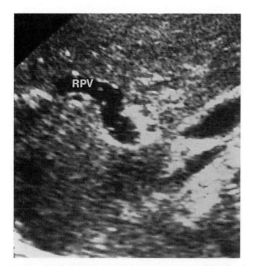

Figure 7-6—Portal Vein Gas. A series of bright dots seen within the right portal vein (RPV) was caused by tiny gas bubbles that were readily seen to move toward the periphery with portal blood flow. The cause of portal vein gas was not ascertained in this elderly, intensive care patient examined because of hyperbilirubinemia.

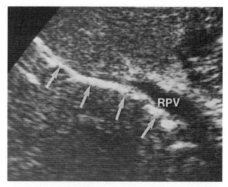

Figure 7-7—Biliary Tract Gas. A row of bright reflections (arrows) caused by biliary tract gas line up adjacent to the right portal vein and one of its branches in this patient who was postcholedochojejunostomy.

tract gas lines up like a string of pearls, *adjacent* to the major portal vein branches (Fig. 7–7). Such collections are stationary (as long as the patient is motionless), as opposed to portal vein gas, which moves quickly to the periphery of the liver.

Gas Versus Calculi

An additional problem germane to the discussion of intrahepatic gas is differentiation between gas and calculi. The bright reflections and acoustic shadows of gas and calculi are identical, but two sonographic findings help differentiate these entities. First, the presence of myriad bright reflections suggests gas, since calculi usually are few in number. Second, gas is supernatant in a fluid medium, whereas stones are dependent. With patient movement, therefore, biliary tract gas can usually be induced to rise to a higher elevation, whereas biliary calculi sink to a lower level (if they are not confined). Radiography also may differentiate between gas and calculi if the gas bubbles or stones are sufficiently large for radiographic detection.

MULTIPLE HEPATIC MICROABSCESSES

Returning now to the subject of hepatic abscesses, it is noteworthy that the liver may be "peppered" with tiny abscesses in immunosuppressed patients (Fig. 7–8), and such abscesses may be sufficiently large for sonographic visualization in some patients.[43–47] Diffuse *Candida albicans* infection may cause multiple small, widely dispersed lesions that either are echogenic or have a "target" appearance (hyperechogenic center and a sonolucent periphery). The echogenic foci are generated by fungal mycelia. Diffuse

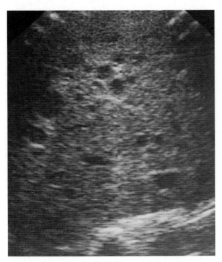

Figure 7-8—Multiple Hepatic Abscesses.
Multiple hypoechoic liver lesions due to *Candida albicans* infection are seen in the liver of an immunocompromised patient.

hepatic infection with *Pneumocystis carinii* in patients with autoimmune deficiency syndrome may generate a mottled appearance similar to that seen with diffuse metastasis (discussed in the following chapter).

PERIHEPATIC ABSCESS

As noted previously, the perihepatic spaces are common locations for the development of pyogenic abscesses. Sonography is an excellent method for diagnosis of these collections, since the liver serves as an effective ultrasonic window. Perihepatic abscesses[48, 49] (Fig. 7–9) tend to be highly transonic, watery collections with a small-to-moderate amount of debris. Although these collections are encapsulated by adhesions, the

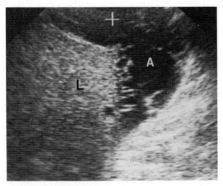

Figure 7-9—Perihepatic Abscess. A loculated abscess (A) surrounds the inferior tip of the right lobe of the liver (L) as seen on this longitudinal scan. The patient had had surgery for a colonic perforation. The cursor marks the depth for percutaneous aspiration.

capsule is not visible. In my experience, most perihepatic abscesses assume a configuration imposed by surrounding structures.

It is important to distinguish between a subphrenic abscess and a pleural fluid collection. This distinction is made easily in most cases (Fig. 7–10) since the diaphragm, which separates the subphrenic and pleural spaces, typically is clearly seen.

It is also important to differentiate between a perihepatic collection and ascites. This distinction depends on two observations. First, ascites usually can be seen at several locations in the peritoneal space—assuming that the sonographer looks for it. Second, ascites often can be displaced from the perihepatic spaces by altering the patient's position. Walled-off perihepatic collections, such as abscesses, cannot be displaced.

AMEBIC ABSCESS

Pathology and Clinical Features

Entamoeba histolytica[50–56] is a protozoan parasite of worldwide distribution, but because of high sanitation standards, human infestation by this organism is uncommon in many Western nations. The organism is transmitted by the fecal-oral route. Ingested cysts change into trophozoites in the colon, invade the colonic mucosa, enter the portal venous system, and are transported to the small portal radicles, where they lodge. The multiplication of the organisms is accompanied by proteolytic tissue destruction, which results in abscess formation.

An amebic abscess is solitary in about 60% of cases, and typically is located in the periphery of the liver.[52–54] Hematogenous spread of *E. histolytica* beyond the liver is rare and usually results in lung or brain abscess formation. Direct extension of the infestation from the liver to adjacent structures is more common than hematogenous spread. Classically, the abscess penetrates the diaphragm and forms an amebic empyema or pulmonary abscess.[51]

A hepatic amebic abscess may be discovered incidentally, for the symptoms of infestation often are mild and nonspecific. Few patients, furthermore, have diarrhea at the time the abscess is discovered, and the organism, in most cases, is no longer present in the stool.

Sonographic Findings

The only finding considered pathognomonic for amebic abscess is disruption of the diaphragm, resulting in a hepatic abscess that is

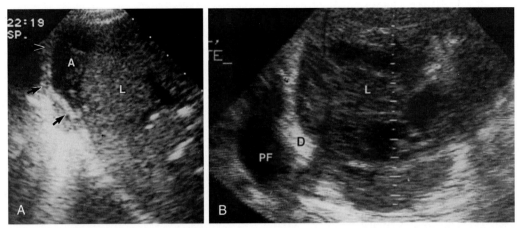

Figure 7-10—Subphrenic vs. Pleural Fluid. (A) A subphrenic abscess (A) related to acute cholecystitis is shown in this longitudinal sonogram. Note that this collection is clearly below the diaphragm (arrows). L = liver. **(B)** A sympathetic (sterile) pleural fluid (PF) collection is seen above the diaphragm (D) in this patient with a liver (L) abscess (same patient as in Figure 7–4A).

contiguous with an empyema or lung abscess.[51–53] Fortunately for amebiasis patients, these findings are uncommon. Several additional findings suggest amebic abscess but are nonspecific. These are (1) peripheral location; (2) fine, homogeneous internal echogenicity; (3) enhanced through-transmission; and (4) a well-defined border without a visible wall.[52–54] Abscess location and echogenicity are particularly important findings; 97% of amebic abscesses abut the liver capsule, and 90% generate fine-grained, low-level echoes at normal or high-gain settings[50–54] (Fig. 7–11). In my experience, pyogenic liver abscesses usually are deep within the parenchyma rather than subcapsular.

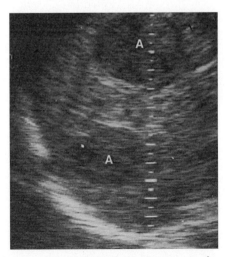

Figure 7-11—Amebic Liver Abscess. Amebic abscesses (A) are seen in the right lobe of the liver on a longitudinal sonogram. These are well defined, homogeneous, and hypoechoic.

Changes Following Therapy

Most amebic abscesses are successfully treated with metronidazole or chloroquine. It is noteworthy that the abscess may actually enlarge transiently during therapy; furthermore, the abscess cavity may persist for months or years in spite of successful treatment (median sonographic disappearance time is 7 months).[55] The adequacy of therapy must be judged, therefore, by clinical and laboratory data, not by sonographic findings.

ECHINOCOCCAL CYSTS

Two species of *Echinococcus* may infest humans, *E. granulosus* and *E. multilocularis.*[57–67] *E. granulosus* is the more common organism, and is classically featured in the medical literature.

Life Cycle

E. granulosus[57–66] is the common dog-sheep tapeworm, for which a carnivore is the definitive host and a ruminant is the intermediate host. Humans serve as an alternate intermediate host.

The adult worms live in the small intestine of the carnivore, which sheds large numbers of eggs with its feces. The eggs subsequently are ingested by the ruminant or by humans, and the embryos within the eggs are released in the duodenum. The embryos enter the portal or lymphatic systems and are disseminated to the liver or the entire body. About 75% of embryos lodge in the sinusoids of the liver, 15% in the lungs, and 10% in the rest of the body. Within the liver, an embryo develops into a cyst that grows slowly over many years. Approximately 60% of patients harbor only one cyst, which almost invariably is located in the right hepatic lobe. The life cycle of *E. granulosus* is completed when the intermediate host is devoured by a carnivore. Fortunately, humans seldom contribute to the completion of the life cycle![57, 60, 61]

Cyst Structure

The echinococcal cyst consists of three layers. The outer layer, called the pericyst, is a thick wall of fibrous tissue contributed by the host in response to the invading organism. The middle, "laminated" layer is about 2 mm thick and is composed of fragile, laminated, acellular material that resembles the white of a hard-boiled egg. The innermost layer is the 1 cell thick germinal layer that generates the scolices that ultimately infect the carnivore. The scolices (actually the "heads" of future tape worms) are formed in tiny brood capsules that project from the inner surface of the germinal layer. When the brood capsules become distended with scolices, they rupture, releasing the scolices into the cyst fluid. Scolices thus released form a layer of sediment described as "hydatid sand." As the cyst ages, "daughter cysts" may bud from the germinal

layer, creating a "cyst-within-a-cyst" appearance. Each daughter produce scolices in the same manner as the mother cyst.[57, 60, 61]

Sonographic Findings

Five sonographic findings strongly suggest the diagnosis of hydatid cyst:

1. Clear-cut visualization of daughter cysts (Fig. 7–12A);
2. A double line or sonolucent cleft at the margin of the cyst, caused by separation of the layers of the cyst wall (Fig. 7–12B);
3. A thin arc of calcification in the cyst wall;
4. The "sonographic water lily sign" (Fig. 7–12C), in which the crumpled, deflated paracytic components lie at the bottom of the pericyst; and
5. The "falling snowflakes sign," in which movement of the patient stirs the hydatid sand, which then settles like falling snow.[58–61, 63–66]

Both the peripheral double line and fine linear calcification are seen in normal, "healthy" cysts, whereas the sonolucent cleft and the water lily sign are evidence of cyst degeneration, with sub-

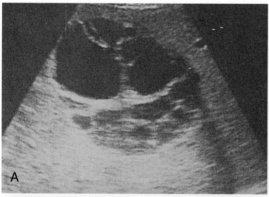

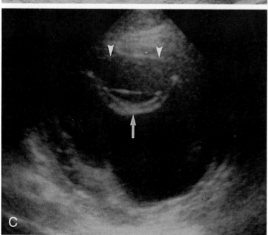

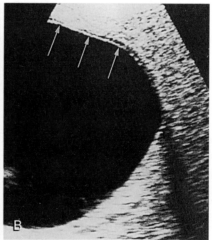

Figure 7-12—Echinococcal Cyst Features. (**A**) Classic multilocular appearance of daughter cysts. (**B**) Double-wall sign (arrows) in a unilocular echinococcal cyst. (**C**) The fallen lily sign in which the endocyst (arrow) has fallen away from the fibrous pericyst (arrowheads). (Parts A and B kindly contributed by Dr Fraydoon Esfahani, Department of Radiology, University of Iowa Hospitals and Clinics; from Esfahani F, Rooholamini SA, Vessal K: Ultrasonography of hepatic hydatid cysts: New diagnostic science. J Ultrasound Med 1:443–450, 1988.)

sequent loss of fluid pressure within the endocyst.

Aging, degenerating, or dead cysts, and those affected by hemorrhage or secondary infection, may be diffusely echogenic or heavily calcified. These lesions often are indistinguishable from other liver lesions, such as abscesses and tumors. A thick rim of calcification is the only sonographic feature that suggests a degenerated echinococcus cyst.[60, 61–64, 66]

Differential Diagnosis

Considering that several of the aforementioned sonographic findings are virtually pathognomonic, one might assume echinococcal cysts are readily identified with ultrasound, but this is not so. In 28% to 65% of cases, *E. granulosus* liver cysts are thin walled, unilocular, and completely anechoic (no daughter cysts or hydatid sand).[63, 64, 66] These cysts resemble idiopathic hepatic cysts or other well-defined fluid-containing lesions. Two findings appear particularly helpful in identifying unilocular hydatid cysts. First, the double peripheral line (Fig. 7–12*B*) can be demonstrated in 92% of cases but is not a feature of any other cystic liver lesions.[66] Second, cyst wall calcification is rare in benign liver cysts, and its presence, therefore, should call *echinococcus* cyst to mind.

Echinococcus Multilocularis

E. multilocularis[67] shares a similar life cycle with *E. granulosus*, but this organism does not incite an effective host response (pericyst) that confines the infestation. Instead, the parasite proliferates as multiple small cysts (1 to 10 mm in diameter) that infiltrate the liver parenchyma in the manner of an invading neoplasm. The sonographic presentation, therefore, is as a poorly marginated, multilocular cystic mass. This interesting parasite is uncommon and does not therefore warrant further mention in this text. Additional details may be found in the article by Dieder and associates.[67]

REFERENCES

1. Lam AH, Shulman L: Ultrasonography in the management of liver trauma in children. J Ultrasound Med 3:199–203, 1984.
2. Kuligowska E: Ultrasound in upper abdominal trauma. Semin Roentgenol 19:281–285, 1984.
3. Athey GN, Rahman SU: Hepatic hematoma following blunt injury: Non-operative management. Injury 13:302–306, 1982.
4. Wick JD, Silver TM, Bree RL: Gray-scale features of hematomas: An ultrasonic spectrum. AJR Am J Roentgenol 131:977–980, 1978.
5. Filly RA, Sommer FG, Minton MJ: Characterization of biological fluids by ultrasound and computed tomography. Radiology 134:167–171, 1980.
6. Coelho JCU, Sigel B, Ryva JC, Machi J, Renigers SA: B-mode sonography of blood clots. J Clin Ultrasound 10:323–327, 1982.
7. Shung KK, Fei D-Y, Yuan Y-W, Reeves WC: Ultrasonic characterization of blood during coagulation. J Clin Ultrasound 12:147–153, 1984.
8. Peters DJ, Flanagan LD, Cranley JJ: Analysis of blood clot echogenicity. J Clin Ultrasound 14:111–116, 1986.
9. Vazquez JL, Thorsen MK, Dodds WJ, et al: Evaluation and treatment of intra-abdominal bilomas. AJR Am J Roentgenol 144:933–938, 1985.
10. Mueller PR, Ferrucci JT, Simeone JF, Cronan JJ, Wittenberg J, Neff CC, van Sonnenberg E: Detection and drainage of bilomas: Special considerations. AJR Am J Roentgenol 140:715–720, 1983.
11. Lorenz R, Beyer D, Peters PE: Detection of intraperitoneal bile accumulations: Significance of ultrasonography, CT, and cholescintigraphy. Gastrointest Radiol 9:213–217, 1984.
12. Sherlock S: Diseases of the Liver and Biliary System. Oxford, Blackwell Scientific Publications, 1985, pp 429–441.
13. Sanfelippo PM, Behrs OH, Weiland LH: Cystic disease of the liver. Ann Surg 179:922–925, 1974.
14. Sanjay S, Mueller PR, Ferrucci JT, et al: Percutaneous aspiration of hepatic cysts does not provide definitive therapy. AJR Am J Roentgenol 141:559–560, 1983.
15. Goldstein HM, Carlyle DR, Nelson RS: Treatment of symptomatic hepatic cysts by percutaneous instillation of Pantopaque. AJR Am J Roentgenol 127:850–853, 1976.
16. Levine E, Cook LT, Grantham JJ: Liver cysts in autosomal-dominant polycystic kidney disease: Clinical and computed tomographic study. AJR Am J Roentgenol 145:229–233, 1985.
17. Weaver RM, Goldstein HM, Green B, Perkins C: Gray-scale ultrasonic evaluation of hepatic cystic disease. AJR Am J Roentgenol 130:849–852, 1978.
18. Jaffe CC, Rosenfield AT, Sommers G, et al: Technical factors influencing the imaging of small anechoic cysts by B-scan ultrasound. Radiology 135:429–433, 1980.
19. Beam WJ, Rodan BA: Hepatic cysts: Treatment with alcohol. AJR Am J Roentgenol 144:237–241, 1985.
20. Athey PA, Lauderman JA, King DE: Massive congenital solitary nonparasitic cyst of the liver in infancy. J Ultrasound Med 5:585–587, 1986.
21. Ergün H, Wolf BH, Hissong SL: Obstructive jaundice caused by polycystic liver disease. Radiology 136:435–436, 1980.
22. Murphy BJ, Casillas J, Ros PR, Morillo G, Albores-Saavedra J, Rolfes DB: The CT appearance of cystic masses of the liver. RadioGraphics 9:307–322, 1989.
23. Pollack HM, Banner MP, Arger PH, Peters J, Mulhern CB, Coleman BG: The accuracy of gray-scale renal ultrasonography in differentiating cystic neoplasms from benign cysts. Radiology 143:741–745, 1982.
24. Santiani B, Davidson ED: Hepatic abscesses: Improvement in mortality with early diagnosis and treatment. Am J Surg 135:647–650, 1978.
25. Cello JP, Sleisenger MH: The liver in systemic conditions. *In* Zakim D, Boyer TD (eds): Hepatology of Liver Disease. Philadelphia, WB Saunders, 1982, pp 817–819.

26. LaMont JT, Iselbacher KJ: Suppurative diseases of the liver. *In* Thorn GW, Adams RD, et al (eds): Harrison's Principles of Internal Medicine. 8th ed. New York, McGraw-Hill, 1977, pp 1617–1618.
27. Hiatt JR, Williams RA, Wilson SE: Intra-abdominal abscess: Etiology and pathogenesis. Semin Ultrasound 4:71–79, 1983.
28. Kuligowska E, Nobel J: Sonography of hepatic abscesses. Semin Ultrasound 4:102–116, 1983.
29. Kuligowska E, Connors SK, Shapiro JH: Liver abscess: Sonography in diagnosis and treatment. AJR Am J Roentgenol 138:253–257, 1982.
30. Subramanyam BR, Balthazar EJ, Raghavendra BN, et al: Ultrasound analysis of solid-appearing abscesses. Radiology 146:487–491, 1983.
31. Freeny PC: Acute pyogenic hepatitis: Sonographic and angiographic findings. AJR Am J Roentgenol 135:388–391, 1980.
32. Powers TA, Jones TB, Karl JH: Echogenic hepatic abscess without radiographic evidence of gas. AJR Am J Roentgenol 137:159–160, 1981.
33. Newlin N, Silver TM, Stuck KJ, et al: Ultrasonic features of liver abscesses. Radiology 139:155–159, 1981.
34. Halvorsen RA, Korobkin M, Foster WL, et al: Variable CT appearance of hepatic abscesses. AJR Am J Roentgenol 142:941–946, 1984.
35. Merritt CRB, Goldsmith JP, Sharp MJ: Sonographic detection of portal venous gas in infants with necrotizing enterocolitis. AJR Am J Roentgenol 143:1059–1062, 1984.
36. Liebman PR, Patten MT, Manny J, et al: Hepatic-portal venous gas in adults: Pathophysiology and clinical significance. Ann Surg 187:281–288, 1989.
37. Gold RP, Seaman WB: Splenic flexure carcinoma as a source of hepatic portal venous gas. Radiology 122:329–330, 1977.
38. Haswell DM, Carsky EW: Hepatic portal venous gas and gastric emphysema with survival. AJR Am J Roentgenol 133:1183–1185, 1979.
39. Gosink BB: Intrahepatic gas: Differential diagnosis. Am J Roentgenol 137:763–767, 1981.
40. Laing FC, Rego JD, Jeffrey RB: Ultrasonographic identification of portal vein gas. J Clin Ultrasound 12:512–514, 1984.
41. Chezmar JL, Nelson RE, Bernardino ME: Portal venous gas after hepatic transplantation: Sonographic detection and clinical significance. AJR Am J Roentgenol 153:1203–1205, 1989.
42. Kriegshauser JS, Reading CC, King BF, Welch TJ: Combined systemic and portal venous gas: Sonographic and CT detection in two cases. AJR Am J Roentgenol 154:1219–1221, 1990.
43. Miller JH, Greenfield LD, Wald BR: Candidiasis of the liver and spleen in childhood. Radiology 142:375–380, 1980.
44. Callen PW, Filly RA, Marcus FS: Ultrasonography and CT in the evaluation of microabscesses in the immunosuppressed patient. Radiology 136:433–434, 1980.
45. Ho B, Cooperberg PL, Li DBK, et al: Ultrasonography and CT in the hepatic candidiasis in immunosuppressed patients. J Ultrasound Med 1:157–159, 1982.
46. Shirkhoda A, Lopez-Berenstein G, Holbert JM, et al: Hepatosplenic fungal infection: CT and pathologic evaluation after treatment with liposomal amphotericin B. Radiology 159:249–253, 1986.
47. Towers MJ, Withers CE, Rachlis AR, Pappas SC, Kolin A: Ultrasound diagnosis of hepatic Kaposi's sarcoma. J Ultrasound Med 10:701–703, 1991.
48. Hiatt JR, Williams RA, Wilson SE: Intraabdominal abscess: Etiology and pathogenesis. Semin Ultrasound 4:71–79, 1983.
49. Rubenstein WA, Auh YH, Whalen JP, Kazam E: The perihepatic spaces: Computed tomographic and ultrasound imaging. Radiology 149:231–239, 1983.
50. Merten EDF, Kirks DR: Ameba liver abscess in children: The role of diagnostic imaging. AJR Am J Roentgenol 143:1325–1329, 1984.
51. Landay MJ, Setiawan H, Hirsch G, et al: Hepatic and thoracic amebiasis. Am J Roentgenol 135:449–454, 1980.
52. Ralls PW, Meyers HI, Lapin SA, et al: Gray-scale ultrasonography of hepatic ameba abscesses. Radiology 132:125–129, 1979.
53. Ralls PW, Colletti PM, Quinn MF, et al: Sonographic findings in hepatic ameba abscess. Radiology 145:123–126, 1982.
54. Ralls PW, Barnes PF, Radin DR, Colletti P, Halls J: Sonographic features of amebic and pyogenic liver abscesses: A blinded comparison. AJR Am J Roentgenol 149:499–501, 1987.
55. Ralls PW, Quinn MF, Boswell WD, et al: Patterns of resolution in successfully treated hepatic ameba abscess. Radiology 149:541–543, 1983.
56. van Sonnenberg E, Mueller PR, Schiffman HR, et al: Intrahepatic ameba abscess: Indications for and results of percutaneous catheter drainage. Radiology 156:631–635, 1985.
57. Marcial MA, Marcial J, Rojas RA: Protozoal and helminthic infections. *In* Kissane JM (ed): Anderson's Pathology. 8th ed. St Louis, CV Mosby, 1985, pp 427–428.
58. Hadidi A: Ultrasound findings in liver hydatid cysts. J Clin Ultrasound 7:365–368, 1979.
59. Itzchak Y, Rubenstein Z, Heyman Z, Gerzof S: Role of ultrasound in the diagnosis of abdominal hydatid disease. J Clin Ultrasound 8:341–345, 1980.
60. Beggs I: The radiology of hydatid disease. AJR Am J Roentgenol 145:630–648, 1985.
61. Lewall DB, McCorkell SJ: Hepatic echinococcal cysts: Sonographic appearance and classification. Radiology 155:773–775, 1985.
62. Barriga P, Cruz F, Lepe V, et al: An ultrasonographically solid, tumor-like appearance of echinococcal cysts in the liver. J Ultrasound Med 2:123–125, 1973.
63. Niron EA, Ozer H: Ultrasound appearance of liver hydatid disease. Br J Radiol 54:335–338, 1981.
64. Gharbi HA, Hassine W, Brauer MW, et al: Ultrasound examination of the hydatid liver. Radiology 139:459–463, 1981.
65. Saint Martin G, Chiesa JC: "Falling snowflakes," an ultrasound sign of hydatid sand. J Ultrasound Med 3:257–260, 1984.
66. Esfahani F, Rooholamini SA, Vessal K: Ultrasonography of hepatic hydatid cysts: New diagnostic signs. J Ultrasound Med 7:443–450, 1988.
67. Dieder D, Weiler S, Rohmer P, et al: Hepatic alveolar echinococcosis: Correlative US and CT study. Radiology 154:179–186, 1985.

Chapter 8

Solid-Appearing Hepatic Masses

William J. Zwiebel

DIFFERENTIAL DIAGNOSIS

The differential diagnosis of solid-appearing hepatic masses is presented in Table 8–1, which is offered as a checklist. As such, it may be culled in individual patients in relation to sonographic findings, patient age, clinical signs and symptoms, and other clinical information. It is noteworthy that this list overlaps that offered in the preceding chapter for cystlike hepatic masses, because some neoplastic lesions are anechoic or fluid-filled, and some fluid-containing lesions are echogenic.

COMPARISON OF IMAGING METHODS

Although this is an ultrasound text, it is useful to compare and contrast the available hepatic imaging techniques with respect to the requirements of newer tumor-management methods, which stress both sensitivity and specificity.[1–49] The following should be regarded as a general outline, for the technology of hepatic imaging is evolving rapidly and certain information no doubt will be dated by the time of publication.

Table 8–1. Differential Diagnosis of Solid-Appearing Hepatic Masses

---

Non-Neoplastic

Complicated benign cyst
Hematoma
Abscess (pyogenic or amebic)
Complicated echinococcal cyst
Regenerative nodule
Focal fatty infiltration

Benign Neoplasms

Focal nodular hyperplasia
Hepatocellular adenoma
Cavernous hemangioma
Rare lesions (see Tables 8–3 and 8–5)

Malignant Neoplasms

Hepatocellular carcinoma
Cholangiocarcinoma
Metastasis
Hepatoblastoma
Infantile hemangioendothelioma

Ultrasound

Ultrasound offers the advantages of low cost, non-invasiveness, portability, and patient comfort. The disadvantages of ultrasound are relatively low sensitivity to hepatic masses, lack of reproducibility from one study to another, and virtual inability to differentiate between malignant and benign lesions. The reported ultrasound detection rates for hepatic masses, on a lesion-by-lesion basis,* range widely,[2, 5–14] but a reasonable figure probably falls between 50% and 80% in patients of Western nations.†[2, 13] Ultrasound performs especially poorly for lesions under 1 cm in size; fewer than 40% of such lesions are detected.[2, 8, 13, 14]

Intraoperative sonography, in contrast to percutaneous sonography, is highly sensitive for hepatic masses (86% to 96%), including subcentimeter lesions, and this technique may be extremely valuable for confirming the resectability of hepatic malignances at operation.[6–8]

Doppler ultrasound has been investigated as a means of differentiating between benign and malignant hepatic lesions,[15–18] but the results of preliminary studies have been mixed. I have doubts about the ultimate value of Doppler sonography for tumor diagnosis.

Computed Tomography

Computed tomography (CT) has been the mainstay of hepatic tumor detection in recent years, but CT is less than ideal in several respects. CT detects roughly 70% to 95% of hepatic masses, which is better than ultrasound. Like ultrasound, however, CT is insensitive for smaller lesions and detects only about 40% to 50% of masses 1 cm or smaller.[2, 6–10, 14, 19–23] The detection rates for both small and large lesions may improve with spiral CT; nevertheless, CT will continue to suffer from limited ability to

---

*The accuracy of imaging methods for liver mass detection is sometimes reported on a patient-by-patient basis. Detection rates are less relevant when tabulated in this way than when tabulated on a lesion-by-lesion basis. All statistics presented herein are based on a lesion-by-lesion correlation.

†The detection rate is higher in Asian series, apparently because patients are smaller and leaner.

Table 8-2. Findings Indicating Intra- or Extrahepatic Location of Mass Lesions

---

Intrahepatic

   Continuity of the liver capsule over the mass
   Bulging of the liver capsule
   Displacement/invasion of portal or hepatic vein radicles
   Posterior displacement of the inferior vena cava

Extrahepatic

   Discontinuity of the liver capsule (invasion by the mass)
   Invagination of the liver capsule
   Fat triangle of wedge between mass and liver
   Anteromedial displacement of inferior vena cava

Based on Graif M, Manor A, Itzchak Y: Sonographic differentiation of extra- and intrahepatic masses. AJR Am J Roentgenol 141:533–556, 1983.

differentiate between benign and malignant masses.

Magnetic Resonance Imaging

Magnetic resonance imaging (MRI) is gaining broader acceptance as a means for detecting and evaluating hepatic neoplasms. MRI appears to be reasonably sensitive for metastases (range of 80% to 100%) and is reported to discriminate between benign and malignant lesions in about 70% to 90% of cases.[2–4, 19, 20, 24–34] The latter ability results from the high level of soft tissue contrast that is inherent in MR images. MRI is noninvasive and risk free, but claustrophobia and patient motion problems preclude the use of this modality for many individuals.

INTRAHEPATIC VERSUS EXTRAHEPATIC LOCATIONS

Whenever a mass is discovered in the vicinity of the liver, it is crucial to determine whether the lesion is intra- or extrahepatic. A number of sonographic findings are helpful in making this distinction, and these are listed in Table 8–2.[50] The most definitive of these are (1) invagination versus bulging of the liver surface, and (2) the presence of a line, wedge, or triangle of fat between the mass and the liver (Fig. 8–1).

BENIGN HEPATIC NEOPLASMS

Benign neoplasms of the liver are encountered frequently in the course of ultrasound, CT, and MR examinations, and their differentiation from malignant lesions has become a formidable diagnostic problem. A histologic classification of benign hepatic neoplasms is presented in Table 8–3.[51, 52] Some of the tumors listed in this table are rare, and only the three most important lesions will be considered in this chapter: focal nodular hyperplasia, hepatocellular adenoma, and cavernous hemangioma. Additional childhood tumors are considered at the end of this chapter.

Focal Nodular Hyperplasia and Hepatocellular Adenoma

Focal nodular hyperplasia (FNH) and hepatocellular adenoma (HCA) are benign hepatic neo-

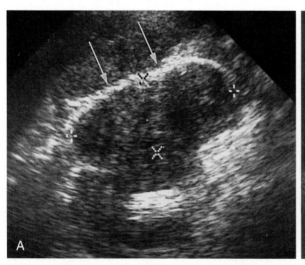
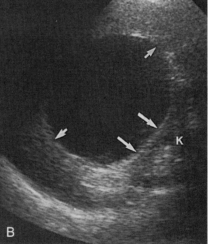

Figure 8-1—Extrahepatic vs. Intrahepatic Location. (A) This extrahepatic mass is separated from the liver by a prominent fat plane (arrows). The bulk of the mass (cursors) is clearly outside the liver. **(B)** This intrahepatic cyst is juxtaposed with the hepatic parenchyma (short arrows), without an intervening fat plane, and the bulk of the mass is intrahepatic. Note that a fat plane (large arrows) separates the cyst and the right kidney.

Table 8-3. Benign Hepatic Neoplasms

Hepatocellular Origin
   Focal nodular hyperplasia
   Hepatocellular adenoma

Cholangiocellular Origin
   Bile duct adenoma
   Bile duct cystadenoma

Blood Vessel Origin
   Cavernous hemangioma
   Infantile hemangioendothelioma

Mesodermal Origin
   Mesenchymal hamartoma

Other
   Fibroma
   Lipoma
   Leiomyoma
   Teratoma
   Adrenal rest
   Pancreatic rest

Based on Ishak KG, Glunz PR: Hepatoblastoma and hepatocellular carcinoma in infancy and childhood. Report of 47 cases. Cancer 20: 396–422, 1967.

plasms that have been encountered more commonly in recent years, in part because of widespread use of ultrasound and CT.[2, 19, 24–28, 44, 45, 51–60] The clinical and pathologic features of FNH and HCA are outlined in Table 8–4. FNH contains all major tissue elements normally occurring in the liver, *including Kupffer cells.* A supporting framework of fibrous tissue is commonly present in FNH, and in some cases there is a distinctive central mass of fibrous tissue, called the "central scar," from which septa radiate toward the periphery of the lesion. HCA, in contrast, is almost totally composed of hepatocytes, with rare fibrous tissue strands and without a consistent supporting framework. Because of these structural differences, intratumor hemorrhage is common in HCA but is rare in FNH.

Intratumor hemorrhage in HCA may be life threatening.

Sonography cannot differentiate between FNH and HCA in most cases, nor may sonography differentiate between these tumors and other solid-appearing hepatic masses. Nonetheless, certain ultrasound findings may suggest the diagnosis of FNH or HCA in the proper clinical setting.[3, 27, 45, 54, 55, 57–60] Both tumors tend to be located in the periphery of the liver, and either may be pedunculated (from the inferior hepatic margin). Both are well-defined and have a smooth border, and both typically are homogeneous. Large tumor size (15 cm or greater) and the visualization of anechoic regions (representing hemorrhagic necrosis) suggest HCA. Much has been made of the detection of the "central scar" of FNH, but this finding is of little value since it is uncommon and is nonspecific. With MRI, a central scar is seen in about 60% of *all* primary hepatic tumors, whether benign or malignant.[3, 27, 54, 57]

When FNH is suspected, the diagnostic procedure of choice is ^{99m}Tc sulfur colloid scintigraphy.[3, 44, 45, 58, 59] Radionuclide uptake equals or exceeds that of normal hepatic parenchyma in approximately 65% of FNH cases, because the tumor contains Kupffer cells that trap sulfur colloid. No other hepatic neoplasm exhibits sulfur colloid uptake. Neither CT nor MRI findings are specific for FNH and HCA.[3, 26, 28]

Cavernous Hemangioma

Cavernous hemangioma[*] is the most common primary hepatic neoplasm. A recent autopsy study revealed an incidence of 20% during the third decade of life,[76] and this tumor has been encountered frequently since the advent of sec-

[*]References 2–4, 19, 24, 25, 27, 29–33, 41–43, 51, 52, 56, and 61–76.

Table 8-4. Clinical and Pathologic Features of Focal Nodular Hyperplasia and Hepatocellular Adenoma

	FNH	HCA
Location	Frequently subcapsular	Frequently subcapsular
Number	Solitary, 80%; two tumors, 14%; >two, 7%	Solitary, 70%; two tumors, 13%; >two, 16%
Size[*]	Usually 4 to 7 cm (maximum reported: 15 cm)	Usually 8 to 15 cm
Histology	Hepatocytes, Kupffer cells, fibrous tissue, and bile ducts. Hemorrhage and necrosis uncommon	Sheets of hepatocytes; rare fibrous tissue septa. Areas of hemorrhage and necrosis common
Gender distribution	86% female. Also occurs in males	Almost exclusively female
Age distribution	Childhood and adulthood	Adulthood only
Symptoms	80% asymptomatic, or vague pain	10% asymptomatic. Symptoms: vague pain, sudden severe discomfort from hemorrhage
Potential for hemorrhage	None	Serious hemorrhage in 23% of cases

[*]At time of clinical diagnosis. Lesions may be smaller when identified incidentally.

tional imaging techniques.[70-72] The tumor develops as a well-defined but nonencapsulated mass of blood-filled chambers. The chambers vary in size but are relatively small in comparison with other angiomatous tumors. Inflow of blood to the tumor is via small, histologically normal arterioles, hence blood flows very slowly, and arteriovenous shunting is not a feature of this tumor. Thrombosis and fibrosis often obliterate the chambers of larger hemangiomas and are thought to be natural processes of tumor aging. Focal calcification also may occur.

Large hemangiomas may cause pain or a palpable mass. Rarely, large lesions may rupture or hemorrhage, causing acute symptoms. Most cavernous hemangiomas detected with imaging procedures are small (less than 5 cm in maximal dimension) and two or more lesions are present in 10% to 61% of cases.[51, 61, 62]

Sonographic Findings. Ninety percent of cavernous hemangiomas[44, 62-67, 71] (Fig. 8–2) are *hyperechoic,* well-defined, and either spherical or ovoid. The remainder may be hypoechoic, lobulated, and/or poorly defined. Approximately 68% of cavernous hemangiomas are homogeneous. The remainder exhibit focal or diffuse heterogeneity that appears to result from thrombosis and subsequent fibrosis of the vascular chambers. A particular diagnostic feature of hemangioma is *enhanced through-transmission* of ultrasound seen in the context of a *hyperechoic* lesion. This combination of findings is seen in 80% of hemangiomas and is said to make other hepatic masses unlikely since hyperechoic lesions typically are strongly attenuating.[62]

Differential Diagnosis of Solitary, Echogenic Masses. The "classic" hemangioma features just described notwithstanding, it is impossible to differentiate between hemangiomas and other hepatic lesions, including malignant neoplasms, with absolute certainty.[63] Hemangiomas can be identified with CT through delayed opacification characteristics, but these features are present in no more than 55% of cases and signify hemangioma with only 75% to 85% reliability.[2, 3, 68, 69] Scintigraphy can also detect the characteristic blood flow pattern of hemangiomas, but only of lesions greater than 3 cm in diameter (unless single photon emission tomography is available).[33, 41-43, 62] MRI appears to be the best technique for identifying hemangiomas. MR signal characteristics suggest hemangioma in approximately 90% of cases, but diagnostic specificity is lower (77% to 90%).[2-4, 19, 24, 33] Hence, some diagnostic uncertainty exists in all cases of apparent hemangioma, and this uncertainty may lead to percutaneous biopsy, which can be carried out safely but with relatively low diagnostic yield.[73-75]

Because of these diagnostic problems, an incidentally discovered echogenic liver lesion can be a significant patient management problem. A conservative approach to such lesions has been advocated by several investigators and now is widely used.[64, 70-72] If the lesion is solitary, echogenic, and less than 3 cm in diameter, and if biochemical tests of hepatic function are normal, then it is reasonable to follow the mass sonographically at 3 months, 6 months, 12 months, and perhaps longer, if desired, from the date of discovery. For larger masses, attempts at definitive diagnosis may be made with CT, MRI, or scintigraphy.

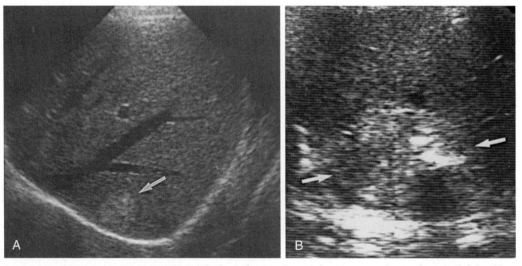

Figure 8–2—Cavernous Hemangioma. (A) Classic features (arrow): homogeneous, hyperechoic, well defined but not encapsulated. **(B)** Variant features (arrows): medium-intensity echogenicity, slight heterogeneity, calcification with shadowing.

An increase in the size of the mass with time, or a change of configuration is an indication for biopsy. If the mass remains stable, then the need for additional follow-up should be reviewed. Gibney and associates[71] followed 68 echogenic lesions in this way for up to 6 years and found that 82% of the lesions did not change, 15% become less distinct or disappeared, 1.5% became smaller, and 1.5% became larger. The results of published series suggest that conservative ultrasound follow-up is a safe method for managing incidentally discovered, echogenic liver lesions.[64, 70–72]

HEPATOCELLULAR CARCINOMA

A variety of malignant primary tumors may arise within the liver (Table 8–5),[56, 77–82] but only hepatocellular carcinoma and cholangiocarcinoma are common in adults. Hepatocellular carcinoma is considered in this section, and cholangiocarcinoma is discussed in Chapter 15.

Epidemiology. Hepatocellular carcinoma (HCC)[56, 77–83] is a frequently fatal malignant neoplasm of hepatocellular origin with peak incidence during the fourth through sixth decades. On a worldwide basis, HCC is one of the most common neoplasms. HCC develops insidiously, and frequently is not diagnosed until the tumor is very large. Survival at 1 year is 21.5% and at 5 years is only 2.4%, regardless of the mode of therapy. Partial hepatectomy may be curative, but only about one fourth of lesions are resectable. Approximately 30% to 60% of hepatocellular carcinomas occur in cirrhotic livers, but HCC also occurs in fibrotic livers without cirrhosis and in normal livers.[56, 77, 78] Exposure to the hepatitis B virus is the most important predisposing factor

in the development of HCC. Numerous other carcinogens also may be causative agents, including alcohol.

Pathology. Four gross pathologic patterns of HCC development have been described, and these govern the sonographic appearance of the tumor.[56, 77, 78] The patterns are (1) solitary, discrete mass, (2) solitary mass with invasion of adjacent hepatic parenchyma, (3) multiple nodules, dispersed widely throughout the liver, and (4) diffuse hepatic infiltration. It is not known whether patterns 3 and 4 result from metastasis or from multicentric origin, but the latter etiology is favored. All hepatomas are primarily composed of small cells that resemble hepatocytes. These cells are organized, to varying degrees, into nonfunctional units resembling hepatic lobules. Large areas of necrosis are uncommon in HCC, and tumor extension into the hepatic or portal veins occurs in about 20% and 30% of cases, respectively.[78]

Sonographic Findings. Roughly 60% to 65% of hepatocellular carcinomas[38, 40, 66, 67, 84–91] (Fig. 8–3) present as homogeneous masses that are more echogenic than surrounding (often cirrhotic) hepatic parenchyma. A sonolucent "halo" or an echogenic rim is seen rarely in these lesions. The remaining 35% to 40% are hypoechoic and/or heterogeneous. The margins of hepatocellular carcinomas may be smooth and clearly defined or irregular and poorly defined.

It appears that tumor size affects the sonographic appearance of HCC. The hyperechoic, heterogeneous, and poorly defined appearance is representative of large tumors. Smaller tumors (3 cm or less) tend to be hypoechoic, homogeneous and better defined.[6, 9, 40] Most HCCs are large at the time of discovery and may replace a sizeable portion, or all, of a hepatic lobe or segment. A solitary lesion is present in 61% of cases, but HCC also may present as multiple, widely separated lesions or as diffuse hepatic infiltration without a focal mass (Fig. 8–3).

Invasion of the portal or hepatic veins (20% and 30% of cases, respectively) is much more common with HCC that with any other hepatic malignancy.[78] Thus, the detection of venous invasion (see Chapter 10) is an important diagnostic clue. Ascites also is present frequently in patients with HCC, and rapid development of ascites may be a presenting feature. Diagnostically, the importance of ascites is tempered by the fact that most patients with hepatoma have cirrhosis, and therefore ample reason to have ascites.

The Problem of Regenerative Nodules. The sonographic differential diagnosis for HCC includes other primary hepatic neoplasms, metastases, inflammatory lesions, and regenerative

Table 8-5. Malignant Hepatic Neoplasms

Primary Neoplasms
Hepatocellular origin
Hepatocellular carcinoma
Hepatoblastoma
Biliary origin
Cholangiocarcinoma
Cystadenocarcinoma
Mesodermal origin
Angiosarcoma
Sarcoma
Secondary Neoplasms
Metastasis
Lymphoma
Leukemia

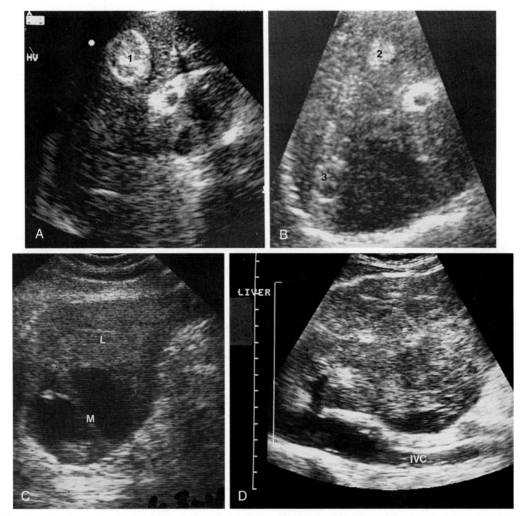

Figure 8-3—Sonographic Patterns of Hepatocellular Carcinoma. (A, B) Multifocal, hyperechoic (three lesions are present, labeled 1 to 3). The posterior hypoechoic region is edema caused by hepatic vein thrombosis. **(C)** Hypoechoic, homogeneous. M = tumor; L = left lobe. **(D)** Massive, heterogeneous, and infiltrating. This longitudinal scan shows tumor replacement of the entire left and caudate lobes. Note mass effect on the inferior vena cava (IVC).

nodules of cirrhosis. In no cases are the sonographic findings sufficient to differentiate among these etiologies. It is particularly noteworthy that small, hypoechoic hepatocellular carcinomas cannot be distinguished from regenerative nodules and hyperplastic adenomatous nodules, both of which may be present in cirrhotic livers. *Regenerative nodules are rarely identified with ultrasound*[40, 92, 93]; therefore, any discrete lesion seen in a cirrhotic liver should be assumed malignant until proved otherwise.

Surveillance for HCC. The only hope of survival for patients with HCC is early diagnosis (particularly of tumors less than 4 or 5 cm in diameter), followed by surgical resection of the affected segment(s); therefore, a mechanism of HCC surveillance is desirable in *selected* patients

with cirrhosis and hepatic fibrosis.* Surveillance probably is not warranted, however, in patients with micronodular (alcohol-related) cirrhosis, since this is a common disorder with a relatively low incidence of HCC (2% to 10%).[56, 78] HCC surveillance is more clearly warranted in patients with posthepatitic, macronodular cirrhosis in whom the estimated incidence of HCC ranges from 10% to 50%.[67, 78]

Alpha-fetoprotein (AFP) is a biochemical marker that may be used for hepatoma surveillance.[8, 78, 82, 83, 94, 95] This marker is highly specific for HCC but is relatively insensitive (29% to 89%). Sonography, CT, and MRI also may be used for HCC surveillance, but each of these

*References 2–5, 24, 25, 27, 29–33, 38–40, 65, 66, 78–81, 84, 85, 91, 94, and 95.

modalities has limitations, as indicated earlier. Ultrasound is not generally recommended as a method of HCC surveillance in inhabitants of western countries, since the detection rate of hepatic masses is relatively low.

HEPATIC METASTASIS

Five sonographic patterns have been described for hepatic metastases[44, 52, 84, 88, 90, 96–105] (Fig. 8–4): (1) discrete, anechoic masses; (2) discrete, hypoechoic masses; (3) discrete, hyperechoic masses; (4) discrete target lesions; and (5) diffuse nonhomogeneity of the hepatic parenchyma. Hypoechoic lesions predominate, but the incidence of each pattern is unknown with respect to current, highly sensitive ultrasound instruments.[88, 96, 97] The pattern of metastasis, unfortunately, is not specific and does not effectively identify the source of metastatic lesions.

Echo Level

The relationship of metastasis echogenicity and histology has been investigated. Echogenicity increases in direct proportion to collagen content, microvascularity, calcification, and tissue heterogeneity. Echogenicity decreases in relation to tissue homogeneity and necrosis.[102, 103] Metastases with very homogeneous histology, such as lymphoma, may be only faintly echoic. Metastases may be truly anechoic if the lesion is principally composed of liquefied material, but a rim of solid tissue typically is visible at the periphery of the tumor.[52, 97, 99–103]

Calcified Metastases

Strong echogenicity in metastatic lesions usually is imparted by diffuse calcification.[52, 98] In most cases, the calcium deposits are microscopic and are not visible as discrete structures, but these tiny particles may dramatically increase echogenicity (Fig. 8–4C). Calcified metastases may or may not cast acoustic shadows, depending on the calcium concentration. Diffusely calcified metastases call to mind gastrointestinal tumors (especially colon and gastric carcinoma), thyroid carcinoma, and malignant carcinoid.

Large, "macroscopic" calcification also may occur in hepatic metastases, either spontaneously or in response to chemotherapy or x-ray therapy. These relatively large calcifications are nonspecific and generate *focal* bright echoes within the lesion, possibly accompanied by acoustic shadows.

Target Metastases

Approximately 13% of hepatic metastases exhibit a target appearance. The center of the target may be hypoechoic and the periphery hyperechoic, or vice versa. The target pattern may be generated in three ways.[88, 96, 97, 101] First, liquefactive or non-liquefactive necrosis produces a central anechoic or hypoechoic zone surrounded by more echogenic solid tissue. Second, compression of surrounding normal hepatic parenchyma produces peripheral sonolucency. Third, for unknown reasons, tumor echogenicity varies from the periphery to the center of lesions, producing an echogenic center and sonolucent periphery, or vice versa.

Diffuse Metastasis

Diffuse hepatic metastasis may be manifested solely by nonhomogeneity of hepatic parenchyma (Fig. 8–4F), usually accompanied by hepatomegaly. This nonhomogeneous appearance may be very subtle and may require considerable scrutiny for detection. A nonhomogeneous appearance may occur with neoplasms that infiltrate the hepatic structure, or with tumors that "pepper" the liver with a multitude of tiny metastases.

LYMPHOMA

Hepatic involvement with Hodgkin and non-Hodgkin lymphoma is detected at staging in 15% and 25% of cases, respectively. Hepatic involvement by either of these neoplasms is found at autopsy in 50% of cases.[106, 107] It is clear that ultrasound usually fails to detect these neoplasms, as hepatic abnormality (other than hepatomegaly) is identified in only 5.2% of lymphoma patients.[108]

When lymphoma is detected sonographically,[108–111] the most common pattern (43% of positive cases) is discrete, homogeneous, hypoechoic masses. The next most common pattern (35% of positive cases) is diffuse nonhomogeneity of the hepatic architecture, which results from pervasive lymphomatous infiltration. The remainder of positive findings (9%) are hyperechoic or target lesions, which are seen only in cases of non-Hodgkin lymphoma. Hepatic nodules in lymphoma patients usually are multiple, and the liver usually is enlarged.[108, 109] Concurrent splenic involvement is invariably present.[107]

HEPATIC MASSES IN INFANCY AND CHILDHOOD

Primary hepatic neoplasms[110–130] constitute 15% of abdominal tumors in the pediatric age

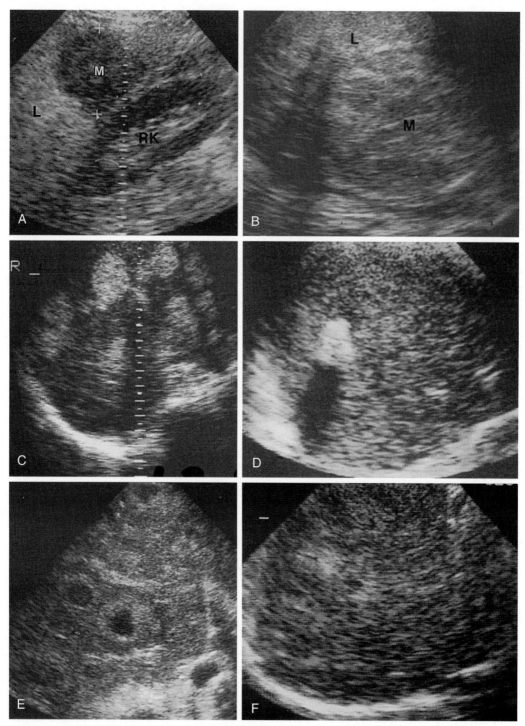

Figure 8-4—Sonographic Patterns of Hepatic Metastases. (**A**) Hypoechoic, homogeneous, well defined. M = metastasis; L = liver; RK = right kidney. (**B**) Isoechoic, heterogeneous. M = metastasis; L = liver. (**C**) Strongly echogenic. (**D**) Echogenic with shadow. (**E**) Target. (**F**) Diffuse heterogeneity—note subtle alteration of the hepatic "texture" caused by innumerable hypoechoic metastases in this longitudinal view of the right lobe. No vessels are visible.

group. Approximately two thirds of these tumors are malignant and one third are benign.[113] Sonography is an expedient method for diagnosis of pediatric abdominal masses, and it should be employed early to direct the diagnostic process properly. The differential considerations for hepatic masses of infancy and childhood are presented in Table 8–6.[113, 114, 116, 118, 120, 125, 128, 130] Many of these lesions have sonographic features identical to their adult counterparts, which are considered elsewhere in this or other chapters. In this section, we will consider only four of these neoplasms: hepatoblastoma, hepatocellular carcinoma, infantile hemangioendothelioma, and mesenchymal hamartoma. These tumors are singled out either because they are relatively common or because they have distinctive sonographic features.

Hepatoblastoma and Hepatocellular Carcinoma

Taken together, hepatoblastoma and hepatocellular carcinoma (HCC)[114–117, 120–122, 125] constitute the third most common form of abdominal neoplasia in pediatric patients, after neuroblastoma and Wilms tumor. Hepatoblastoma is an embryonal neoplasm that presents exclusively during the *first two years* of life. Pediatric HCC is identical histologically with adult HCC and virtually always presents at or beyond 5 *years of*

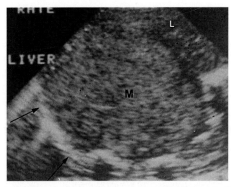

Figure 8–5—Hepatoblastoma. This 18 month old patient presented with an abdominal mass (hepatomegaly). The right lobe of the liver (L) contains a homogeneous, hyperechoic mass (M) that abuts the diaphragm (arrows). The mass is about 7 cm in its largest dimension.

age. No predisposing factors, such as cirrhosis, have been detected for pediatric hepatoblastoma or HCC.

As seen with ultrasound, hepatoblastoma (Fig. 8–5) most commonly is a hyperechoic, rounded or lobulated mass that frequently exhibits a heterogeneous echo texture, due to calcification and/or liquefactive necrosis. HCC usually presents as a well-defined, hyperechoic mass similar to adult HCC. A range of sonographic appearances is possible, however, with both these tumors. Hepatic and/or portal venous invasion occurs commonly with both lesions. Venous invasion is an important finding, since it confirms the malignant nature of the lesion and may affect resectability.

Infantile Hemangioendothelioma

Infantile hemangioendothelioma[110, 111, 114, 117, 122–127] is a benign but aggressive tumor of blood vessel origin that occurs in fetal life and infancy. The mass consists of vascular spaces of various sizes, supported by a fibrous stromal network. The tumor may be localized or may extend throughout the liver. The striking diagnostic feature of this neoplasm is arteriovenous shunting, which varies in degree from case to case. If the shunt is large, it causes high-output congestive heart failure. Infantile hemangioendothelioma regresses spontaneously over a period of months and leaves no sequelae; hence, treatment generally is confined to supportive measures. In some cases, however, death results from high-output heart failure. Consumptive coagulopathy and hepatic dysfunction are other causes of death.[123, 125]

Infantile hemangioendothelioma is characterized by the following findings: (1) sonolucency predominates, although the mass is mixed in

Table 8–6. Hepatic Masses in Children

Cysts
    Idiopathic congenital cysts
    Choledochal cysts
    Caroli disease

Infectious Diseases and Parasites
    Pyogenic abscesses
    Amebic abscesses
    Fungal and granulomatous lesions
    Hydatid cyst

Neoplasms
    Cavernous hemangioma
    Focal nodular hyperplasia
    Liver cell adenoma
    Hepatoblastoma
    Hepatocellular carcinoma
    Sarcomas
    Hemangioendothelioma
    Mesenchymal hamartoma
    Metastases

Traumatic Lesions
    Focal necrosis
    Hematoma

Adapted from Jabra AA, Fishman EK, Taylor GA: Hepatic masses in infants and children: CT evaluation. AJR Am J Roentgenol 158: 143–149, 1992.

echogenicity; (2) various-sized fluid-filled chambers are present; (3) Doppler examination reveals blood flow in the vascular chambers; and (4) secondary effects of arteriovenous shunting are evident, including dilatation of the heart, hepatic veins, and inferior vena cava, and Doppler evidence of high-volume flow in abdominal vessels.[110, 111, 117, 122, 124, 126, 127] Scintigraphy with [99mTc]-labeled red blood cells may be diagnostic.

Mesenchymal Hamartoma

The rare hepatic tumor called mesenchymal hamartoma[110, 111, 113, 114, 117, 124, 128–130] usually presents during the first year of life as a large, asymptomatic epigastric mass. Histologically, the mass is composed of mesenchyme and bile ducts, with *abundant* pseudocyst formation. The presence of these pseudocysts imparts a characteristic multilocular, cystic configuration. The mass may be so large that hepatic origin cannot be confirmed, and in such cases, the differential diagnosis includes other large cystic neoplasms.[128–130]

REFERENCES

1. Adson MA: Hepatic metastases in perspective. AJR Am J Roentgenol 140:695–700, 1983.
2. Ferrucci JT: Liver tumor imaging: Current concepts. AJR Am J Roentgenol 155:473–484, 1990.
3. Thoeni RF: Clinical applications of magnetic resonance imaging of the liver. Invest Radiol 3:266–273, 1991.
4. Reinig JW: Differentiation of hepatic lesions with MR imaging: The last word? Radiology 179:601–602, 1991.
5. Kanematsu T, Sonoda T, Takenaka K, et al: The value of ultrasound in the diagnosis and treatment of small hepatocellular carcinoma. Br J Surg 72:23–25, 1985.
6. Hayashi N, Yamamoto K, Tamaki N, Shibata T, Itoh K, Fujisawa I, Nakano Y, Yamaoka Y, Kobayashi N, Mori K, Ozawa K, Torizuka K: Metastatic nodules of hepatocellular carcinoma: Detection with angiography, CT, and US. Radiology 165:61–63, 1987.
7. Yoshimatsu S, Inoue Y, Ibukuro K, Suzuki S: Hypovascular hepatocellular carcinoma undetected at angiography and CT with iodized oil. Radiology 171:343–347, 1989.
8. Takayasu K, Moriyama N, Muramatsu Y, Makuuchi M, Hasegawa H, Okazaki N, Hirohashi S: The diagnosis of small hepatocellular carcinomas: Efficacy of various imaging procedures in 100 patients. AJR Am J Roentgenol 155:49–54, 1990.
9. Shibata T, Kubo S, Itoh K, Sagoh T, Nishimura K, Nakano Y, Yamaoka Y, Ozawa K, Konishi J: Recurrent hepatocellular carcinoma: Usefulness of ultrasonography compared with computed tomography and AFP assay. J Clin Ultrasound 19:463–469, 1991.
10. Miller WJ, Federle MP, Campbell WL: Diagnosis and staging of hepatocellular carcinoma: Comparison of CT and sonography in 36 liver transplantation patients. AJR Am J Roentgenol 157:303–306, 1991.
11. Alderson PO, Adams DF, McNeil BJ, et al: Computed tomography, ultrasonography, and scintigraphy of the liver in patients with breast carcinoma: A prospective comparison. Radiology 149:225–230, 1983.
12. Schölmerich J, Volk BA, Neuer J, et al: Aussagefähigkeit der Sonographie bei Lebermetastasen. Dtsch Med Wschr 109:326–329, 1984.
13. Suramo I, Paivansalo M, Pamilo M: Unidentified liver metastases at ultrasonography or computed tomography. Acta Radiol Diagn 25:385–389, 1984.
14. Wernecke K, Rummeny E, Bongartz G, Vassallo P, Kivelitz D, Wiesmann W, Peters PE, Reers B, Reiser M, Pircher W: Detection of hepatic masses in patients with carcinoma: Comparative sensitivities of sonography, CT, and MR imaging. AJR Am J Roentgenol 157:731–739, 1991.
15. Tanaka S, Kitamura T, Fujita M, Nakanishi K, Okuda S: Color Doppler flow imaging of liver tumors. AJR Am J Roentgenol 154:509–514, 1990.
16. Tanaka S, Kitamura T, Fujita M, Kasugai H, Inoue A, Ishiguro S: Small hepatocellular carcinoma: Differentiation from adenomatous hyperplastic nodule with color Doppler flow imaging. Radiology 182:161–165, 1992.
17. Shimamoto K, Sakuma S, Ishigaki T, Ishiguchi T, Itoh S, Fukatsu H: Hepatocellular carcinoma: Evaluation with color Doppler US and MR imaging. Radiology 182:149–153, 1992.
18. Dock W, Grabenwöger F, Metz V, Eibenberger K, Farrés MT: Tumor vascularization: Assessment with duplex sonography. Radiology 181:241–244, 1991.
19. Stark DD, Wittenberg J, Butch RJ, Ferrucci JT: Hepatic metastases: Randomized, controlled comparison of detection with MR imaging and CT. Radiology 165:399–406, 1987.
20. Reinig JW, Dwyer AJ, Miller DL, White M, Frank JA, Sugarbaker PH, Chang AE, Doppman JL: Liver metastasis detection: Comparative sensitivities of MR imaging and CT scanning. Radiology 162:43–47, 1987.
21. Itoh K, Nishimura K, Tagashi K, Fujisawa I, Noma S, Minami S, Sagoh T, Nakano Y, Itoh H, Mori K, Ozawa K, Torizuka K: Hepatocellular carcinoma: MR imaging. Radiology 164:21–25, 1987.
22. Freeny PC, Marks WM, Ryan JA, et al: Colorectal carcinoma evaluation with CT: Preoperative staging and detection of postoperative recurrence. Radiology 158:347–353, 1968.
23. Freeny PC, Baron RL, Teefey SA: Hepatocellular carcinoma: Reduced frequency of typical findings with dynamic contrast-enhanced CT in a non-Asian population. Radiology 182:143–149, 1992.
24. Brown JJ, Lee JM, Lee JKT, Van Lom KJ, Malchow SC: Focal hepatic lesions: Differentiation with MR imaging at 0.5T. Radiology 179:675–679, 1991.
25. Rummeny E, Weissleder R, Stark DD, Saini S, Compton CC, Bennett W, Hahn PF, Wittenberg J, Malt RA, Ferrucci JT: Primary liver tumors: Diagnosis by MR imaging. AJR Am J Roentgenol 152:63–72, 1989.
26. Mattison GR, Glazer GM, Quint LE, Francis IR, Bree RL, Ensminger WD: MR imaging of hepatic focal nodular hyperplasia: Characterization and distinction from primary malignant hepatic tumors. AJR AM J Roentgenol 148:711–715, 1987.
27. Rummeny E, Weissleder R, Sironi S, Start DD,

Compton CC, Hahn PF, Saini S, Wittenberg J, Ferrucci JT: Central scars in primary liver tumors: MR features, specificity, and pathologic correlation. Radiology 171:323–326, 1989.

28. Lee MJ, Saini S, Hamm B, Taupitz M, Hahn PF, Seneterre E, Ferrucci JT: Focal nodular hyperplasia of the liver: MR findings in 35 proved cases. AJR Am J Roentgenol 156:317–320, 1991.

29. Li KC, Glazer GM, Quint LE, Francis IR, Aisen AM, Ensminger WD, Bookstein FL: Distinction of hepatic cavernous hemangioma from hepatic metastases with MR imaging. Radiology 169:409–415, 1988.

30. Ohtomo K, Itai Y, Yoshida H, Kokubo T, Yoshikawa K, Lio M: MR differentiation of hepatocellular carcinoma from cavernous hemangioma: Complementary roles of FLASH and T2 values. AJR Am J Roentgenol 152:505–507, 1989.

31. Yoshida H, Itai Y, Ohtomo K, Kokubo T, Minami M, Yashiro N: Small hepatocellular carcinoma and cavernous hemangioma: Differentiation with dynamic FLASH MR imaging with Gd-DTPA. Radiology 171:339–342, 1989.

32. Itoh K, Saini S, Hahn PF, Imam N, Ferrucci JT: Differentiation between small hepatic hemangiomas and metastases on MR images: Importance of size-specific quantitative criteria. AJR Am J Roentgenol 155:61–66, 1990.

33. Birnbaum BA, Weinreb JF, Megibow AJ, Sanger JJ, Lubat E, Kanamuller H, Noz ME, Bosniak MA: Definitive diagnosis of hepatic hemangiomas: MR imaging versus Tc-99m-labeled red blood cell SPECT. Radiology 176:95–101, 1990.

34. Rummeny E, Saini S, Stark DD, Weissleder R, Compton CC, Ferrucci JT: Detection of hepatic metastases with MR imaging: Spin-echo vs. phase-contrast pulse sequences at 0.6T. AJR Am J Radiol 153:1207–1211, 1989.

35. Snow JH, Goldstein HM, Wallace S: Comparison of scintigraphy, sonography, and computed tomography in the evaluation of hepatic neoplasms. AJR Am J Roentgenol 132:915–918, 1979.

36. Smith TJ, Kemeny MM, Sugarbaker PH, et al: A prospective study of hepatic imaging in the detection of metastatic disease. Ann Surg 195:486–491, 1982.

37. Bondestam S, Lahde S, Annala R, et al: Scintigraphy and sonography in the investigation of liver metastases. Diagn Imag 49:339–342, 1980.

38. Broderick TW, Gosink B, Menuk L, et al: Echographic and radionuclide detection of hepatoma. Radiology 135:149–151, 1980.

39. Takashima T, Osamu M, Suzuki M: Diagnosis and screening of small hepatocellular carcinomas. Radiology 145:635–638, 1982.

40. Maringhini A, Cottone M, Sciarrino E, et al: Ultrasonographic and radionuclide detection of hepatocellular carcinoma in cirrhotics with low alpha-fetoprotein levels. Cancer 54:2924–2926, 1984.

41. Wiener SN, Parulekar SG: Scintigraphy and sonography of hepatic hemangioma. Radiology 132:149–153, 1979.

42. Front D, Royal HD, Israel O: Scintigraphy of hepatic hemangiomas: The value of Tc-99m-labeled red blood cells: Concise communication. J Nucl Med 22:684–687, 1981.

43. Moinuddin M, Allison JR, Montgomery JH, et al: Scintigraphic diagnosis of hepatic hemangioma: Its role in the management of hepatic mass lesions. AJR Am J Roentgenol 145:223–228, 1985.

44. Rogers JV, Mack LA, Freeny PC, et al: Hepatic focal nodular hyperplasia: Angiography, CT, sonography, and scintigraphy. AJR Am J Roentgenol 137:983–990, 1981.

45. Casarella WJ, Knowles DM, Wolff M, et al: Focal nodular hyperplasia and liver cell adenoma: Radiologic and pathologic differentiation. AJR Am J Roentgenol 131:393–402, 1978.

46. Kudo M, Tomita S, Tochio H, Mimura J, Okabe Y, Kashida H, Hirasa M, Ibuki Y, Todo A: Small hepatocellular carcinoma: Diagnosis with US angiography with intraarterial CO_2 microbubbles. Radiology 182:155–160, 1992.

47. Sumida M, Ohto M, Ebara M, Kimura K, Okuda K, Hirooka N: Accuracy of angiography in the diagnosis of small hepatocellular carcinoma. AJR Am J Roentgenol 147:531–536, 1986.

48. Takayasu K, Shima Y, Muramatsu Y, Goto H, Moriyama N, Yamada T, Makuuchi M, Yamasaki S, Hasegawa H, Okazaki N, Hirohashi S, Kishi K: Angiography of small hepatocellular carcinomas: Analysis of 105 resected tumors. AJR Am J Roentgenol 147:525–529, 1986.

49. Takahashi K, Saito K, Tamura K, Honda M, Touei K, Sakai O, Kawashima Y, Kuji T, Ohtani M, Kawamoto T, Ohsawa T: Hepatic neoplasms: Detection with hepatoportal subtraction angiography—a new technique of DSA. Radiology 177:243–248, 1990.

50. Graif M, Manor A, Itzchak Y: Sonographic differentiation of extra- and intrahepatic masses. AJR Am J Roentgenol 141:553–556, 1983.

51. Ishak KG, Rabin L: Benign tumors of the liver. Med Clin North Am 59:995–1013, 1975.

52. Edmondson HA, Peters RL: Tumors of the liver: Pathologic features. Semin Roentgenol 18:75–83, 1983.

53. Scott LD, Katz AR, Duke JH, et al: Oral contraceptives, pregnancy, and focal nodular hyperplasia of the liver. JAMA 251:1461–1463, 1984.

54. Bowerman RA, Samuels BI, Silver TM: Ultrasonographic features of hepatic adenomas in type I glycogen storage disease. J Ultrasound Med 2:51–54, 1983.

55. Crossman H, Ram PC, Colemal RA, et al: Hepatic ultrasonography in type I glycogen storage disease (von Gierke disease). Detection of hepatic adenoma and carcinoma. Radiology 141:752–756, 1981.

56. Oberfield RA, Steele G, Gollan JL, Sherman D: Liver cancer. Cancer J Clinicians 39:206–218, 1989.

57. Scatarige JC, Fishman EK, Sanders RC: The sonographic "scar sign" in focal nodular hyperplasia of the liver. J Ultrasound Med 1:275–278, 1982.

58. Sandlerm MA, Petrocelli RD, Marks DS, et al: Ultrasonic features and radionuclide correlation in liver cell adenoma and focal nodular hyperplasia. Radiology 135:393–397, 1980.

59. Majewski A, Geastz KF, Brölsch C, et al: Sonographic pattern of focal nodular hyperplasia of the liver. Eur J Radiol 4:52–57, 1984.

60. Bruneton JN, Mathieu D, Drouillard J, et al: Diagnostic ultrasound of adenoma and nodular hyperplasia of the liver. Presented at the AIUM/SDMS Annual Convention, Dallas, Oct 8–11, 1985.

61. Ochsner JL, Halpert B: Cavernous hemangioma of the liver. Surgery 43:577–582, 1958.

62. Taboury J, Porcel A, Tubiana JM, et al: Cavernous hemangiomas of the liver studied by ultrasound. Radiology 149:781–785, 1983.
63. Freeny PC, Vimont TR, Barnett DC: Cavernous hemangioma of the liver: Ultrasonography, arteriography and computed tomography. Radiology 132:143–148, 1979.
64. Bruneton JN, Drouillard J, Fenart D, et al: Ultrasonography of hepatic cavernous hemangiomas. Br J Radiol 56:791–795, 1983.
65. Itai Y, Ohtomo K, Araki T, et al: Computed tomography and sonography of cavernous hemangioma of the liver. AJR Am J Roentgenol 141:315–320, 1983.
66. Onodera H, Ohta K, Oikawa M, et al: Correlation of real time sonographic appearance of hepatic hemangiomas with angiography. J Clin Ultrasound 11:421–425, 1983.
67. Sheu JC, Sung JL, Chen DS, et al: Ultrasonography of small hepatocellular tumors using high-resolution linear-array real-time instruments. Radiology 150:797–802, 1984.
68. Johnson CM, Sheedy PF, Stanson AW, et al: Computed tomography and angiography of cavernous hemangiomas of the liver. Radiology 138:115–121, 1981.
69. Barnett PH, Zerhouni EA, White RI, et al: Computed tomography of the diagnosis of cavernous hemangioma of the liver. AJR Am J Roentgenol 134:439–447, 1980.
70. Bruneton JN: Solitary hyperechoic hepatic nodules smaller than 3 cm diameter. Diagnostic procedure. JEMU (Paris) 6:47–48, 1985.
71. Gibney RG, Hendin AP, Cooperberg PL: Sonographically detected hepatic hemangiomas: Absence of change over time. AJR Am J Roentgenol 149:953–957, 1987.
72. Bree RL, Schwab RE, Reiman HL: Solitary echogenic spot in the liver: Is it diagnostic of a hemangioma? AJR Am J Roentgenol 104:41–45, 1983.
73. Cronan JJ, Esparza AR, Dorfman GS, Ridlen MS, Paolella LP: Cavernous hemangioma of the liver: Role of percutaneous biopsy. Radiology 166:135–138, 1988.
74. Solbiati L, Livraghi T, DePra L, et al: Fine-needle biopsy of hepatic hemangioma with sonographic guidance. AJR Am J Roentgenol 144:471–474, 1985.
75. van Sonnenberg E, Wittenberg J, Ferrucci JT, et al: Triangulation method for percutaneous needle guidance: The angled approach to upper abdominal masses. AJR Am J Roentgenol 137:757–761, 1981.
76. Karhunen PJ: Benign hepatic tumors and tumor-like conditions in men. J Clin Pathol 39:183–188, 1986.
77. Ruebner BH, Montgomery CK: Pathology of the Liver and Biliary Tract. New York, John Wiley & Sons, 1982, pp 245–252.
78. Okuda K, Peters RL (eds): Hepatocellular Carcinoma. New York, John Wiley & Sons, 1976, pp 387–436.
79. Okuda K, Liver Cancer Study Group of Japan: Primary liver cancer in Japan. Cancer 45:2663–2669, 1980.
80. Lim RC, Bongard FS: Hepatocellular carcinoma: Changing concepts in diagnosis and management. Arch Surg 119:637–642, 1984.
81. Tsuzuki T, Ogata Y, Iida S, et al: Hepatic resection in 125 patients. Arch Surg 119:1025–1032, 1984.
82. Wands JR, Blum HE: Primary hepatocellular carcinoma. N Engl J Med 325:729–731, 1991.
83. Colombo M, de Franchis R, Del Ninno E, Sangiovanni A, de Fazio C, Tommasini M, Donato MF, Piva A, di Carlo V, Dioguardi N: Hepatocellular carcinoma in Italian patients with cirrhosis. N Engl J Med 325:675–680, 1991.
84. Kawisaki M, Sakaguchi S, Irisa T, et al: Value of B-scan ultrasonography in the diagnosis of liver cancer. Am J Gastroenterol 69:436–442, 1978.
85. Cottone M, Marceno MP, Maringhini A: Ultrasound in the diagnosis of hepatocellular carcinoma associated with cirrhosis. Radiology 147:517–519, 1983.
86. Tanaka S, Tsugio K, Shingi I, et al: Hepatocellular carcinoma: Sonographic and histological correlation. AJR Am J Roentgenol 140:701–707, 1983.
87. Boultbee JF: Grey scale ultrasound appearance of hepatocellular carcinoma. Clin Radiol 30:547–552, 1979.
88. Green B, Bree RL, Goldstein HM, Stanley C: Gray scale ultrasound evaluation of hepatic neoplasms: Patterns and correlations. Radiology 124:203–208, 1977.
89. Kamin PD, Bernadion ME, Green B: Ultrasound manifestations of hepatocellular carcinoma. Radiology 131:459–461, 1979.
90. Raylor KJW, Richman TS: Diseases of the liver. Semin Roentgenol 18:94–101, 1983.
91. Dubbins PA, O'Riordan D, Melia WM: Ultrasound in hepatoma—can a specific diagnosis be made? Br J Radiol 54:307–311, 1981.
92. Freeman MP, Vick CW, Taylor KJW, et al: Regenerative nodules in cirrhosis: Sonographic appearance with anatomic correlation. AJR Am J Radiol 146:533–536, 1986.
93. Giorgio A, Francica G, de Stefano G, et al: Sonographic recognition of intraparenchymal regenerating nodules using high-frequency transducers in patients with cirrhosis. J Ultrasound Med 10:355–359, 1991.
94. Okazaki N, Yoshida T, Yoshino M, et al: Screening of patients with chronic liver disease for hepatocellular carcinoma by ultrasonography. Clin Oncol 10:241–246, 1984.
95. Shinagawa T, Ohto M, Kimura K, et al: Diagnosis and clinical features of small hepatocellular carcinoma with emphasis on the utility of real-time ultrasonography. Gastroenterology 86:495–502, 1984.
96. Hillman BJ, Smith EH, Gammelgaard J, et al: Ultrasonographic-pathologic correlation of malignant hepatic masses. Gastrointest Radiol 4:361–365, 1979.
97. Scheible W, Gosink BB, Leopold GR: Gray scale echographic patterns of metastatic disease. AJR Am J Roentgenol 129:983–987, 1977.
98. Katragadda CS, Goldstein HM, Green B: Gray scale ultrasound of calcified liver metastases. AJR Am J Roentgenol 129:591–593, 1977.
99. Bree RL, Green B: The gray scale appearance of intra-abdominal mesenchymal sarcomas. Radiology 128:193–197, 1978.
100. Federle MP, Filly RA, Moss AA: Cystic hepatic neoplasms: Complementary roles of CT and sonography. AJR Am J Roentgenol 136:345–348, 1981.
101. Wooten WB, Green B, Goldstein HM: Ultrasonography of necrotic hepatic metastases. Radiology 128:447–450, 1978.

102. Marchal GJ, Plyser K, Tshibwabwa-Tumba EA, et al: Anechoic halo in solid liver tumors: Sonographic, microangiographic, and histologic correlation. Radiology 156:479–483, 1985.

103. Marchal G, Tshibwabwa-Tumba E, Oyen R, et al: Correlation of sonographic patterns in liver metastasis with histology and microangiography. Invest Radiol 22:79–84, 1985.

104. Paling MR, Shawker TH, Love IL: The sonographic appearance of metastatic malignant melanoma. J Ultrasound Med 1:75–78, 1982.

105. Stutte H, Müller PH, d'Hoedt B, Stroebel W: Ultrasonographic diagnosis of melanoma metastases in liver, gallbladder, and spleen. J Ultrasound Med 8:541–547, 1989.

106. Bragg DG, Colby TV, Ward JH: New concepts in non-Hodgkin's lymphoma: Radiologic implications. Radiology 159:298–304, 1968.

107. Castellino RA: Hodgkin's disease: Practical concepts for the diagnostic radiologist. Radiology 159:305–310, 1986.

108. Ginaldi S, Bernardini ME, Jing BS, et al: Ultrasonographic patterns of hepatic lymphoma. Radiology 136:427–431, 1980.

109. Honda H, Franken EA, Barloon TJ, Smith JL: Hepatic lymphoma in cyclosporine-treated transplant recipients: Sonographic and CT findings. AJR Am J Roentgenol 152:501–503, 1989.

110. Miller JH, Greenspan BS: Integrated imaging of hepatic tumors in childhood. Part I: Malignant lesions (primary and metastatic). Radiology 154:83–90, 1985.

111. Miller JH, Greenspan BS: Integrated imaging of hepatic tumors in childhood. Part II: Benign lesions (congenital, reparative, and inflammatory). Radiology 154:91–100, 1985.

112. Macpherson RE, Saldana JA, Cone RM, et al: Primary liver masses in infants. J Can Assoc Radiol 32:81–87, 1981.

113. de Lorimer AA: Hepatic tumors of infancy and childhood. Surg Clin North Am 57:443–448, 1977.

114. Jabra AA, Fishman EK, Taylor GA: Hepatic masses in infants and children: CT evaluation. AJR Am J Roentgenol 158:143–149, 1992.

115. Brunelle F, Chaumont P: Hepatic tumors in children: Ultrasonic differentiation of malignant from benign lesions. Radiology 150:695–699, 1984.

116. Dachman AH, Lichtenstein JE, Friedman AC, et al: Infantile hemangioendothelioma of the liver: A radiologic-pathologic-clinical correlation. AJR Am J Roentgenol 140:1091–1096, 1983.

117. Miller JH, Gates GF, Stanley P: The radiologic investigation of hepatic tumors in childhood: Radiology 124:451–458, 1977.

118. Clatworthy HW, Schiller M, Grossfield JL: Primary liver tumors in infancy and childhood. Arch Surg 109:143–147, 1974.

119. Madigan SM, Teele RL: Ultrasonography of the liver and biliary tree in children. Semin Ultrasound CT MRI 5:68–84, 1984.

120. Ishak KG, Glunz PR: Hepatoblastoma and hepatocellular carcinoma in infancy and childhood. Report of 47 cases. Cancer 20:396–422, 1967.

121. Diament MJ, Parvey LS, Tonkin ILD, et al: Hepatoblastoma: Technetium sulfur colloid uptake simulating focal nodular hyperplasia. AJR Am J Roentgenol 139:168–171, 1982.

122. Korobkin M, Kirks D, Sullavin DC, et al: Computed tomography of primary liver tumors in children. Radiology 139:431–435, 1981.

123. Burrows PE, Rossemberg HC, Chuang HS: Diffuse hepatic hemangiomas: Percutaneous transcatheter embolization with detachable silicone balloons. Radiology 156:85–88, 1985.

124. Kaude JV, Felman AH, Hawkins IF: Ultrasonography in primary hepatic tumors in early childhood. Pediatr Radiol 9:77–83, 1982.

125. Dachman AH, Pakter RL, Ros PR, Fishman EK, Goodman ZD, Lichtenstein JE: Hepatoblastoma: Radiologic-pathologic correlation in 50 cases. Radiology 164:15–19, 1987.

126. Rumack CM, Saunders EL, Manco-Johnson ML: Ultrasound of hemangiomas. Presented at the AIUM/SDMS Annual Convention, Dallas, Oct 8–11, 1985.

127. Abramson SJ, Lack EE, Teele RL: Benign vascular tumors of the liver in infants: Sonographic appearance. AJR Am J Roentgenol 138:629–632, 1982.

128. Rosenbaum DM, Mindell HJ: Ultrasonographic findings in mesenchymal hamartoma of the liver. Radiology 138:425–427, 1981.

129. Foucar E, Williamson RA, Yiu-Chiu V, et al: Mesenchymal hamartoma of the liver identified by fetal sonography. AJR Am J Roentgenol 140:970–972, 1983.

130. Ros PR, Goodman ZD, Ishak KG, et al: Mesenchymal hamartoma of the liver: Radiologic-pathologic correlation. Radiology 158:619–624, 1986.

Chapter 9

Diffuse Liver Disease

William J. Zwiebel

TEXTURE AND SPECKLE

It is common to refer to tissue "texture" in describing the ultrasound features of solid organs. For example, the texture of the pancreas is described as "coarse" compared with the liver. It is important to realize, however, that the tiny "dots" that constitute soft tissue texture do not actually represent discrete anatomic structures. Instead, these dots represent something that engineers call "speckle."[1] Each speckle dot seen on the screen is the *net* result of interaction between the ultrasound beam and multiple tiny elements within the tissue. Although each dot does not represent a discrete anatomic structure per se, the speckle pattern does nonetheless represent the tissue in a general way.

The speckle pattern that characterizes normal hepatic parenchyma (Fig. 9–1) emanates from tiny (0.1 to 1.0 mm) architectural boundaries that are thought to be interfaces between tissues with high collagen content (stroma) and high water content (hepatocytes).[2, 3] This hypothesis nicely accounts for the tissue texture alterations that occur with diffuse liver disease. For instance, the formation of intracellular fat globules in fatty liver dramatically increases hepatic echogenicity because the boundaries between these globules and cellular water are highly reflective. The converse is true in conditions that cause edema, such as severe acute viral hepatitis. The increased water content of the edematous liver appears to "dilute" the collagen/water interfaces, decreasing hepatic echogenicity.[4, 5]

METHODS FOR ASSESSING HEPATIC ECHOGENICITY

Quantitative methods for measuring tissue echogenicity[2, 3, 6–10] are used in experimental settings, but these methods are laborious and are not used in clinical ultrasound departments. Clinical assessment of echogenicity is based almost exclusively on subjective comparison of the echo "brightness" of the liver with the "brightness" of the renal cortex and the pancreas.[4, 5, 11–20] Normally, liver echogenicity equals

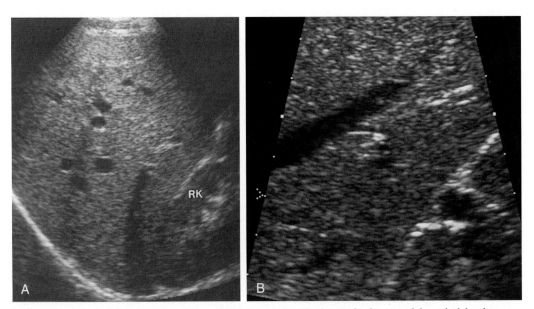

Figure 9-1—Normal Hepatic Parenchymal "Texture." (**A**) This longitudinal image of the right lobe shows normal features of the hepatic parenchyma: (1) the liver is slightly more echogenic than the right kidney (RK); (2) the speckle elements are of medium size and homogeneous; and (3) multiple vessels are visible. (**B**) A magnified view of the right hepatic lobe illustrates the medium-sized speckle of the normal liver.

or slightly exceeds renal cortical echogenicity (Fig. 9–1A), and the liver is slightly less echogenic than the pancreas[11] (see Chapter 6). With liver disease, these relationships may change, as discussed later.

The subjective assessment of hepatic echogenicity is useful clinically but is error prone for three reasons. First, disease processes may alter the echogenicity of kidney or pancreas, invalidating these organs as "standards" of comparison; second, interobserver variability is considerable; and third, instrument variables (inherent or operator-controlled) may diminish or accentuate differences in echogenicity.

DIFFUSE DISEASES THAT ALTER HEPATIC ECHOGENICITY

The disease processes that alter the sonographic texture of the liver fall into four categories: (1) neoplastic infiltration, (2) infection, (3) fatty liver, and (4) fibrosis. Neoplastic infiltration, which causes diffuse nonhomogeneity of the liver, was discussed in the preceding chapter and will not be considered further. Infectious processes are considered briefly herein, but the bulk of this chapter is devoted to fatty liver, fibrosis, and cirrhosis, which are of considerable importance from a clinical and sonographic perspective.

Infectious Hepatitis

Sonography does not play a prominent role in the clinical evaluation of acute hepatitis, except to search for bile duct obstruction when the cause of jaundice is unclear. Hepatomegaly probably is the most common manifestation of acute hepatitis. Clinical experience indicates that hepatic echogenicity remains normal in most acute hepatitis cases (no published data exist on this point). Uncommonly, however, acute infectious hepatitis causes an appreciable *decrease* of hepatic echogenicity attributed to hydropic swelling of liver cells and increased extracellular fluid.[4, 5] In these instances, periportal collagenous tissue stands out with exceptional brightness in contrast to the hypoechoic parenchyma (Fig. 9–2). This appearance is described as the "starry night liver." The gallbladder also is edematous in severe, acute hepatitis cases, and the fluid-laden wall may be massively thickened, as illustrated in Chapter 14. Ascites may be present in severe cases.

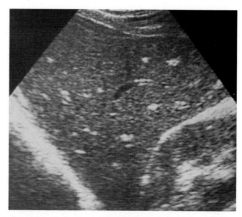

Figure 9-2—Starry Night Liver (Acute Hepatitis A). Marked contrast is evident between the periportal fibrous tissue and the hypoechoic hepatic parenchyma (the starry night appearance) in this longitudinal scan through the right lobe. The liver is slightly *less* echogenic than the kidney, but this finding is difficult to appreciate on this reproduction.

Diffuse Opportunistic Infection

In patients with the autoimmune deficiency syndrome, and in other immunosuppressed individuals, the liver may be studded with innumerable microscopic abscesses. In some cases, these abscesses merely cause an inhomogeneous appearance similar to that seen with diffuse metastasis. In other cases, small, discrete lesions are seen that usually are hypoechoic. This subject is discussed further in Chapter 7.

FATTY LIVER AND FIBROSIS

Both fatty liver and fibrosis are nonspecific responses of the liver to hepatocellular injury. The potential causes of such injury are numerous (Table 9–1).[21] The characteristic histologic feature of fatty liver (fatty infiltration or steatosis)

Table 9-1. Causes of Fatty Liver and Hepatic Fibrosis

Fatty Liver	Fibrosis
Viral hepatitis	Viral hepatitis
Alcohol abuse	Alcohol abuse
Toxins (including medications)	Toxins (including medications)
Metabolic disorders	Metabolic disorders
Obesity	Prolonged cholestasis
Nutritional disorders	Hepatic venous obstruction
Systemic disease	Immune disorders
Cryptogenic	Intestinal bypass
	Cryptogenic

Based on Sherlock S, Dooley J: Diseases of the Liver and Biliary Systems. London, Blackwell Scientific Publications, 1993, pp 322–356.

is the accumulation of fat globules within the hepatocytes. Fatty liver is a reversible condition that may resolve quickly. Hepatic fibrosis, in contrast, represents irreversible, diffuse scarring that results from necrosis of hepatocytes and other cellular elements.

Sonographic Findings in Fatty Liver

Table 9–2 lists the ultrasound findings associated with fatty liver.[2–19] The severity of these abnormalities correlates roughly with hepatocellular fat content and with biochemical dysfunction.[2, 14, 16]

The sonographic hallmark of fatty liver (Fig. 9–3) is diffusely increased parenchymal echogenicity (the so-called "bright liver"). Increased echogenicity often is accompanied by an unusually "fine" liver texture.

The second notable feature of fatty liver is increased attenuation of the ultrasound beam. This feature of fatty liver goes hand-in-hand with increased echogenicity. The greater the brightness of the liver, the greater the attenuation, and the harder it is to penetrate the liver with the ultrasound beam.

The third readily detectable feature of fatty liver is decreased sonographic visualization of portal and hepatic veins. Normally, four to six

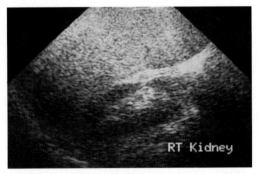

Figure 9-3—Fatty Liver. A longitudinal scan through the right hepatic lobe demonstrates markedly increased parenchymal echogenicity (compare with the right kidney). No hepatic vessels are visible. Note that distal (posterior) structures are poorly seen because of excessive attenuation by the fat-laden liver.

portal or hepatic veins are visible in every longitudinal section of the right hepatic lobe. Fewer vessels are visible in patients with moderate hepatocellular disease, and in severe disease, only the main right portal branch is seen. The disappearance of hepatic vessels appears to result from compression by the surrounding fat-laden parenchyma.

Sonographic Findings in Hepatic Fibrosis

The ultrasound literature on hepatic fibrosis is confusing, because earlier studies did not differentiate between the effects of fatty infiltration and fibrosis, which frequently coexist. More recent studies have revealed that hepatic fibrosis, of and by itself, has little or no effect on hepatic echogenicity. At most, hepatic fibrosis may increase echogenicity slightly (Table 9–2), and in most instances, diffuse hepatic fibrosis cannot be detected in the course of clinical ultrasound examination.[7–10] When fibrosis progresses to cirrhosis, however, ultrasound may demonstrate a coarsened hepatic texture and characteristic changes in hepatic morphology, as discussed later.

Table 9-2. Sonographic Findings in Fatty Liver, Hepatic Fibrosis, and Cirrhosis

Fatty Liver
>   Increased strength (brightness) of echoes
>   Increased number of echoes
>   Fine parenchymal texture
>   Increased attenuation (diminished through-transmission)
>   Decreased number of vessels
>   Hepatomegaly
>   Regional differences in echogenicity

Fibrosis
>   Normal appearance of liver
>   Slight increase in echogenicity
>   Changes related to cirrhosis (below)
>   Increased periportal echogenicity (schistosomiasis—rare, Western nations)

Cirrhosis
>   Normal or slightly increased echogenicity
>   Good through-transmission of ultrasound
>   Coarse parenchymal texture
>   Nodularity
>   Small (shrunken) liver
>   Small right lobe, enlarged left and/or caudate lobe
>   Decreased number of vessels
>   Regenerative nodules (rare)
>   Manifestations of portal hypertension

Based on references 24 to 30.

Diagnostic Accuracy

Ultrasound is not a very accurate means for diagnosing fatty liver and hepatic fibrosis. Subjective assessment of liver echogenicity has a positive predictive value of 67% to 100% and a negative predictive value of 59% to 94% for these conditions.[5, 12–19] The wide spread of these statistics stems from the subjective nature of ultrasound findings, variation in experimental design, and the variable mixture of fatty liver (easily detected) and fibrosis (not detected readily) in any patient population. In general, ultrasound "rules in" hepatocellular disease better than it rules it out, and ultrasound detects moderate or severe hepatocellular disease much better than it detects mild abnormality.[2, 9, 14, 19, 20]

Nonhomogeneous Fatty Liver

One might reasonably assume that fatty infiltration is always a uniform process, but this is not the case. Nonhomogeneous fatty liver (focal fatty infiltration) is common and may cause considerable diagnostic confusion.[22–30] *Hyperechoic,* fat-laden areas may mimic echogenic neoplasms (Fig. 9–4). Alternatively, "spared" normal areas may be mistaken for focal *hypoechoic* lesions, since they are less echogenic than surrounding fat-laden tissue (Fig. 9–5). Most sonographic errors fall into the latter category.

The following observations assist with correct identification of focal fatty infiltration or focal spared areas: (1) nonspherical shape, (2) sharply angulated boundaries, (3) interdigitization of fatty and normal areas, (4) absence of mass effect, (5) absence of vascular displacement or distortion, and (6) lobar or segmental distribution. Computed tomography is the suggested method for confirming the diagnosis of focal fatty infiltration. Echogenic, fatty areas seen with ultrasound correspond to low attenuation regions on computed tomograms (Figs. 9–4, 9–5).[22, 25, 26, 29] Focal fat accumulation also may be confirmed with magnetic resonance imaging.[30]

CIRRHOSIS
Pathology

Cirrhosis[31] is the nonspecific, end-stage manifestation of hepatocyte injury, which leads, ultimately, to tissue necrosis, fibrosis, and attempted regeneration of liver tissue. In general terms, the causes of cirrhosis are the same as those listed in Table 9–1 for hepatic fibrosis. In Western nations, alcoholism is the principal etiology, but in Asia, Africa, and most Third World countries, viral hepatitis is the usual cause. Although cirrhosis is an advanced form of hepatic fibrosis, *these disorders are not synonymous* and have markedly different clinical implications. Cirrhosis should be diagnosed with ultrasound only when specific findings are identified, as discussed later. Cirrhosis is classified as micronodular or macronodular, depending on the size of regenerative nodules present. Macronodular cirrhosis is simply an advanced stage that has gone beyond the micronodular form.

Sonographic Diagnosis

The sonographic findings that characterize cirrhosis[7, 12, 18, 32–39] are listed in Table 9–2 and illustrated in Figure 9–6. The following manifestations of cirrhosis are particularly noteworthy:

1. The attenuation of the cirrhotic liver is *similar* to normal hepatic parenchyma. The cirrhotic liver may be slightly more echogenic than a normal liver, but the cirrhotic liver is not strongly echogenic and is easily penetrated by the ultrasound beam. (An exception to this rule occurs if fatty infiltration is superimposed on cirrhotic changes.)

2. In patients with advanced cirrhosis, the texture of the liver is coarser than normal, and the surface is irregular due to the presence of regenerative nodules. Surface nodularity is most easily detected when ascites surrounds the liver and highlights its surface. Even fine

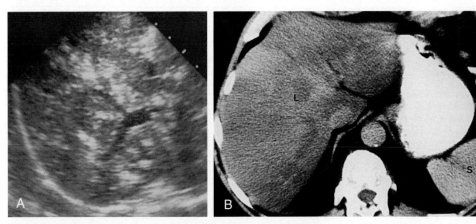

Figure 9-4—Nonhomogeneous Fatty Infiltration. (**A**) A bizarre pattern of increased parenchymal echogenicity is seen in this longitudinal view of the right lobe of the liver. (**B**) Corresponding CT scan shows a geographic pattern of low density consistent with heterogeneous fatty infiltration. Note that the low-density portions of the liver are less dense than the spleen.

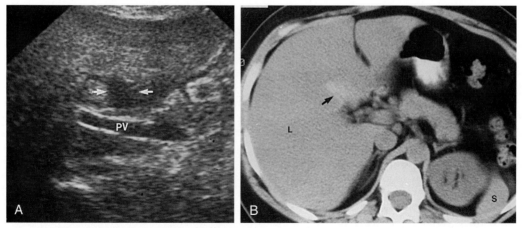

Figure 9-5—Focal Sparing from Fatty Infiltration. (A) This oblique scan of the liver shows a hypoechoic area (arrows) ventral to the portal vein (PV). Note that the hypoechoic region is irregularly shaped and does not exhibit mass effect. (B) A noncontrast computed tomogram obtained the same day shows that the liver (L) is slightly less dense, overall, than the spleen(s), consistent with fatty infiltration. The area corresponding to the hypoechoic region (arrow) is denser than the rest of the liver, indicating that it is a "spared" area.

surface nodularity is abnormal and strongly suggests the diagnosis of cirrhosis.[33] Furthermore, nodularity is associated with sinusoidal obstruction and resultant portal hypertension. *By identifying parenchymal nodules, one may distinguish between cirrhosis and other forms of liver disease, such as uncomplicated hepatic fibrosis and fatty liver.*

3. Large, regenerative nodules may occasionally be visualized as discrete, rounded structures within the liver parenchyma.[36–39] These nodules either are isoechoic or slightly hypoechoic relative to the surrounding hepatic tissue. Regenerative nodules are extremely numerous in cirrhotic livers, yet their visualization with ultrasound is *rare*. Therefore, "regenerative

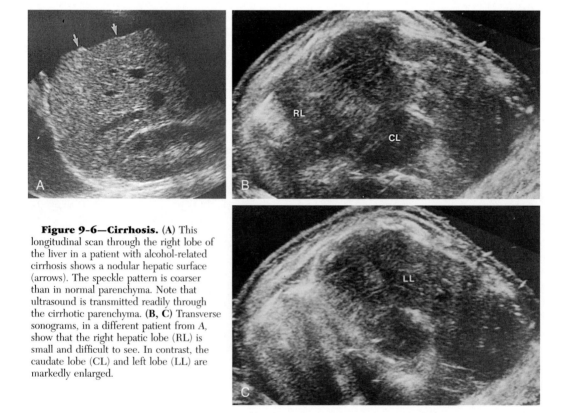

Figure 9-6—Cirrhosis. (A) This longitudinal scan through the right lobe of the liver in a patient with alcohol-related cirrhosis shows a nodular hepatic surface (arrows). The speckle pattern is coarser than in normal parenchyma. Note that ultrasound is transmitted readily through the cirrhotic parenchyma. (B, C) Transverse sonograms, in a different patient from A, show that the right hepatic lobe (RL) is small and difficult to see. In contrast, the caudate lobe (CL) and left lobe (LL) are markedly enlarged.

nodule" should not be the first thought when a discrete lesion is seen in a cirrhotic liver. Instead, the sonologist should think of neoplasia, and particularly of hepatocellular carcinoma (Chapter 8).

4. The number of visible portal or hepatic veins is reduced in cirrhotic livers, in proportion to the severity of disease. The loss of visible vessels appears to be a compressive phenomenon, as mentioned previously.

5. Portal hypertension is an important concomitant finding in patients with diffuse liver disease. The presence of portal hypertension confirms the diagnosis of cirrhosis, and vice versa, as discussed in the following chapter.

6. Cirrhosis may be accompanied by nonspecific, generalized shrinkage of the liver. In many cases, the right lobe shrinks more than the other lobes, and the caudate and left lobes enlarge as the right lobe shrinks.[33–35] The cause of these morphologic changes is unknown. Cirrhosis may be diagnosed in some patients simply by comparing the maximal transverse dimension of the caudate and right lobes of the liver, as seen on transverse scans just below the portal bifurcation. If the caudate/right lobe ratio exceeds 0.65, cirrhosis may be diagnosed with 90% to 100% certainty.[32, 35] Unfortunately, this ratio is only 43% sensitive for cirrhosis.[35]

SCHISTOSOMIASIS, A SPECIAL CASE

Although schistosomiasis is rare in Western nations, it is a common disorder worldwide, with vast public health implications. Brief mention of this disorder is warranted since it has characteristic ultrasound findings.[40–42] *Schistosoma mansoni* is the most common of several schistosomes that may infect humans. The embryonic parasites enter the portal system from the gut and lodge in the portal veins, where they develop into adult worms that can live for many years. Ova shed by the worms lodge in portal vein radicles and cause chronic granulomatous periphlebitis, which leads in turn to fibrosis and portal hypertension. Morbidity and mortality result principally from portal hypertension.[40–42]

The sonographic finding that characterizes chronic schistosomiasis is a thick band of highly echogenic fibrous tissue that surrounds the portal vein branches, from the porta hepatis to the periphery of the liver. Scans transverse to the portal branches demonstrate a bull's eye appearance, with the anechoic portal vein surrounded by an echogenic mantle of fibrous tissue. Typical sonographic manifestations of portal hyperten-

sion, as presented in the following chapter, occur in virtually all patients.

REFERENCES

1. Beach KW: 1975–2000: A quarter century of ultrasound technology. Ultrasound Med Biol 18:377–388, 1992.
2. Shawker TH, Moran B, Linzer M, et al: B-scan echo-amplitude measurement in patients with diffuse infiltrative liver disease. J Clin Ultrasound 9:293–301, 1981.
3. Behan M, Kazam E: The echogenic characteristics of fatty tissues and tumors. Radiology 129:143–151, 1978.
4. Kurtz AB, Rubin CS, Cooper HS, Nisenbaum HL, Cole-Beuglet C, Medoff J, Goldberg BB: Ultrasound findings in hepatitis. Radiology 136:717–723, 1980.
5. Needleman L, Kurtz AB, Rifkin MD, et al: Sonography of diffuse benign liver disease: Accuracy of pattern recognition and grading. AJR Am J Roentgenol 146:1011–1015, 1986.
6. Ralls PW, Johnson MB, Kanel G, Dobalian DM, Colletti PM, Boswell WD, Radin DR, Halls JM: FM sonography in diffuse liver disease: Prospective assessment and blinded analysis. Radiology 161:451–454, 1986.
7. Taylor KJW, Riely CA, Hammers L, Flax S, Weltin G, Garcia-Tsao G, Conn HO, Kuc R, Barwick KW: Quantitative US attenuation in normal liver and in patients with diffuse liver disease: Importance of fat. Radiology 160:65–71, 1986.
8. Garra BS, Insana MF, Shawker TH, Russell MA: Quantitative estimation of liver attenuation and echogenicity: Normal state versus diffuse liver disease. Radiology 162:61–67, 1987.
9. Lin T, Ophir J, Potter G: Correlation of ultrasonic attenuation with pathologic fat and fibrosis in liver disease. Ultrasound Med Biol 14:729–734, 1988.
10. Kuni CC, Johnson TK, Crass JR, Snover DC: Correlation of Fourier spectral shift-determined hepatic acoustic attenuation coefficients with liver biopsy findings. J Ultrasound Med 8:631–634, 1989.
11. Platt JF, Rubin JM, Bowerman RA, Marn CS: The inability to detect disease on the basis of renal echogenicity. AJR Am J Roentgenol 151:317–19, 1988.
12. Debongnie JC, Pauls C, Fieves M, et al: Prospective evaluation of the diagnostic accuracy of liver ultrasonography. Gut 22:130–135, 1981.
13. Dewbury KC, Clark B: The accuracy of ultrasound in the detection of cirrhosis of the liver. Br J Ultrasound 52:945–948, 1979.
14. Foster KL, Dewbury KC, Griffith AH, et al: The accuracy of ultrasound in the detection of fatty infiltration of the liver. Br J Radiol 53:440–442, 1980.
15. Gosink BB, Lemon SK, Scheible W, et al: Accuracy of ultrasonography in diagnosis of hepatocellular disease. AJR Am J Roentgenol 133:19–23, 1979.
16. Scatrige JC, Scott WW, Donovan PJ, et al: Fatty infiltration of the liver. Ultrasound and computed tomographic correlation. J Ultrasound Med 3:9–14, 1984.
17. Scott WW, Donovan PJ, Sanders RJ: The sonography of diffuse liver disease. Semin Ultrasound II:219–225, 1981.
18. Taylor KJW, Gorelick FS, Rosenfeld AT, et al: Ultrasonography of alcoholic liver disease with

histological correlation. Radiology 141:157–161, 1981.

19. Pamilo M, Sotaniemi EA, Suramo I, et al: Evaluation of liver steatotic and fibrous content by computerized tomography and ultrasound. Scand J Gastroenterol 18:743–747, 1983.

20. Levenson H, Greensite F, Hoefs J, Friloux L, Applegate G, Silva E, Kanel G, Buxton R: Fatty infiltration of the liver: Quantification with phase-contrast MR imaging at 1.5 T vs. biopsy. AJR Am J Roentgenol 156:307–312, 1991.

21. Sherlock S, Dooley J: Diseases of the Liver and Biliary System. London, Blackwell Scientific Publications, 1993, pp 322–356.

22. Halvorssen RA, Korbokin M, Ram PC, et al: CT appearance of focal fatty infiltration of the liver. AJR Am J Roentgenol 139:277–281, 1982.

23. Quinn SF, Gosink BB: Characteristic sonographic signs of hepatic fatty infiltration. AJR Am J Roentgenol 145:753–755, 1985.

24. Swobodnik W, Wechsler JG, Manne W, Ditschuneit H: Multiple regular circumscript fatty infiltrations of the liver. J Clin Ultrasound 13:577–580, 1985.

25. Baker MK, Wenker JC, Cockerill EM, Ellis JH: Focal fatty infiltration of the liver: Diagnostic imaging. RadioGraphics 5:923–939, 1985.

26. Yates CK, Streight RA: Focal fatty infiltration of the liver simulating metastatic disease. Radiology 159:83–84, 1986.

27. Sauerbrei EE, Lopez M: Pseudotumor of the quadrate lobe in hepatic sonography: A sign of generalized fatty infiltration. AJR Am J Roentgenol 147:923–927, 1986.

28. White EM, Simeone JF, Mueller PR, Grant EG, Choyke PL, Zeman RK: Focal periportal sparing in hepatic fatty infiltration: A cause of hepatic pseudomass on US. Radiology 162:57–59, 1987.

29. Yoshikawa J, Matsui O, Takashima T, Sugiura H, Katayama K, Nishida Y, Tsuji M: Focal fatty change of the liver adjacent to the falciform ligament: CT and sonographic findings in five surgically confirmed cases. AJR Am J Roentgenol 149:491–494, 1987.

30. Dao TH, Mathieu D, Nguyen-tan T, Derby S, Vasile N: Value of MR imaging in evaluating focal fatty infiltration of the liver: Preliminary study. RadioGraphics 11:1003–1012, 1991.

31. Sherlock S, Dooley J: Diseases of the Liver and Biliary System. London, Blackwell Scientific Publications, 1993, pp 357–369.

32. Harbin WP, Robert NJ, Ferrucci JT: Diagnosis of cirrhosis based on regional changes in hepatic morphology. Radiology 135:273–283, 1980.

33. Di Lelio A, Cestari C, Lomazzi A, Beretta L: Cirrhosis: Diagnosis with sonographic study of the liver surface. Radiology 172:389–392, 1989.

34. Gore RM, Ghahremani GG, Joseph AE, Nemcek AA, Marn CS, Vogelzang RL: Acquired malposition of the colon and gallbladder in patients with cirrhosis: CT findings and clinical implications. Radiology 171:739–742, 1989.

35. Giorgii A, Amoroso P, Lettieri G, Fico P, de Stefano G, Finelli L, Scala V, Tarantino L, Pierri P, Pesce G: Cirrhosis: Value of caudate to right lobe ratio in diagnosis with US. Radiology 161:443–445, 1986.

36. Freeman MP, Vick CW, Taylor KJW, Carithers RL, Brewer WH: Regenerating nodules in cirrhosis: Sonographic appearance with anatomic correlation. AJR Am J Roentgenol 146:533–536, 1986.

37. Day DL, Letourneau JG, Allan BT, Sharp HL, Ascher N, Dehner LP, Thompson WM: Hepatic regenerating nodules in hereditary tyrosinemia. AJR Am J Roentgenol 149:391–393, 1987.

38. Murakami T, Kuroda C, Murakawa T, Harada K, Wakasa K, Sakurai M, Monden M, Kasahara A, Kawata S, Kozuka T: Regenerating nodules in hepatic cirrhosis: MR findings with pathologic correlation. AJR Am J Roentgenol 155:1227–1231, 1990.

39. Giorgio A, Francica G, de Stefano G, Aloisio T, Pierri P, Amoroso P, Tarantino L: Sonographic recognition of intraparenchymal regenerating nodules using high-frequency transducers in patients with cirrhosis. J Ultrasound Med 10:355–359, 1991.

40. Fattar S, Bassiony H, Satyanath S, et al: Characteristic sonographic features of schistosomal periportal fibrosis. AJR Am J Roentgenol 143:69–71, 1984.

41. Cerri GG, Alves VA, Magalhaes A: Hepatosplenic *Schistosomiasis mansoni:* Ultrasound manifestations. Radiology 153:777–780, 1984.

42. Hussain S, Hawass ND, Zaidi AJ: Ultrasonographic diagnosis of schistosomal periportal fibrosis. J Ultrasound Med 3:449–452, 1984.

Chapter 10

Vascular Disorders of the Liver

William J. Zwiebel

The discussion of cirrhosis in the preceding chapter leads naturally into the subject of vascular disorders of the liver, for many of these conditions are seen in association with cirrhosis. The disorders that will be considered here are portal hypertension, portal thrombosis, and hepatic vein occlusion. Please see Chapter 6 for details concerning the normal vascular anatomy of the liver.

PORTAL HYPERTENSION

The term "portal hypertension" refers to elevated pressure in the portal venous system, which results from impedance of blood flow through the liver. Increased splanchnic blood flow also contributes to portal hypertension in some cases.[1-56] Cirrhosis is the usual cause of portal hypertension in Western nations. Other causes include hepatic vein occlusion, portal vein occlusion, and schistosomiasis.

Advances in duplex° ultrasound instrumentation have made possible direct, noninvasive interrogation of portal vein flow. The following duplex ultrasound parameters are of value for diagnosis of portal hypertension: (1) portal vein diameter, (2) the response of the portal, splenic, or superior mesenteric veins to respiration, (3) portal flow direction, (4) portal flow velocity and waveforms, and (5) spleen size. Each of these parameters will be discussed in turn.

Portal Vein Diameter

In normal individuals (Fig. 10–1), the portal vein diameter does not exceed 13 mm in quiet respiration and 16 mm in deep inspiration, as measured where the portal vein crosses anterior to the inferior vena cava.[6, 12–21] Respiration and patient position greatly affect the size of the portal vein and its tributaries; therefore, diagnostic measurements must be standardized by using a supine patient position and a state of quiet respiration. Under these circumstances, a portal vein diameter exceeding 13 mm (Fig. 10–2A) indicates portal hypertension with a high degree of specificity (100% reported), but with low sensitivity (45% to 50%).[20, 21] Sensitivity is increased

by evaluating the response of the splenic or superior mesenteric veins to respiratory maneuvers. In normal individuals, the diameter of these veins increases by 20% to 100% from quiet respiration to deep inspiration (Fig. 10–1C,D). An increase of less than 20% (Fig. 10–2B,C) indicates portal hypertension with 81% sensitivity and 100% specificity.[21]

Portal Flow Direction and Velocity

In normal individuals, portal flow is hepatopedal (toward the liver) throughout the entire cardiac cycle. Mean flow velocity is about 15 to 18 cm/sec,[15, 16, 22–24] but the normal range is wide. Portal flow velocity varies with cardiac activity and respiration, giving the portal waveform an undulating appearance (Fig. 10–1B).

With the development of portal hypertension, flow velocity decreases and velocity fluctuations disappear (i.e., flow becomes "continuous"). As portal pressure increases, the flow in the portal vein may become to-and-fro (biphasic), or the flow direction may reverse (hepatofugal flow) in either the portal vein or the splenic vein (Fig. 10–2D).

Flow reversal in the portal or splenic veins is a variable finding in portal hypertension, since flow direction in these vessels is influenced by collateral development. For instance, if splenorenal collaterals are the primary mode of portal decompression, then flow may reverse in the portal vein. If, on the other hand, a large umbilical vein collateral is the primary mode of decompression, then splenic vein and portal vein flow may well be normal (hepatopedal), since the umbilical vein originates in the left portal system (discussed later). For the same reason, it is possible for flow to be reversed in the right portal vein and normally directed in the left portal vein in the same patient.

The Congestive Index

Portal hypertension also may be recognized with the "congestive index," which is the ratio of the portal vein area (cm²) divided by the mean portal flow velocity (cm/sec).[22, 23] This ratio,

---

°Doppler plus B-mode; see Chapter 1.

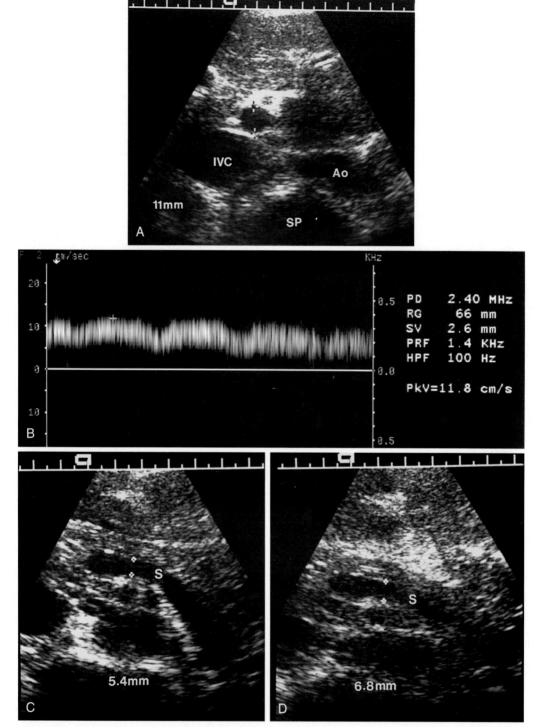

Figure 10-1—Normal Portal Vein Features. (A) The portal vein (cursors) is measured where it crosses anterior to the inferior vena cava (IVC). With the patient supine and breathing quietly, portal vein diameter does not normally exceed 13 mm. Ao = aorta; SP = spine. **(B)** Portal flow velocity undulates slightly in response to cardiac pulsation and respiration. **(C, D)** In this normal individual, the diameter of the splenic vein (S) increases more than 26% from quiet respiration **(C)** to deep inspiration **(D)**.

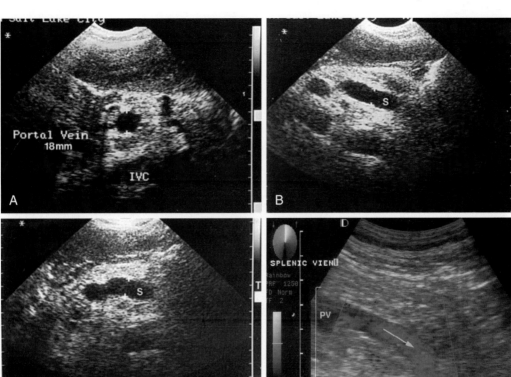

Figure 10-2—Features of Portal Hypertension. (**A**) The portal vein diameter (cursors) is 18 mm with the patient supine and breathing quietly. In the same patient, the diameter of the splenic vein (S) increases only 8% (from 13 mm to 14 mm) from quiet respiration (**B**) to deep inspiration (**C**). (**D**) Splenic vein flow (arrow) is reversed (toward the spleen) in this transverse scan obtained in another patient with portal hypertension. (The spleen is not visible in this view.) PV = portal vein. (See Color Figure 10–2 *D* following page 108.)

which does not exceed 0.7 in normal individuals, is attractive because it takes into account two intersecting physiologic changes that occur in portal hypertension: portal vein dilatation and diminished flow velocity.

Spleen Size

An important manifestation of portal hypertension is splenomegaly. The size of the spleen does not correlate well with the level of portal pressure; nonetheless, splenomegaly is a common feature of portal hypertension.[1, 2] The spleen is best measured in a coronal plane. A maximal cephalocaudal measurement exceeding 13 cm indicates enlargement with a high degree of reliability (Chapter 11).

Pitfalls of Portal Flow Assessment

Duplex ultrasound examination of the portal venous system (portal vein, splenic vein, and superior mesenteric vein) is successful in 95% of patients with suspected portal hypertension, but portions of the portal system may be obscured by bowel gas in up to 10% of successful studies.[8] Even in successful studies errors may be made, and the following pitfalls are particularly noteworthy:*

1. The direction of flow in the portal vein may be ambiguous or may spuriously appear to be reversed for technical reasons. Abnormal flow direction, therefore, should be confirmed with several interrogations of the portal vein, preferably from different transducer positions.
2. Splenic vein occlusion or splenic flow reversal may be overlooked if only hilar branches are visualized and the splenic vein per se is not examined. This error occurs because blood flow, of necessity, must exit from the spleen. Hence, flow in the hilar branches always is normally directed to the point where these branches communicate with collaterals.
3. Portal vein dilatation may be caused by severe congestive heart failure (CHF), owing to transmission of back-pressure from the right

---

*References 2, 4–6, 10, 24, 25, 32, 34–36, 50–71.

atrium through the hepatic circulation to the portal circulation.[25, 26] Such dilatation may be attributed mistakenly to cirrhosis. Two findings help differentiate between CHF and "true" portal hypertension: in CHF, portal flow is markedly pulsatile, and the inferior vena cava is dilated. Neither of these findings is a feature of portal hypertension related to liver disease.

PORTOSYSTEMIC COLLATERALS

Portosystemic venous collaterals[2, 3, 6, 27–49] are a very important finding, for in most cases their presence is a clear indication of portal hypertension. The exception to this rule is collateralization related to venous occlusive disease, such as portal or splenic vein thrombosis. Portosystemic collaterals develop of necessity in patients with portal hypertension, for blood from the gut must have an alternative means of reaching the heart when passage through the liver is blocked. The major portosystemic collateral routes are illustrated in Figure 10–3.

A systematic search is required for detecting portosystemic collaterals, as outlined in Table 10–1. Sonography is reported to visualize 65% to 90% of portosystemic collaterals,[35, 36, 40, 41, 53] and virtually every collateral that may occur has been seen with ultrasound.[6, 27–49] Only a few portosystemic collaterals are identified regularly, and these are described in Table 10–2 and Figures 10–3 through 10–8. Please review this material before proceeding, as it is not repeated in the text.

Several caveats are noteworthy with respect to portosystemic collaterals:

1. The effectiveness of large collaterals in decompressing the portal system is subject to debate.[27, 33, 38, 41, 46] Large collaterals do not clearly protect a patient from gastroesophageal hemorrhage.
2. The *coronary vein* may be seen in some normal individuals; therefore, the mere presence of a coronary vein does not indicate portal hypertension. The diameter of normal coronary veins does not exceed 4 mm, whereas a diameter exceeding 7 mm is evidence of an abnormal portal/systemic pressure gradient (exceeding 10 mm Hg).[36, 42]

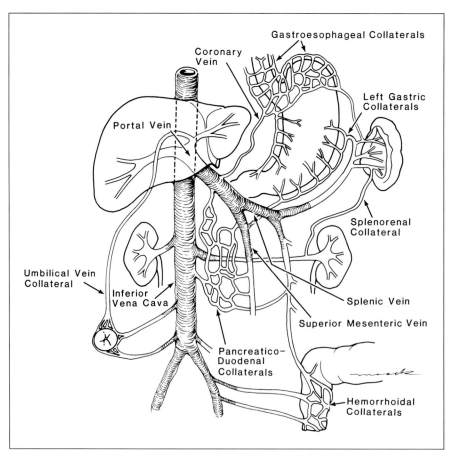

Figure 10-3—Major Portosystemic Collaterals.

Table 10-1. How to Search for Portosystemic Collaterals

Step 1. Begin with the splenic vein and note the direction of flow in this vessel. If flow is reversed (toward the spleen), splenogastric or splenorenal collaterals are likely to exist.

Step 2. Look for a dilated coronary vein by locating the superior mesenteric vein–portal junction on longitudinal images. Move the scan plane slightly to the right and left until a *cephalad-directed* vessel is identified, as seen in Figure 10–4. (See Figure 10–4 following page 108.)

Step 3. Look for varices in the gallbladder wall and bed (Fig. 10–5).

Step 4. Return to the portal vein and follow it to the vicinity of the falciform ligament, where an umbilical vein collateral may be visible (Fig. 10–6).

Step 5. With longitudinal scans, sweep along the left lobe of the liver, looking for left gastric collaterals adjacent to the posterior surface of the liver (Fig. 10–7).

Step 6. With longitudinal scans, look for collaterals in the vicinity of the gastroesophageal junction (Fig. 10–8). (See Figure 10–8 following page 108.)

Step 7. With the patient in the right lateral decubitus position and using coronal or transverse scans, look for splenorenal and splenogastric collaterals in the area between the spleen and upper pole of the left kidney (Fig. 10–8).

3. *Umbilical vein collateral flow* is an important feature of portal hypertension, for it carries a diagnostic specificity of 100%.[47, 48] An artery or vein of up to 2 mm in diameter may be present normally in the ligamentum teres; therefore, *the mere presence of a vessel in the ligamentum teres does not imply umbilical vein collateralization.*[43–48] The diagnosis of collateral flow requires documentation of *venous flow away from* the liver (Fig. 10–6).

4. Portosystemic collaterals may develop in response to venous occlusive disease unrelated to portal hypertension. The most common example is splenic vein occlusion, which is the most likely diagnosis when large splenosystemic collaterals are detected[49] (Fig. 10–8). (See Figure 10–8 following page 108.) Differentiation between splenic vein thrombosis and portal hypertension generally is not a problem, since splenic vein flow usually can be documented with color Doppler examination.

5. Large portosystemic collaterals at the esophagogastric junction (Fig. 10–8) may be mistaken for neoplastic masses if color Doppler examination is not performed.[32]

THERAPEUTIC PORTOSYSTEMIC SHUNTS

Portosystemic shunts may be created by transvascular or surgical means to decompress the portal venous system and thereby protect patients with portal hypertension from gastroesophageal bleeding. Duplex sonography is a routine and effective method for postprocedure assessment of shunt patency and function.[2, 6, 50–56]

Percutaneous Transhepatic Stents

Intrahepatic portocaval stents, installed percutaneously via the jugular vein, have become an important alternative to surgical portocaval shunts as a means of decompressing the portal venous system. The acronym TIPS is used for these shunts: *T*ransvenous (or Transjugular) *I*ntrahepatic *P*ortocaval *S*hunt. The shunt is created with a metallic vascular stent, which is readily seen and easily evaluated with duplex ultrasound[57, 58] (Fig. 10–9). (See Figure 10–9 following page 108.) The goals of duplex examination are to confirm that the shunt is patent and to search for stenosis.

The following examination protocol has been recommended.[57] A preprocedure scan is per-

Table 10-2. The Sonographic Appearance of Portosystemic Collaterals

Collateral	Appearance
Coronary vein	Prominent, *cephalad-directed* vessel that arises from the portal vein approximately opposite to the superior mesenteric vein; visible on longitudinal images
Left gastric veins	Cephalad-directed vessels seen along the inferior border of the left lobe of the liver on longitudinal images
Short gastric and gastroesophageal veins	Tortuous vessels near the upper pole of the spleen and the gastroesophageal junction, seen primarily on coronal images
Splenorenal collaterals	Tortuous, inferiorly directed vessels located between the spleen and the upper pole of the left kidney, possibly accompanied by left renal vein enlargement; primarily seen on coronal images
Umbilical vein	Solitary vessel that may be large, which originates from the ascending portion of the left portal vein. It courses inferiorly through the falciform ligament and along the anterior abdominal wall to the umbilicus. Seen on longitudinal or transverse images

Data from Pollard JJ, Nebesar RA: Altered hemodynamics in the Budd-Chiari syndrome demonstrated by selective hepatic and splenic angiography. Radiology 89:236–243, 1967; and Menu Y, Alison D, Lorphelin J-M, et al: Budd-Chiari syndrome: US evaluation. Radiology 157: 761–764, 1985.

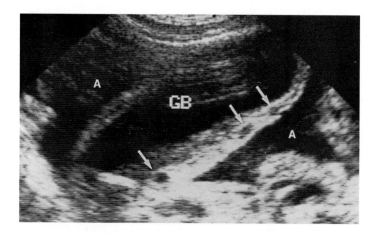

Figure 10-5—Gallbladder Wall Collateral. A longitudinal sonogram in a patient with cirrhosis shows large varices (arrows) within the gallbladder (GB) wall. Flow in these vessels was visualized on a computed tomogram (not shown). A = ascites surrounding the gallbladder.

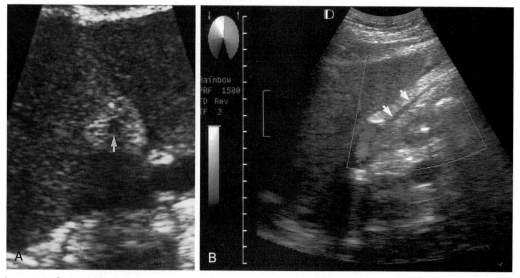

Figure 10-6—Umbilical Vein Collateral. (A) A transverse sonogram through the ligamentum teres shows a central vessel (arrow) that could be either normal or abnormal. (B) A longitudinal color Doppler sonogram demonstrates that flow in this vessel (arrows) is hepatopedal (away from the liver), indicating that the umbilical vein is functioning as a portosystemic collateral. (See Color Figure 10–6B following page 108.)

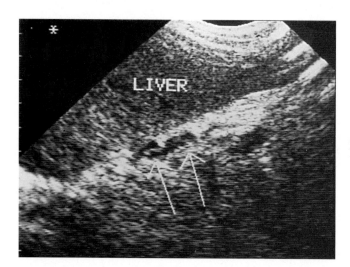

Figure 10-7—Left Gastric Collaterals. Collateral veins (arrows) are seen ventral to the left lobe of the liver.

formed to document patency and flow direction in the portal vein, the splenic vein, and the superior mesenteric vein (SMV), and to confirm that the hepatic veins are patent. The shunt is then scanned 24 hours after stent placement to document shunt patency and to establish baseline flow velocities in the shunt and the portal vein. Follow-up examinations then are conducted at the discretion of the interventional radiologist. Regular follow-up is advisable, as shunt stenosis is fairly common and may be treatable with balloon angioplasty if detected before the shunt becomes occluded.

Normal shunt findings are the following:

1. Slight protrusion of the proximal and distal ends of the shunt into the portal and hepatic veins (respectively).
2. Flow filling the stent from "wall to wall."
3. Flow continuously toward the heart, usually with some pulsatility.
4. Moderate-to-marked spectral broadening (turbulence) is the rule.
5. Peak systolic velocity ranging from 70 to 200 cm/sec (occasionally higher).
6. Fairly uniform velocity throughout the shunt.
7. Hepatopedal flow in the portal vein in 40% to 60% of individuals.
8. An increase in portal flow velocity, compared with pre-procedure findings.

As of this writing, TIPS shunts are considered by some clinicians to be a temporizing measure, as there is a high incidence of shunt stenosis and failure within 2 years of placement (due primarily to intimal hyperplasia). The identification of shunt stenosis helps prolong shunt life through timely intervention with angioplasty. Once the shunt has occluded, there is no possibility of re-establishing flow.

The most common location for shunt stenosis is in the portal vein branch immediately adjacent to the stent, but stenosis also can occur at the hepatic vein end of the stent, or within the stent itself. Shunt stenosis may be diagnosed directly with Doppler ultrasound, through detection of *localized* high-velocity flow and severe turbulence. Stenosis-related velocities as high as 400 cm/sec have been reported. The usual way to identify a stenotic shunt, however, is by detection of reduced flow velocity *throughout* the stent, compared with baseline values. Alternatively, a marked drop in velocity may be detected in the portal vein.

Shunt occlusion is indicated by absence of flow in the shunt, and return of portal flow velocity and direction to preprocedure status. Caution is advised in assessing the apparently occluded

shunt as low-flow velocity in a highly stenosed stent may be difficult to detect with ultrasound. If flow is not detected with color Doppler imaging, then try spectral Doppler (which generally is more sensitive) before concluding that the shunt is occluded. Shunt occlusion should be confirmed angiographically, because a "trickle" of flow may be present that cannot be detected with ultrasound. A highly stenosed stent may be treated with balloon angioplasty, whereas an occluded stent cannot be repaired by any means.

In summary, bad signs for TIPS shunts include (1) a drop in velocity from baseline values; (2) a drop in velocity in the portal vein; (3) a peak velocity less than 70 cm/sec; (4) Absence of flow in the shunt; and (5) a return to hepatofugal flow in the portal system.

Surgical Shunts

The patency of surgically created portosystemic shunts may be confirmed directly, through the detection of flow in the shunt itself, or indirectly, through the assessment of flow direction and waveform characteristics in vessels that communicate with the shunt. For example, in a patient with a portocaval shunt, the direction of splenic vein flow should be normal (away from the spleen) if the shunt is patent, and reversed if the shunt is occluded.

A great variety of surgical shunts exist, and duplex examination of surgical shunts is difficult regardless of the shunt type. Therefore, foreknowledge of the shunt anatomy generally is a prerequisite for successful duplex examination.

PORTAL VEIN OCCLUSION

Pathology

Portal vein occlusion[2, 4–6, 10, 59–74] is principally caused by thrombosis or tumor invasion. Thrombosis may be precipitated by stagnant portal flow in patients with cirrhosis. Other causes include hypercoagulable states, surgery, or intraperitoneal inflammatory processes such as pancreatitis and appendicitis. In the latter case, the inflammatory process causes portal phlebitis, which in turn causes thrombus to form. Tumor invasion of the portal vein occurs most frequently with hepatocellular carcinoma and pancreatic carcinoma.[59–64, 70, 72–74]

Portal vein occlusion usually is permanent, but recanalization may occur in some cases of thrombosis. Portal flow also may be re-established via "cavernous transformation" (discussed later). If portal flow is not adequately re-established, decompression of the portal system occurs via

Acute Findings

The sonographic manifestations of acute portal vein occlusion[2, 6, 62–64, 66–74] are illustrated in Figure 10–10. These include failure to visualize the portal vein, detection of echogenic intraluminal material, absence of flow on color Doppler examination, and other color Doppler abnormalities to be discussed.

The main portal vein is seen on 97% of upper abdominal sonograms[65]; therefore, when a normal-appearing portal vein is not *readily* seen, portal vein occlusion should come to mind. The most important findings that corroborate the diagnosis of portal vein occlusion are absence of portal flow accompanied by echogenic material within the portal vein lumen. Occluding material, whether thrombus or tumor, generally is low or moderate in echogenicity. Recently formed thrombosis may be almost anechoic, and it may be overlooked in the absence of Doppler interro-

gation of flow. On color Doppler examination, flow may be absent in an occluded portal vein, or a "trickle" of flow may be seen around the obstruction. If the portal vein is only partially blocked (Fig. 10–A), increased flow velocity and disturbed flow may be apparent at the site of obstruction. The occluding material frequently dilates the portal vein and its branches noticeably (Fig. 10–10B). In some cases, a massively dilated vein may be mistaken for a neoplastic mass. Thrombus may extend into the splenic or superior mesenteric veins (Fig. 10–10C), and these tributaries should be evaluated to confirm the extent of occlusion.

Patent segments of the portal system distal* to an occluded portal vein often are dilated, and low-velocity, continuous flow may be present in these segments, rather than the normal phasic flow pattern. Flow may be reversed in the splenic or superior mesenteric veins.

---

*The terms "distal" and "proximal" are used with respect to the heart. Proximal means closer to the heart, and distal means farther from the heart.

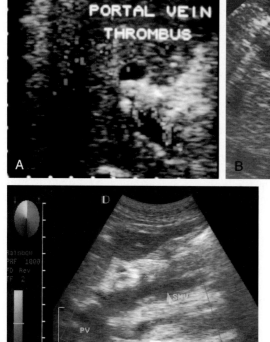

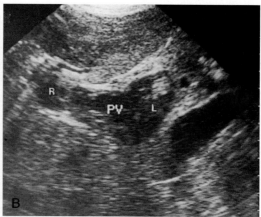

Figure 10-10—Examples of Portal Vein Occlusion. (A) Blood (blue color) flows around a thrombus within the portal vein in this patient with a hypercoagulable state and abdominal pain. Note that the portal vein is at most slightly dilated. (Findings confirmed with portal venography.) (See Color Figure 10–10A on the following page.) **(B)** An oblique sonogram in a patient with cirrhosis shows massive thrombotic distention of the portal vein (PV) and the right (R) and left (L) portal branches. The portal vein measured 4 cm in maximum diameter. **(C)** No flow is evident in the portal vein (PV) and the superior mesenteric vein (SMV, arrow) in this patient with acute pancreatitis. Note that flow is visible in other vessels at an equal depth. The splenic vein (not shown) also was thrombosed. (See Color Figure 10–10C.)

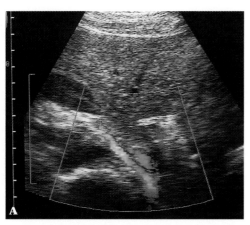

Figure 1-17A. Color Doppler sonography refers to the representation of blood flow in color on a two-dimensional ultrasound image, as shown here.

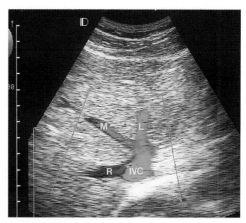

Figure 6-5. Convergence of the hepatic veins at the diaphragm. The right (R), middle (M), and left (L) hepatic vein trunks converge on the inferior vena cava (IVC), as seen on a transverse sonogram. Note that the middle and left trunks join shortly before entering the IVC. Flow is less evident in the right trunk than in the other branches, as the right trunk is almost perpendicular to the ultrasound beam (hence the Doppler shift is minimal).

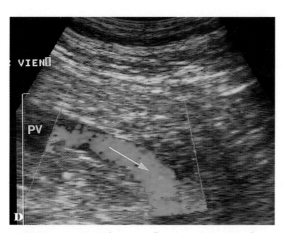

Figure 10-2D. Splenic vein flow (arrow) is reversed (toward the spleen) in this transverse scan obtained in another patient with portal hypertension. (The spleen is not visible in this view.) PV = portal vein.

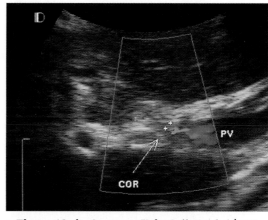

Figure 10-4—Coronary Vein Collateral. A longitudinal sonogram shows a coronary vein (COR, arrow) at its attachment to the portal vein (PV), near the portosplenic junction. This coronary vein is not dilated (3-mm diameter), but portal hypertension is evident since flow is cephalad (hepatofugal), as indicated by the blue color.

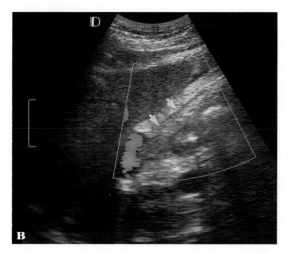

Figure 10-6B. Umbilical Vein Collateral. A longitudinal color Doppler sonogram demonstrates that flow in this vessel (arrows) is hepatopedal (away from the liver), indicating that the umbilical vein is functioning as a portosystemic collateral.

PLATE I

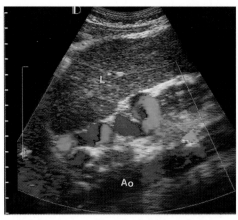

Figure 10-8—Splenogastroesophageal Collaterals. Large, tortuous collateral veins (mixed red and blue) are seen in the vicinity of the gastroesophageal junction on this longitudinal scan through the left lobe of the liver (L). These collaterals arose from the splenic hilum in this patient with chronic splenic vein occlusion. Ao = aorta.

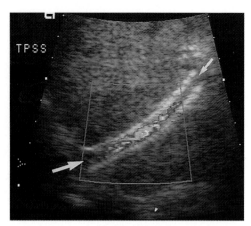

Figure 10-9—Transhepatic Portosystemic Shunt. Both the portal and hepatic venous ends of the shunt (arrrows) are visualized. Color Doppler examination demonstrated uniform flow throughout the shunt as well as normal flow velocity (not shown).

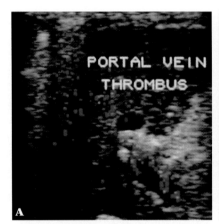

Figure 10-10A. Blood (blue color) flows around a thrombus within the portal vein in this patient with a hypercoagulable state and abdominal pain. Note that the portal vein is at most slightly dilated. (Findings confirmed with portal venography.)

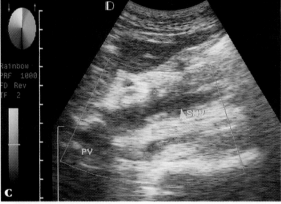

Figure 10-10C. No flow is evident in the portal vein (PV) and the superior mesenteric vein (SMV, arrow) in this patient with acute pancreatitis. Note that flow is visible in other vessels at an equal depth. The splenic vein (not shown) also was thrombosed.

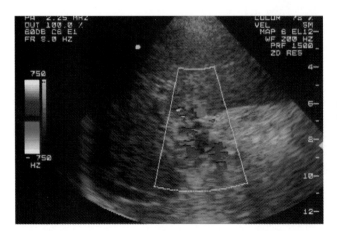

Figure 10-11B. Color Doppler examination confirms the presence of hepatofugal flow in these collaterals.

PLATE II

Chronic Findings

If portal vein thrombosis persists without substantial lysis, the portal vein undergoes fibrosis and may vanish from a sonographic perspective. Cavernous transformation of the portal vein is the principal manifestation of chronic portal vein thrombosis. Cavernous transformation produces a distinctive tangle of tortuous vessels in the porta hepatis (Fig. 10–11). The uninitiated sonographer may mistake these vessels for other pathology, including biliary dilatation. Duplex sonographic examination should prevent such errors, however, by demonstrating venous flow in the collateral vessels. A secondary sign of chronic portal vein occlusion is the development of portosystemic collaterals. These are identical in location and appearance to those described previously (Table 10–1, Fig. 10–3).

Diagnostic Accuracy

The sonographic diagnosis of portal vein occlusion is highly accurate (sensitivity, 94% to 100%, and specificity, 96%).[70-77] Although diagnostic errors are uncommon, three pitfalls are particularly noteworthy. First, recently formed thrombus that is virtually anechoic may remain undetected, as noted earlier. Second, patients with portal hypertension may have low velocity or to-and-fro portal flow that is difficult to detect with Doppler ultrasound, causing a false-positive impression of occlusion. Third, an inadequate Doppler angle may preclude detection of portal flow, leading to a false-positive diagnosis.

HEPATIC VEIN OCCLUSION

A second venous occlusive disorder that may be detected sonographically is hepatic vein occlusion, which results in a clinical complex called the Budd-Chiari syndrome.[2, 5, 75-88]

Pathology

The term "Budd-Chiari syndrome" refers to clinical and histologic abnormalities occurring in response to acute obstruction of hepatic vein flow.[76-79] The clinical abnormalities are hepatomegaly (due to congestion), abdominal pain (due to hepatomegaly) and abrupt development of ascites, and hepatocellular dysfunction (evidenced by biochemical tests). The histologic findings specific for the Budd-Chiari syndrome are centrizonal sinusoidal distention and pooling of blood in the sinusoids.

The causes of the Budd-Chiari syndrome are numerous and vary in relation to the primary site of obstruction, which may be sinusoids, at the hepatic vein level, or in the inferior vena cava (IVC). These three locations of venous occlusion are noteworthy:

1. With sinusoidal occlusion,* the major hepatic veins may remain patent, or they may become occluded *secondarily,* as a result of sluggish blood flow. Sonography can diagnose the sinusoidal form of the Budd-Chiari syndrome only when the hepatic veins undergo secondary thrombosis. Fortunately, the potential for false-negative studies is low since sinusoidal occlusion is rare.

2. *Primary* hepatic vein occlusion results either from thrombosis or tumor invasion. Thrombosis usually is related to cirrhosis (20% of cases)[75] or to hypercoagulable disorders. Neoplastic invasion is most often seen with hepatoma.

3. IVC occlusion or stenosis *cephalad to* the hepatic veins causes the Budd-Chiari syndrome by inducing hepatic vein congestion (backpressure) or secondary hepatic vein throm-

---

*Centrilobular venous occlusion sometimes is referred to by the confusing term "veno-occlusive disease of the liver."

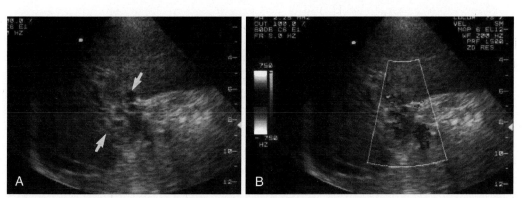

Figure 10-11—Cavernous Transformation of the Portal Veins. (A) An irregular tangle of vessels (arrows) is seen at the porta hepatis in this patient with a remote history of portal vein thrombosis due to abdominal sepsis. **(B)** Color Doppler examination confirms the presence of hepatofugal flow in these collaterals. (See Color Figure 10–11*B* following page 108.)

bosis. IVC obstruction may have a variety of causes, including congenital stenosis or occlusion,* thrombosis from hypercoagulable states, and neoplastic invasion. A Budd-Chiari-like syndrome may occur with excessive high right atrial pressure, as occurs with severe congestive heart failure or pericardial tamponade.

Sonographic Findings

The sonographic findings associated with hepatic vein obstruction fall into three categories: (1) direct manifestations of hepatic vein or IVC

---

*This rare condition is attributed to congenital causes; nevertheless, the Budd-Chiari syndrome frequently does not occur until the fifth decade of life (40+ years).

occlusion; (2) secondary morphologic changes in the liver; and (3) secondary extrahepatic findings.

Direct Sonographic Findings

The direct ultrasound manifestations of hepatic vein obstruction[2, 5, 6, 75, 76, 79–87] (Fig. 10–12) are the following:

1. Echogenic intraluminal material (thrombus or tumor).
2. Absence of hepatic vein flow.
3. Localized flow disturbances due to partial obstruction.
4. Continuous flow (Fig. 10–12C), to-and-fro flow, or reversed flow (rather than the normal, hepatofugal, pulsatile flow pattern) in the por-

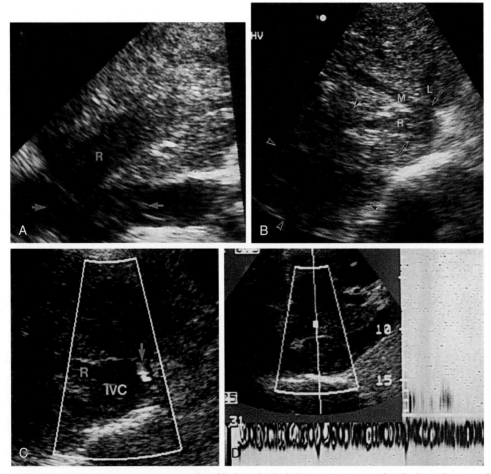

Figure 10-12—Hepatic Vein Occlusion. This elderly male alcoholic patient presented with classic features of the Budd-Chiari syndrome. **(A)** A coronal image of the right lobe of the liver shows a dilated, tumor-filled right hepatic vein (R), and tumor (arrows) within the IVC. **(B)** A transverse scan shows the tumor-filled right hepatic vein (R) and IVC (arrows). A poorly defined hypoechoic area (arrowheads), representing hepatic edema, is seen in the posterior portion of the right hepatic lobe. The middle (M) and left (L) hepatic veins were patent but exhibited sluggish flow. **(C)** Blood flow (arrow) from the middle and left hepatic veins passes through a narrow residual lumen between the tumor mass and the wall of the IVC. (Black-and-white representation of a transverse color Doppler image.) R = right hepatic vein. **(D)** Doppler flow signals in the middle and left hepatic veins are continuous, consistent with significant obstruction.

tions of the hepatic veins deep within the liver that remain patent.

5. Visualization of intrahepatic collateral veins° (under 1 cm and not following the usual course of hepatic vessels) that connect hepatic vein branches or connect the hepatic veins with portal or systemic veins.

6. Portal flow abnormalities, including biphasic or reversed portal flow, decreased flow velocity, or secondary portal occlusion.

When IVC occlusion causes the Budd-Chiari syndrome[2, 5, 6, 76–79, 82–85, 87, 88] (Fig. 10–12), the direct sonographic findings include the visualization of thrombus or tumor within the IVC lumen, accompanied by absence of flow, Doppler manifestations of stenosis, and abnormal flow patterns in the patient portion of the IVC and the iliac veins.

The occluding material in the IVC generates low-level echogenicity regardless of whether it is tumor or thrombus. Flow may be either absent or disturbed (in cases of stenosis) in the obstructed segment. Caudal portions of the IVC and the iliac veins typically remain patent. These vessels are dilated, and demonstrate flow abnormalities that may include a continuous flow pattern, flow reversal, and absence of the normal Valsalva response.

The hepatic veins usually become occluded secondarily in patients with IVC obstruction, either from stasis-related thrombosis or from tumor extension (Fig. 10–12). In some patients, however, the hepatic veins remain patent, and low-velocity antegrade flow is present in the hepatic veins, accompanied by *retrograde* flow in the patent portions of the IVC.

Secondary Morphologic Changes

Striking morphologic changes may occur in the liver in association with hepatic vein obstruction. Acutely, the portions of the liver subtended by obstructed veins are enlarged (swollen) and hypoechoic (Fig. 10–12B). In the subacute and chronic phases, the affected areas become fibrosed and shrink in size, and these areas may be relatively echogenic compared with normal hepatic parenchyma. The caudate or left lobes of the liver may undergo striking compensatory enlargement, since these portions of the liver are relatively spared from the effects of venous backpressure.

Secondary Extrahepatic Manifestations

Ascites, pleural effusion, and gallbladder edema are commonly seen in the acute stage of the Budd-Chiari syndrome. Splenomegaly and portosystemic collaterals may be evident in chronic cases, in relation to persistent portal hypertension.

The Problem of Nonvisualization

Empiric observations suggest that nonvisualization of the hepatic veins is of little diagnostic value when the Budd-Chiari syndrome is suspected, since the hepatic veins may sometimes be patent but invisible sonographically. *In my opinion, the Budd-Chiari syndrome can be excluded only when the patency of the major hepatic vein branches can be confirmed unequivocally.* If large segments of the hepatic veins cannot be seen clearly (from the IVC to deep within the liver), then no comment can be made with respect to the Budd-Chiari syndrome. It is easy to locate and follow the hepatic veins in a young, healthy individual, but this task may be difficult or impossible in a patient with a shrunken, cirrhotic liver.

REFERENCES

1. Sherlock S, Dooley J: Diseases of the Liver and Biliary System. 9th ed. London, Blackwell Scientific Publications, 1993, pp 132–178.
2. Koslin DB, Mulligan SA, Berland LL: Duplex assessment of the splanchnic vasculature. Semin Ultrasound CT MRI 13:34–39, 1992.
3. Zwiebel WJ, Fruechte D: Basics of abdominal and pelvic duplex: Instrumentation, anatomy, and vascular Doppler signatures. Semin Ultrasound CT MRI 13:3–21, 1992.
4. Ralls PW: Color Doppler sonography of the hepatic artery and portal venous system. AJR Am J Roentgenol 155:517–525, 1990.
5. Becker CD, Cooperberg PL: Sonography of the hepatic vascular system. AJR Am J Roentgenol 150:999–1005, 1988.
6. Bolondi L, Mazziotti A, Arienti V, Casanova P, Gasbarrini G, Cavallari A, Bellusci R, Gozzetti G, Possati L, Labo G: Ultrasonographic study of portal venous system in portal hypertension and after portosystemic shunt operations. Surgery 95:261–269, 1984.
7. Taylor KJW, Burns PN: Duplex Doppler scanning in the pelvis and abdomen. Ultrasound Med Biol 11:643–658, 1985.
8. Patriquin H, Lafortune M, Burns PN, Dauzat M: Duplex Doppler examination in portal hypertension: Technique and anatomy. AJR Am J Roentgenol 149:71–76, 1987.
9. Zierler BK, Horn JR, Bauer LA, Reiss WG, Strandness DE: Hepatic blood flow measurements

---

°These intrahepatic collaterals may communicate with non-occluded hepatic veins, the portal vein, or even systemic veins.

by duplex ultrasound: How to minimize variability. J Vasc Technol 15:16–22, 1991.

10. Parvey HR, Eisenberg RL, Giyanani V, Krebs CA: Duplex sonography of the portal venous system: Pitfalls and limitations. AJR Am J Roentgenol 152:765–770, 1989.

11. Bolondi L: The value of Doppler US in the study of hepatic hemodynamics (Consensus Conference Report, Bologna, Italy, 12 Sept 1989). J Hepatol 10:353–355, 1990.

12. Strohm VWD, Wehr B: Korrelation zwischen Lebervenverchylubfrick und sonographich bestimmtem Durchmesser von Pfortader und Milz bei Leberkranken. Z Gastroenterol 17:695–703, 1979.

13. Rahim N, Adam EJ: Ultrasound demonstration of variations in normal portal vein diameter with posture. Br J Radiol 58:313–314, 1985.

14. Weinreb J, Kumari S, Phillips G, Pochaczevski R: Portal vein measurements by real-time sonography. AJR Am J Roentgenol 139:497–499, 1982.

15. Rabinovici N, Narot N: The relationship between respiration, pressure and flow distribution in the vena cava and portal and hepatic veins. Surg Gynecol Obstet 151:753–763, 1980.

16. Moriyasu F, Ban N, Nishida O, Nakamura T, Miyake T, Uchino H, Kanematsu Y, Koizumi S: Clinical application of an ultrasonic duplex system in the quantitative measurement of portal blood flow. J Clin Ultrasound 14:579–588, 1986.

17. Zoli M, Dondi C, Marchesini G, et al: Splanchnic vein measurements in patients with liver cirrhosis: A case-control study. J Ultrasound Med 4:641–646, 1985.

18. Goyal AK, Pokharna DS, Sharma SK: Ultrasonic measurements of portal vasculature in diagnosis of portal hypertension. A controversial subject reviewed. J Ultrasound Med 9:45–48, 1990.

19. Cottone M, D'Amico G, Maringhini A, et al: Predictive value of ultrasonography in the screening of non-ascitic cirrhotic patients with large varices. J Ultrasound Med 5:189–192, 1965.

20. Bolondi L, Gamrolfi L, Arienti V, et al: Ultrasonography in the diagnosis of portal hypertension: Diminished response of portal vessels to respiration. Radiology 142:167–172, 1982.

21. Bolondi L, Mazziotti A, Arienti V, et al: Ultrasonographic study of portal venous system in portal hypertension and after portosystemic shunt operations. Surgery 95:261–269, 1984.

22. Moriyasu F, Ban N, Nishida O, Nakamura T, Soh Y, Miura K, Sakai M, Miyake T, Uchino H: Portal hemodynamics in patients with hepatocellular carcinoma. Radiology 161:707–711, 1986.

23. Moriyasu F, Nishida O, Ban N, Nakamura T, Sakai M, Miyake T, Ochino H: "Congestion Index" of the portal vein. AJR Am J Roentgenol 146:735–739, 1986.

24. Gaiani S, Bolondi L, Li Bassi S, Santi V, Zironi G, Barbara L: Effect of meal on portal hemodynamics in healthy humans and in patients with chronic liver disease. Hepatology 9:815–819, 1989.

25. Hosoki T, Arisawa J, Marukawa T, Tokunaga K, Kuroda C, Kozuka T, Nakano S: Portal blood flow in congestive heart failure: Pulsed duplex sonographic findings. Radiology 174:733–736, 1990.

26. Duerinckx A, Grant EG, Perrella RR, Szeto A, Tessler FN: The pulsatile portal vein in cases of congestive heart failure: Correlation of duplex Doppler findings with right atrial pressures. Radiology 176:655–658, 1990.

27. DeCandio G, Campstelli A, Mosca F, et al: Ultrasound detection of unusual spontaneous portosystemic shunts associated with uncomplicated portal hypertension. J Ultrasound Med 4:297–305, 1985.

28. Patriquin H, Tessier G, Grignon A, Boisvert J: Lesser omental thickness in normal children: Baseline for detection of portal hypertension. AJR Am J Roentgenol 145:693–696, 1985.

29. Neumaier CE, Cicco GR, Derchi LE, Biggi E: The patent ductus venosus: An additional ultrasonic finding in portal hypertension. J Clin Ultrasound 11:231–233, 1983.

30. West MS, Garra BS, Horii SC, Hayes WS, Cooper C, Silverman PM, Zeman RK: Gallbladder varices: Imaging findings in patients with portal hypertension. Radiology 179:179–182, 1991.

31. Marchal GF, Van Holsbeeck M, Tschibwabwa-Ntumba E, Goddeeris PG, Fevery J, Oyen RH, Adisoejoso B, Baert AL, Van Steenbergen W: Dilatation of the cystic veins in portal hypertension: Sonographic demonstration. Radiology 154:187–189, 1985.

32. Brady TM, Gross BH, Glazer GM, Williams DM: Adrenal pseudomasses due to varices: Angiographic-CT-MRI-pathologic correlations. AJR Am J Roentgenol 145:301–304, 1985.

33. Di Candio G, Campatelli A, Mosca F, Santi V, Casanova P, and Bolondi L: Ultrasound detection of unusual spontaneous portosystemic shunts associated with uncomplicated portal hypertension. J Ultrasound Med 4:297–305, 1985.

34. Jüttner H-U, Jenney JM, Ralls PW, Goldstein LI, Reynolds TB: Ultrasound demonstration of portosystemic collaterals in cirrhosis and portal hypertension. Radiology 142:459–463, 1982.

35. Dökmeci AK, Kimura K, Matsutani S, Ohto M, Ono T, Tsuchiya Y, Saisho H, Okuda K: Collateral veins in portal hypertension: Demonstration by sonography. AJR Am J Roentgenol 137:1173–1177, 1981.

36. Dach JL, Hill MC, Palaez JC, LePage JR, Russell E: Sonography of hypertensive portal venous system: Correlation with arterial portography. AJR Am J Roentgenol 137:511–517, 1981.

37. Mori H, Hayashi K, Fukuda T, Matsunaga N, Futagawa S, Nagasaki M, Mutsukura M: Intrahepatic portosystemic venous shunt: Occurrence in patients with and without liver cirrhosis. AJR Am J Roentgenol 149:711–714, 1987.

38. Sie A, Johnson MB, Lee KP, Ralls PW: Color Doppler sonography in spontaneous splenorenal portosystemic shunts. J Ultrasound Med 10:167–169, 1991.

39. Subramanyam BR, Balthazar EJ, Raghavenadra BN, Lefleur RS: Sonographic evaluation of patients with portal hypertension. Am J Gastroenterol 78:369–373, 1983.

40. Subramanyam BR, Balthazar EJ, Madamba MR, Raghavendra BN, Horii SC, and Lefleur RS: Sonography of porto-systemic collaterals in portal hypertension. Radiology 146:161–166, 1983.

41. Takayasu K, Moriyama N, Shima Y, Yamada T, Kobayashi C, Musha H, Okuda K: Sonographic detection of large spontaneous spleno-renal shunts and its clinical significance. Br J Radiol 57:565–570, 1984.

42. Lafortune M, Marleau D, Breton G, Vaillet A, Lavoie P, Huet P-M: Portal venous system measurements in portal hypertension. Radiology 151:27–30, 1984.

43. Schabel S, Rittenberg GM, Javid LH, Cunningham J, Ross P: The "bull's-eye" falciform ligament: A sonographic finding of portal hypertension. Radiology 136:157–159, 1980.

44. Saddekni S, Hutchinson DE, Cooperberg PL: The sonographically patent umbilical vein in portal hypertension. Radiology 145:441–443, 1982.

45. Aagaard J, Jensen LI, Sørensen TIA, Christensen U, Burcharth F: Recanalized umbilical vein in portal hypertension. AJR Am J Roentgenol 139:1107–1109, 1982.

46. Lafortune M, Constantin A, Breton G, Légaré AG, Lavoie P: The recanalized umbilical vein in portal hypertension: A myth. AJR Am J Roentgenol 144:549–553, 1985.

47. Gibson RN, Gibson PR, Donlan JD, Clunie DA: Identification of a patent paraumbilical vein by using Doppler sonography: Importance in the diagnosis of portal hypertension. AJR Am J Roentgenol 153:513–516, 1989.

48. Mostbeck GH, Wittich GR, Herold C, Vergesslich KA, Walter RM, Frotz S, Sommer G: Hemodynamic significance of the paraumbilical vein in portal hypertension: Assessment with duplex US. Radiology 170:339–342, 1989.

49. Marn CS, Glazer GM, Williams DM, Francis IR: CT-angiographic correlation of collateral venous pathways in isolated splenic vein occlusion: New observations. Radiology 175:375–380, 1990.

50. Rice S, Lee KP, Johnson MB, Korula J, Ralls PW: Portal venous system after portosystemic shunts or endoscopic sclerotherapy: Evaluation with Doppler sonography. AJR Am J Roentgenol 156:85–89, 1991.

51. O'Connor SE, LaBombard E, Musson AM, Zwolak RM: Duplex imaging of distal splenorenal shunts. J Vasc Technol 15:28–31, 1991.

52. Chezmar JL, Bernardino ME: Mesoatrial shunt for the treatment of Budd-Chiari syndrome: Radiologic evaluation in eight patients. AJR Am J Roentgenol 149:707–710, 1987.

53. Lafortune M, Patriquin H, Pomier G, Huet PM, Weber A, Lavoie P, Blanchard H, Breton G: Hemodynamic changes in portal circulation after portosystemic shunts: Use of duplex sonography in 43 patients. AJR Am J Roentgenol 149:701–706, 1987.

54. Patriquin H, Lafortune M, Weber A, Blanchard H, Garel L, Roy C: Surgical portosystemic shunts in children: Assessment with duplex Doppler US. Radiology 165:25–28, 1987.

55. Grant EG, Tessler FN, Gomes AS, Holmes CL, Perrella RR, Duerinckx AJ, Busuttil RW: Color Doppler imaging of portosystemic shunts. AJR Am J Roentgenol 154:393–397, 1990.

56. Bolondi L, Gaiani S, Mazziotti A, Casanova P, Cavallari A, Gozzetti G, Barbara L: Morphological and hemodynamic changes in the portal venous system after distal splenorenal shunt: An ultrasound and pulsed Doppler study. Hepatology 8:652–657, 1988.

57. Khedkar N, Traverso L, Walat S, et al: Transjugular intrahepatic portosystemic shunt (TIPS) duplex imaging. Presented at the 17th Annual Conference of the Society for Vascular Technology. J Vasc Technology 17:192, 1993.

58. Chong WK, Malisch TW, Mazer MJ: Sonographic transjugular intrahepatic portosystemic shunts. Semin Ultrasound CT MRI 16:69–80, 1995.

59. Grendell JH, Ockner RK: Mesenteric venous thrombosis. *In* Sleisinger MH, Fordtran JS (eds): Gastrointestinal Disease. Philadelphia, WB Saunders, 1983, pp 1557–1558.

60. Johnson CC, Baggenstoss AH: Mesenteric vascular occlusion: Study of 99 cases of occlusion of veins. Mayo Clin Proc 24:628–636, 1949.

61. North JP, Wollenman OJ: Venous mesenteric occlusion in the course of migratory thrombophlebitis. Surg Gynecol Obstet 95:665–671, 1952.

62. Babcock DS: Ultrasound diagnosis of portal vein thrombosis as a complication of appendicitis. AJR Am J Roentgenol 133:317–319, 1979.

63. Verbanck JJ, Rutgeerts LJ, Haerens MH, Tytgat JH, Segaert MF, Tytgat HJ, Afschrift MB: Partial splenoportal and superior mesenteric venous thrombosis. Gastroenterology 86:949–952, 1984.

64. Papanicolaou N, Harmatz P, Simeone JF, Truman JT, Ferrucci JT: Sonographic demonstration of reversible portal vein thrombosis following splenectomy in an adolescent. J Clin Ultrasound 12:575–577, 1984.

65. Merritt CBR: Ultrasonographic demonstration of portal vein thrombosis. Radiology 133:425–427, 1979.

66. Marx M, Scheible W: Cavernous transformation of the portal vein. J Ultrasound Med 1:167–169, 1982.

67. Subramanyam BR, Balthazar EJ, Lefleur RS, Horii SC, Hulnick DH: Portal venous thrombosis: Correlative analysis of sonography, CT, and angiography. Am J Gastroenterol 79:773–776, 1984.

68. Kauzlaric D, Petrovic M, Barmeir J: Sonography of cavernous transformation of the portal vein. AJR Am J Roentgenol 142:383–384, 1984.

69. Weltin G, Taylor KJW, Carter AR, Taylor CR: Duplex Doppler: Identification of cavernous transformation of the portal vein. AJR Am J Roentgenol 144:999–1001, 1985.

70. Gansbeke FV, Avni EF, Delcour C, Engelholm L, Struyven J: Sonographic features of portal vein thrombosis. AJR Am J Roentgenol 144:749–752, 1985.

71. Tessler FN, Gehring BJ, Gomes AS, Perrella RR, Ragavendra N, Busuttil RW, Grant EG: Diagnosis of portal vein thrombosis: Value of color Doppler imaging. AJR Am J Roentgenol 157:293–296, 1991.

72. Wang L-Y, Lin Z-Y, Chang W-Y, Chen S-C, Chuang W-L, Hsieh M-Y, Tsai J-F, Okuda K: Duplex pulsed Doppler sonography of portal vein thrombosis in hepatocellular carcinoma. J Ultrasound Med 10:265–269, 1991.

73. Subramanyam BR, Balthazer EJ, Hilton S, et al: Hepatocellular carcinoma with venous invasion. Radiology 150:793–796, 1984.

74. Atri M, de Stempel J, Bret PM, Illescas FF: Incidence of portal vein thrombosis complicating liver metastasis as detected by duplex ultrasound. J Ultrasound Med 9:285–289, 1990.

75. Pollard JJ, Nebesar RA: Altered hemodynamics in the Budd-Chiari syndrome demonstrated by selective hepatic and splenic angiography. Radiology 89:236–243, 1967.

76. Chopra S: Budd-Chiari syndrome and veno-occlusive disease. Disorders of the Liver. Philadelphia, Lea & Febiger, 1988, pp 156–162.

77. Stanley P: Budd-Chiari syndrome. Radiology 170:625–627, 1989.

78. Cho KJ, Geisinger KR, Shields JJ, Forrest ME: Collateral channels and histopathology in hepatic vein occlusion. AJR Am J Roentgenol 139:703–709, 1982.

79. Murphy FB, Steinberg HV, Shires GT, Martin LG,

Bernardino ME: The Budd-Chiari syndrome: A review. AJR Am J Roentgenol 147:9–15, 1986.

80. Mathieu D, Vasile N, Menu Y, Van Beers B, Lorphelin JM, Pringot J: Budd-Chiari syndrome: Dynamic CT. Radiology 165:409–413, 1987.

81. Harter LP, Gross BH, St Hilaire J, Filly RA, Goldberg HI: CT and sonographic appearance of hepatic vein obstruction. AJR Am J Roentgenol 139:176–178, 1982.

82. Baert AL, Fevery J, Marchal G, Goddeeris P, Wilms G, Ponette E, De Groote J: Early diagnosis of Budd-Chiari syndrome by computed tomography and ultrasonography: Report of five cases. Gastroenterology 84:587–595, 1983.

83. Makuuchi M, Hasegawa H, Yamazaki S, Moriyama N, Takayasu K, Okazaki M: Primary Budd-Chiari syndrome: Ultrasonic demonstration. Radiology 152:775–779, 1984.

84. Menu Y, Alison D, Lorphelin J-M, Valla D, Belghiti J, Nahum H: Budd-Chiari syndrome: US evaluation. Radiology 157:761–764, 1985.

85. Grant EG, Perrella R, Tessler FN, Lois J, Busuttil R: Budd-Chiari syndrome: The results of duplex and color Doppler imaging. AJR Am J Roentgenol 152:377–381, 1989.

86. Brown BP, Abu-Yousef M, Farner R, LaBrecque D, Gingrich R: Doppler sonography: A noninvasive method for evaluation of hepatic veno-occlusive disease. AJR Am J Roentgenol 154:721–724, 1990.

87. Hosoki T, Kuroda C, Tokunaga K, Marukawa T, Masuike M, Kozuka T: Hepatic venous outflow obstruction: Evaluation with pulsed duplex sonography. Radiology 170:733–737, 1989.

88. Takayasu K, Moriyama N, Muramatsu Y, Goto H, Shima Y, Yamada T, Makuuchi M, Yamasaki S, Hasegawa H, Hojo K: Intrahepatic venous collaterals forming via the inferior right hepatic vein in 3 patients with obstruction of the inferior vena cava. Radiology 154:323–328, 1985.

Chapter 11
The Spleen

William J. Zwiebel

The spleen is included in most upper abdominal sonograms; furthermore, the spleen serves as a convenient "window" for visualization of the left subphrenic space, the left pleural space, and the upper lesser sac. Although splenic examination is seldom a *primary* sonographic objective, sonographers should be familiar with normal and abnormal features of the spleen since this organ may exhibit important pathologic findings.

NORMAL FEATURES

The spleen is a lymphoreticular organ that has hematopoietic, hemolytic, immune, and detoxification functions.[1] It is situated posterolaterally within the left upper quadrant of the abdominal cavity, adjacent to the diaphragm and the lateral abdominal wall (Fig. 11–1). The shape of the spleen is variable, but in all cases it is more or less bean shaped, with a convex outer border (posterolateral) and a flat or concave inner border (anteromedial). The spleen lies in close proximity to the stomach, the left kidney, the left adrenal gland, and the pancreatic tail.

The splenic artery and vein are attached at the slitlike hilum, located on the inner (convex) splenic border. The artery and the vein branch *before* entering the hilum, and it is noteworthy that the coalescence of the vein branches may be up to 6 cm from the hilum. This anatomic feature may have important imaging consequences in patients with portal vein thrombosis or portal hypertension, as discussed in Chapter 10.

On sonographic examination, the spleen is smoothly marginated and lies *adjacent* to the diaphragm and body wall. Displacement of the spleen from these structures suggests pathologic fluid accumulation. The splenic parenchyma is less echogenic than the liver and has a homogeneous, fine-grained sonographic "texture" (Fig. 11–2).

SIZE ASSESSMENT

Splenic size may be assessed in a variety of ways. I prefer a simple yet accurate method: measurement of the maximal longitudinal dimension of the organ, either in the parasagittal or coronal plane (Fig. 11–2). The normal spleen does not exceed 13 cm in length in adults aged 50 years or less, or 11 cm in older adults.[1] Table 11–1 lists normal splenic lengths in children in relation to age.[2]

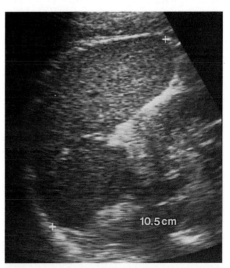

Figure 11-2—Normal Sonographic Features (coronal view). The normal spleen is homogeneous in texture and is slightly less echogenic than the liver (not shown). The cursors (+) illustrate the method for measuring splenic length (10.5 cm in this case).

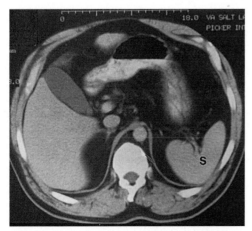

Figure 11-1—Splenic Location. A computed tomogram illustrates the posterolateral position of the spleen (S) and its relationship to surrounding viscera.

Table 11-1. Splenic Length in Children in Relation to Age

Age	Median Length (cm)	Suggested Maximum Length (cm)
At birth	4.5	6.0
1 yr	6.9	8.0
2 and 3 yr	7.4	9.0
4 and 5 yr	7.8	9.5
6 and 7 yr	8.2	10.0
8 and 9 yr	9.2	11.0
10 and 11 yr	9.9	11.5
12–14 yr	10.1	12.0
15–19 yr	10.0 (female)	12.0 (female)
	11.2 (male)	13.0 (male)

Adapted from Rosenberg HK, Markowitz RI, Kolberg H, et al: Normal splenic size in infants and children: Sonographic measurement. AJR Am J Roentgenol 157:119–121, 1991.

EXAMINATION TECHNIQUE

The spleen is best visualized with ultrasound with the patient in a right lateral decubitus position (left side up), using coronal or near-coronal images obtained from a lateral or posterolateral transducer position. Transverse or oblique splenic images also may be useful and are obtained from a similar patient and transducer position.

ANOMALIES

Accessory spleens probably are the most common splenic anomaly.[1, 3–5] One or more foci of accessory splenic tissue (Fig. 11–3) are present in 10% to 25% of normal individuals.[1, 3] Most accessory spleens are less than 1 cm in size, but they may occasionally be as large as 4 cm in

diameter.[1, 3] When larger accessory spleens are visualized sonographically, they may be mistaken for lymphadenopathy or neoplastic masses. The location of accessory spleens is variable, but most are adjacent to the *medial* border of the spleen.

Congenital clefts occur commonly in the spleen,[1, 4] and these may be mistaken for lacerations or fractures in trauma patients. Two varieties occur: (1) narrow fissures along the outer, convex surface, and (2) wider clefts along the medial border.

The "wandering spleen"[1, 3, 6] is an unusually mobile spleen that moves from its usual left upper quadrant location as the patient changes position. Both ligamentous laxity and emaciation may contribute to the wandering tendency. The errant spleen may lie anterior to the left kidney or at more distant locations, such as the left iliac fossa or even the true pelvis. The wandering spleen usually is mistaken for a neoplastic mass and is subject to infarction because of torsion of the vascular pedicle.

Splenic agenesis[1] is a rare but important condition. In 25% of cases, splenic agenesis is an isolated anomaly or is associated only with gastric hypoplasia. In the remaining 75% of cases, splenic agenesis is a component of the asplenia syndrome, and it is, therefore, associated with cardiac malformations (frequently major) and defects of body symmetry. The latter may include midline position of the liver, bowel malrotation, cardiac malposition, and situs abnormalities.

SPLENOMEGALY

Splenomegaly, or enlargement of the spleen,[7–9] may result from a wide variety of diseases. As an aid to differential diagnosis, it is useful to group the causes of splenomegaly into a few general categories, as listed in Table 11–2.

Reactive Splenomegaly

Reactive splenomegaly connotes splenic enlargement in response to systemic disease. Stimuli for reactive splenomegaly include immune, hematopoietic, hemolytic, or infectious disorders. Examples include infectious mononucleosis,

Table 11-2. General Causes of Splenomegaly

Reaction to systemic disease
Primary neoplasms
Secondary neoplasms
Portal hypertension
Trauma
Cysts
Abscesses

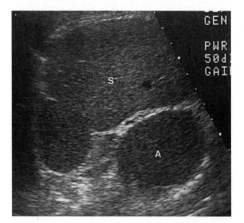

Figure 11-3—Accessory Spleen. A large accessory spleen (A) is seen adjacent to the medial aspect of the spleen (S) in a patient with idiopathic polysplenia.

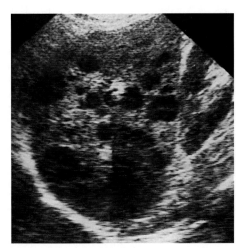

Figure 11-4—Splenic Metastases. Multiple hypoechoic and slightly heterogeneous metastases are present in the spleen in a patient with widely disseminated uroepithelial carcinoma.

juvenile rheumatoid arthritis, hemolytic anemias, and myelofibrosis with extramedullary hematopoiesis.

PRIMARY NEOPLASMS

Lymphoma[8, 10] is by far the most common primary neoplasm affecting the spleen. One third of all patients with lymphoma (regardless of cell type) exhibit splenic involvement at some time during the course of the illness. In 90% of such cases, however, the tumor infiltrates the spleen without producing discrete masses. Therefore, splenomegaly is the only sonographic abnormality in most cases of splenic lymphoma. In the remaining cases, lymphoma produces discrete, rounded, hypoechoic masses similar to those shown in Figure 11–4. Typically, these masses are multiple and are accompanied by splenomegaly.

Other primary tumors of the spleen[8, 10] are rare and include hemangiomas, dermoids, and sarcomas. Hemangiomas generally have the same ultrasound and computed tomographic features as their hepatic analogues (chapter 8). Dermoids may resemble ovarian dermoids, and sarcomas tend to produce bulky masses with large areas of necrosis.

SECONDARY NEOPLASMS

Splenic metastases[8] are found at autopsy in 50% to 67% of patients with *disseminated* neoplasms of thoracic or abdominal origin. These metastases are only rarely visualized sonographically, however, since they generally are small, and the spleen is seldom examined in great detail.

Splenic metastases (Fig. 11–4) seen with ultrasound are either well defined or poorly defined, round or irregular, and homogeneous or inhomogenous.[8, 10] They typically are less echogenic than the normal splenic parenchyma, but echogenicity varies. Multiplicity of lesions is the rule, and the spleen usually is enlarged.

PORTAL HYPERTENSION

Elevated portal venous pressure may cause the spleen to enlarge, and splenomegaly is a significant manifestation of portal hypertension. This subject is considered further in Chapter 10.

TRAUMA

The spleen has been likened in structure to a "vascular sponge."[7] The structural components of this sponge are relatively sparse, and the spleen, therefore, is subject to damage from concussive as well as penetrating trauma. Computed tomography is the preferred means for evaluating trauma patients; nonetheless, sonologists should be aware of the ultrasound manifestations of acute trauma, in the event that these are encountered incidentally. Splenic trauma may produce any of the following findings:[7]

1. Splenomegaly
2. Free intraperitoneal blood, adjacent to or distant from the spleen
3. Curved or crescentic subcapsular hematomas
4. Rounded, linear, or irregular intrasplenic hematomas (Fig. 11–5)

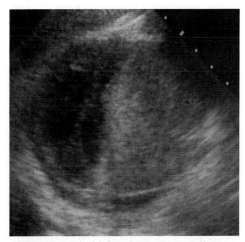

Figure 11-5—Splenic Hematoma. A large hypoechoic hematoma is visible in the spleen adjacent to the diaphragm. Linear echogenicity is present in the collection, consistent with clot retraction. Etiology: blunt trauma from a motor vehicle accident.

5. A nonhomogeneous splenic texture, due to diffuse contusion and hematoma formation
6. A normal-appearing spleen accompanied by free intraperitoneal blood

Splenic hematomas, like hematomas at other locations, vary in echogenicity in relation to the state of thrombus evolution.[7, 11] This subject is considered in detail in Chapter 7. Splenic hematomas are reabsorbed slowly, typically over a period of weeks-to-months.[7, 11, 12] Uncommonly, a splenic hematoma fails to resolve and persists as a post-traumatic pseudocyst (a cyst without an epithelial lining). Splenic pseudocysts may be very large and may cause symptoms by compressing adjacent organs. They also are subject to rupture.

On ultrasound examination, splenic pseudocysts generally are anechoic and well defined, but they may contain clumped or layered echogenic material, or they may be diffusely echogenic.[7, 10–12] No ultrasound features differentiate with certainty between pseudocysts and other fluid-containing lesions, such as abscesses, true cysts, and echinococcal cysts (discussed later).

Splenic Infarction

Infarction of a portion of the spleen[9, 13, 14] is an infrequent complication of sepsis, hemolytic anemia, and myeloproliferative disorders. Splenomegaly is a usual concomitant of infarction.

During the acute and subacute stages, splenic infarcts are hypoechoic on ultrasound examination (Fig. 11–6). The margins of the lesion vary from poorly defined to well defined. Splenic infarcts may be complicated by subcapsular hematoma formation, splenic rupture, and free intraperitoneal fluid (blood). Differentiation from

Table 11-3. Cysts and Cystslike Lesions of the Spleen

Idiopathic serous (simple) cysts
Neoplastic cysts of epithelial, mesothelial or endothelial origin (e.g., dermoid)
Pseudocysts (post-traumatic or postinfarction)
Hematoma
Infarct
Abscess
Parasitic cysts

traumatic hematomas, abscesses, or other hypoechoic lesions is not possible. Splenic infarcts gradually resolve over weeks to months, in a fashion similar to hematomas, and may leave a residual area of echogenicity attributed to scarring.

Cysts and Cystlike Lesions

True cysts, pseudocysts (discussed earlier), parasitic cysts, and abscesses of the spleen are conveniently lumped together in this section, since they have similar sonographic features and often are indistinguishable on the basis of ultrasound findings. Cysts and cystlike lesions are classified in Table 11–3. The following caveats are noteworthy concerning sonographic differentiation among these lesions:[9, 10, 12, 15–17]

1. The benign, endothelium-lined, "simple" cyst of the spleen (Fig. 11–7) has ultrasound features identical to simple cysts of the liver and kidney as described in Chapter 7.
2. Simple splenic cysts may occur sporadically or in conjunction with polycystic kidney disease.
3. Primary splenic cysts other than simple cysts occur rarely and may originate from epithelial, mesothelial, or endothelial elements. The sonographic features of these cysts vary from

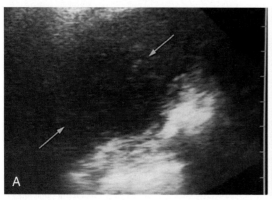
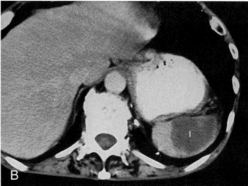

Figure 11-6—Splenic Infarct. (A) A poorly defined, hypoechoic splenic infarct (arrows) is barely visible in this patient with a hypercoagulable state. Note how difficult it is to visualize the abnormal area. **(B)** The infarct (I) is seen much more clearly on a contrast-enhanced computed tomogram. Note the absence of mass effect.

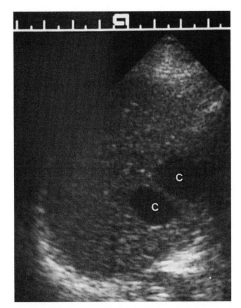

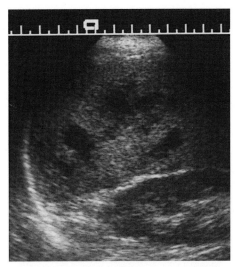

Figure 11-9—Splenic Abscess. A cluster of poorly defined abscesses is visible in the spleen in this patient with autoimmune deficiency syndrome.

Figure 11-7—Simple Cyst. Two anechoic splenic cysts (C) are visible in the sonogram of this elderly woman with biliary tract obstruction. Enhanced through-transmission is not clearly seen in this view because of difficulties with scanning through the intercostal spaces. Typical cyst features were seen with computed tomography.

classic simple cyst features to an apparently solid appearance.

4. Parasitic cysts of the spleen may occur with amebic and echinococcal infestation as well as a variety of other parasites not included in this text. The splenic manifestations of amebic and echinococcal cysts are analogous to those described in Chapter 7.

5. About 10% of nonparasitic splenic cysts are heavily calcified.[8] The differential diagnosis of a heavily calcified splenic lesion (Fig. 11–8) includes primary neoplastic cyst (e.g., dermoid), chronic hematoma, post-traumatic pseudocyst, and calcified echinococcal cyst.

6. Splenic abscesses[16, 17] (Fig. 11–9) have sonographic features similar to those seen in cases of liver abscess (Chapter 7). It is noteworthy that abscesses of the spleen may be poorly defined and difficult to appreciate sonographically.

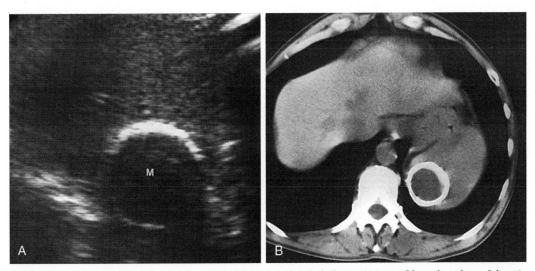

Figure 11-8—Calcified Splenic Mass. (A) A circular, heavily calcified mass (M) is visible in the spleen of this 48 year old man examined for possible cholelithiasis. **(B)** A computed tomogram shows that the lesion is a calcified "cyst." The etiology remains obscure as the lesion was asymptomatic and the patient did not agree that our curiosity warranted splenectomy.

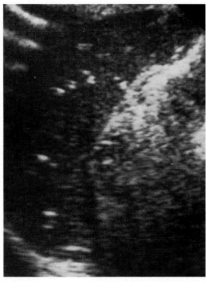

Figure 11-10—Multiple Splenic Granulomas.
Multiple highly reflective foci are seen incidentally in the spleen of an elderly man examined for possible urinary tract obstruction.

Diffuse Calcification

Diffuse, punctate splenic calcification (Fig. 11–10) is seen fairly commonly during splenic examination. The most common cause of such calcification in the United States is systemic *Histoplasma capsulatum* infection. This organism is confined by means of granuloma formation, and the granulomas subsequently calcify. The patient almost always is unaware of the *H. capsulatum* infection. Identical splenic calcification may develop in response to *Mycobacterium tuberculosis* infection. Additional, less common causes of diffuse splenic calcification are *Brucella* species and the formation of phleboliths in splenic veins.[18]

REFERENCES

1. Senecail B: Sonographic anatomy of the normal spleen, normal anatomic variants, and pitfalls. *In* Bruneton JN (ed): Ultrasonography of the Spleen. Berlin, Springer-Verlag, 1988, pp 1–13.
2. Rosenberg HK, Markowitz RI, Kolberg H, et al: Normal splenic size in infants and children: Sonographic measurement. AJR Am J Roentgenol 157:119–121, 1991.
3. Tran-Minh V, Pracros JP, Deffrenne P, Morin de Fine CH: Congenital anomalies of the spleen. *In* Bruneton JN (ed): Ultrasonography of the Spleen. Berlin, Springer-Verlag, 1988, pp 14–32.
4. Dodds WJ, Taylor AJ, Erickson SJ, Stewart ET, Lawson TL: Radiologic imaging of splenic anomalies. AJR Am J Roentgenol 155:805–810, 1990.
5. Subramanyam BR, Balthazar EJ, Horii SC: Sonography of the accessory spleen. AJR Am J Roentgenol 143:47–49, 1984.
6. Tait NP, Young JR: The wandering spleen: An ultrasonic diagnosis. J Clin Ultrasound 13:141–144, 1985.
7. Benozio M: Splenic trauma. *In* Bruneton JN (ed): Ultrasonography of the Spleen. Berlin, Springer-Verlag, 1988, pp 33–45.
8. Bruneton JN, Balu-Maestro C, Drouillard J, Normand F, Fuzibet JG: Splenic tumors. *In* Bruneton JN (ed): Ultrasonography of the Spleen. Berlin, Springer-Verlag, 1988, pp 46–62.
9. Anagnostoupoulos C, Jacquenod P, Chagnon S, Blery M: Splenic abscess and infarction. *In* Bruneton JN (ed): Ultrasonography of the Spleen. Berlin, Springer-Verlag, 1988, pp 63–69.
10. Goerg C, Schwerk WB, Goerg K: Sonography of focal lesions of the spleen. AJR Am J Roentgenol 156:949–953, 1991.
11. Lupien C, Sauerbrei EE: Healing in the traumatized spleen: Sonographic investigation. Radiology 151:181–185, 1984.
12. Dachman AH, Ros PR, Murari PJ, Olmsted WW, Lichtenstein JE: Nonparasitic splenic cysts: A report of 52 cases with radiologic-pathologic correlation. AJR Am J Roentgenol 147:537–542, 1986.
13. Maresca G, Mirk P, De Gaetano AM, Barbaro B, Colagrande C: Sonographic patterns in splenic infarct. J Clin Ultrasound 14:23–28, 1986.
14. Goerg C, Schwerk WB: Splenic infarction: Sonographic patterns, diagnosis, follow-up, and complications. Radiology 174:803–807, 1990.
15. Gharbi HA, Marbot P, Ben Cheikh M: Splenic involvement in parasitoses. *In* Bruneton JN (ed): Ultrasonography of the Spleen. Berlin, Springer-Verlag, 1988, pp 70–85.
16. Pawar S, Kay CJ, Gonzalez R, Taylor KJW, Rosenfield AT: Sonography of splenic abscess. AJR Am J Roentgenol 138:259–262, 1982.
17. Hertzanu Y, Mendelsohn DB, Goudie E, Butterworth A: Splenic abscess: A review of the value of ultrasound. Clin Radiol 34:661–667, 1983.
18. Eisenberg RL: Clinical Imaging: An Atlas of Differential Diagnosis. 2nd ed. Gaithersberg, MD, Aspen Publishers, Inc, 1992, pp 396–397.

Section 4
The Biliary System

INTRODUCTION

Those of you who are old enough to remember the cephalin flocculation test and oral cholecystography can appreciate the impact ultrasound has had on medical diagnosis. In case you are not that old, cephalin flocculation was one of a battery of tests used to try to determine whether a jaundiced patient was suffering from biliary obstruction or hepatocellular disease. Oral cholecystography was used to visualize the gallbladder radiographically and detect gallstones. The biliary tract examination became much easier and much more accurate when ultrasound came along, and the pioneers in the field were quick to appreciate the potential of ultrasound biliary imaging. In the days of static ultrasound scanners, we did pretty well examining the biliary tract, but biliary sonography really came into its own with high resolution real-time imaging. Presently, ultrasound is by far the most common imaging method used for biliary tract diagnosis.

As an ultrasound practitioner, it is likely that you will examine the biliary tract as often as anything else in the abdomen, and it is important, therefore, that you acquire the essentials of this examination. To this end we present the biliary tract in four parts dealing with anatomy, calculi, gallbladder pathology, and biliary obstruction.

Chapter 12

The Biliary System: Sonographic Technique and Anatomy

William J. Zwiebel

GALLBLADDER ANATOMY

The gallbladder (Figs. 12–1, 12–2) is an ovoid, sonolucent structure that projects inferiorly from the major interlobar fissure of the liver (between the right and left lobes).[1-4] The neck of the gallbladder is funnel-like and trails off into the interlobar fissure, where it communicates with the cystic duct. The fundus of the gallbladder (the rounded, caudal portion) hangs freely within the peritoneal space. The cystic duct, which connects the gallbladder with the bile duct, has a serpen-tine shape, caused by the valves of Heister within its muscular wall. Because of this serpentine configuration, and its small size, the cystic duct is not often visualized during *routine* sonographic examination. With a detailed search, however, the cystic duct can be seen in about 50% of normal individuals and does not exceed 5 mm in diameter.[5] The cystic duct may be visualized more easily when the biliary system is dilated (Fig. 12–2*B*).

Gallbladder Size

The size and shape of the gallbladder are extremely variable, as indicated by volume measurements that range from 2.4 to 40 ml (5th to 95th percentile) in normal individuals.[6-10] Gallbladder size, therefore, generally is not a good parameter for defining normality or abnormality. Nonetheless, gallbladder size and shape should not be disregarded out-of-hand. Most normal gallbladders do not exceed 4 cm in diameter[11]; therefore, a very large gallbladder (greater than 6 cm in diameter or over 12 cm long) should at least call to mind the possibility of pathologic dilatation. Likewise, an inordinately small gallbladder should be viewed with suspicion for pathology. For example, a 3-cm-long gallbladder should not be passed over as unremarkable in an adult man who has been fasting for 12 hours. Chronic cholecystitis (Chapter 14) is the primary consideration when the gallbladder is inordinately small, but there are other potential causes, including reduced bile production in severe liver disease, bile duct obstruction proximal to the gallbladder, and recent ingestion of food.

The Gallbladder Wall

The interior surface of the normal gallbladder wall is smooth; therefore, any irregularity should be regarded with concern. The normal gallbladder wall does not exceed 2 mm in thickness on postmortem measurements,[12] and the reported maximal *sonographic* thickness for a *well-distended* gallbladder is 2 to 3 mm.[10, 12-18] The thick-

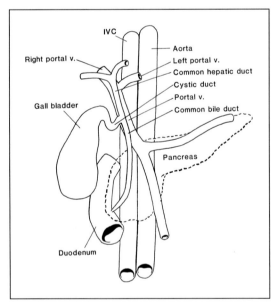

Figure 12-1—Biliary System Anatomy. The common hepatic duct begins at the junction of the right and left hepatic ducts and ends at the cystic duct. The common bile duct begins at the cystic duct and extends to the duodenum. The common bile duct lies in the free edge of the hepatoduodenal ligament (lesser omentum), which is not shown in this drawing.[29] Note that the upper portion of the common bile duct parallels the portal vein, whereas the lower portion bends slightly to parallel (roughly) the inferior vena cava (IVC). This bend often makes it difficult to show the entire bile duct in a single ultrasound image.[31] The lower portion of the bile duct passes through the pancreatic head. The very distal end of the duct often is slightly enlarged (the ampulla of Vater) and takes an abrupt lateral turn.

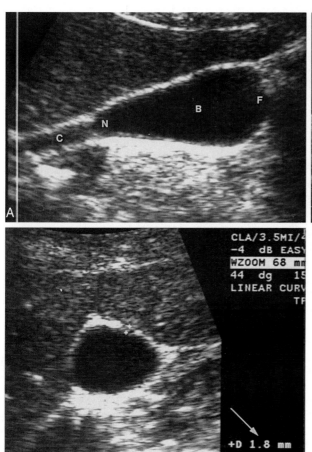

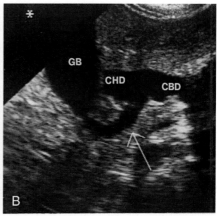

Figure 12-2—Sonographic Anatomy of the Gallbladder. (A) Longitudinal view through the neck (N), body (B), and fundus (F) of the gallbladder. C = cystic duct. (B) The cystic duct (arrow) is unusually well seen in this dilated biliary system. Also seen is the junction of the cystic and common hepatic ducts (CHD), forming the common bile duct (CBD). GB = gallbladder. (C) Transverse view of the gallbladder. The wall thickness measures 1.8 mm.

ness of the gallbladder wall is inversely related to the degree of gallbladder distention. Poorly distended gallbladders always are thick walled[13, 18] (Fig. 12–3), and for that reason, gallbladder wall thickness can be appraised only in patients who are fasting (at least 4 hours, and preferably longer).

For accurate measurement of gallbladder wall

Figure 12-3—Effects of Distention on Gallbladder Wall Appearance. After I ingested a cheeseburger and fried onion rings at the hospital cafeteria, the wall of my contracted gallbladder is thick (3.8 mm) and indistinct. Compare with fasting appearance in Figure 12–2A. (The author survived the experiment.)

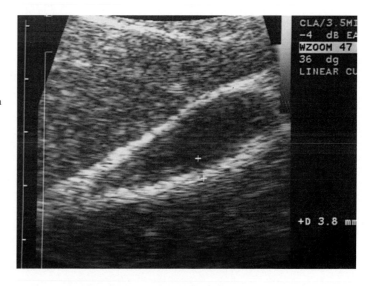

thickness, the ultrasound beam must be perpendicular to the wall at the point of measurement. Nonperpendicular measurements will exaggerate wall thickness, as illustrated in Figure 12–4. I prefer to measure gallbladder wall thickness from short axis* sections (Fig. 12–2C), to avoid the problem shown in Figure 12–4.

Echogenic Bile

Echogenic material is frequently present in dependent portions of the gallbladder and sometimes this material is called "sludge." I prefer the term "echogenic bile," since this material bears no resemblance to the sludge found in other fluids, such as motor oil. Echogenic bile (Fig. 12–5) is normal bile that happens to be highly concentrated. Echoes in this concentrated bile emanate from precipitated bile pigment (bilirubinate) crystals and cholesterol crystals.[1, 2, 19–23]

In certain settings, an association has been postulated between echogenic bile and calculus formation[21–23]; furthermore, echogenic bile has been indicted as a cause of calculous cholecystitis (Chapter 14). It must be emphasized, however,

---

*"Long axis" means along the longest plane of the gallbladder, from the neck to the fundus. "Short axis" means perpendicular to the gallbladder axis.

that echogenic bile, of and by itself, is not pathologic and is merely an indication of stasis. For example, the gallbladder of a patient who has fasted for an extended period (such as an intensive care patient) may be filled with echogenic bile (Fig. 12–5B), yet the gallbladder and bile ducts are normal. To assess the significance of echogenic bile, one must relate the *quantity* of echogenic bile to the *length* of fasting. For example, after 12 hours of fasting, the gallbladder normally contains only a small amount of echogenic bile. The detection of a large quantity of echogenic bile after a 12-hour fast, therefore, should raise concern about pathologic stasis, perhaps due to obstruction.

Echogenic bile typically produces uniform, low- to medium-level echoes, as seen in Figure 12–5. *Coarse intraluminal material and nonhomogeneous echogenicity suggest something other than echogenic bile, such as purulent debris or blood clots.* Occasionally, echogenic bile may "ball up" and form echogenic clumps (so-called "sludge balls") that may be confused with calculi or polyps,[20, 21] as discussed in the following chapter. Aggregates of echogenic bile are less reflective (bright) than calculi, do not cast acoustic shadows, and move sluggishly when the patient changes position. Cholesterol or adenomatous polyps may have about the same echogenicity as echogenic bile aggregates, but they are stationary (do not move with changes in patient position).

Anatomic Variants

Ultrasound practitioners should be aware of several variants of gallbladder anatomy and position that can be confusing or can lead to misdiagnosis.

Agenesis. Gallbladder agenesis occurs rarely but is likely to be confused with chronic cholecystitis, both of which cause nonvisualization of the gallbladder. The result of this error may be an unnecessary attempt at cholecystectomy.

Ectopia. Gallbladder ectopia is significant because it is relatively common and makes it difficult to locate the gallbladder sonographically, leading to diagnostic error. The usual cause of gallbladder ectopia is atypical liver configurations (see Chapter 6), which shift the position of the major interlobar fissure of the liver (where the gallbladder is located). The causes of atypical liver configuration include congenital variation, surgical resection, cirrhosis, and neoplastic masses. Contrary to popular belief, the gallbladder is not always a right upper quadrant structure; in fact, it may be located anywhere from a right lateral position to the left upper quadrant. When the gallbladder is ectopic, the signs and

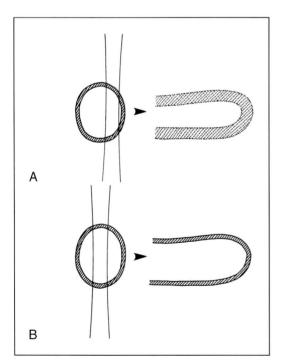

Figure 12-4—Effect of Plane of Section on Wall Thickness. (A) An off-axis image plane makes the gallbladder wall appear thickened and indistinct. **(B)** A correct image plane (through the diameter) produces a sharply defined, thin-walled appearance.

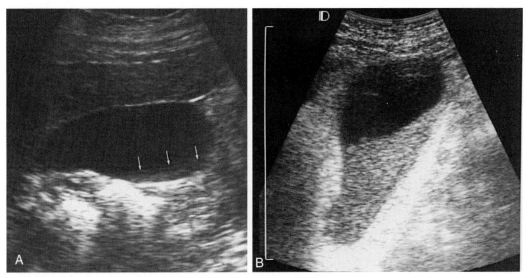

Figure 12-5—Echogenic Bile. (A) A small amount of echogenic bile (arrows) is seen at the dependent portion of this normal gallbladder. **(B)** The gallbladder of this intensive care patient receiving total parenteral nutrition contains a large amount of echogenic bile.

symptoms of cholecystitis may be ectopic as well.*

To locate a difficult-to-find gallbladder, systematically review hepatic anatomy to find the major interlobar fissure (between the right and left lobes) or the porta hepatis (Chapter 6). The gallbladder *must* communicate with the bile ducts in the general location of the major fissure and porta hepatis; hence it can almost always be found (even if it is empty) through careful anatomic analysis.

Folds. Normally occurring folds or septa in the gallbladder wall may cause confusion during sonographic examination by generating bright reflections (and sometimes shadows) mimicking gallstones.[24, 25] A prominent fold often is present near the gallbladder neck (Fig. 12–6).

The Phrygian Cap. A prominent fold in the gallbladder near the fundus produces the so-called "phrygian cap" deformity. The fundus (the rounded caudad end) folds upon the body of the gallbladder in a configuration that resembles a Greek hat[25, 26] (Fig. 12–6B). This gallbladder variant may be difficult to recognize sonographically, which is a significant problem since it is quite easy to overlook calculi trapped within the phrygian cap.

BILE DUCT ANATOMY
The Extrahepatic Ducts

The anatomy of the biliary tree[27–32] is illustrated in Figure 12–1. Please review this figure

---

*For example, I once examined a patient with epigastric pain in whom the gallbladder was nowhere to be found. Finally, the patient said, "Would it help if I told you where it hurts?" She then pointed to the *left* hypochondrium, which was where her gallbladder, and gallstones, were located.

before proceeding as the contents of this illustration are not repeated in the text.

Because the cystic duct, as noted earlier, is infrequently seen with ultrasound, there seldom is a sonographic landmark to show where the common hepatic duct ends and the common bile duct begins. This lack of a landmark creates a semantic problem that can lead to miscommunication. My solution is to skirt the issue entirely with the term "extrahepatic bile duct." Although this is a vague term, its use avoids anatomic miscommunication that may be significant. The term "common duct" should be avoided, since most clinicians equate common duct with "common bile duct." Take, for example, the case in which obstruction of the common duct was described sonographically. Surgery, in this case, was misdirected to the area of the pancreatic head, while the actual point of obstruction was much higher.

The Sandwich View

The classic sonographic view of the extrahepatic bile duct is the so-called "sandwich view." With this view, the bile duct and the portal vein are visualized as side-by-side, parallel "tubes" (Fig. 12–7).[28, 30, 32] The more superficial tube is the bile duct, and the deeper tube is the portal vein. A circular structure is "sandwiched" between the bile duct and the portal vein. This usually is the right hepatic artery, but in some cases it may be a "knuckle" of a tortuous proper hepatic artery.[30] *Demonstration of the hepatic artery is essential*, since it ensures, by a process of elimination, that the anechoic tube anterior to

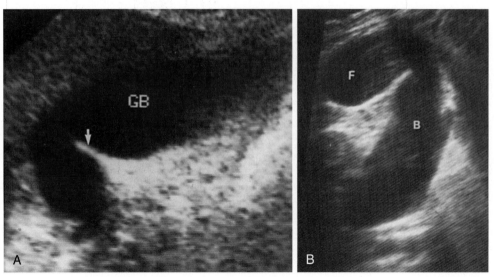

Figure 12-6—Normal Gallbladder Folds. (A) A prominent fold is seen near the neck of the gallbladder (GB). **(B)** In the phrygian cap deformity, the fundus (F) of the gallbladder folds upon the body (B).

the portal vein is the bile duct and not the hepatic artery. In elderly patients, the hepatic artery commonly enlarges and may easily be mistaken for a dilated bile duct.[30] This error can be avoided through critical assessment of porta hepatis anatomy, and through the routine use of color Doppler sonography to confirm the identity of the hepatic artery and bile duct (Fig. 12–7B).

The Mickey Mouse View

I prefer the "Mickey Mouse" view, illustrated in Figure 12–8, for identifying and examining the extrahepatic bile duct.[23] With this view, the bile duct is represented as Mickey's laterad ear, and the hepatic artery as the mediad* ear. Color Doppler demonstrates flow in the hepatic artery, further differentiating this vessel from the bile duct.

The Mickey Mouse view is usually obtained with the patient supine or in a left lateral decubitus position (Fig. 12–8A). To get Mickey in view, first align the scan plane *with the long axis of the portal vein*, just below the porta hepatis. Then *look at the scanhead* (not at the viewing monitor) and *rotate the scanhead exactly 90 degrees*. Look back at the viewing monitor and you should see the portal vein as a circular structure (Mickey's head). Adjust the position of the scanhead slightly to bring Mickey into full view. Once Mickey is in view, the bile duct usually can be followed caudad into the pancreatic head, or cephalad to the porta hepatis.

Mickey Mouse view pitfalls:

1. If you scan too high, you can mistake the right portal branch for the main portal vein, and you will not be able to find Mickey. If the portal vein is surrounded only by liver, then you are too high and you need to move inferiorly until Mickey is surrounded by echogenic fat.
2. Mickey's ears both happen to lie to the right of the portal vein (a normal anatomic variant). Solve this problem by pretending that Mickey is lying on his right side (Fig. 12–9).
3. Mickey has three ears! This occurs when the right hepatic artery arises from the superior mesenteric artery (so-called "replaced" right hepatic artery). The farthest right (posterolateral) ear is the replaced right hepatic artery (Fig. 12–10). Color Doppler examination helps determine which of Mickey's ears is which, and if necessary, the replaced right hepatic artery may be traced to its origin from the superior mesenteric artery (Fig. 12–10C). Mickey also may have three ears if the image plane passes through a bend in a tortuous hepatic artery.[30] Once again, color Doppler examination assists in identifying the bile duct and arteries.

Extrahepatic Bile Duct Size

Measurements reported in the literature for the caliber of the normal extrahepatic bile duct[33–45] vary widely because of several factors: (1) differences in measurement technique; (2) measurement of different portions of the extra-

---

*"Laterad" means toward the lateral side, and "mediad" toward the midline.

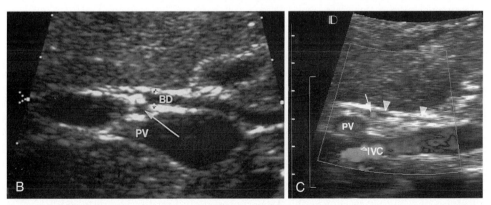

Figure 12-7—"Sandwich" View of the Extrahepatic Bile Ducts. (A) Anatomic drawing illustrating the scan plane used for obtaining the sandwich view. **(B)** Gray scale sonogram of the sandwich view. The right hepatic artery (arrow) is sandwiched between the bile duct (BD) and the portal vein (PV). **(C)** Color Doppler sonogram showing flow in the right hepatic artery (arrow) and portal vein (PV). IVC = inferior vena cava. (See Color Figure 12–7C following page 164.)

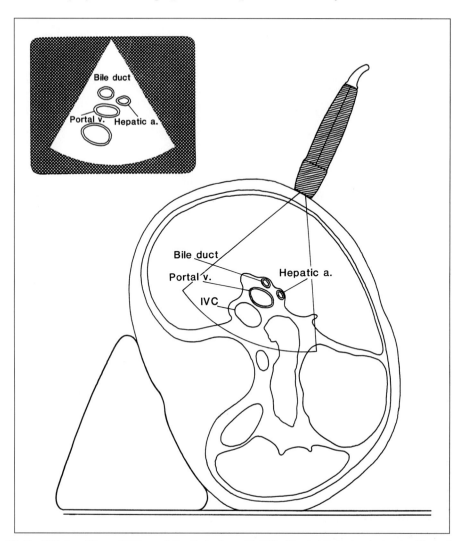

Figure 12-8—"Mickey Mouse" View of the Extrahepatic Bile Duct. (A) Anatomic drawing illustrating the scan plane used to obtain the Mickey Mouse view.

hepatic duct; (3) normal physiologic variation in ductal distention; and (4) age-related change in duct caliber.°[33–39] In spite of these variables, reliable normal standards of bile duct size have been established.

An *internal* ductal diameter of 6 mm or less generally is accepted as normal *at or near the porta hepatis* (i.e., in the vicinity of the right hepatic vein). An internal diameter of 7 mm at or near the porta hepatis is considered equivocal, and a diameter of 8 mm or greater at this location very likely indicates ductal dilatation.[36, 40–44] The maximal internal ductal diameter *below the porta hepatis* normally ranges from 7 to 10 mm, and a diameter exceeding 10 mm *anywhere*

along the extrahepatic duct strongly suggests ductal dilatation.[39, 44, 45] These measurements are summarized in Table 12–1.

The accurate diagnosis of ductal dilatation requires technical consistency. Be sure to measure only the duct lumen, and always be aware of whether you are measuring the smaller portion of the duct, at the porta hepatis, or the potentially larger distal portion.[35] Finally, be sure to examine the entire duct, not just the portion at the porta hepatis. The distal portion of the duct may dilate before the proximal portion, as discussed in Chapter 15.

Intrahepatic Ducts

The intrahepatic ductal branches parallel the portal veins, and the nomenclature for the intrahepatic bile ducts is analogous to that of the

---

°The extrahepatic duct has been noted to dilate with age, and it may be as large as 10 mm sonographically in elderly patients without biliary obstruction.[37–39]

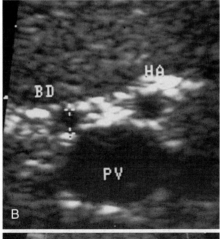

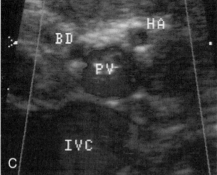

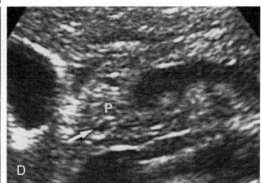

Figure 12-8 *Continued* **(B)** Gray scale Mickey Mouse sonogram showing the bile duct (BD) (measuring 3.2 mm), the proper hepatic artery (HA), and the portal vein (PV). **(C)** Color Doppler Mickey Mouse view. Note that flow is absent in the bile duct (BD) and present in the portal vein (PV), hepatic artery (HA), and inferior vena cava (IVC). (See Color Figure 12–8C following page 164.) **(D)** Transverse view of the bile duct (arrow) in the pancreatic head (P). Note that it has a relatively posterior position.

portal branches (e.g., right hepatic duct and left hepatic duct). Normal intrahepatic ducts may be visualized sonographically near the porta hepatis (Fig. 12–11); therefore, merely visualizing bile ducts at this location does not imply ductal dilatation unless the ducts are unusually large. The inside diameter of these ducts should not exceed 5 mm,[45] and ductal diameter should not exceed 40% of the adjacent portal vein diameter.[46] Normal intrahepatic bile ducts, furthermore, are not seen more than a few centimeters beyond the porta hepatis. Therefore, the visualization of *any* bile duct deeper within the liver suggests dilatation, as described in Chapter 15. Intrahepatic bile duct size is summarized in Table 12–1.

It is an unfortunate fact that the relationship of the intrahepatic bile ducts and portal branches is inconstant. Sometimes the ducts are anterior to the portal veins and sometimes they are posterior to the veins.[47–49] To make matters worse, the right and left hepatic arteries are sometimes visible at the porta hepatis, and these arteries may be confused with dilated bile ducts.[46, 47] Considerable potential exists, therefore, for diagnostic error, and color Doppler sonography is essen-

Figure 12-9—Tilted Mickey Mouse View. Arrow = bile duct; HA = hepatic artery; PV = portal vein.

Table 12-1. Bile Duct Size

Extrahepatic Ducts	Intrahepatic Ducts
Porta hepatis	Near porta hepatis
≤6 mm: Normal	≤5 mm: Normal
>6 to <8 mm: Equivocal	>5 mm: Dilated
≥8 mm: Dilated	≤40% portal: Normal
Below porta hepatis	>40% portal: Dilated
7 to 10 mm: Normal	Deep intrahepatic
At any location	Not visible: Normal
>10 mm: Dilated	Visible: Dilated

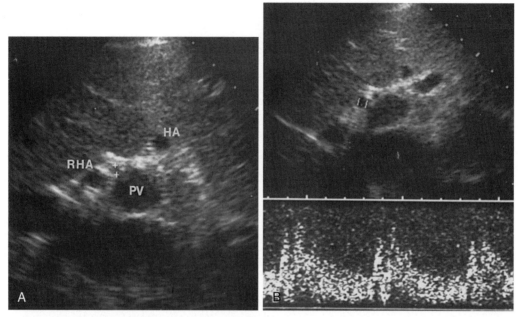

Figure 12-10—Replaced Right Hepatic Artery. (A) The cursors mark the bile duct, which is quite small (3 mm). Farther to the left is a replaced right hepatic artery (RHA). HA = proper hepatic artery; PV = portal vein. **(B)** A Doppler sample volume (cursors) has been placed in the replaced right hepatic artery, clearly demonstrating arterial flow signals.

tial for preventing such confusion. The anatomic identity of the bile ducts should be confirmed with color Doppler (through absence of flow) before a diagnosis of intrahepatic biliary dilatation is made.[50]

BILIARY EXAMINATION PROTOCOL

Haphazard scanning represents an accuracy liability, regardless of the area of examination. Sonographic assessment of the biliary tree, therefore, should follow a well-defined technical pro-

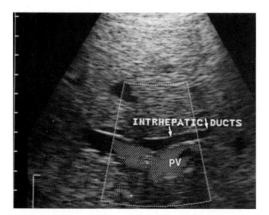

Figure 12-11—Normal Intrahepatic Bile Duct.
A normal left hepatic duct (arrows) is seen adjacent to the portal vein (PV) on this color Doppler view.

tocol, such as that listed in Chapter 6, which includes both the biliary system and the liver. The biliary tree and liver are always examined as a unit, hence the protocols for these areas are combined.

REFERENCES

1. Kane RA: Ultrasonographic evaluation of the gallbladder. Crit Rev Diagn Imaging 11:107–159, 1982.
2. Cooperberg PL, Gibney RG: Imaging of the gallbladder, 1987. Radiology 163:605–613, 1987.
3. Burrell MI, Zeman RK, Simeone JF, Dachman AH, McGahan JP, vanSonnenberg E, Zimmon DS, Torres W, Laufer I: The biliary tract: Imaging for the 1990's. AJR Am J Roentgenol 157:223–233, 1991.
4. Callen PW, Filly RA: Ultrasonographic localization of the gallbladder. Radiology 133:687–691, 1979.
5. Parulekar SG: Sonography of the distal cystic duct. J Ultrasound Med 8:367–373, 1989.
6. Kishk SMA, Darweesh RMA, Dodds WJ, Lawson TL, Stewart ET, Kern MK, Hassanein EH: Sonographic evaluation of resting gallbladder volume and postprandial emptying in patients with gallstones. AJR Am J Roentgenol 148:875–879, 1987.
7. Wedmann B, Schmidt G, Wegener M, Coenen C, Ricken D, Dröge C: Sonographic evaluation of gallbladder kinetics: In vitro and in vivo comparison of different methods to assess gallbladder emptying. J Clin Ultrasound 19:341–349, 1991.
8. Nino-Murcia M, Burton D, Chang P, Stone J, Perkash I: Gallbladder contractility in patients with spinal cord injuries: A sonographic investigation. AJR Am J Roentgenol 154:521–524, 1990.

9. Donald JJ, Fache JS, Buckley AR, Burhenne HJ: Gallbladder contractility: Variation in normal subjects. AJR Am J Roentgenol 157:753–756, 1991.

10. Giorgio A, Francica G, Amoroso P, Fico P, de Stefano G, Pierri P, Lettieri G, Aloisio T, Finelli L, Pierri G: Morphologic and motility changes of the gallbladder in response to acute liver injury. A prospective real-time sonographic study in 255 patients with acute viral hepatitis. J Ultrasound Med 8:499–506, 1989.

11. Raghavendra BN, Feiner HD, Subramanyam BR, et al: Acute cholecystitis: Sonographic-pathologic analysis. AJR Am J Roentgenol 137:327–332, 1981.

12. Handler SJ: Ultrasound of gallbladder wall thickening and its relation to cholecystitis. AJR Am J Roentgenol 132:581–585, 1979.

13. Marchal G, Van de Voorde P, Van Dooren W, et al: Ultrasonic appearance of the filled and contracted normal gallbladder. J Clin Ultrasound 8:439–442, 1980.

14. McGahan JP, Phillips HE, Cox KL: Soography of the normal pediatric gallbladder and biliary tract. Radiology 144:873–875, 1982.

15. Finberg HJ, Birnholz JC: Ultrasound evaluation of the gallbladder wall. Radiology 133:693–698, 1979.

16. Engle JM, Deitch EA, Sikkema W: Gallbladder wall thickness: Sonographic accuracy and relation to disease. AJR Am J Roentgenol 134:907–909, 1980.

17. Ralls PW, Quinn MF, Juttner HU, et al: Gallbladder wall thickening: Patients without intrinsic gallbladder disease. AJR Am J Roentgenol 137:65–68, 1981.

18. Wegener M, Borsch G, Schneider J, et al: Gallbladder wall thickness: A prospective study. J Clin Ultrasound 15:307–312, 1978.

19. Filly RA, Allen B, Minton MJ, Bernhoft R, Way LW: In vitro investigation of the origin of echoes within biliary sludge. J Clin Ultrasound 8:193–200, 1980.

20. Fakhry J: Sonography of tumefactive biliary sludge. AJR Am J Roentgenol 139:717–719, 1982.

21. Britten JS, Golding RH, Cooperberg PL: Sludge balls to gallstones. J Ultrasound Med 3:81–82, 1984.

22. Matos C, Avni EF, Van Gansbeke D, Pardou A, Struyven J: Total parenteral nutrition (TPN) and gallbladder diseases in neonates. Sonographic assessment. J Ultrasound Med 6:243–248, 1987.

23. Pfeiffer WR, Robinson LH, Balsara VJ: Sonographic features of bile plug syndrome. J Ultrasound Med 5:161–163, 1986.

24. Meilstrup JW, Hopper KD, Thieme GA: Imaging of gallbladder variants. AJR Am J Roentgenol 157:1205–1208, 1991.

25. Murayama S, Mizushima A, Russell WJ, Higashi Y: Sonographic diagnosis of bicameral gallbladders: A report of three cases. J Ultrasound Med 4:539–543, 1985.

26. Edell S: A comparison of the "Phrygian Cap" deformity with bistable and gray scale ultrasound. J Clin Ultrasound 6:1–72, 1978.

27. Grant JCB, Basmajian JV: Grant's Method of Anatomy, 7th ed. Baltimore, Williams & Wilkins, 1965, pp 242–254.

28. Kane RA: Ultrasonographic anatomy of the liver and biliary tree. Semin Ultrasound 1:78–95, 1980.

29. Weinstein JB, Heiken JP, DiSantis DJ, Balfe DM, Weyman PJ, Peterson RR: High resolution CT of the porta hepatis and hepatoduodenal ligament. RadioGraphics 6:55–74, 1986.

30. Berland LL, Lawson TL, Foley WD: Porta hepatis: Sonographic discrimination of bile ducts from arteries with pulsed Doppler with new anatomic criteria. AJR Am J Roentgenol 138:833–840, 1982.

31. Jacobson JB, Brodey PA: The transverse common duct. AJR Am J Roentgenol 136:91–95, 1981.

32. Bartrum RJ, Crow HC: Inflammatory diseases of the biliary system. Semin Ultrasound 1:102–112, 1980.

33. Glazer GM, Filly RA, Laing FC: Rapid change in caliber of the nonobstructed common duct. Radiology 140:161–162, 1981.

34. Mueller PR, Ferrucci JT, Simeone JF, vanSonnenberg E, Hall DA, Wittenberg J: Observations on the distensibility of the common bile duct. Radiology 142:467–472, 1982.

35. Sauerbri EE, Cooperberg PL, Gordon P, et al: The discrepancy between radiographic and sonographic bile-duct measurements. Radiology 137:751–755, 1980.

36. Freise J, Gebel M, Kleine P, Weyand C: The diameter of the common bile duct determined by ultrasound and ERCP is not necessarily comparable. Ann Radiol (Paris) 28:5–8, 1984.

37. Bodvall B: Late results following cholecystectomy in 1930 cases and special studies on postoperative biliary distress. Acta Chir Scand Suppl 329:83–88, 1964.

38. Mahour GH, Wakim KG, Ferris DO: The common bile duct in man: Its diameter and circumference. Ann Surg 165:415–419, 1967.

39. Wu C-C, Ho Y-H, Chen C-Y: Effect of aging on common bile duct diameter: A real-time ultrasonographic study. J Clin Ultrasound 12:473–478, 1984.

40. Parulekar SG: Ultrasound evaluation of bile duct size. Radiology 133:703–707, 1979.

41. Cooperberg PL: High-resolution real-time ultrasound in the evaluation of the normal and obstructed biliary tract. Radiology 129:477–480, 1979.

42. Cooperberg PL, Li R, Wong P, et al: Accuracy of common hepatic duct size in evaluation of extrahepatic biliary obstruction. Radiology 135:141–144, 1980.

43. Parulekar SG, McNamara MP Jr: Ultrasonography of choledocholithiasis. J Ultrasound Med 2:395–400, 1983.

44. Niederau C, Müller J, Sonnenberg A, Scholten T, Erckenbrecht J, Fritsch W-P, Brüster T, Strohmeyer G: Extrahepatic bile ducts in healthy subjects, in patients with cholelithiasis, and in postcholecystectomy patients: A prospective ultrasonic study. J Clin Ultrasound 11:23–27, 1983.

45. Deitch EA: The reliability and clinical limitations of sonographic scanning of the biliary ducts. Ann Surg 127:167–170, 1981.

46. Bressler EL, Rubin JM, McCracken S: Sonographic parallel channel sign: A reappraisal. Radiology 164:343–346, 1987.

47. Wing VW, Laing FC, Jeffrey RB, Guyon J: Sonographic differentiation of enlarged hepatic arteries from dilated intrahepatic bile ducts. AJR Am J Roentgenol 145:57–61, 1985.

48. Lim JH, Rya KN, Ko YT, Lee DH: Anatomic relationship of intrahepatic bile ducts to portal veins. J Ultrasound Med 9:137–143, 1990.

49. Bret PM, de Stempel JV, Atri M, Lough JO, Illescas FF: Intrahepatic bile duct and portal vein anatomy revisited. Radiology 169:405–407, 1988.

50. Ralls PW, Mayekawa DS, Lee KP, Johnson MB, Halls J: The use of color Doppler sonography to distinguish dilated intrahepatic ducts from vascular structures. AJR Am J Roentgenol 152:291–292, 1989.

Chapter 13

Gallstones and Their Mimics

William J. Zwiebel

The gallbladder may be adequately examined with ultrasound in more than 97% of patients,[1] and gallstones may be detected sonographically with considerable accuracy. Because sonography is both effective and accurate, it is the procedure of choice for evaluating patients with suspected cholelithiasis.

PATHOLOGY

Most gallstones are mixtures of cholesterol, calcium carbonate, and calcium bilirubinate. Seventy percent of gallstones are composed principally of cholesterol, and 30% are composed principally of bile pigments (bilirubinate stones).[2] Overall, only about 10% to 20% of gallstones contain enough calcium to be radiopaque,[2–6] but virtually all gallstones located within the gallbladder are visible sonographically, since sonographic detection does not depend on calcium content. Gallstones located within the bile ducts are less reliably detected, as will be discussed.

Gallstones accrete° from normal bile components. The factors that contribute to their accretion remain somewhat mysterious. Current theory emphasizes the importance of "lithogenic bile" in which cholesterol (insoluble in water) cannot be maintained in micellar form. A number of additional biochemical and physiologic factors also affect the development of gallstones. The interrelationship of these factors is complex and poorly understood.[4, 5]

EPIDEMIOLOGY

The overall incidence of gallstones among adults in the United States is 2.6% to 6.2% in men and 2.3% to 12% in women. The incidence of gallstones varies greatly with age, sex, and race.[7–11] Overall, the incidence in women is about twice that for men, and by age 60 years, about 25% of women have gallstones.[4, 7, 9, 11] Although many gallstones are asymptomatic, the onset of symptoms portends complications of cholelithiasis that virtually always require cholecystectomy.[4]

SONOGRAPHIC ACCURACY

The accuracy of real time sonography for the diagnosis of *gallbladder* calculi is truly exquisite. Sensitivity ranges from 92% to 100% in pathologically proved series, and specificity ranges from 86% to 95%.[5, 12–21] The specificity of ultrasound is subject to question, since patients with negative studies generally are excluded from pathologic confirmation. Nonetheless, sonography is clearly the best available means for detecting gallstones located in the gallbladder. In comparison, the sensitivity of oral cholecystography may be as low as 65%, and the sensitivity of computed tomography is about 80%.[12, 13, 16, 21]

CLASSIC ULTRASOUND FINDINGS

Classically, gallstones located within the gallbladder are *strongly reflective*, generate clearly defined *acoustic shadows*, and *move* rapidly with changes in patient position[17, 19–25] (Figs. 13–1, 13–2). I call these features the "cardinal" gallstone findings. If all three findings cannot be demonstrated, then an intracholecystic object may not be a gallstone.

The high reflectivity of gallstones results from a massive acoustic impedance mismatch at the stone/bile interface. This mismatch is very great regardless of the composition of the calculus; hence a strong reflection occurs with all stones, even those that are not calcified.

Acoustic shadowing occurs distal to virtually all† gallstones, regardless of composition.[23, 26–30] Therefore, when a shadow cannot be demonstrated, the intracholecystic object either is not a gallstone, or technical factors are preventing the demonstration of the shadow. The technical factors that may affect gallstone shadowing are illustrated in Figure 13–3.

Gallstones assume a dependent position in the gallbladder and move promptly in response to changes in patient position.‡ Rapid movement

---

° The terms "accrete" and "accretion" refer to the process in which an object, such as a gallstone, is built up over time from the repeated or continuous application of material.

---

†Rare cases of nonshadowing, poorly compacted gallstones have been reported in patients with chronic biliary stasis and bile inspissation.

‡Rarely, gallstones may be of sufficiently low density to float on a layer of concentrated bile or a layer of oral gallbladder contrast.[30] Such calculi appear suspended in the gallbladder lumen on sonographic examination.

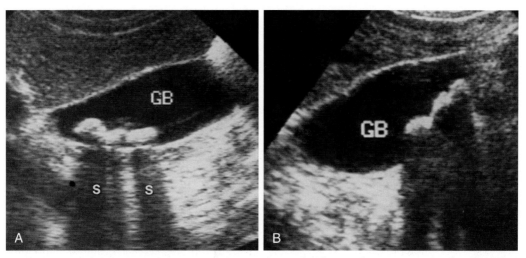

Figure 13-1—Classic Gallstone Features. (**A**) Discrete, strongly echogenic foci are seen within the gallbladder (GB) lumen. These cast prominent acoustic shadows (S). (**B**) The calculi move with altered patient position (as compared with **A**).

occurs because gallstones are denser, for the most part, than bile. Other intracholecystic material, such as echogenic bile, may "ball up" in spherical masses that resemble calculi, but this material moves sluggishly with changes in patient position.[19, 20, 22, 31, 32] Polyps are adherent to the gallbladder wall and do not move at all.

OTHER MANIFESTATIONS OF CHOLELITHIASIS

The Packed Bag

The cardinal gallstone signs just described are the most reliable evidence of cholelithiasis. The second most reliable finding is the "packed bag," which is characterized by a broad area of strong reflection and acoustic shadowing in the gallbladder fossa.[25] As the name implies, the packed bag (Fig. 13–4) is a gallbladder completely filled with stones, with little or no surrounding fluid. With

diligent scanning, the wall usually is visible as a moderately echogenic structure adjacent to the mass of calculi. In such cases, the wall and the stones have a "double arc" configuration,[33] as illustrated in Figure 13–4. Visualization of the gallbladder wall is of utmost importance for confirming the diagnosis of a packed bag. If only strong reflections and acoustic shadowing are seen, there is potential for error, as these findings may be generated by bowel gas as well as a packed bag.

Gallbladder Nonvisualization

The third sonographic finding that may be encountered in cholelithiasis is nonvisualization of the gallbladder, which is caused by marked scarring and small gallbladder size.[25] I feel that

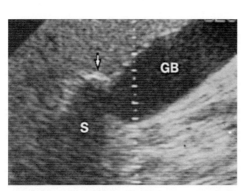

Figure 13-2—Impacted Gallstone. A prominent acoustic shadow (S) is seen distal to a gallstone impacted in the gallbladder (GB) neck. The surface of the stone (arrow) is indicated by a curvilinear reflection.

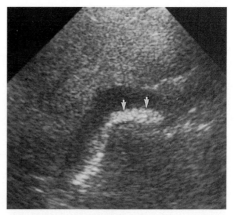

Figure 13-3—Tiny Gallstones. Very small gallstones are indicated by small bright reflections (arrows) seen in the dependent portion of the gallbladder.

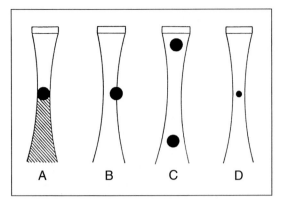

Figure 13-4—Technical Factors Affecting Gallstone Shadowing. Shadowing occurs if the calculus substantially blocks the ultrasound beam (**A**). Shadowing does not occur if the calculus is not squarely within the sound beam (**B**); if the calculus is outside the focal region (**C**); or if the calculus is too small to block a substantial portion of the ultrasound beam (**D**).

it is unwise to place very much credence on nonvisualization, since a normal gallbladder may, in fact, be present but overlooked sonographically for a variety of reasons. The causes of gallbladder nonvisualization include (1) obscuration by bowel gas; (2) ectopic location; (3) agenesis; and (4) small size due to normal (physiologic) contraction or diminished bile output (severe liver disease).[19–22]

Impacted Gallstones

Whereas calculi are easily identified in the echo-free gallbladder lumen, calculi impacted in the gallbladder neck (Fig. 13–5) or in the cystic duct may be difficult to detect with ultrasound because the surrounding structures also are echogenic and do not provide sonographic contrast. Small calculi in the neck or cystic duct are particularly apt to be overlooked, but even larger stones may be passed over. To help identify im-

Table 13-1. Noncalculous Intracholecystic Material

Hyperplastic polyp
Adenomatous polyp
Cholesterol polyp
Echogenic bile
Thrombus
Parasites
Debris from empyema
Gallbladder carcinoma
Metastasis

pacted calculi, the sonographer should always trace the gallbladder proximally as far as possible into the porta hepatis. To ensure visualization of the neck area, an image should be obtained that shows both the gallbladder and the adjacent portal vein.

DIFFERENTIAL DIAGNOSIS OF CHOLELITHIASIS

A variety of noncalculous material may produce rounded echogenic masses within the gallbladder lumen, as listed in Table 13–1.[4, 20, 22, 31, 32, 34–37] The diagnosis of cholelithiasis must be made, therefore, only when intraluminal objects exhibit *all* the cardinal features of gallstones described earlier! The differential diagnosis of intraluminal material includes the following.

Cholesterol Polyp

Cholesterol polyps are masses of intracellular cholesterol (see Chapter 14) that are characterized sonographically by the following findings (Fig. 13–6): (1) uniform, strong echogenicity that exceeds hepatic echogenicity but is less intense than a calculus of equivalent size; (2) immobility; and (3) a weak acoustic shadow or no acoustic shadow at all.[19, 22, 35] The strong echogenicity of cholesterol polyps deserves emphasis, as this fea-

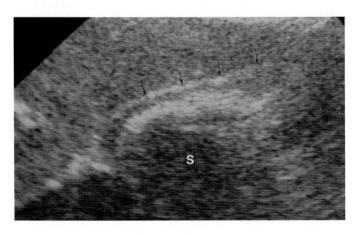

Figure 13-5—Packed Bag. The gallbladder is contracted about a collection of calculi, which is represented by a bright curvilinear reflection and prominent acoustic shadows (S). The thickened wall of the gallbladder (arrows) is barely visible adjacent to the calculi.

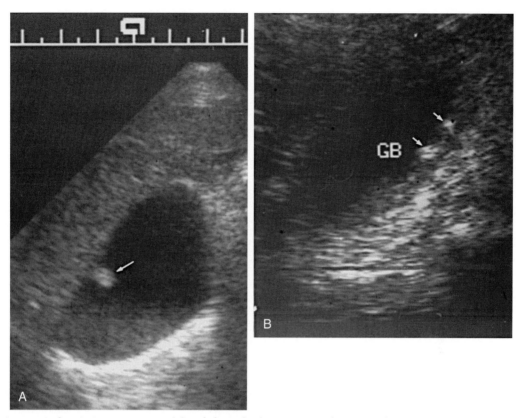

Figure 13-6—Cholesterol Polyp. (A) A cholesterol polyp generates a discrete, moderately echogenic focus, *without an acoustic shadow*, in a nondependent location. **(B)** Cholesterol crystals (arrows) deposited in the gallbladder (GB) wall (chronic cholecystitis) produce strong reflections. Note the comet tail artifact behind one of the crystals.

ture differentiates these polyps from all the other masses listed in Table 13–1. Only adherent, non-mobile gallstones (which are uncommon) are apt to be mistaken for cholesterol polyps, but these should be *more* reflective than polyps and should cast prominent acoustic shadows.

Hyperplastic or Adenomatous Polyp

Little information exists about the sonographic features of hyperplastic or adenomatous polyps arising from the gallbladder mucosa.[4, 22] This type of polyp should be considered diagnostically when a fixed mass is seen that resembles a cholesterol polyp but is not strongly echogenic. Adenomatous polyps may be premalignant; thus, to mistake this lesion for a cholesterol polyp could be a serious error.

Balls of Echogenic Bile

Balls of echogenic bile (Fig. 13–7) are probably the intraluminal objects most commonly confused with gallstones.[19, 20, 22, 31, 32, 36] In most cases, however, these globs of viscid bile can be cor-

rectly identified on the basis of the following features: (1) they are low or medium in echogenicity; (2) they do not have a shadow; (3) they move very slowly; and (4) they change size and shape as they "ooze" from one location to another (in response to altered patient position). These features usually serve to differentiate between balls of echogenic bile and calculi, but when doubt remains, differentiation can be made

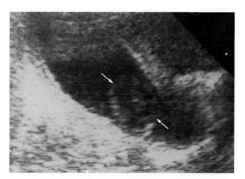

Figure 13-7—Echogenic Bile. A ball of echogenic bile (arrows) is seen within the gallbladder lumen. Note that it is low in echogenicity and heterogeneous in texture. It changed shape in response to altered patient position.

with oral cholecystography or with a repeat sonographic examination on another day. Balls of echogenic bile are not likely to be present on consecutive days if the patient is eating normally.

Other Intraluminal Material

Thrombus within the gallbladder lumen (from acute cholecystitis or hematobilia) can produce mobile masses identical to echogenic bile.[19, 22, 36, 37] Alternatively, thrombus can produce a fluid-fluid layer, tumor-like masses, or diffuse irregular thickening of the gallbladder wall reminiscent of gallbladder carcinoma.[37] As you might have gleaned from this description, no features specifically identify biliary thrombus.

Among the remaining lesions listed in Table 13–1, empyema and gallbladder carcinoma are considered in Chapter 14. Parasitic infestation and metastasis are rare and will not be considered further.

REFERENCES

1. Raptopoulos V, Moss L, Reuter K, Kleinman P: Comparison of real-time and gray-scale static ultrasonic cholecystography. Radiology 140:152–154, 1981.
2. Bring JA, Ferrucci JT: CT imaging of gallstones: What does it really add? Appl Radiol 29:22–25, 1990.
3. Simeone JF, Mueller PR, Ferrucci JT: Nonsurgical therapy of gallstones: Implications for imaging. AJR Am J Roentgenol 152:11–17, 1989.
4. DeSchryver-Kecskemeti K: Gallbladder and biliary ducts. *In* Kissane JM (ed): Anderson's Pathology, 8th ed. St Louis, CV Mosby, 1985, pp 1213–1232.
5. Maglinte DDT, Torres WE, Laufer I: Oral cholecystography in contemporary gallstone imaging: A review. Radiology 178:49–58, 1991.
6. Berk RN, Maglinte DDT: Conventional radiology of the biliary tract. *In* Berk JE, Haubrich WS, Kalser MH, Roth JLA, Schaffner F (eds): Bockus' Gastroenterology, 4th ed. Philadelphia, WB Saunders, 1985, pp 3518–3534.
7. Williamson SL, Williamson MR: Cholecysto-sonography in pregnancy. J Ultrasound Med 3:329–331, 1984.
8. Bartoli E, Calonaci N, Nenci R: Ultrasonography of the gallbladder in pregnancy. Gastrointest Radiol 9:35–38, 1984.
9. Fein AB, Rauch RF, Bowie JD, Pryor DB, Grufferman S: Value of sonographic screening for gallstones in patients with chest pain and normal coronary arteries. AJR Am J Roentgenol 146:337–339, 1986.
10. Schuster JJ, Raptopoulos V, Baker SP: Increased prevalence of cholelithiasis in patients with abdominal aortic aneurysm: Sonographic evaluation. AJR Am J Roentgenol 152:509–511, 1989.
11. Friedman GD, Hannel WB, Sawber TR: The epidemiology of gallbladder disease: Observations of the Framingham study. J Chronic Dis 19:273–276, 1966.
12. Bartrum RJ, Crow HC, Foote SR: Ultrasound examination of the gallbladder. An alternative to "double-dose" oral cholecystography. JAMA 236:1147–1148, 1987.
13. Bartrum RJ, Crow HC, Foote SR: Ultrasonic and radiographic cholecystography. N Engl J Med 296:538–541, 1977.
14. Lee JKT, Melson GL, Koehler RE, Stanley RJ: Cholecystosonography: Accuracy, pitfalls, and unusual findings. Am J Surg 139:223–228, 1980.
15. McIntosh DMF, Penney HF: Gray-scale ultrasonography as a screening procedure in the detection of gallbladder disease. Radiology 136:725–727, 1980.
16. Cooperberg PL, Burhenne HJ: Real-time ultrasonography. Diagnostic technique of choice in calculous gallbladder disease. N Engl J Med 302:1277–1279, 1980.
17. Hessler PC, Hill DS, Detorie FM, Rocco AF: High-accuracy sonographic recognition of gallstones. AJR Am J Roentgenol 136:517–520, 1981.
18. Elyaderani MK: Accuracy of cholecystosonography with pathologic correlation. W V Med J 80:111–115, 1984.
19. Kane RA: Ultrasonographic evaluation of the gallbladder. Crit Rev Diagn Imaging 11:107–159, 1982.
20. Cooperberg PL, Gibney RG: Imaging of the gallbladder, 1987. Radiology 163:605–613, 1987.
21. Burrell MI, Zeman RK, Simeone JF, Dachman AH, McGahan JP, vanSonnenberg E, Zimmon DS, Torres W, Laufer I: The biliary tract: Imaging for the 1990's. AJR Am J Roentgenol 157:223–233, 1991.
22. Rosenthal SJ, Cox GG, Wetzel LH, Batnitzky S: Pitfalls and differential diagnosis in biliary sonography. RadioGraphics 10:285–311, 1990.
23. King W, Kimme-Smith C, Winter J: Renal stone shadowing: An investigation of contributing factors. Radiology 154:191–196, 1985.
24. Crow HC, Bartrum RJ, Foote SR: Expanded criteria for the ultrasonic diagnosis of gallstones. J Clin Ultrasound 4:289–292, 1976.
25. Simeone JF, Ferrucci JT: New trends in gallbladder imaging. JAMA 246:380–383, 1980.
26. Sommer FG, Taylor JW: Differentiation of acoustic shadowing due to calculi and gas collections. Radiology 135:399–403, 1980.
27. Gonzalez L, MacIntyre WJ: Acoustic shadow formation by gallstones. Radiology 135:217–218, 1980.
28. Filly RA, Moss AA, Way LW: In vitro investigation of gallstone shadowing with ultrasound tomography. J Clin Ultrasound 7:255–262, 1979.
29. Rubin JM, Adler RS, Bude RO, Fowlkes JB, Carson PL: Clean and dirty shadowing at US: A reappraisal. Radiology 181:231–236, 1991.
30. Libensart P, Bloom RA, Meretyk S, Landau E, Shiloni E: Oral cholecystosonography: A method for facilitating the diagnosis of cholesterol gallstones. Radiology 153:255–256, 1984.
31. Fakhry J: Sonography of tumefactive biliary sludge. AJR Am J Roentgenol 139:717–719, 1982.
32. Filly RA, Allen B, Minton MJ, Bernhoft R, Way LW: In vitro investigation of the origin of echoes within biliary sludge. J Clin Ultrasound 8:193–200, 1980.
33. Raptopoulos V, D'Orsi C, Smith E, Reuter K, Moss

L, Kleinman P: Dynamic cholecystosonography of the contracted gallbladder: The double-arc-shadow sign. AJR Am J Roentgenol 138:275–278, 1982.

34. Worrell JA, Fleischer AC, Kaufman AJ, Lind CD, Richards WO, Josephs LG, Arnold JH, Dietrich MS, Williams LF: Variation in the size and number of stone fragments after gallbladder lithotripsy. J Ultrasound Med 10:509–512, 1991.

35. Cover KL, Slasky BS, Skolnick ML: Sonography of cholesterol in the biliary system. J Ultrasound Med 4:647–653, 1985.

36. Jeanty P, Ammann W, Cooperberg P, Gooding GAW, Kunstlinger F, LeClercq F, van Gansbeke D: Mobile intraluminal masses of the gallbladder. J Ultrasound Med 2:65–71, 1983.

37. Grant EG, Smirniotopoulos JG: Intraluminal gallbladder hematoma: Sonographic evidence of hemobilia. J Clin Ultrasound 11:507–509, 1983.

Chapter 14

Gallbladder Pathology

William J. Zwiebel

This chapter considers the primary pathologic processes that affect the gallbladder. Our attention will focus mainly on acute and chronic cholecystitis. In addition, we will briefly consider cholesterolosis, which is a common but not serious condition; gallbladder carcinoma, which is uncommon but deadly; and adenomyomatosis, which is common but seldom recognized.

ACUTE CHOLECYSTITIS

Pathology

It is widely accepted that gallstone formation precedes and causes cholecystitis, and not vice versa. The pathogenesis of acute cholecystitis is not entirely understood, but in about 85% to 95% of cases, this condition is associated with calculous obstruction of the cystic duct or the gallbladder neck.[1-3] Calculi are absent in the remaining 5% to 15% of cases. The usual symptoms of a "gallbladder attack": right upper quadrant pain and tenderness, are caused by (1) contraction of the gallbladder against the blocked outlet; (2) distention of the gallbladder; and (3) inflammation of the gallbladder wall and surrounding tissues. The cause of gallbladder distention is unclear. Possibilities include transudation of inflammatory fluid, or a "ball-valve effect," in which bile can enter the gallbladder but cannot leave. The immediate cause of inflammation in acute cholecystitis also is unclear, but a combination of factors probably comes into play, including the toxic effects of trapped bile salts, ischemia from overdistention, and the overgrowth of bacteria native to the biliary system. Gross infection of the gallbladder or its contents occurs in about three fourths of acute cholecystitis cases. Untreated gallbladder infection may lead to significant complications, including empyema (intracholecystic abscess), gangrene, and local or distant abscess.

Sonographic Findings

A spectrum of sonographic abnormalities is associated with acute cholecystitis,[4-20] as listed in Table 14–1 and illustrated in Figure 14–1. Please review this material and then proceed with the discussion of these important findings.

Gallstones. As noted, acute cholecystitis is caused by calculous obstruction of the gallbladder neck in 85% to 95% of cases.[1-3] Gallstones, therefore, are very important diagnostically, and one must be cautious when making a diagnosis of acute cholecystitis if a gallstone cannot be demonstrated. Calculi may sometimes be lost from view when they are impacted in the cystic duct; furthermore, acalculous acute cholecystitis is a recognized pathologic entity. The absence of a calculus, therefore, does not preclude the diagnosis of acute cholecystitis.

Gallstones Do Not Equal Cholecystitis. Although gallstones are an important diagnostic feature of acute cholecystitis, the mere presence of a gallstone does not equate with acute cholecystitis. The prevalence of gallstones in adults is great, and the incidence of acute cholecystitis is small by comparison. As Shakespear* once said, "Gallstones do not a diagnosis of cholecystitis make"!

The Impacted Calculus. Impaction of a calculus in the gallbladder neck (Fig. 14–1C) is strongly suggestive of acute cholecystitis. Impaction can be documented sonographically if the stone does not move when the patient is in a steep left decubitus or upright position. Virtually all stones impacted in the gallbladder neck can be visualized sonographically, but sonography is not uniformly unsuccessful in detecting calculi lodged within the cystic duct.[16]

Gallbladder Wall Thickening. The accumulation of inflammatory fluid in and around the gallbladder wall[4-8, 10, 13, 16-20] increases the thickness of the wall beyond the normal 2- to 3-mm limit and separates the layers of the wall, producing a striated appearance (Fig. 14–1A). Gallbladder wall thickening is an extremely im-

---

*Joseph Shakespear, an ancient sonologist.

Table 14–1. Sonographic Findings in Acute Cholecystitis

Calculi (usually)
Calculus impacted in gallbladder neck
Gallbladder wall thickening
Edema (sonolucency) in or surrounding the gallbladder wall
Gallbladder distention
Point tenderness over gallbladder

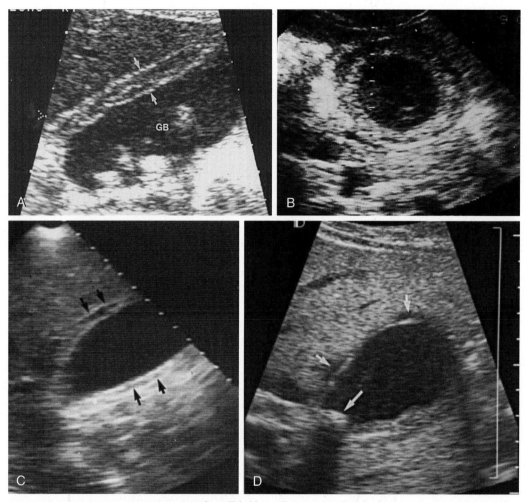

Figure 14-1—Acute Cholecystitis. (A) The gallbladder wall (arrows) is thickened (6 to 8 mm) and has a sonolucent, striated appearance. Gallstones are apparent in the lumen. **(B)** A short axis view in another patient demonstrates marked wall thickening (1 cm or more), and sonolucency due to edema. **(C)** The only evidence of acute cholecystitis in this patient is pericholecystic edema (arrows). Note that the gallbladder wall is sharp and thin. **(D)** An impacted calculus (large arrow) is seen in the gallbladder neck. This could not be displaced with changes in patient position. Pericholecystic edema (small arrows) is present.

portant finding, but thickening should never be the sole diagnostic basis for acute cholecystitis. A wide range of pathologic processes may thicken the gallbladder wall, as listed in Table 14–2.[18–30] Viral hepatitis is particularly noteworthy, since it may cause massive wall edema (Fig. 14–2) that is indistinguishable from the inflammatory thickening of acute cholecystitis.

Note also that solid-appearing gallbladder wall thickening is *not* a feature of acute cholecystitis. Solid thickening suggests chronic cholecystitis and other conditions, as discussed later.

Pericholecystic Fluid. Inflammatory fluid related to acute cholecystitis may accumulate adjacent to the gallbladder, and such fluid may be visible sonographically. This "pericholecystic" fluid usually is accompanied by other findings, but in some cases, pericholecystic fluid may be the sole manifestation of acute cholecystitis (Fig. 14–1*B*). In the proper clinical setting, therefore, pericholecystic fluid suggests acute cholecystitis, but this finding, like wall thickening, is nonspecific.

Gallbladder Distention. Normal variability makes gallbladder size a poor sign of acute cholecystitis. Most normal gallbladders do not exceed 4 cm in maximal transverse diameter, however, and a dimension greater than this should at least raise the possibility of distention.[31] This finding, however, should not be the sole diagnostic criterion for acute cholecystitis.

The Sonographic Murphy Sign. Point tenderness over the gallbladder (the "sonographic Murphy sign") is a useful finding in acute chole-

Table 14–2. Conditions Associated with Gallbladder Wall Thickening

Chronic cholecystitis
Acute cholecystitis
Adenomyomatosis
Sclerosing cholangitis
Gallbladder carcinoma
Portal hypertension*
Varices related to portal hypertension
Renal failure
Autoimmune deficiency syndrome
Acute hepatitis
Giardiasis
Lymphatic obstruction

*Wall thickening in cirrhosis is related to portal hypertension and is a direct result of transudative edema, not hypoalbuminemia as previously believed.[28, 30]

cystitis, but care must be taken to ensure that the gallbladder is in fact the source of tenderness.[5–7, 32, 33] I suggest the following method for evaluating gallbladder tenderness: Place the transducer in the midline, adjacent to the costal margin, and tell the patient to let you know when pain occurs. Then, *watch the patient's face* as you move the transducer toward the right, along the costal margin. When the patient grimaces or indicates with a verbal expletive that the painful spot has been reached, look at the image monitor and see whether the gallbladder is in view. Then repeat this maneuver from another direction to confirm that the pain localizes directly to the gallbladder. In any event, do *not* localize the gallbladder first and then mash down on it while saying "Does that hurt?" You are guaranteed to have false-positive Murphy signs with that method.

The Normal-Appearing Gallbladder. In about 3% of acute cholecystitis cases, gallbladder

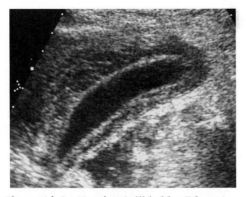

Figure 14–2—Massive Gallbladder Edema is present in this patient with acute viral hepatitis. The gallbladder wall measures 15 mm or more in thickness. A discontinuous, striated appearance is seen, illustrating the fact that such an appearance is not pathognomonic of acute cholecystitis.

sonography is entirely normal.[18] Even gangrenous gallbladders may appear normal on ultrasound examination![18, 33] A normal ultrasound study should always be followed with cholescintigraphy, therefore, if there is strong clinical suspicion of acute cholecystitis.

The Three-Finding Rule

As the preceding discussion indicates, many of the acute cholecystitis findings listed in Table 14–1 are nonspecific. Therefore, the diagnosis of acute cholecystitis must be made with caution. In some cases, the sonologist can say unequivocally: "This patient has acute cholecystitis, go to the operating room." Unfortunately, these cases are rare, and in most instances the sonologist can say only that the findings suggest acute cholecystitis but are not diagnostic.

Before an unequivocal ("go to the operating room") diagnosis of acute cholecystitis is made, I feel that *several abnormalities* should be present, and that these should include *gallstones, sonolucency* in or adjacent to the gallbladder wall, and *point tenderness* over the gallbladder—the three-finding rule. Alternatively, acute cholecystitis may be diagnosed with great certainty when findings of empyema or gangrene are present, as discussed later.

Sonographic Accuracy

Sonography is 85% to 94% sensitive and 85% to 96% specific for acute cholecystitis, if strict diagnostic criteria are utilized, including wall abnormality, gallstones, and point tenderness.[5, 16, 18, 34] Furthermore, in patients presenting with right upper quadrant pain, the source of pain may be identified with ultrasound in about 65% of cases, regardless of whether it is the gallbladder or another structure.[12, 15, 16]

Cholescintigraphy boasts sensitivity and specificity exceeding 95% for acute cholecystitis and clearly is more accurate than sonography.[12, 35–40] But cholescintigraphy may take several hours to perform, is considerably more expensive, and provides little or no information about disorders outside the biliary tract. In comparison, sonographic results are available immediately, and sonography provides anatomic information about the entire upper abdomen. Hence, I feel that sonography is a reasonable first choice in patients with signs and symptoms of acute cholecystitis, but caution is advisable when sonographic findings are equivocal.

COMPLICATIONS OF ACUTE CHOLECYSTITIS

The capacity to identify serious complications of acute cholecystitis is a somewhat unappreciated benefit of sonography. Complications that may be identified include empyema, pericholecystic abscess, and distant abscess.[4–8, 33, 41–50]

Empyema

Gallbladder empyema is, in essence, an intracholecystic abscess. As such, it is a harbinger of perforation, septicemia, or other dire effects. The following sonographic findings suggest empyema[20, 33, 41–45, 49]:

1. Coarse debris within the gallbladder lumen
2. Irregular and discontinuous striation of the gallbladder wall
3. Delamination of the wall
4. Gas within the gallbladder lumen or wall
5. Total disorganization of the gallbladder

Intracholecystic debris in empyema is shown in Figure 14–3A. *Note that this debris is fairly coarse in "texture," is nonlayering, and is heterogeneous in echogenicity.* This appearance is quite different from that of echogenic bile, which is fine-grained, homogeneous, and low in echogenicity (see Figure 12–5B in Chapter 12). Clumps of echogenic thrombus also may be present within the gallbladder lumen in empyema.

The disorganized, striated pattern of the gallbladder wall seen in empyema results from loss of structural integrity.[20, 43–45] The striated pattern is not specific and can be seen with other forms of gallbladder wall edema. With more advanced gallbladder wall disruption, sloughed wall components may fall into the gallbladder lumen (Fig. 14–3B), and the wall may become indistinct or grossly perforated.[41, 43–45]

Subacute or chronic empyema may lead to disintegration of the gallbladder wall and the formation of a gallbladder bed abscess. In such instances, the gallbladder fossa may contain a fluid collection or a nonhomogeneous mass. The latter finding may be indistinguishable from gallbladder carcinoma.

The presence of gas in the gallbladder lumen or wall (Fig. 14–4) is virtually proof-positive of empyema, as long as an iatrogenic source of biliary tract gas is excluded. The presence of gas implies gangrene, or frank necrosis of the gallbladder. Differentiation between wall gas and calcification may be difficult, but two findings are helpful. First, features that support the diagnosis of empyema (e.g., coarse debris, wall thickening, point tenderness) usually are present. Second, gas tends to *move* within the wall to a supernatant location, whereas calcification is stationary.[48]

The presence of a large amount of gas within the gallbladder lumen occasionally may complicate empyema diagnosis, since gas may obscure the gallbladder entirely or may cause the gallbladder to be mistaken for a bowel loop. Nonetheless, the presence of intracholecystic gas usually is obvious sonographically.[41, 46–48]

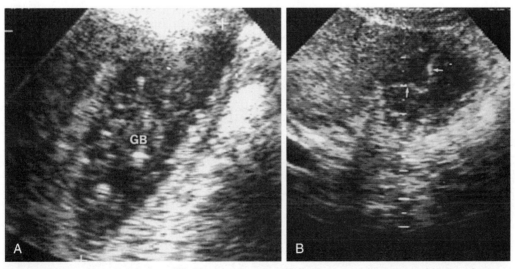

Figure 14-3—Empyema. (A) The gallbladder (GB) lumen is filled with coarse debris. Scattered bright reflections accompanied by comet-tail artifacts are seen. These probably represent tiny gas bubbles. Note that the debris within the gallbladder lumen is heterogeneous in texture and much coarser than echogenic bile, which is illustrated in Chapter 13. **(B)** In another patient with empyema, sloughed components of the wall (arrows) droop into the gallbladder lumen. Note the poor definition of the gallbladder wall.

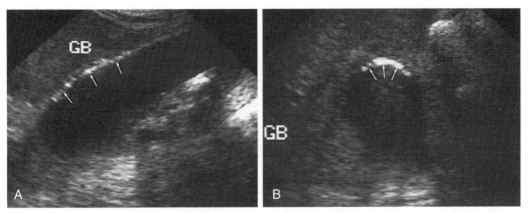

Figure 14-4—Emphysematous Cholecystitis. Longitudinal (**A**) and transverse (**B**) views of the gallbladder (GB) demonstrate bright reflections within the gallbladder wall (arrows) in a supernatant position. Debris, including gallstones, is present in the dependent portion of the gallbladder lumen.

When sonographic findings in empyema are uncertain, radiography and computed tomography are convenient ways to confirm the presence of gas and to differentiate between gas and calcification.

Pericholecystic and Distant Abscess

Gallbladder perforation in acute cholecystitis may lead to abscess formation adjacent to the gallbladder or elsewhere within the peritoneal space (typically subphrenic or subhepatic).[4, 20, 41, 44, 49, 50] With pericholecystic abscess, a fluid collection that may contain dependent debris or loculations is seen adjacent to or surrounding the gallbladder (Fig. 14–5). More distant intraperitoneal abscesses related to acute cholecystitis exhibit features described elsewhere in this text (Chapters 7 and 24). These abscesses are not always readily apparent; therefore, the perihepatic spaces (where they commonly accumulate) should be carefully examined for fluid collections in patients with suspected acute cholecystitis.

ACUTE ACALCULOUS CHOLECYSTITIS

The pathogenesis of gallbladder inflammation in the absence of gallstones (acalculous cholecystitis) remains mysterious.[3, 5] There are two forms of acalculous cholecystitis, chronic and acute, but we shall concern ourselves only with the acute form. Acute acalculous cholecystitis is prone to occur in seriously ill intensive care patients, in whom it may be unrecognized until late in its course, with the result that sepsis, gangrene, and rupture are common complications.[3, 5, 42, 51]

The diagnostic criteria for acute acalculous cholecystitis are the same as those described pre-

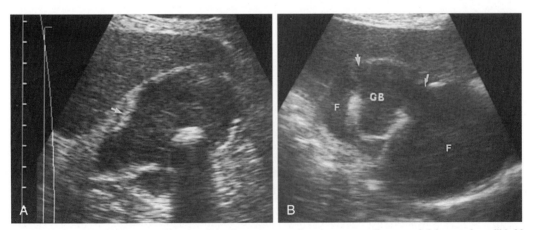

Figure 14-5—Pericholecystic Abscess. (**A**) A long axis view demonstrates a gallstone and debris in the gallbladder lumen. A portion of the wall is sloughing (arrow). (**B**) Two pericholecystic fluid collections (F) are apparent on this short axis view. Defects in the wall (arrows) are clearly apparent in relation to the collections. GB = gallbladder.

viously for acute calculous cholecystitis, with the exception that gallstones are absent. The sonographic Murphy sign also may be absent in intensive care patients who are unresponsive.[5, 51, 52] Seriously ill intensive care patients often have many reasons for gallbladder wall edema, including acute hepatitis and congestive heart failure. The potential for false-positive diagnosis of acute cholecystitis is high, therefore, in these patients.

The diagnostic accuracy of ultrasound for acute acalculous cholecystitis is poor. A sensitivity level of only 56% was reported in the only sizable series in the medical literature.[51] Cholescintigraphy appears to be the best means for diagnosing this condition, as the reported sensitivity is 93% to 100%.[35, 38, 51, 53–55]

ACUTE CHOLECYSTITIS IN CHILDREN

A predisposing cause of cholelithiasis is identified in as many as 80% of pediatric patients with gallstones, and in about 20% of patients the predisposing factor is a hemolytic anemia.[56–60] Other predisposing conditions include liver disease, bowel resection, lysis of hematoma after extensive orthopedic surgery, cardiac shunts, and pregnancy.

About 50% of acute cholecystitis cases in children are of the acalculous variety, as compared with about 10% in adults.[2, 60] The cause of this high incidence of acalculous disease is unknown. Since cholecystitis is relatively uncommon in children, the symptoms of gallbladder disease frequently are attributed to other disorders, particularly appendicitis. The sonographer would do well, therefore, to examine the gallbladder in all pediatric patients with unexplained abdominal pain.

The previously described sonographic features of gallstones and acute cholecystitis apply to children as well as adults.[56, 57, 59]

CHRONIC CHOLECYSTITIS

Pathologic-Sonographic Correlation

Chronic cholecystitis[1, 4–8, 17, 61–65] results from repeated episodes of acute cholecystitis, and it is characterized histologically by fibrous thickening of the gallbladder wall. Most calculi-containing gallbladders demonstrate some histologic evidence of chronic cholecystitis, but the degree of abnormality is quite varied. The mere presence of gallstones, therefore, should not be equated with chronic cholecystitis.

Sonographic Findings

The ultrasound findings in chronic cholecystitis are solid-appearing wall thickening (Fig. 14–6), reduced gallbladder size, gallstones, and calcification. The packed bag illustrated in Chapter 13 represents the ultimate scarred, contracted gallbladder.[4–8, 17, 61, 62, 64] An additional uncommon manifestation of chronic cholecystitis is the presence of small crypts within the gallbladder wall that result from inflammatory destruction of the muscular layer. These crypts may contain strongly reflective cholesterol deposits (see Figure 13–6B in Chapter 13) or calculi.[64, 65]

The Porcelain Gallbladder

Dystrophic gallbladder wall calcification may occur focally or diffusely in chronic cholecystitis.[1, 4, 5, 61–63] Such calcification causes strong wall reflections and distal acoustic shadowing that is relatively easy to recognize when it is diffuse but may go unnoticed when it is localized.

A diffusely calcified gallbladder is called a "porcelain" gallbladder in view of its radiographic and pathologic appearance. Three principal sonographic findings identify a porcelain gallbladder:

1. A prominent arcuate reflection accompanied by an acoustic shadow (Fig. 14–7). This resembles the packed bag described previously, except that a thickened gallbladder wall is *not* present extrinsic to the arcuate reflection;
2. Two *opposing*, highly echogenic arcs, one emanating from the near gallbladder wall and the other from the far wall,* accompanied by an acoustic shadow; or

---

*"Near," as used here, means nearer to the transducer. "Far" means farther from the transducer.

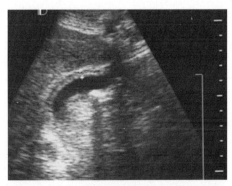

Figure 14–6—Chronic Cholecystitis. A long axis view shows that the gallbladder is inordinately small (about 4 cm long on two occasions with the patient fasting) and the wall (cursors) is both thick (4 mm) and solid-appearing. A gallstone is evident.

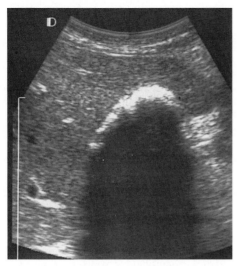

Figure 14-7—Porcelain Gallbladder. A long axis view shows strong reflections in the gallbladder wall and dramatic acoustic shadowing from "solid" wall calcification. Note that the strong reflections arise *within* the gallbladder wall; i.e., no wall is visible extrinsic to the bright reflection.

3. Focal reflective foci within the gallbladder wall associated with localized calcification.

Other manifestations of chronic cholecystitis may accompany a porcelain gallbladder, including wall thickening, reduced gallbladder size, and gallstones. An obstructing stone may be visible in the gallbladder neck, as a porcelain gallbladder invariably is obstructed.

The final sonographic manifestation of chronic cholecystitis is milk of calcium bile, which is uncommon but distinctive. Bile may be replaced, in a chronically obstructed gallbladder, by a colorless mucoid fluid, called "white bile," that typically is rich in calcium salts. These salts may precipitate as milk of calcium,[1, 62, 63] which produces a strongly echogenic, dependent layer within the gallbladder lumen, accompanied by distal acoustic shadowing. Other findings of chronic cholecystitis also are present, including, perhaps, an impacted calculus. Sonographic differentiation between milk of calcium and tiny, dependent calculi may be difficult.

HYPERPLASTIC CHOLECYSTOSES

The term "hyperplastic cholecystoses" was coined to describe noninflammatory, non-neoplastic disorders of the gallbladder wall characterized by hyperplasia.[65–69] Two entities are included in this diagnostic category: cholesterolosis and adenomyomatosis. The most important hyperplastic gallbladder disorder, from a sono-

graphic perspective, is cholesterolosis, but this disorder is not believed to be symptomatic. Adenomyomatosis is less important sonographically, but it may be a cause of epigastric pain. Only brief mention of adenomyomatosis can be included herein.

At the onset of this discussion, it should be recalled that the inner surface of the gallbladder normally is smooth. Nodularity or irregularity of the wall should always be viewed with suspicion and should call to mind the hyperplastic cholecystoses as well as other gallbladder disorders.

Cholesterolosis and Cholesterol Polyps

Cholesterolosis[65–72] typically is a diffuse disorder characterized by the deposition of esterified cholesterol beneath the epithelial lining of the gallbladder. Although these deposits may be present in great numbers, they may be invisible sonographically due to their small size. Alternatively, they may be manifested solely by irregularity of the inner surface of the gallbladder, perhaps accompanied by slight wall thickening. *Remember, the inner surface of the normal gallbladder is smooth. A rough inner surface implies pathology.*

Larger, polypoid deposits of esterified cholesterol are called cholesterol polyps. These are visible sonographically as fixed, rounded, echogenic masses that may be sessile or pedunculated (see Figure 13–6A in Chapter 13). The features that differentiate cholesterol polyps from gallstones were described in Chapter 13: (1) cholesterol polyps are not as strongly echogenic as calculi of similar size; (2) cholesterol polyps are fixed in place, whereas stones are mobile; and (3) cholesterol polyps cast only faint shadows, or no shadow at all, whereas calculi generate profound acoustic shadows.[66–72] Differentiation between gallstones and cholesterol polyps is extremely important, since cholesterolosis is generally an asymptomatic condition that does not warrant cholecystectomy.

Large cholesterol crystals are among the most echogenic objects seen with ultrasound in humans (see Figure 13–6B in Chapter 13), yet cholesterol polyps, which contain the same material, are nowhere near as echogenic and often do not even cast acoustic shadows. Two factors account for these differences.[72] First, the concentration of crystalline material is relatively low in cholesterol polyps,* since the crystalline material

---

*In the case of cholesterol polyps, the crystalline material is cholesterol, whereas in gallstones the crystalline material may include cholesterol, bile pigment salts, or calcium salts.

is dispersed in a cellular (protein) matrix. Second, crystal size is much smaller in cholesterol polyps than in other cholesterol deposits. These factors decrease reflectivity and permit through-transmission of ultrasound.

Adenomyomatosis

Adenomyomatosis of the gallbladder[1, 63–69, 73–76] is commonly found at autopsy but is seldom recognized sonographically. This disorder is characterized pathologically by muscular hypertrophy of the gallbladder wall and by the development of diverticulum-like outpouchings that project into the muscular layer (it is similar, in a sense, to colonic diverticulosis). Adenomyomatosis may develop focally as a sessile, polypoid lesion, circumferentially (in a bandlike fashion) or diffusely. Adenomyomatosis is sometimes symptomatic, and surgery is warranted in selected cases. The cause of this disorder is unknown.

A characteristic sonographic finding identifies adenomyomatosis: a thickened gallbladder wall containing intramural diverticula.[65, 73–76] These diverticula may contain anechoic bile; echogenic inspissated bile; large cholesterol crystals (which

cast distinctive V-shaped artifacts as seen in Figure 13–6B in Chapter 13); or calculi, which show typical bright reflections and acoustic shadows. In severe cases, the gallbladder lumen may be occluded by massive wall thickening. In less severe cases, slight wall thickening and irregularity may be the only findings.

GALLBLADDER CARCINOMA

Pathology

Gallbladder carcinoma[1, 2, 77, 78] is an uncommon neoplasm of elderly people that is almost always fatal (5-year survival is less than 5%). This tumor frequently presents at an advanced, incurable stage; jaundice, due to metastatic obstruction of the bile duct, is a common presenting sign. Other signs and symptoms may mimic chronic cholecystitis. Gallstones are present in about 80% of cases and are thought to be pathogenic by an unidentified mechanism.

Sonographic Findings

The sonographic appearance of gallbladder carcinoma is variable and depends on both the

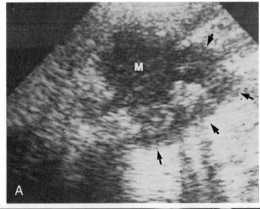

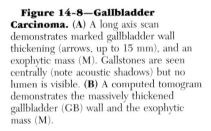

Figure 14-8—Gallbladder Carcinoma. (A) A long axis scan demonstrates marked gallbladder wall thickening (arrows, up to 15 mm), and an exophytic mass (M). Gallstones are seen centrally (note acoustic shadows) but no lumen is visible. (B) A computed tomogram demonstrates the massively thickened gallbladder (GB) wall and the exophytic mass (M).

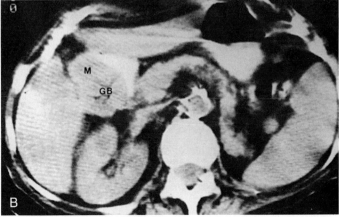

extent and pattern of tumor growth.[79–82] Recognized patterns include the following:

1. Focal or diffuse infiltration, and resultant thickening, of the gallbladder wall (Fig. 14–8). Infiltrating tumors may be confused sonographically with chronic cholecystitis or adenomyomatosis.
2. Formation of a homogeneous, moderately echogenic mass that projects either extrinsically (Fig. 14–8) or into the gallbladder lumen.
3. Replacement of the gallbladder by a nonhomogeneous mass that may extend to adjacent organs. The latter appearance may be similar to that seen with a subacute or chronic gallbladder bed abscess.[64]

Gallstones are evident in virtually all cases of gallbladder carcinoma, either within the residual gallbladder lumen (Fig. 14–8) or embedded within the tumor mass. In addition, the biliary system may be dilated, and metastases may be evident (usually in the liver, porta hepatis, or parapancreatic area).

REFERENCES

1. DeSchryver-Kecskemeti K: Gallbladder and biliary ducts. *In* Kissane JM (ed): Anderson's Pathology, 8th ed. St Louis, CV Mosby, 1985, pp 1213–1232.
2. Sherlock S, Dooley J: Diseases of the Liver and Biliary System. London, Blackwell Scientific Publications, 1993, pp 562–591.
3. Howard RJ: Acute acalculous cholecystitis. Am J Surg 141:194–198, 1981.
4. Kane RA: Ultrasonographic evaluation of the gallbladder. Crit Rev Diagn Imaging 11:107–159, 1982.
5. Cooperberg PL, Gibney RG: Imaging of the gallbladder, 1987. Radiology 163:605–613, 1987.
6. Burrell MI, Zeman RK, Simeone JF, Dachman AH, McGahan JP, vanSonnenberg E, Zimmon DS, Torres W, Laufer I: The biliary tract: Imaging for the 1990's. AJR Am J Roentgenol 157:223–233, 1991.
7. Rosenthal SJ, Cox GG, Wetzel LH, Batnitzky S: Pitfalls and differential diagnosis in biliary sonography. RadioGraphics 10:285–311, 1990.
8. Bartrum RJ, Crow JC: Inflammatory diseases of the biliary system. Semin Ultrasound 1:102–112, 1980.
9. Handler SJ: Ultrasound of gallbladder wall thickening and its relation to cholecystitis. AJR Am J Roentgenol 132:581–585, 1979.
10. Finberg HJ, Birnholz JC: Ultrasound evaluation of the gallbladder wall. Radiology 133:693–698, 1979.
11. Engle JM, Deitch EA, Sikkema W: Gallbladder wall thickness: Sonographic accuracy and relation to disease. AJR Am J Roentgenol 134:907–909, 1980.
12. Shuman WP, Mack LA, Rudd TG, Rogers JV, Gibbs P: Evaluation of acute right upper quadrant pain: Sonography and 99mTc-PIPIDA cholescintigraphy. AJR Am J Roentgenol 139:61–64, 1982.
13. Sanders RC: The significance of sonographic gallbladder wall thickening. J Clin Ultrasound 8:143–146, 1980.
14. Ralls PW, Colletti PM, Lapin SA, Chandrasoma P, Boswell WD, Ngo C, Radin DR, Halls JM: Real-time sonography in suspected acute cholecystitis. Prospective evaluation of primary and secondary signs. Radiology 155:767–771, 1985.
15. Philbrick TH, Kaude JV, McInnis AN, Wright PG: Abdominal ultrasound in patients with acute right upper quadrant pain. Gastroint Radiol 6:251–256, 1981.
16. Laing FC, Federle MP, Jeffrey RB, Brown TW: Ultrasonic evaluation of patients with acute right upper quadrant pain. Radiology 140:449–455, 1981.
17. Raghavendra BN, Feiner HD, Subramanyam BR, Ranson JHC, Toder SP, Horii SC, Madamba MR: Acute cholecystitis: Sonographic-pathologic analysis. AJR Am J Roentgenol 137:327–332, 1981.
18. Croce F, Montali G, Solbiati L, Marinoni G: Ultrasonography in acute cholecystitis. Br J Radiol 54:927–931, 1981.
19. Cohan RH, Mahony BS, Bowie JD, Cooper C, Baker ME, Illescas FF: Striated intramural gallbladder lucencies on US studies: Predictors of acute cholecystitis. Radiology 164:31–35, 1987.
20. Teefey SA, Baron RL, Bigler SA: Sonography of the gallbladder: Significance of striated (layered) thickening of the gallbladder wall. AJR Am J Roentgenol 156:945–947, 1991.
21. Shlaer WJ, Leopold GR, Scheible FW: Sonography of the thickened gallbladder wall: A nonspecific finding. AJR Am J Roentgenol 136:337–339, 1981.
22. Ralls PW, Quinn MF, Jüttner HU, Halls JM, Boswell WD: Gallbladder wall thickening: Patients without intrinsic gallbladder disease. AJR Am J Roentgenol 137:65–68, 1981.
23. Jüttner HU, Ralls PW, Quinn MF, Jenney JM: Thickening of the gallbladder wall in acute hepatitis: Ultrasound demonstration. Radiology 142:465–466, 1982.
24. Carroll BA: Gallbladder wall thickening secondary to focal lymphatic obstruction. J Ultrasound Med 2:89–91, 1983.
25. Patriquin HB, DiPietro M, Barber FE, Teele RL: Sonography of thickened gallbladder wall: Causes in children. AJR Am J Roentgenol 141:57–60, 1983.
26. Maresca G, De Gaetano AM, Mirk P, Cauda R, Federico G, Colagrande C: Sonographic patterns of the gallbladder in acute viral hepatitis. J Clin Ultrasound 12:141–146, 1984.
27. Saigh J, Williams S, Cawley K, Anderson JC: Varices: A cause of focal gallbladder wall thickening. J Ultrasound Med 4:371–373, 1985.
28. Kaftori JK, Pery M, Green J, Gaitini D: Thickness of the gallbladder wall in patients with hypoalbuminemia: A sonographic study of patients on peritoneal dialysis. AJR Am J Roentgenol 148:1117–1118, 1987.
29. Romano AJM, vanSonnenberg E, Casola G, Gosink BB, Withers CE, McCutchan JA, Leopold GR: Gallbladder and bile duct abnormalities in AIDS: Sonographic findings in eight patients. AJR Am J Roentgenol 150:123–127, 1988.
30. Colli A, Cocciolo M, Buccino G, Parravicini R, Martinez E, Rinaldi G, Scaltrini G: Thickening of the gallbladder wall in ascites. J Clin Ultrasound 19:357–359, 1991.
31. Raghavendra BN, Feiner HD, Subramanyam BR, et al: Acute cholecystitis: Sonographic-pathologic analysis. AJR Am J Roentgenol 137:327–332, 1981.
32. Ralls PW, Halls J, Lapin SA, Quinn MF, Morris UL,

Boswell W: Prospective evaluation of the sonographic Murphy sign in suspected acute cholecystitis. J Clin Ultrasound 10:113–115, 1982.

33. Simeone JF, Brink JA, Mueller PR, Compton C, Hahn PF, Saini S, Silverman SG, Tung G, Ferrucci JT: The sonographic diagnosis of acute gangrenous cholecystitis: Importance of the Murphy sign. AJR Am J Roentgenol 152:289–290, 1989.

34. Mirvis SE, Wainright JR, Nelson AW, Johnston GS, Sher R, Rodriguez A, Whitley NO: The diagnosis of acute acalculous cholecystitis: A comparison of sonography, scintigraphy, and CT. AJR Am J Roentgenol 147:1171–1175, 1986.

35. Weissman HS, Frank MS, Bernstein LH, et al: Rapid and accurate diagnosis of acute cholecystitis with 99m-Tc-IDA cholescintigraphy. AJR Am J Roentgenol 132:523–528, 1979.

36. Hall AW, Hutchinson WF, Wood RAB, Cuschieri A: The place of hepatobiliary isotope scanning in the diagnosis of gallbladder disease. Br J Surg 68:85–90, 1981.

37. Worthen NJ, Uszler JM, Funamura JL: Cholecystitis: Prospective evaluation of sonography and ^{99m}Tc-HIDA cholescintigraphy. AJR Am J Roentgenol 137:973–978, 1981.

38. Mauro MA, McCartney WH, Melmed JR: Hepatobiliary scanning with ^{99m}Tc-PIPIDA in acute cholecystitis. Radiology 142:193–197, 1982.

39. Samuels BI, Freitas JE, Bree BL, Schwab BE, Heller ST: A comparison of radionuclide hepatobiliary imaging and real-time ultrasound for the detection of acute cholecystitis. Radiology 147:207–210, 1983.

40. Fajman WA: Acute right upper quadrant abdominal pain: Radionuclide approach. J Clin Ultrasound 11:193–200, 1983.

41. Kane RA: Ultrasonographic diagnosis of gangrenous cholecystitis and empyema of the gallbladder. Radiology 134:191–194, 1980.

42. Smith JP, Bodai BI: Empyema of the gallbladder—potential consequence of medical intensive care. Crit Care Med 10:451–452, 1982.

43. Wales LR: Desquamated gallbladder mucosa: Unusual sign of cholecystitis. AJR Am J Roentgenol 139:810–811, 1982.

44. Teefey SA, Baron RL, Radke HM, Bigler SA: Gangrenous cholecystitis: New observations on sonography. J Ultrasound Med 10:603–606, 1991.

45. Jeffrey RB, Laing FC, Wong W, Callen PW: Gangrenous cholecystitis: Diagnosis by ultrasound. Radiology 148:219–221, 1983.

46. Parulekar SG: Sonographic findings in acute emphysematous cholecystitis. Radiology 145:117–119, 1982.

47. Blaquiere RM, Dewbury KC: The ultrasound diagnosis of emphysematous cholecystitis. Br J Radiol 55:114–116, 1982.

48. Bloom RA, Fisher A, Pode D, Asaf Y: Shifting intramural gas—a new ultrasound sign of emphysematous cholecystitis. J Clin Ultrasound 12:40–42, 1984.

49. Fleischer AC, Muhletaler CA, Jones TB: Sonographic detection of gallbladder perforation. South Med J 75:606–607, 1982.

50. Takada T, Yasuda H, Uchiyama K, Hasegawa H, Asagoe T, Shikata J: Pericholecystic abscess: Classification of US findings to determine the proper therapy. Radiology 172:693–697, 1989.

51. Shuman WP, Rogers JV, Rudd TG, Mack LA, Plumley T, Larson EB: Low sensitivity of sonography and cholescintigraphy in acalculous cholecystitis. AJR Am J Roentgenol 142:531–534, 1984.

52. Deitch EA, Engel JM: Acute acalculous cholecystitis. Ultrasonic diagnosis. Am J Surg 142:290–292, 1981.

53. Weissman HS, Berkowitz D, Fox MS, Gliedman ML, Rosenblatt R, Sugarman LA, Freeman LM: The role of technetium-99m iminodiacetic acid (IDA) cholescintigraphy in acute acalculous cholecystitis. Radiology 146:177–180, 1983.

54. Swayne LC: Acute acalculous cholecystitis: Sensitivity in detection using technetium-99m iminodiacetic acid cholescintigraphy. Radiology 160:33–38, 1986.

55. Ramanna L, Brachman MB, Tanasescu DE, Berman DS, Waxman AD: Cholescintigraphy in acute acalculous cholecystitis. Am J Gastroenterol 79:650–653, 1984.

56. Henschke CI, Teele RL: Cholelithiasis in children: Recent observations. J Ultrasound Med 2:481–484, 1983.

57. Garel L, Lallemand D, Montagne J, et al: The changing aspects of cholelithiasis in children through a sonographic study. Pediatr Radiol 11:75–80, 1981.

58. Harned RK, Babbitt DP: Cholelithiasis in children. Radiology 117:391–393, 1975.

59. Greenberg M, Kangarloo H, Cochran ST, et al: The ultrasonographic diagnosis of cholecystitis and cholelithiasis in children. Radiology 137:745–749, 1980.

60. Pieretti R, Auldist AW, Stephens CA: Acute cholecystitis in children. Surg Gynecol Obstet 140:16–18, 1975.

61. Kane RA, Jacobs R, Katz J, Costello P: Porcelain gallbladder: Ultrasound and CT appearance. Radiology 152:137–141, 1984.

62. Love MB: Sonographic features of milk of calcium bile. J Ultrasound Med 1:325–327, 1982.

63. Rubner BH, Montgomery CK: Pathology of the Liver and Biliary Tract. New York, John Wiley & Sons, 1982, pp 312–332.

64. Bluth EI, Katz MM, Merritt CRB, Sullivan MA, Mitchell WT: Echographic findings in xanthogranulomatous cholecystitis. J Clin Ultrasound 7:213–214, 1979.

65. Jutras JA, Longtin JM, Levescue HP: Hyperplastic cholecystoses. AJR Am J Roentgenol 5:795–827, 1960.

66. Lafortune M, Gariepy G, Dumont A, Breton G, Lapointe R: The V-shaped artifact of the gallbladder wall. AJR Am J Roentgenol 147:505–508, 1986.

67. Galloni SS, Gervasio M, Saguatti G, Lipparini M, Stamati R, Miceli R: Ecotomografia real-time ad alta definizione e colecistografia per via orale nello studio delle colecistosi iperplastiche. Radiol Med 69:533–537, 1983.

68. Berk RN, van der Vegt JH, Lichtenstein JE: The hyperplastic cholecystoses: Cholesterolosis and adenomyomatosis. Radiology 146:593–601, 1983.

69. Jenett M, Dohrmann E: Adenomyomatose und Cholesterinpolypen der Gallenblase. Rofo Fortschr Geb Rontgenstr Neuen Bildgeb Verfahr 140:524–531, 1984.

70. Ruhe AH, Zachman JP, Mulder BD, Rime AE: Cholesterol polyps of the gallbladder: Ultrasound demonstration. J Clin Ultrasound 7:386–388, 1979.

71. Päivänsalo M, Myllylä V: Sonographic and cholecystographic diagnosis of cholesterolosis of the gallbladder. Röntgenpraxis 38:357–358, 1984.

72. Cover KL, Slasky BS, Skolnick ML: Sonography of

cholesterol in the biliary system. J Ultrasound Med 4:647–653, 1985.

73. Hidalgo HJ, Lewicki AM: Adenomyomatosis of the gallbladder. Am J Gastroenterol 73:81–84, 1980.

74. Rice J, Sauerbrei EE, Semogas P, Cooperberg PL, Burhenne HJ: Sonographic appearance of adenomyomatosis of the gallbladder. J Clin Ultrasound 9:336–337, 1981.

75. Raghavendra BN, Subramanyam BR, Balthazar EJ, Horii SC, Megibow AJ, Hilton S: Sonography of adenomyomatosis of the gallbladder: Radiologic-pathologic correlation. Radiology 146:747–752, 1983.

76. Kidney M, Goiney R, Cooperberg PL: Adenomyomatosis of the gallbladder: A pictorial exhibit. J Ultrasound Med 5:331–333, 1986.

77. Shieh CJ, Dunn E, Standard JE: Primary carcinoma of the gallbladder: A review of a 16-year experience at the Waterbury Hospital Health Center. Cancer 47:996–1004, 1981.

78. Kelly TR, Chamberlain TR: Carcinoma of the gallbladder. Am J Surg 143:737–741, 1982.

79. Dalla Palma L, Rizzatto G, Pozzi-Mucelli RS, Bazzocchi M: Grey-scale ultrasonography in the evaluation of carcinoma of the gallbladder. Br J Radiol 53:662–667, 1980.

80. Lampmann LEH, Meijer JG, Stroucken AAHM: Sonographic detection of early gallbladder cancer. Diagn Imag Clin Med 53:99–103, 1984.

81. Lane J, Buck JL, Zeman RK: Primary carcinoma of the gallbladder: A pictorial essay. RadioGraphics 9:209–228, 1989.

82. Tsuchiya Y: Early carcinoma of the gallbladder: Macroscopic features and US findings. Radiology 179:171–175, 1991.

Chapter 15

Bile Duct Pathology

William J. Zwiebel

This chapter considers sonographic findings that are associated with bile duct pathology. Biliary obstruction and choledocholithiasis are the principal focus of this chapter, for these conditions most frequently are the subject of sonographic examination. Sclerosing cholangitis, cholangiocarcinoma, choledochal cyst, Caroli disease, and neonatal jaundice also are included in this chapter, but these subjects receive less emphasis as they are less common.

INTRAHEPATIC DILATATION

As noted in Chapter 12, normal intrahepatic bile ducts are visible only in the vicinity of the porta hepatis, and they do not exceed 5 mm in diameter, or 40% of the adjacent portal vein diameter. Bile ducts are not seen normally *deep* within the liver; therefore, the detection of *any* bile duct *deep* within the liver suggests ductal obstruction.

Traditionally, intrahepatic biliary dilatation has been detected with the "parallel channel" or "shotgun" signs, in which the dilated bile duct is seen parallel to the right or left portal vein[1, 2] (Fig. 15-1). These signs are useful, but they are not as reliable as once believed, because hepatic artery branches or non-dilated bile ducts may produce a parallel channel appearance (see Figure 12–11 in Chapter 12). Before rendering a

diagnosis of biliary dilatation based on parallel channels, therefore, the diameter of the dilated intrahepatic duct should exceed 5 mm and 40% of the adjacent portal vein,[3, 4] and the identity of the hepatic artery should be confirmed with color Doppler sonography.

Marked Dilatation—Too Many Tubes

Markedly dilated intrahepatic ducts generally are easily detected with ultrasound, and differentiation from hepatic blood vessels usually is not a problem. Markedly dilated ducts are tortuous and resemble a "tangle of worms" as they converge at the porta hepatis. They produce a distinctive appearance called the *"too many tubes"* sign (Fig. 15–2).

Less Severe Dilatation

In contrast, minimal-to-moderate intrahepatic dilatation may be difficult to detect with ultrasound. In many cases, the dilated ducts can be recognized only by exclusion—that is, by the absence of blood flow in the ducts and the presence of flow in adjacent blood vessels (Fig. 15–3). The recognition of mildly dilated intrahepatic ducts is further complicated by the absence of a consistent anatomic relationship among the portal vein branches, the bile ducts, and the hepatic

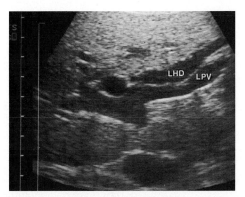

Figure 15-1—Parallel Channel Sign. A dilated left hepatic duct (LHD) is visible adjacent to the left portal vein (LPV) on this transverse image. Note that the duct is *larger* than the portal vein branch.

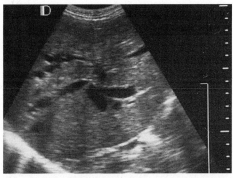

Figure 15-2—Too Many Tubes. A longitudinal scan of the right hepatic lobe demonstrtes a cluster of dilated, tortuous ducts at the porta hepatis.

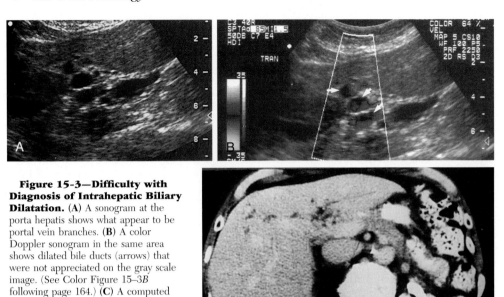

Figure 15-3—Difficulty with Diagnosis of Intrahepatic Biliary Dilatation. (A) A sonogram at the porta hepatis shows what appear to be portal vein branches. (B) A color Doppler sonogram in the same area shows dilated bile ducts (arrows) that were not appreciated on the gray scale image. (See Color Figure 15–3*B* following page 164.) (C) A computed tomogram in the same patient readily demonstrates intrahepatic ductal dilatation (black structures).

artery branches.[3] In some individuals, the bile ducts are anterior to the veins; in others, they are posterior to the veins, creating problems of identity.

Localized Dilatation

Localized or segmental dilatation deep within the liver is particularly difficult to detect sonographically, since such dilatation is apt to be overlooked on a routine survey of the liver. Even with careful examination, regional dilatation is apt to be overlooked.[5]

Accuracy for Intrahepatic Dilatation

Owing to the aforementioned difficulties, the sensitivity of ultrasound for *intrahepatic* dilatation is relatively poor (50% to 85%°), but specificity for intrahepatic dilatation is reported at 95%.[1–4] Thus, when intrahepatic dilatation is identified sonographically, this diagnosis may be relied upon.

EXTRAHEPATIC DILATATION

The sonographic diagnosis of extrahepatic biliary dilatation is based on careful measurement of the extrahepatic portions of the biliary ductal system. Grossly dilated extrahepatic ducts are

°Regardless of whether extrahepatic ducts are dilated.

quite easily seen with ultrasound (Fig. 15–4), both with the classic "sandwich" view and the "Mickey Mouse" views. The extrahepatic ducts are considered normal if the inside diameter is 6 mm or less, possibly dilated if the inside diameter is 7 mm, and dilated if the inside diameter equals or exceeds 8 mm *at the porta hepatis.* The ducts also may be considered dilated when the inside diameter exceeds 10 mm *at any extrahepatic location* (from the porta hepatis to the duodenum). Ductal dilatation implies obstruction, and the probability of *obstruction* increases with the degree of *dilatation.* For instance, a diameter of 7 mm at the porta hepatis *suggests* obstruction, but a diameter of 10 mm at the same location is virtually diagnostic of obstruction.[4, 6–12]

Ostensibly, the diagnosis of biliary obstruction with ultrasound should be a simple matter of measuring the bile duct diameter; however, the following pitfalls may cause diagnostic error.

Misidentification of the Duct

Accurate diagnosis depends on correct identification of the bile duct! This may appear to be an overstatement of an obvious fact, but misidentification of the duct is a common error, especially among inexperienced sonographers. To identify the extrahepatic bile duct accurately, one must clearly demonstrate classic sonographic anatomy with the "sandwich" or "Mickey Mouse" views, as described in Chapter 12. The use of color Doppler also may be necessary to identify

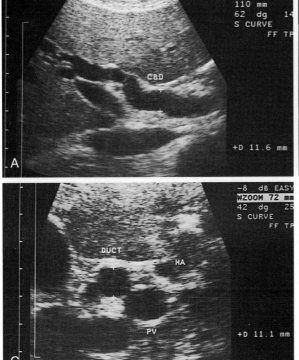

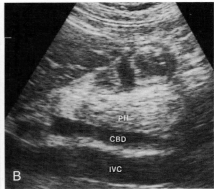

Figure 15-4—Extrahepatic Bile Duct Dilatation. (A) The classic "sandwich" view shows an 11-mm extrahepatic duct (CBD). **(B)** The distal portion of the extrahepatic duct (CBD) is seen within the pancreatic head (PH) on this longitudinal view. IVC = inferior vena cava. **(C)** A "Mickey Mouse" view at the porta hepatis shows the dilated duct (DUCT, cursors), the portal vein (PV) and the hepatic artery (HA).

the portal vein, the hepatic artery, and the bile duct (through absence of flow).

Obstructed but Nondilated Ducts

Three phases of ductal obstruction have been noted: (1) a pre-dilatory phase in which liver function studies and scintigraphy are abnormal but bile duct size may remain within normal limits; (2) a dilatory phase characterized by progressive ductal dilatation; and (3) an icteric phase characterized by ductal dilatation, bilirubin elevation, and gross clinical jaundice.[13–25] The pre-dilatory phase may extend for a day or two after an abrupt obstruction occurs (e.g., calculus-related obstruction). During this phase, the bile ducts may be normal sonographically, even though the ductal system is completely obstructed.[15–20, 23] Ductal dilatation also may be absent if obstruction occurs intermittently, as may occur in patients with small intraductal calculi.

Dilated but Nonobstructed Ducts

Extrahepatic ductal dilatation may occur in the *absence* of obstruction or jaundice.[1, 12, 21–23] Such dilatation is uncommon but may lead to a false-positive diagnosis of obstruction. Non-obstructive dilatation results from loss of ductal elasticity (due to prior obstruction), or it may be idiopathic.

Postcholecystectomy Dilatation

Contrary to traditional beliefs, the extrahepatic bile duct *does not* assume a reservoir function and dilate following cholecystectomy. On average, the caliber of the extrahepatic duct increases slightly after cholecystectomy, but if the bile duct is intrinsically normal (i.e., no retained calculi or stricture), it will assume a normal caliber postcholecystectomy in about 85% of cases, even if it was dilated prior to surgery.[12, 26–28] Postcholecystectomy ductal dilatation, therefore, is a harbinger of obstruction and should not be passed over as a normal physiologic alteration. A pathologic cause of biliary dilatation is found in approximately 80% of patients with postcholecystectomy biliary dilatation.[28]

Ascending Dilatation

Dilatation in the biliary tree begins at the point of obstruction and proceeds *cephalad*.[24, 25] In cases of distal obstruction (i.e., in the pancreatic head), dilatation may be present near the pancreatic head but absent at the porta hepatis. Obstruction may be unrecognized, therefore, if the ducts are examined only at the porta hepatis or in the liver. Ductal dilatation should always be sought distally, in the head of the pancreas, as well as at the porta hepatis and in the liver.

Borderline Ductal Dilatation

A diagnostic dilemma occurs with a porta hepatis duct measurement of 7 mm, which *suggests* obstruction but is not definitive. The administration of a fatty meal or a cholecystokinin analogue has been advocated in this situation to relax the sphincter of Oddi and reduce the caliber of the unobstructed duct.[29-31] The physiologic response of these maneuvers is quite variable, however, and most sonologists have tried and abandoned these methods. When ultrasound findings are equivocal, one generally must resort to cholescintigraphy for further diagnostic information.

The Ectatic Hepatic Artery

The hepatic artery commonly is ectatic in elderly patients (a diameter of 10 mm is not unusual). Hepatic artery dilatation, therefore, may mimic extrahepatic ductal dilatation in an older patient. Because of this possibility, the identity of the hepatic artery and the bile duct should be confirmed with color duplex sonography whenever porta hepatis anatomy is unclear.

SONOGRAPHIC ACCURACY

Sonography is frequently the first imaging procedure requested when biliary obstruction is suspected, because ultrasound is reasonably accurate, the results of the examination are available without delay, and ultrasound often can pinpoint the level and cause of obstruction. In spite of these merits, it is noteworthy that ultrasound diagnosis of obstruction is merely inferential. Obstruction is *inferred* sonographically when the

bile ducts are dilated, but in some instances obstructed ducts are not dilated, and in others, dilated ducts are not obstructed.

In some series, the sensitivity and specificity of ultrasound for biliary obstruction exceeds 90%. It is difficult, nonetheless, to pinpoint the accuracy of ultrasound, since published figures vary widely and many of the studies are out of date (Table 15–1).[4, 9, 18, 26, 32-35] The apparent causes of this wide range include the evolution of ultrasound instrumentation and the identification, over time, of the diagnostic pitfalls cited previously. Furthermore, the statistics cited in Table 15–1 refer to the detection of ductal obstruction *at any level* within the biliary tree. Accuracy figures would probably be greater if only extrahepatic obstruction were considered.

ACCURACY OF OTHER IMAGING STUDIES

In contrast to sonography, cholescintigraphy detects obstruction *directly*, through the visualization of bile flow. As a result, this method, with sensitivity and specificity exceeding 90%, is the most accurate noninvasive method for identifying or excluding biliary obstruction.[32, 34] The use of scintigraphy is encouraged, therefore, when sonography is limited technically, when duct size is equivocal, and when the duct size is normal but acute obstruction is strongly suspected clinically (i.e., during the "predilatory" phase).

Computed tomography (Figure 15–3C) appears to be considerably better then sonography for detecting intrahepatic biliary dilatation, but it is not considered accurate for detection of extrahepatic obstruction.[36] Computed tomography is very useful, however, for determining the location and cause of biliary obstruction, as addressed next.

DETERMINING THE LOCATION AND CAUSE OF OBSTRUCTION

Think location and cause! Whenever biliary dilatation is detected, the sonographer should

Table 15-1. Biliary Obstruction: Reported Diagnostic Accuracy of Sonographic Assessment

Reference #	32	9	33	18	4	34	35	26
Date	1979	1980	1981	1981	1981	1984	1984	1991
Number of cases	31	203	84	54	85	49	108	91
Sensitivity (%)	43	99	81	90	86	55	75	96
Specificity (%)	96	96	89	60	85	93	81	96
PPV° (%)	75	86	97	60	50	85	87	89
NPV† (%)	85	99	84	97	97	73	60	95

°Positive predictive value.
†Negative predictive value.

Table 15-2. Some Masses That May Cause Biliary Tract Obstruction

Intrahepatic metastases
Hepatocellular carcinoma
Porta hepatitis nodal metastases°
Parapancreatic nodal metastases°
Pancreatic carcinoma
Gallbladder carcinoma
Cholangiocarcinoma
Bile duct polyp

°Including lymphoma.

seek the location and the cause of obstruction. At the least, this information may affect the selection of additional diagnostic studies, and in some cases this information may influence the entire therapeutic plan.

Ultrasound correctly identifies the level of obstruction in 92% to 95% of cases,[37, 38] and in 71% to 88% of cases the cause can be narrowed to three broad categories: neoplastic mass, pancreatitis, and calculi.[37, 38]

Masses

Most masses that obstruct the bile ducts are quite large by the time icterus is apparent clinically; therefore, ultrasound correctly identifies about 90% of obstructing neoplasms.[38] Pancreatic carcinoma is the primary neoplastic cause of biliary obstruction (Chapter 5), but a variety of other neoplasms also may obstruct the biliary tree, as listed in Table 15-2. The sonologist, therefore, should consider all possibilities.

Pancreatitis

Bile duct obstruction may *result from* acute pancreatitis (pancreatic head edema), or it may *cause* pancreatitis (distal bile duct calculus). Therefore, when biliary dilatation is present in a pancreatitis patient, the distal bile duct should be scrutinized for a calculus that may be blocking both the bile duct and the pancreatic duct.

Intraductal Calculi

The accurate detection of intraductal calculi[37–43] requires clear visualization of the distal, intrapancreatic portion of the duct, since most obstructing calculi lodge there. Transverse images through the pancreatic head are particularly valuable in this respect, but longitudinal scans also may demonstrate distal ductal calculi.

The ultrasound detection rates for ductal calculi range widely in literature reports,[37–43] but a reasonable figure appears to be about 60%, which is not outstanding.[43] The principal cause for this disappointing performance is lack of echo-contrast between an impacted ductal calculus and surrounding tissues. A calculus is easily visualized when it is surrounded by bile in a widely dilated duct (Fig. 15–5A), but a stone in a non-dilated duct or a stone impacted in the pancreatic head "fades" into the echogenic background of surrounding tissues.[40, 44] This brings up an important point: choledocholithiasis cannot be excluded on the basis of a normal ultrasound examination. In 21% to 36% of cases, calculus-containing ducts are *not* dilated. In most of these cases, the intraductal calculi are small, obstruction is intermittent,[40, 42, 44] and the calculi will not

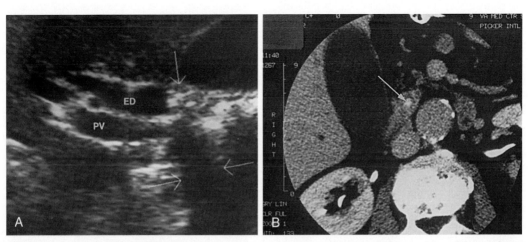

Figure 15-5—Choledocholithiasis. (A) A calculus (vertical arrow) is visible in the lower portion of the extrahepatic bile duct (ED) on this "sandwich" ultrasound view. Note the acoustic shadow (horizontal arrows). PV = portal vein. (B) A computed tomogram in a different patient shows a calculus (arrow) impacted in the lower portion of the pancreatic head. This calculus was not visible sonographically.

be found with ultrasound. Endoscopic retrograde cholangiography is the procedure of choice for identifying small intraductal calculi that obstruct intermittently.

It is heartening to note that ultrasonic specificity for choledocholithiasis exceeds 95%.[37–43] So, if we cannot find ductal calculi too often, at least we can be sure of the diagnosis when we do find duct stones. False-positives include gas bubbles, surgical clips, parasites, and other echogenic material.[44]

CT Determination of the Cause of Obstruction

When ultrasound fails to determine the cause of biliary obstruction, computed tomography (CT) is often a logical next choice. CT appears to be superior to sonography for detecting both the level and cause of obstruction.[39, 45–49] CT determines the cause of obstruction in 94% of cases and visualizes ductal calculi directly in 50% to 90% of cases[39, 45–49] (Fig. 15–5*B*); furthermore, CT is highly accurate for the diagnosis of neoplastic obstruction and provides valuable staging information in patients with tumors.

CHOLANGIOCARCINOMA

Cholangiocarcinoma[50–57] is a malignant neoplasm that originates in the bile duct epithelium. The tumor may arise either in an intra- or extrahepatic location and may grow linearly along the bile duct, with little mass effect; as a localized, bulky mass; or (rarely) as an intraluminal polyp. The "Klatskin tumor" is a bulky, slow-growing, late-metastasizing form of cholangiocarcinoma located at the junction of the right and left hepatic ducts.[51, 52, 57] The outlook is poor for patients with cholangiocarcinoma. Overall, average survival is only 185 days postdiagnosis[50]; for the Klatskin variety, average survival is about 16 months.

Cholangiography is the principal mode of diagnosis, but the potential is relatively good for sonographic diagnosis of cholangiocarcinoma (by an astute sonographer), because sonography is used initially in most jaundiced patients. Sonographic diagnosis may be accomplished in about 50% of cases, with proper attention to ductal detail.[52]

The sonographic findings relate directly to the mode of tumor development.[50–56] Tumors at the porta hepatis are manifested by a distinctive sonographic observation: dilated ducts are seen in the right and left lobes, but the dilated ducts cannot be traced to the common hepatic duct (i.e., do not converge), because the tumor intervenes. Close scrutiny may demonstrate the intervening tumor mass. Tumors that grow linearly or intraluminally are manifested by the following: ductal narrowing and irregularity; thickening of the duct wall (greater than 5 mm); and a low echogenicity mass *centered* on the bile duct (Fig. 15–6). It is noteworthy that a duct wall thickness exceeding 5 mm strongly suggests cholangiocarcinoma, rather than a cicatricial process such as sclerosing cholangitis.[56]

It is not surprising that the most common and prominent sonographic finding in cholangiocarcinoma is generalized ductal dilatation. Differentiation between dilatation from cholangiocarcinoma and sclerosing cholangitis is considered in the next section.

SCLEROSING CHOLANGITIS

Sclerosing cholangitis[58] is a diffuse process of biliary scarring affecting both the extra- and intrahepatic bile ducts, which ultimately results in biliary cirrhosis and death. The disease usually affects men less than 40 years of age. In some cases, chronic pyogenic infection (especially following biliary diversion), or *Clonorchis sinensis* infestation is identified as the cause of the cicatricial process. Alternatively, sclerosing cholangitis may occur as a primary disorder of unknown etiology. The primary form is associated epidemiologically with inflammatory bowel disease (particularly Crohn disease), and oriental cholangitis. The relationship of the latter condition to *Clonorchis sinensis* infestation is debated.[59, 60]

In sclerosing cholangitis, fibrous tissue overgrowth obliterates the ductal lumen and pro-

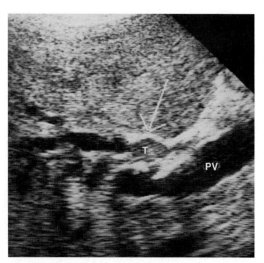

Figure 15–6—Cholangiocarcinoma. In this case, the tumor mass (T, arrow) is seen to fill the extrahepatic duct on a "sandwich" view. PV = portal vein.

duces numerous areas of stenosis or occlusion. Biliary tract sclerosis is pervasive, affecting both the small and large biliary radicals and both the intra- and extrahepatic ducts. Even the gallbladder may be affected. Ductal narrowing typically is circumferential and involves short segments, with intervening "skip areas" that may be normal in caliber or dilated. The result is a "string of beads" cholangiographic appearance (Fig. 15–7A).

The sonographic hallmark of sclerosing cholangitis[59-64] is ductal dilatation that is multifocal, affects relatively short segments, and is discontinuous (Fig. 15–7B). Characteristically, both the extra- and intrahepatic ducts are involved. The duct walls may be markedly thickened or irregular, and the gallbladder wall also may be thickened. Reactive enlargement of regional lymph nodes may occur in response to the inflammatory process, and enlarged nodes may be mistaken for neoplastic masses.[61] Dilated portions of the ductal system may contain echogenic bile, nonshadowing "soft" calculi, typical shadowing calculi,

or proteinaceous debris. The presence of large, poorly shadowing calculi and extensive intraductal debris is suggestive of *Clonorchis* cholangitis or its close relative, oriental cholangitis.[59, 60, 64, 65] Debris is a less prominent feature in other types of sclerosing cholangitis.

The following points are useful for differentiating between sclerosing cholangitis and cholangiocarcinoma: Sclerosing cholangitis causes multifocal dilatation, intra- and extrahepatic ductal involvement, possible gallbladder involvement, and in some cases extensive stone and debris formation. In contrast, cholangiocarcinoma causes a single area of obstruction, dilatation of the entire ductal system proximal to the tumor, and an extrinsic tumor mass (in most cases); furthermore, calculi and intraductal debris are uncommon.

CHOLEDOCHAL CYST

A choledochal "cyst" is not, in fact, a cyst but is a congenital dilatation of the extrahepatic

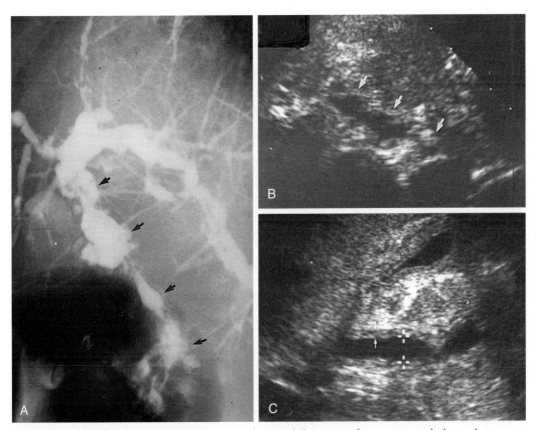

Figure 15-7—Sclerosing Cholangitis. (A) A transhepatic cholangiogram demonstrates marked irregularity (narrowing and dilatation) of the extrahepatic (arrows) and intrahepatic bile ducts. (B) Sonography shows thickening and irregularity of the extrahepatic portion of the bile duct (arrows). (C) In another patient with AIDS-related cholangitis, the extrahepatic bile duct wall (arrows) is visibly thickened (about 4 mm). The wall normally is not visible. Cursors = bile duct lumen.

portion of the biliary tree.[66-72] This rare disorder usually presents with pain or biliary obstruction during the first few years of life, but some cases do not present until adulthood. Choledochal cysts are complicated by bile stasis, calculus formation, and cholangitis.

Three primary types of choledochal cysts have been described. Type I is most common; it consists of *diffuse* and massive biliary ectasia proximal to a stenotic or atretic distal common bile duct segment. Ectasia may extend into the cystic duct or the main intrahepatic branches. Type II is a *localized*, diverticulum-like outpouching from the ductal system (usually the common duct). The cyst may compress and obstruct a normal portion of the extrahepatic duct, causing generalized biliary dilatation and icterus. Type III is the rarest form and consists of dilatation of the common duct *within* the wall of the duodenum, forming a "choledochocele" that may obstruct the biliary system or the duodenum.[66, 67, 70, 71] Type I (diffuse dilatation) may be diagnosed with certainty on ultrasound examination if a massively dilated, cystlike duct segment is seen to communicate directly with the remainder of the biliary system. The diverticulum-like Type II cyst (Fig. 15–8) is less likely to be diagnosed conclu-

sively, since the point of communication between the cyst and the ductal system generally is not demonstrable. Thus, other cystlike lesions fall into the differential diagnosis. The diagnosis of choledochal cyst can be confirmed scintigraphically through uptake of tracer in the cystic segment. Generalized biliary dilatation is an ancillary finding that is present in about 60% of choledochal cyst cases.

The sonographic differential diagnosis for choledochal cyst includes duplication cyst, renal cyst, abscess, pancreatic pseudocyst, hepatic artery or portal vein aneurysm, and cavernous transformation of the portal vein.

CAROLI DISEASE

Communicating cavernous ectasia of the intrahepatic biliary ducts (Caroli disease)[66, 67, 73-75] is a rare disorder. It is included herein only because it has characteristic sonographic findings. This developmental disorder is characterized by saccular dilatation of the *intrahepatic* ducts.

The sonographic pattern that characterizes Caroli disease is saccular, *grossly dilated* intrahepatic duct segments that *converge* toward the porta hepatis.[66, 67, 73-75] Convergence is sufficiently

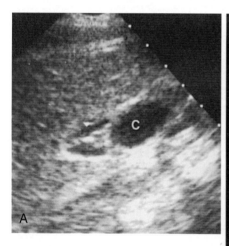

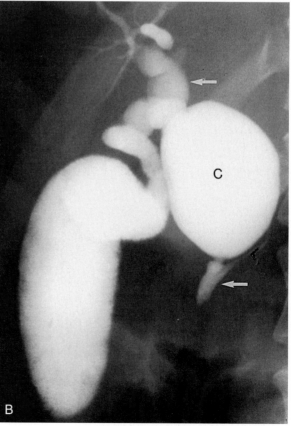

Figure 15-8—Choledochal Cyst. (A) An oblique sonogram shows a cyst (C) in the porta hepatis in this adult Asian woman with epigastric pain. Other views confirmed that this cyst was separate from the gallbladder. **(B)** A transhepatic cholangiogram shows cystic dilatation (C) of the common bile duct. The proximal and distal portions of the bile duct are indicated by arrows.

characteristic to allow for sonographic diagnosis. Also characteristic is the visualization of saccular ducts "wrapping around" adjacent portal blood vessels, with the vessels either protruding into or enveloped completely by the dilated duct. The gallbladder is normal in Caroli disease. The extrahepatic ducts may be normal; alternatively, ductal dilatation or a choledochal cyst may accompany the intrahepatic abnormalities.

PERSISTENT NEONATAL CHOLESTASIS

Etiology

Neonatal cholestasis is diagnosed when the conjugated fraction exceeds 20% of the total bilirubin.[76] Virtually all cases of *persistent* cholestasis in the neonatal period result from biliary atresia, neonatal hepatitis, or the bile plug syndrome.[66, 67, 72, 76–85]

It is hypothesized that biliary atresia is related etiologically to neonatal hepatitis, since both conditions appear to have an infectious origin (possibly viral). In neonatal hepatitis, the biliary tree remains normal, whereas in biliary atresia a sclerotic process occurs that obliterates part or all of the biliary system. A choledochal cyst may occur in association with biliary atresia, and these conditions are thought to have a common etiology *when seen concurrently.*[72, 76, 82] In the bile plug syndrome, the ductal system is normal but is filled with viscid bile that causes obstruction.[76–78] This condition usually is precipitated by dehydration, sepsis, prolonged hyperalimentation, or cystic fibrosis.

Therapeutic Differentiation

The accurate and prompt differentiation among biliary atresia, the bile plug syndrome, and neonatal hepatitis may be crucial for the survival of a cholestatic infant. Biliary atresia must be treated surgically, and prompt surgical treatment appears to be advantageous. Success in achieving bile drainage decreases from 91% before 2 months of age to only 17% in infants older than 3 months.[79] The bile plug syndrome may be treated supportively (e.g., hydration) in some instances, but surgical intervention is sometimes required to dissolve or remove the inspissated material. Unfortunately, neonatal hepatitis can be treated only with supportive measures.

Sonographic Findings

Ultrasound is a first-line examination in the cholestatic neonate. The crucial sonographic finding is generalized ductal dilatation, which directs the inquiry away from biliary atresia and neonatal hepatitis and instead focuses the investigation on the bile plug syndrome, or other causes of biliary obstruction. When biliary dilatation is encountered, the extrahepatic ducts should be scrutinized for low-to-moderately echogenic material indicative of a bile plug.[76–78] Less commonly, sonographic findings in the cholestatic neonate may point directly to choledochal cyst or Caroli disease, as discussed earlier.

It is noteworthy that *ductal dilatation does not occur in biliary atresia* even though ductal obstruction usually is localized (at porta, 75% to 85% of cases; at distal common duct, 15% to 25% of cases), and the remainder of the ductal system is patent. The lack of biliary dilatation is attributed to the diffuse nature of the inflammatory process that characterizes biliary atresia.[76] Although only portions of the ductal system are obliterated, the ducts are abnormal throughout and do not dilate. The diffuse nature of the disorder permits definitive diagnosis by liver biopsy, when noninvasive methods are inconclusive.

The gallbladder almost always is affected in biliary atresia; it either is small and irregular or cannot be found sonographically (in spite of fasting). Caution is advised in the interpretation of gallbladder findings, however.[76, 80–82] Infants with atresia may occasionally have a normal-sized gallbladder; conversely, the gallbladder may be small in neonatal hepatitis due to reduced bile output. Before the gallbladder is deemed normal, a typical ovoid or "tear-drop" shape should be noted, the maximum dimension should be at least 1.5 cm, and a substantial decrease in size should occur after feeding.

The Role of Scintigraphy

Once diffuse ductal dilatation and choledochal cyst have been excluded with ultrasound in the cholestatic infant, scintigraphy should be used to distinguish between biliary atresia and neonatal hepatitis. The absence of tracer excretion into the bowel at 24 hours is diagnostic of biliary atresia with a high level of accuracy, particularly if the infant is pretreated with phenobarbital to enhance conjugation and excretion of the tracer.[76, 80, 83, 85] Tracer excretion is evident by 24 hours in cases of neonatal hepatitis.

Other Studies

Differential diagnosis of neonatal cholestasis can almost always be accomplished with a combination of laboratory tests, ultrasound, and scintigraphy.[76] In some cases, however, percutaneous liver biopsy is required to differentiate between biliary atresia and neonatal hepatitis.

Intraoperative cholangiography is used routinely immediately prior to attempted surgical repair of atresia, both to confirm the diagnosis of atresia and to define the atretic segment(s).[76]

REFERENCES

1. Weill F, Eisencher A, Zeltner F: Ultrasonic study of the normal and dilated biliary tree. The "shotgun" sign. Radiology 127:221–224, 1978.

2. Willi UV, Teele RL: Hepatic arteries and the parallel-channel sign. J Clin Ultrasound 7:125–127, 1979.

3. Bressler EL, Rubin JM, McCracken S: Sonographic parallel channel sign: A reappraisal. Radiology 164:343–346, 1987.

4. Deitch EA: The reliability and clinical limitations of sonographic scanning of the biliary ducts. Ann Surg 193:167–170, 1981.

5. Miller WJ, Federle MP, Campbell WL: Diagnosis and staging of hepatocellular carcinoma: Comparison of CT and sonography in 36 liver transplantation patients. AJR Am J Roentgenol 157:303–306, 1991.

6. Parulekar SG: Ultrasound evaluation of bile duct size. Radiology 133:703–707, 1979.

7. Parulekar SG, McNamara MP Jr: Ultrasonography of choledocholithiasis. J Ultrasound Med 2:395–400, 1983.

8. Cooperberg PL: High-resolution real-time ultrasound in the evaluation of the normal and obstructed biliary tract. Radiology 129:477–480, 1979.

9. Cooperberg PL, Li R, Wong P, et al: Accuracy of common hepatic duct size in evaluation of extrahepatic biliary obstruction. Radiology 135:141–144, 1980.

10. Freise J, Gebel M, Kleine P, Weyand C: The diameter of the common bile duct determined by ultrasound and ERCP is not necessarily comparable. Ann Radiol 28:5–8, 1984.

11. Wu C-C, Ho Y-H, Chen C-Y: Effect of aging on common bile duct diameter: A real-time ultrasonographic study. J Clin Ultrasound 12:473–478, 1984.

12. Niederau C, Müller J, Sonnenberg A, Scholten T, Erckenbrecht J, Fritsch W-P, Brüster T, Strohmeyer G: Extrahepatic bile ducts in healthy subjects, in patients with cholelithiasis, and in postcholecystectomy patients: A prospective ultrasonic study. J Clin Ultrasound 11:23–27, 1983.

13. Burrell MI, Zeman RK, Simeone JF, Dachman AH, McGahan JP, vanSonnenberg E, Zimmon DS, Torres W, Laufer I: The biliary tract: Imaging for the 1990s. AJR Am J Roentgenol 157:223–233, 1991.

14. Ralls PW, Quinn MF, Halls J: Biliary sonography: Ventral bowing of the dilated common duct. AJR Am J Roentgenol 137:1127–1129, 1981.

15. Muhletaler CA, Gerlock AJ, Fleischer AC, James AE: Diagnosis of obstructive jaundice with nondilated bile ducts. AJR Am J Roentgenol 134:1149–1152, 1980.

16. Floyd JL, Collins TL: Discordance of sonography and cholescintigraphy in acute biliary obstruction. AJR Am J Roentgenol 140:501–502, 1983.

17. Scheske GA, Cooperberg PL, Cohen MM, Burhenne HJ: Dynamic changes in the caliber of the major bile ducts, related to obstruction. Radiology 135:215–216, 1980.

18. Klingensmith WC, Johnson ML, Kuni CC, et al: Complementary role of Tc-99m-diethyl-IDA and ultrasound in large and small duct biliary tract obstruction. Radiology 138:177–184, 1981.

19. Miller DR, Egbert RM, Braunstein P: Comparison of ultrasound and hepatobiliary imaging in the early detection of acute common bile duct obstruction. Arch Surg 119:1233–1238, 1984.

20. Taylor KJW, Rosenfield AT, Spiro HM: Diagnostic accuracy of gray scale ultrasonography for the jaundiced patient. A report of 275 cases. Arch Intern Med 139:60–63, 1979.

21. Zeman R, Taylor KJW, Burrell MJ, Gold J: Ultrasound demonstration of anicteric dilatation of the biliary tree. Radiology 134:689–692, 1980.

22. Weinstein BJ, Weinstein DP: Biliary tract dilatation in the nonjaundiced patient. AJR Am J Roentgenol 134:899–906, 1980.

23. vanSonnenberg E, Ferrucci JT, Neff CC, Mueller PR, Simeone JF, Wittenberg J: Biliary pressure: Manometric and perfusion studies at percutaneous transhepatic cholangiography and percutaneous biliary drainage. Radiology 148:41–50, 1983.

24. Shawker TH, Jones BL, Girton ME: Distal common bile obstruction: An experimental study in monkeys. J Clin Ultrasound 9:77–82, 1981.

25. Zeman RK, Dorfman GS, Burrell MI, Stein S, Berg G, Gold JA: Disparate dilatation of the intrahepatic and extrahepatic bile ducts in surgical jaundice. Radiology 138:129–136, 1981.

26. Stott MA, Farrands PA, Guyer PB, Dewbury KC, Browning JJ, Sutton R: Ultrasound of the common bile duct in patients undergoing cholecystectomy. J Clin Ultrasound 19:73–76, 1991.

27. Mueller PR, Ferrucci JT, Simeone JF, Wittenberg J, vanSonnenberg E, Polansky A, Isler RJ: Postcholecystectomy bile duct dilatation: Myth or reality? AJR Am J Roentgenol 136:355–358, 1981.

28. Graham MF, Cooperberg PL, Cohen MM, Burhenne HJ: Ultrasonographic screening of the common hepatic duct in symptomatic patients after cholecystectomy. Radiology 138:137–139, 1981.

29. Fein AB, Rauch RF, Bowie JD, Halvorsen RA, Rosenberg ER: Intravenous cholecystokinin octapeptide: Its effect on the sonographic appearance of the bile ducts in normal subjects. Radiology 153:499–501, 1984.

30. Simeone JF, Butch RJ, Mueller PR, vanSonnenberg E, Ferrucci JT, Hall DA, Kopans DB, Dawson SL, Wittenberg J, McCarthy K: The bile ducts after a fatty meal: Further sonographic observations. Radiology 154:763–768, 1985.

31. Willson SA, Gosink BB, vanSonnenberg E: Unchanged size of a dilated common bile duct after a fatty meal: Results and significance. Radiology 160:29–31, 1986.

32. Cheng TH, Davis MA, Seltzer SE, et al: Evaluation of hepatobiliary imaging by radionuclide scintigraphy, ultrasonography, and contrast cholangiography. Radiology 133:761–767, 1979.

33. Haubek A, Pedersen JH, Burcharth F, et al: Dynamic sonography in the evaluation of jaundice. AJR Am J Roentgenol 136:1071–1074, 1981.

34. O'Connor KW, Snodgrass PJ, Swonder JE, Mahoney S, Burt R, Cockerill EM, Lumeng L: A blinded prospective study comparing four current noninvasive approaches in the differential diagnosis

of medical versus surgical jaundice. Gastroenterology 84:1498–1504, 1983.

35. Lassegue A, Deschamps J-P, Ottignon Y, Rohmer P, Didier D, Weill F, Carayon P, Miguel J-P: Valeur diagnostique pragmatique de l'échographie hépato-biliaire chez 193 malades ictériques consécutifs adressés dans un centre de cholangiographie rétrograde endoscopique (CRE). Gastroenterol Clin Biol 8:512–517, 1984.

36. Egbert RN, Braunstein P, Lyons KP, et al: Total bile duct obstruction. Arch Surg 118:709–712, 1983.

37. Laing FC, Jeffrey RB, Wing VW, Nyberg DA: Biliary dilatation: Defining the level and cause by real-time US. Radiology 160:39–42, 1986.

38. Gibson RN, Yeung E, Thompson JN, Carr DH, Hemingway AP, Bradpiece HA, Benjamin IS, Blumgart LH, Allison DJ: Bile duct obstruction: Radiologic evaluation of level, cause and tumor resectability. Radiology 160:43–47, 1986.

39. Mitchell SE, Clark RA: A comparison of computed tomography and sonography in choledocholithiasis. AJR Am J Roentgenol 142:729–733, 1984.

40. Einstein DM, Lapin SA, Ralls PW, Halls JM: The insensitivity of sonography in the detection of choledocholithiasis. AJR Am J Roentgenol 142:725–728, 1984.

41. Espinoza P, Kunstlinger F, Liguory C, Meduri B, Pelletier G, Etienne J-P: Valeur de l'échotomographie pour le diagnostic di lithiase de la voie biliare principale. Gastroenterol Clin Biol 8:42–46, 1984.

42. Laing FC, Jeffrey RB, Wing VW: Improved visualization of choledocholithiasis by sonography. AJR Am J Roentgenol 143:949–952, 1984.

43. Cronan JJ: US diagnosis of choledocholithiasis: A reappraisal. Radiology 161:133–134, 1986.

44. Lewandowski B, French G, Winsberg F: The normal post-cholecystectomy sonogram: Gas vs. clips. J Ultrasound Med 4:7–12, 1985.

45. Pedrosa CS, Casanova R, Rodriguez R: Computed tomography in obstructive jaundice. Part I: The level of obstruction. Radiology 139:627–634, 1981.

46. Pedrosa CS, Casanova R, Lezana AH, Fernandez MC: Computed tomography in obstructive jaundice. Part II: The cause of obstruction. Radiology 139:635–645, 1981.

47. Jeffrey RB, Federle MP, Laing FC, Wall S, Rego J, Moss AA: Computed tomography of choledocholithiasis. AJR Am J Roentgenol 140:1179–1183, 1983.

48. Baron RL: Common bile duct stones: Reassessment of criteria for CT diagnosis. Radiology 162:419–424, 1987.

49. Deyoe LA, Cronan JJ: Noninvasive imaging of common duct stones. Appl Radiol 20:13–15, 1991.

50. Norton RA, Foster EA: Bile duct cancer. CA Cancer J Clin 40:225–233, 1990.

51. Meyer DG, Weinstein BJ: Klatskin tumors of the bile ducts: Sonographic appearance. Radiology 148:803–804, 1983.

52. Machan L, Müller NL, Cooperberg PL: Sonographic diagnosis of Klatskin tumors. AJR Am J Roentgenol 147:509–512, 1986.

53. Marchal G, Gelin J, Van Steenbergen W, Fevery J, Vanneste A, Geboes K, Kerremans R, Ponette E, Baert AL: Sonographic diagnosis of intraluminal bile duct neoplasm: A report of 3 cases. Gastrointest Radiol 9:329–333, 1984.

54. Subramanyam BR, Raghavendra BN, Balthazar EJ, Horii SC, LeFleur RS, Rosen RJ: Ultrasonic features of cholangiocarcinoma. J Ultrasound Med 4:405–408, 1984.

55. Pastakia B, Shawker TH, Horvath K: Biliary neoplasms simulating dilated bile ducts. J Ultrasound Med 6:333–338, 1987.

56. Schulte SJ, Baron RL, Teefey SA, Rohrmann CA, Freeny PC, Shuman WP, Foster MA: CT of the extrahepatic bile ducts: Wall thickness and contrast enhancement in normal and abnormal ducts. AJR Am J Roentgenol 154:79–85, 1990.

57. Tsuzuki T, Ogata Y, Iida S, Nakanishi I, Takenaka Y, Yoshii H: Carcinoma of the bifurcation of the hepatic ducts. Arch Surg 118:1147–1151, 1983.

58. LaRusso NF, Wiesner RH, Ludwig J, MacCarty RL: Primary sclerosing cholangitis. N Engl J Med 310:899–903, 1984.

59. vanSonnenberg E, Casola G, Cubberley DA, Halasz NA, Cabrera OA, Wittich GR, Mattrey RF, Scheible FW: Oriental cholangiohepatitis: Diagnostic imaging and interventional management. AJR Am J Roentgenol 146:327–331, 1986.

60. Lim JH: Radiologic findings of clonorchiasis. AJR Am J Roentgenol 155:1001–1008, 1990.

61. Carroll BA, Oppenheimer DA: Sclerosing cholangitis: Sonographic demonstration of bile duct wall thickening. AJR Am J Roentgenol 139:1016–1018, 1982.

62. Rahn NJ, Koehler RE, Weyman PJ, Truss CD, Sagel SS, Stanley JJ: CT appearance of sclerosing cholangitis. AJR Am J Roentgenol 141:549–552, 1983.

63. Teefey SA, Baron RL, Rohrmann CA, Shuman WP, Freeny PC: Sclerosing cholangitis: CT findings. Radiology 169:635–639, 1988.

64. Lim JH, Ko YT, Lee DH, Kim SY: Clonorchiasis: Sonographic findings in 59 proved cases. AJR Am J Roentgenol 152:761–764, 1989.

65. Lim JH, Ko YT, Lee DH, Hong KS: Oriental cholangiohepatitis: Sonographic findings in 48 cases. AJR Am J Roentgenol 155:511–514, 1990.

66. Haller JO: Sonography of the biliary tract in infants and children. AJR Am J Roentgenol 157:1051–1058, 1991.

67. Gates GF, Sinatra FR, Thomas DW: Cholestatic syndromes in infancy and childhood. AJR Am J Roentgenol 134:1141–1148, 1980.

68. Savader SJ, Benenati JF, Venbrux AC, Mitchell SE, Widlus DM, Cameron JL, Osterman FA: Choledochal cysts: Classification and cholangiographic appearance. AJR Am J Roentgenol 156:327–331, 1991.

69. Wiedmeyer DA, Stewart ET, Dodds WJ, et al: Choledochal cyst: Findings on cholangiopancreatography with emphasis on ectasia of the common channel. AJR Am J Roentgenol 153:969–972, 1989.

70. Kangarloo H, Sarti DA, Sample WF, Amundson G: Ultrasonographic spectrum of choledochal cysts in children. Pediatr Radiol 9:15–18, 1980.

71. Richardson JD, Grant EG, Barth KH, Arnstein N, Jacobs N, DeRosa R, Chun BK: Type II choledochal cyst: Diagnosis using real-time sonography. J Ultrasound Med 3:37–39, 1984.

72. Torrisi JM, Haller JO, Velcek FT: Choledochal cyst and biliary atresia in the neonate: Imaging findings in five cases. AJR Am J Roentgenol 155:1273–1276, 1990.

73. Mittelstaedt CA, Volberg FM, Fischer GJ, McCartney WH: Caroli's disease: Sonographic findings. AJR Am J Roentgenol 134:585–587, 1980.

74. Marchal GJ, Desmet VJ, Proesmans WC, Moerman

PL, Van Roost WW, Van Holsbeeck MT, Baert AL: Caroli disease: High-frequency US and pathologic findings. Radiology 158:507–511, 1986.

75. Toma P, Lucigrai G, Pelizza A: Sonographic patterns of Caroli's disease: Report of 5 new cases. J Clin Ultrasound 19:155–161, 1991.

76. Paltiel HJ: Imaging in neonatal cholestasis. Semin Ultrasound CT MRI 15:290–305, 1994.

77. Davies C, Daneman A, Stringer DA: Inspissated bile in a neonate with cystic fibrosis. J Ultrasound Med 5:335–337, 1986.

78. Oppenheimer DA, Carroll BA: Spontaneous resolution of hyperalimentation-induced biliary dilatation: Ultrasonic description. J Ultrasound Med 1:213–214, 1982.

79. Kasai M, Suzuki H, Ohashi E, et al: Technique and results of operative management of biliary atresia. World J Surg 2:571–580, 1978.

80. Kirks DR, Coleman RE, Filston HC, Rosenberg ER, Merten DF: An imaging approach to persistent neonatal jaundice. AJR Am J Roentgenol 142:461–465, 1984.

81. Carroll BA, Oppenheimer DA, Muller HH: High-frequency real-time ultrasound of the neonatal biliary system. Radiology 145:437–440, 1982.

82. Green D, Carroll BA: Ultrasonography in the jaundiced infant: A new approach. J Ultrasound Med 5:323–329, 1986.

83. Miller JH, Sinatra FR, Thomas DW: Biliary excretion disorders in infants: Evaluation using ^{99m}Tc PIPIDA. AJR Am J Roentgenol 135:47–52, 1980.

84. Gerhold JP, Klingensmith WC, Kuni CC, Lilly JR, Silverman A, Fritzberg AR, Nixt TL: Diagnosis of biliary atresia with radionuclide hepatobiliary imaging. Radiology 146:499–504, 1983.

85. Wells RG, Sty JR, Starshak RJ: Hepatobiliary imaging in neonatal jaundice. Appl Radiol 16:57–85, 1987.

The Urinary Tract

INTRODUCTION

Ultrasound is commonly used to examine the urinary tract, both in adults and in pediatric patients. It is worthwhile, therefore, to consider urinary tract sonography in considerable detail. The indications for urinary tract sonography include the assessment of anomalies, renal failure, renal masses, urinary tract infection, urinary tract calculi, bladder pathology, and renal allografts. Each of these areas will be considered in detail in Chapters 16 to 23. Transrectal sonographic examination of the prostate will not be considered, as this subject, although important, is beyond the scope of this text.

Chapter 16

The Urinary Tract: Embryology, Anatomy, and Sonographic Technique

William J. Zwiebel

URINARY TRACT EMBRYOLOGY

The definitive urinary tract, the metanephros, begins to develop during the 6th week of gestation.[*][1, 2] The first part of the metanephros to develop is the ureteric bud (Fig. 16–1) (also called the metanephric duct), which forms as a "diverticulum" from a more primitive fetal kidney called the mesonephros. The ureteric bud grows cephalad as a blind-ended tube, and as it does so, a mass of mesoderm (the metanephrogenic cap) forms around its upper end. This cap of mesoderm undergoes a series of changes (beginning at about 9 weeks) leading to the development of nephrons, the formation of the kidney, and the establishment of vascular connections. During the developmental period, the ureteric bud branches to form the renal pelvis, calyces, and the collecting tubules. The branching process typically generates 12 to 14 calyces, each of which drains a discrete unit of parenchyma called a "lobe." As the metanephros develops, the mesonephros (primitive kidney) regresses and disappears.

The initial stages of kidney development occur within the fetal pelvis. Through a process of differential growth, the developing kidneys "ascend" into the abdomen and eventually achieve their adult location, at the approximate level of the first lumbar vertebra. During their "ascent," the vasculature of the kidneys is transferred from the hypogastric vessels to the common iliac vessels, and finally to the aorta.

The bladder and urethra develop from the cloaca and allantois during the 6th through 14th weeks of gestation. The union of these components, forming the lower urinary tract, is illustrated in Figure 16–1.

SONOGRAPHIC ANATOMY

The anatomy of the kidneys[3–5] is illustrated in Figures 16–2 and 16–3. Not shown in these figures is the fibrous capsule that surrounds the kidneys. This thin but tough layer is only rarely visible sonographically—as a fine, echogenic line that follows the kidney contour. The capsule is best demonstrated when it is stripped away by a subcapsular hematoma. Please review Figures 16–2 and 16–3 before proceeding, as this material is not repeated in the text.

The kidneys are obliquely oriented relative to the body axis, with the lower poles farther apart than the upper poles. This orientation is imposed by their juxtaposition to the psoas muscles, which are wider inferiorly. Accurate longitudinal views of the kidneys, therefore, require image planes that are oblique to the sagittal axis of the body. As shown in Figure 16–4, the renal hilum and the renal pelvis project anteromedially. Because of this orientation, the most useful views of the kidneys generally are obtained from a posterolateral transducer approach, with the patient in a decubitus position, as shown in Figure 16–5.

Age-Related Changes in Kidney Appearance

It is important to note that the kidneys in childhood (Figure 16–6) have a much different appearance than in adults. These differences can be summarized as follows.

- First, infantile kidneys[5–9] are large relative to overall body size (typically 4 to 5 cm long at birth).
- Second, during the first three years of life, the renal cortex is much more echogenic than it is in adulthood, and echogenicity during this period normally *exceeds* hepatic echogenicity. Enhanced cortical echogenicity is attributed to increased cortical cellularity and a large con-

---

[*]Gestational age, as used herein, is menstrual age; i.e., the elapsed time since the start of the last menstrual period.

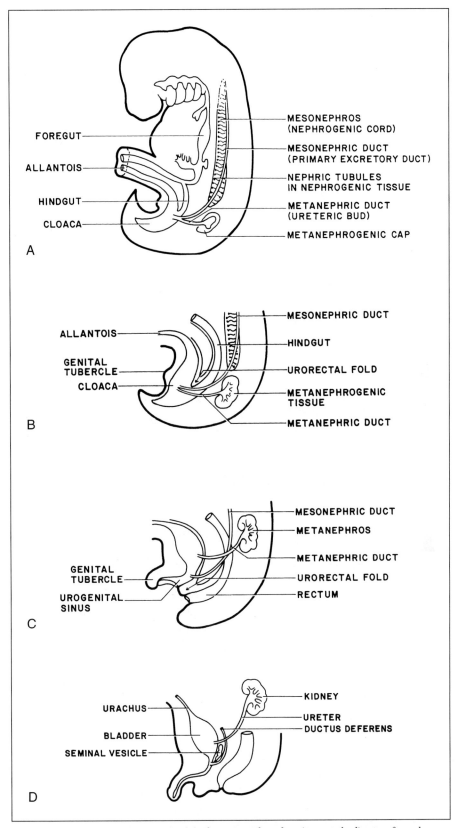

Figure 16-1—Urinary Tract Embryology. (**A**) The metanephric duct (ureteric bud) arises from the more primitive mesonephric duct. Note the position of the metanephros (definitive kidney) and the mesonephros (more primitive kidney). (**B**) At a slightly later stage, the meso- and metanephric ducts (ureteric bud) insert separately into the cloaca, and the metanephrogenic tissue is better developed. At this stage, the urorectal fold has begun to separate the hindgut and the allantois. (**C**) Still later, the metanephros is well developed, and the urorectal fold has separated the rectum and urogenital sinus. (**D**) In the final stage of development, the kidney has achieved its definitive form, the urogenital tract and rectum have separated, the urachus has closed, and the mesonephric duct has become the ductus deferens.

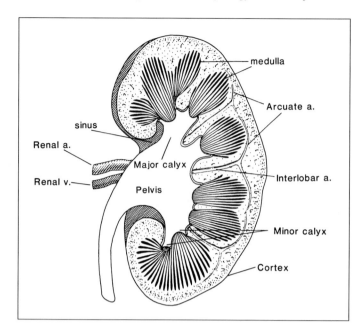

Figure 16-2—Illustrated Kidney Anatomy. Each kidney is bean shaped and consists of a mantle of parenchyma (functional tissue) surrounding a cavity called the renal sinus, which contains fat, blood vessels, and structures that collect the urine. The parenchyma has two components: the cortex, which contains the glomeruli that makes the urine, and the medulla (medullary rays or medullary pyramids), which contains the collecting tubules that drain into the calyces. The renal hilum is the opening through which the vessels and collecting structures pass. Note the location of the interlobar and arcuate arteries, as well as the difference between major and minor calyces.

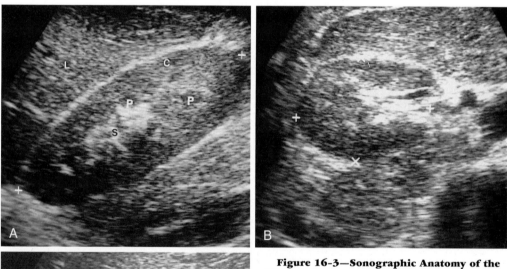

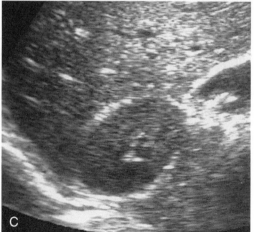

Figure 16-3—Sonographic Anatomy of the Kidney. (**A**) Sonograms in the long axis of the kidney (as shown here) generally show the kidney as an ovoid structure. The renal cortex (C), the renal pyramids (P) (medullary rays), and the renal sinus (S) are visibly different in echogenicity. Note that the echogenicity of the renal cortex, *in adults,* normally equals or is less than liver (L) echogenicity. The sinus (S) is the most echogenic portion of the adult kidney, because it contains a large amount of echogenic fat interspersed among the renal collecting structures and vessels. Cursors at the upper (left) and lower (right) poles mark the location for measuring kidney length. (**B**) The kidney is "U" shaped on transverse sections that pass through the renal hilum. Cursors mark the location for measurement of the anteroposterior (X) and transverse (+) dimensions of the kidney. (**C**) The kidney is doughnut-shaped on sections nearer the upper and lower poles.

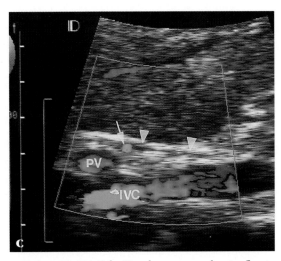

Figure 12-7C. Color Doppler sonogram showing flow in the right hepatic artery (arrow) and portal vein (PV). IVC = inferior vena cava.

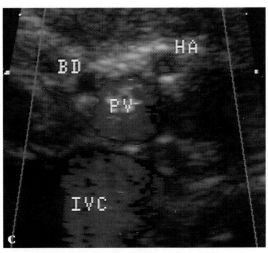

Figure 12-8C. Color Doppler Mickey Mouse view. Note that flow is absent in the bile duct (BD) and present in the portal vein (PV), hepatic artery (HA), and inferior vena cava (IVC).

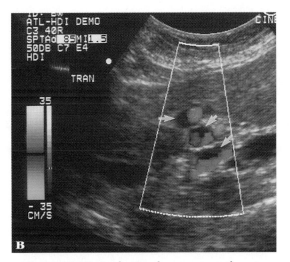

Figure 15-3B. A color Doppler sonogram in the same area shows dilated bile ducts (arrows) that were not appreciated on the gray scale image.

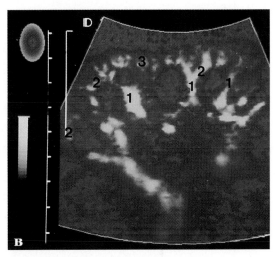

Figure 16-8B. A power Doppler image shows the interlobar arteries (1), the arcuate arteries (2), and cortical branches (3). (Reproduced with the kind permission of the Diasonics Corporation, Milpitas, CA.)

PLATE III

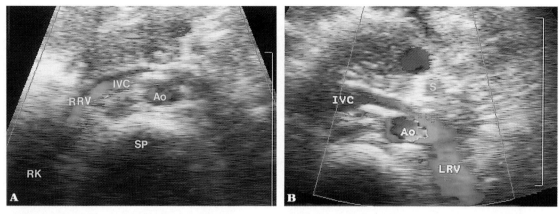

Figure 16-9—The Renal Veins. (A) The right renal vein (RRV) extends posterolaterally from the inferior vena cava (IVC). RK, right kidney; Ao, aorta; SP, spine. **(B)** The left renal vein (LRV) lies between the aorta (Ao) and the superior mesenteric artery (S). IVC, inferior vena cava.

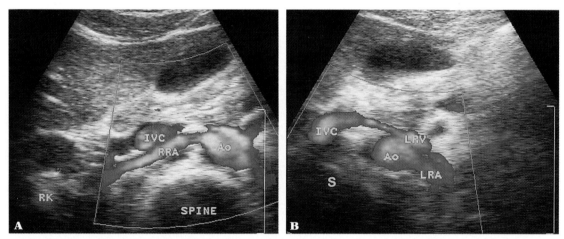

Figure 16-10—The Renal Arteries. (A) Transverse power Doppler image showing the right renal artery (RRA). Note that this vessel arises anterolaterally from the aorta (Ao) and then passes posterior to the inferior vena cava (IVC) as it proceeds to the right kidney (RK). **(B)** Transverse power Doppler image of the left renal artery (LRA). Note that this vessel is adjacent to the left renal vein (LRV) and appears to merge with the vein in this image. Care must be taken to identify the vein and artery correctly. Ao = aorta; IVC = inferior vena cava; S = spine.

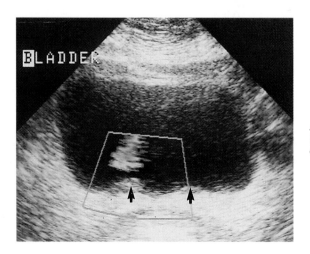

Figure 16-15A.—The Urinary Bladder Anatomy. Transverse image demonstrating small bumps (arrows) on the inner surface of the bladder at the ureteral orifices, and a ureteral jet (color).

PLATE IV

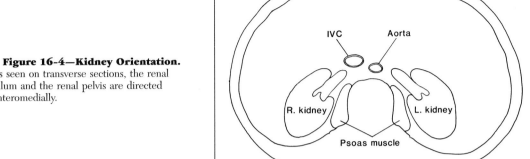

Figure 16-4—Kidney Orientation.
As seen on transverse sections, the renal hilum and the renal pelvis are directed anteromedially.

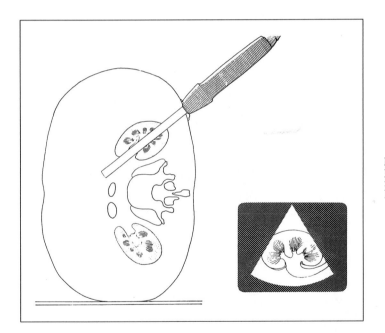

Figure 16-5—The decubitus position and a posterolateral transducer position are used to obtain longitudinal images of the kidney (as shown at the lower right).

Figure 16-6—Normal Infant Kidney (age 5 months).
The cortex is thin and hyperechoic compared with the adjacent liver (L). The pyramids are very large, and renal sinus fat is inapparent. Kidney length is measured at 4.9 cm. Compare with adult appearance in Figure 16–3.

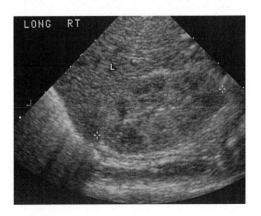

centration of glomeruli in the immature cortex (as compared with older children and adults). Cortical echogenicity assumes adult characteristics when the child is about 3 years of age as glomeruli become more dispersed and overall cellularity decreases.

- Third, the renal pyramids are *relatively* large in infants, and they stand out in striking contrast to the hyperechoic cortex. The pyramids are not really enlarged, but they appear large because the cortex is relatively thin. Pyramidal/cortical proportions gradually assume an adult relationship during the 1st year of life, as the cortex develops.

- Fourth, the renal sinus in infants and children contains relatively little fat, and as a result the sinus is *not* the most echogenic portion of the kidney, as it is in older children and adults. Fat accumulation occurs gradually, and sinus echogenicity achieves adult proportions by about age 10 years.

- Finally, the boundaries between the renal lobes (described earlier) may be visible early in infancy as prominent indentations on the surface of the kidney. These lobar boundaries are clearly visible in fetal life, but they usually disappear by birth or shortly thereafter.[9] They occasionally persist into adult life, as illustrated in the following chapter.

Age-related changes also occur in the kidneys throughout adult life,[16–25] but these are less obvious than the changes that occur in childhood. The thickness of the renal parenchyma decreases at about 10% per decade after age 20 years.[10] The overall size of the kidneys also decreases gradually, but this decrease is only apparent in elderly people, for it is overshadowed by measurement variability and a relative increase in the volume of renal sinus fat.[20] Perhaps the most easily recognized sign of aging is loss of contrast between the cortex and pyramids caused by interstitial fibrosis. This "normal" aging process increases cortical and pyramidal echogenicity, but the effect is more obvious in the pyramids, which gradually fade from view as their echogenicity increases.[5]

Renal Collecting Structures

The renal pelvis is the most commonly visualized portion of the normal renal collecting system, but on good-quality scans portions of the calyces and the infundibula also can be seen with ultrasound[4, 5, 11–13] (Figs. 16–3, 16–7). Calyces usually do not exceed 5 mm in diameter, but they may occasionally measure as much as 10 mm.[11] These large calyces generally are located

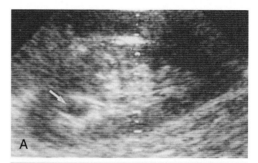
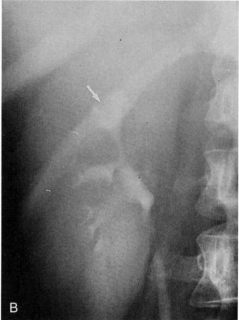

Figure 16-7—Prominent, but Normal Calyx. (A) A rounded sonolucency (arrow) is visible in the upper pole of the kidney. This might be mistaken for a dilated calyx, or for other pathology. **(B)** Intravenous pyelography shows a prominent but normal upper pole calyx (arrow).

in the upper or lower poles (Fig. 16–7) and may be mistaken for hydronephrosis, cysts, or other pathology. Calyceal visualization is enhanced by diuresis or back pressure, both of which distend the collecting system.

Blood Vessels

Portions of blood vessels are seen commonly with ultrasound in the renal sinus, or even in the renal parenchyma. Vessels are particularly apt to be seen in pediatric patients or in renal allografts (transplants), where image quality is excellent. Care must be taken not to mistake blood vessels for calyceal dilatation[12]; this error can be prevented with color Doppler identification of blood flow.

The arcuate arteries are seen occasionally as brightly echogenic structures located at the bases of the medullary pyramids (Fig. 16–8*A*). These arteries, which define the corticomedullary junction, should not be mistaken for calcifications.

Segmental and interlobar vessels (arteries and veins) are visible on good-quality color Doppler images, and even small cortical vessels are visible on power Doppler images (Fig. 16–8*B*). The arborization of these vessels in the renal parenchyma should be uniform. Patchy arborization suggests arterial occlusion.

The main renal veins are seen frequently between the kidneys and the inferior vena cava, as shown in Figure 16–9. Note the position of the left renal vein. It lies *between* the superior mesenteric artery and the aorta, as opposed to the splenic vein, which crosses *anterior to* the superior mesenteric artery. The left renal vein frequently is quite distended in supine individuals, and this distended vein should not be mistaken for a fluid collection or periaortic mass.

The main renal arteries[14, 15] can be identified with diligent scanning in sonogenic individuals (Fig. 16–10). The renal arteries arise *anterolaterally* from the aorta and then curve posterolaterally toward the kidneys. The origin of the renal arteries is no more than 2 cm below the superior mesenteric artery; therefore, the best way to find the renal arteries is to visualize the superior mesenteric artery origin in the transverse plane and then carefully move the scan plane inferiorly until the renal arteries are located. Identification of the right renal artery is aided by its unique location, *posterior* to the inferior vena cava. In infants and small children, the renal artery origins can be seen readily on coronal images through the aorta, and this should be the first approach to imaging these vessels.

The renal artery and vein lie close to each other, and care must be taken not to mistake one for the other. Differentiation is aided by Doppler ultrasound, as the venous signals (Fig. 16–9*C*) have a "windstorm" pattern that is quite different from the pulsatile signals of the renal arteries. Note that the renal arteries exhibit low resistance flow features (low pulsatility), as illustrated in Figure 16–10*C*. A high resistance pattern suggests pathology such as urinary tract obstruction or renal transplant rejection, as discussed elsewhere.[14, 15]

Kidney Size in Adults

Sonography has generally replaced radiography as a means for assessing kidney size.[4, 5, 10, 16–20] The size of the kidneys is affected by age, sex (greater in men than in women), and body size; furthermore, the left kidney is slightly larger than the right in most individuals. The median renal length in adult men and women aged 30 to 70 years approximates 11 cm (10.9 cm for the right kidney and 11.2 cm for the left kidney). The normal range (10th to 90th percentile) is 9.5 to 12.1 cm for women and 10.1 to 12.6 cm for men.[20] Body habitus and age should be considered whenever kidney size is evaluated. A 10-cm-long kidney may fall within the normal statistical range, but a kidney of this size is likely to be abnormal for a 20 year old man who is 6 feet tall and weighs 200 pounds!

Kidney volume[17] may be calculated easily with ultrasound from measurements of length, width, and height:

$$\text{volume} = \text{length} \times \text{width} \times \text{height} \times 0.49$$

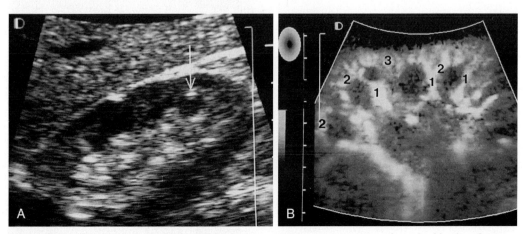

Figure 16-8—Intrarenal Arterial Vasculature. (**A**) An arcuate artery (arrow) produces focal bright reflections at the base of a pyramid. These reflections should not be mistakenly attributed to calcification. (**B**) A power Doppler image shows the interlobar arteries (1), the arcuate arteries (2), and cortical branches (3). (See Color Figure 16–8*B* following page 164.) (**B** reproduced with the kind permission of the Diasonics Corporation, Milpitas, CA.)

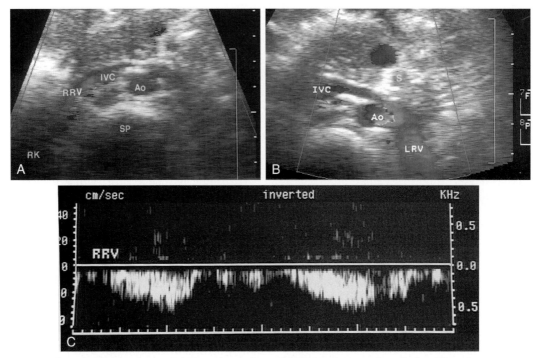

Figure 16-9—The Renal Veins. (**A**) The right renal vein (RRV) extends posterolaterally from the inferior vena cava (IVC). RK = right kidney; Ao = aorta; SP = spine. (**B**) The left renal vein (LRV) lies between the aorta (Ao) and the superior mesenteric artery (S). IVC = inferior vena cava. (See Color Figure 16–9A and B following page 164.) (**C**) The renal vein Doppler signal undulates with respiration and has a "windstorm" sound.

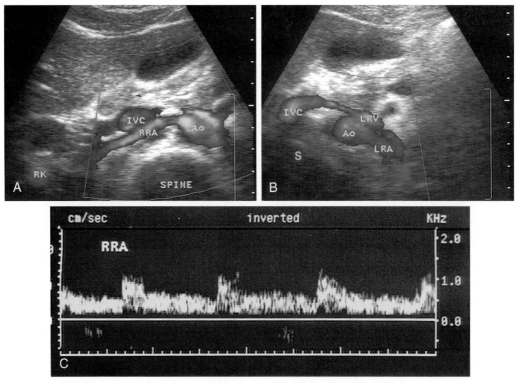

Figure 16-10—The Renal Arteries. (**A**) Transverse power Doppler image showing the right renal artery (RRA). Note that this vessel arises anterolaterally from the aorta (Ao) and then passes posterior to the inferior vena cava (IVC) as it proceeds to the right kidney (RK). (**B**) Transverse power Doppler image of the left renal artery (LRA). Note that this vessel is adjacent to the left renal vein (LRV) and appears to merge with the vein in this image. Care must be taken to identify the vein and artery correctly. Ao = aorta; IVC = inferior vena cava; S = spine. (See Color Figure 16–10A and B following page 164.) (**C**) The normal renal artery Doppler signal exhibits the following low-resistance flow characteristics: broad systolic peaks; continuous flow throughout diastole; and continuous forward flow in diastole (no flow reversal).

Accurate volume measurements depend on correct width and height measurements. Measurements of median renal volume in adults range from 134 to 159 ml, again with men larger than women and the left kidney larger than the right.[17, 18, 20] The normal range is presented in Table 16–1.[17, 18]

Kidney Size in Children

Kidney growth in childhood is generally assessed sonographically. It is customary to relate renal length to age,[21] but this comparison is somewhat imprecise because body habitus varies widely in children at all ages. Kidney length correlates more closely with height, weight, or surface area[21–23] (Fig. 16–11), but even these correlations lack precision. As a result, interobserver measurement variability may be greater than the expected annual increase in kidney length (2.5 ± 5.7 mm in children).[22, 25] For maximum precision, renal volume measurements are recommended, and these should be correlated with the weight of the child (Fig. 16–12).[22] Such detailed measurements generally are needed, however, only for children with known or suspected parenchymal renal disease.

The Perirenal and Pararenal Spaces

Well-developed fascial planes surround the kidneys, and these divide the retroperitoneum into distinct spaces,[26–29] as illustrated in Figure 16–13. Please review this figure with respect to the location of the peri- and pararenal spaces. As an aid to memorization, note that the prefix "peri" means around, and that the space immediately surrounding each kidney is the *peri*renal space. Note also that the prefix "para" is the root of the word parallel, and the spaces anterior and posterior to each kidney are called the *para*renal spaces. If you remember this analogy, it is easy to remember the anatomy of the posterior fossa! The fascial planes that form the peri- and pararenal spaces are visualized rarely with ultrasound, but they are seen routinely with computed tomography.

Note in Figure 16–13 that the anterior pararenal space contains the pancreas, the duodenum, and portions of the ascending and descending colon, all of which may contribute pathology that spreads through the anterior pararenal space. Pathology within the perirenal space almost always arises from the kidney. Pathology is relatively uncommon in the posterior pararenal space and usually arises from the spine or psoas muscles.

With rare exceptions, the right and left peri- and pararenal spaces do not communicate with one another across the midline, and pathology, therefore, does not spread beyond the midline in these spaces. Pathology may spread among ipsilateral peri- and pararenal spaces, however, since the bottom "ends" of these spaces intercommunicate low in the abdomen.

The Bladder

The urinary bladder lies within the true pelvis and is readily examined sonographically when it is distended with urine (Fig. 16–14*A, B*). The wall of the bladder is smoothly marginated, and the bladder contents are anechoic. With careful scanning, the muscular wall of the bladder may be visualized as a medium-echogenicity layer (Fig. 16–14 *C*). The adventitia of the bladder wall is the highly echogenic layer external to the muscular portion. The thickness of the bladder wall varies greatly with the degree of bladder distention. In children, the maximum lumen-to-adventitial thickness is 3 mm with the bladder distended and 5 mm with the bladder empty.[30] The 3- and 5-mm values probably apply to adults as well, but this has not been determined conclusively.[30] Pathologic thickening of the muscular layer often cannot be differentiated sonographically from mucosal thickening.

With careful scanning, the ureterovesical junctions can be seen on transverse sonograms as small bumps that project into the bladder lumen (Fig. 16–15*A*). If the distal ureters are sufficiently distended, they may be visualized within the bladder wall, near the ureterovesical bumps (Fig. 16–15*B*). Streams of urine are expelled into the bladder lumen from the distal ureters at intervals ranging from about 2 to 12 minutes.[31–33] These streams (or jets) are readily visualized on gray scale or color Doppler images (Fig. 16–15*A*). Visualization of a jet indicates that the corresponding ureter is patent but does not exclude partial obstruction. Absence of a jet suggests ureteral obstruction. It is noteworthy that visualization of ureteral jets is somewhat quixotic, and their presence or absence should be considered only in the context of other findings of obstruction. The orientation of the jet does not

Text continued on page 174

Table 16-1. Renal Volume in Adults (Sum of Both Kidneys)

	ml/kg	ml/m²
5th percentile	4.3	153
Median	5.7	220
95th percentile	8.0	295

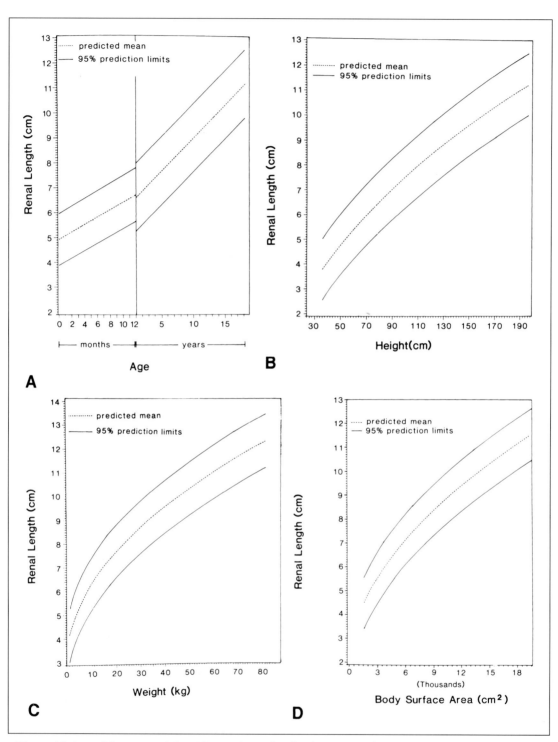

Figure 16-11—Kidney Length in Children. (Reproduced with permission from Han DK, Babcock DS: Sonography of Kidneys in Childhood. AJR Am J Roentgenol 145:611, 1985.)

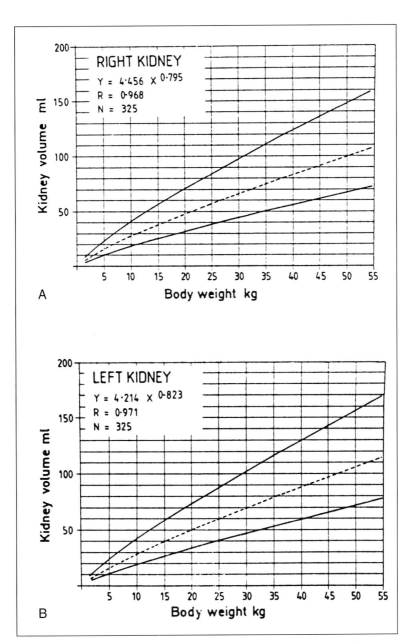

Figure 16-12—Kidney Volume Versus Weight in Children. (**A**) Right kidney. (**B**) Left kidney. Y = y axis; X = x axis; R = regression coefficient; N = number of subjects. (Reproduced with permission from Dinkel E, Ertel M, Dittrich M, et al: Kidney size in childhood. Pediatr Radiol 15:38, 1985.)

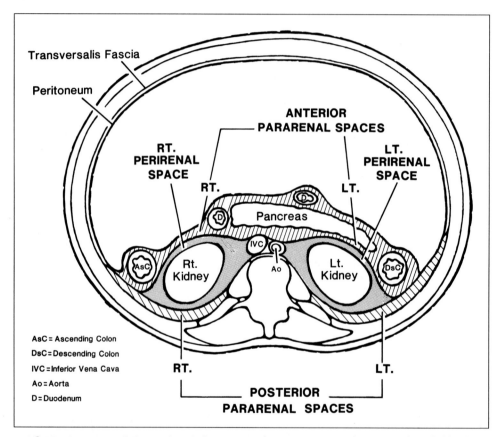

Figure 16-13—Anatomy of the Perinephric Spaces. The anterior *para*renal spaces are bounded by the peritoneum and the anterior pararenal fascia. The *peri*renal spaces are bounded by the anterior and posterior perirenal fascia. The posterior *para*renal spaces are bounded by the posterior perirenal fascia and the posterior musculature.

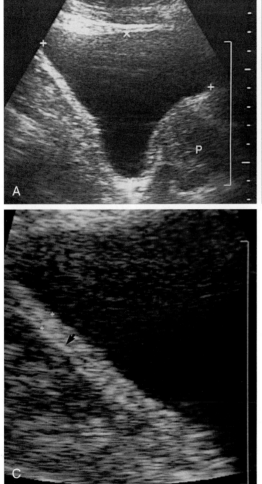

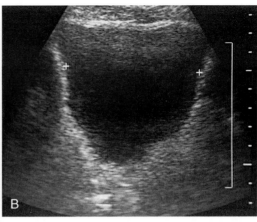

Figure 16-14—Sonographic Anatomy of the Urinary Bladder. Representative longitudinal (**A**) and transverse (**B**) views of the bladder are shown. Cursors are measurement points for bladder volume, as discussed in Chapter 23. The prostate (P) is visible inferiorly. (**C**) Magnified view showing the muscular wall of the bladder (cursors) and the adventitia (arrow).

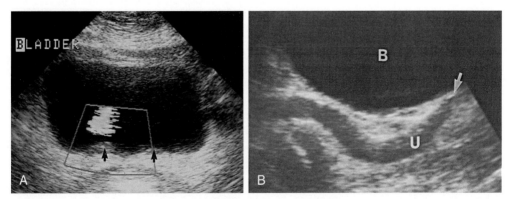

Figure 16-15—The Urinary Bladder Anatomy. (**A**) Transverse image demonstrating small bumps (arrows) on the inner surface of the bladder at the ureteral orifices, and a ureteral jet (color). (See Color Figure 16–15A following page 164.) (**B**) Longitudinal view of the distal ureter (U) coursing posterior to the bladder and into the bladder wall (arrow). B = bladder.

Table 16-2. Protocol for Urinary Tract Sonography

A Longitudinal images of each kidney
  • Hard copy of images through renal hilum

B Transverse views of each kidney
  • Hard copy of images at upper pole, hilum, lower pole

C Color and spectral Doppler assessment of renal artery, renal vein, and parenchymal blood flow (as needed)

D Longitudinal and transverse images of the bladder
  • Representative hard copy images
  • Postvoid images to confirm emptying (as needed)

E Renal-time search for ureteral dilatation and calculi (as needed)
  • Near lower pole of kidney
  • Near iliac vessels
  • Posterior to bladder

seem helpful for determining whether the ureteral orifice is normally located or ectopic. Some investigators believe that ureteral jets are interesting phenomena that provide little diagnostic information.

In men, the prostate and seminal vesicles may be visualized sonographically on longitudinal (Fig. 16–14A) and on inferiorly angulated transverse scans. The seminal vesicles also can be seen on transverse images. The prostate and seminal vesicles are best examined transrectally. This subject is beyond the scope of this text.

EXAMINATION PROTOCOL

Sonographic examinations performed in a given ultrasound department should be conducted in a consistent way by all personnel. Consistency can be achieved only if a protocol is followed, and the protocol I suggest for urinary tract examination is presented in Table 16–2.

REFERENCES

1. Warwick R, Williams PL (eds): Gray's Anatomy, 35th British ed. Philadelphia, WB Saunders, 1973, p 183.
2. Touvey TW: The early development of the human nephros. Embryology Carnegie Inst 35:159–197, 1954.
3. Platt JF, Rubin JM, Bowerman RA, Marn CS: The inability to detect disease on the basis of renal echogenicity. AJR Am J Roentgenol 151:317–319, 1988.
4. Huntington DK, Hill SC, Hill MC: Sonographic manifestations of medical renal disease. Semin Ultrasound CT MR 12:290–307, 1991.
5. Marchal G, Verbeken E, Oyen R, Moerman F, Baert AL, Lauweryns J: Ultrasound of the normal kidney: A sonographic anatomic and histologic correlation. Ultrasound Med Biol 12:999–1009, 1986.
6. Han BK, Babcock DS: Sonographic measurements and appearance of normal kidneys in children. AJR Am J Roentgenol 145:611–616, 1985.
7. Cramer BC, Jequier S, de Chadarevian JP: Factors associated with renal parenchymal echogenicity in the newborn. J Ultrasound Med 5:633–638, 1986.
8. Hricak H, Slovis TL, Callen CW, Callen PW, Romanski RN: Neonatal kidneys: Sonographic anatomic correlation. Radiology 147:699–702, 1983.
9. Patriquin H, Lefaivre J-F, Lafortune M, Russo P, Boisvert J: Fetal lobation: An anatomic-ultrasonographic correlation. J Ultrasound Med 9:191–197, 1990.
10. Gourtsoyiannis N, Prassopoulos P, Cavouras D, Pantelidis N: The thickness of the renal parenchyma decreases with age: A CT study of 360 patients. AJR Am J Roentgenol 155:541–544, 1990.
11. Peak SL, Roxburgh HB, Langlais SLP: Ultrasound assessment of hydronephrosis of pregnancy. Radiology 196:167–170, 1983.
12. Scola FH, Cronan JJ, Schepps B: Grade I hydronephrosis, pulsed Doppler evaluation. Radiology 171:519–520, 1989.
13. Kamholtz RG, Cronan JJ, Dorfman GS: Obstruction and the minimally dilated renal collecting system: US evaluation. Radiology 170:51–53, 1989.
14. Rifkin MD, Pasto ME, Goldberg BB: Duplex Doppler examination in renal disease: Evaluation of vascular involvement. Ultrasound Med Biol 11:341–346, 1985.
15. Greene ER, Venters MD, Avasthi PS, Conn RL, Jahnke RW: Noninvasive characterization of renal artery blood flow. Kidney Int 20:523–529, 1981.
16. Jones TB, Riddick LR, Harpen MD, Dubuisson RL, Samuels D: Ultrasonographic determination of renal mass and renal volume. J Ultrasound Med 2:151–154, 1983.
17. Rasmussen SN, Haase L, Kjeldsen H, Hancke S: Determination of renal volume by ultrasound scanning. J Clin Ultrasound 6:160–164, 1978.
18. Hricak H, Lieto RP: Sonographic determination of renal volume. Radiology 148:311–312, 1983.
19. Brandt TD, Neiman HL, Dragowski MJ, Bulawa W, Claykamp G: Ultrasound assessment of normal renal dimensions. J Ultrasound Med 1:49–52, 1982.
20. Ememian SA, Nielsen MB, Pedersen JF, Ytte L: Kidney dimensions at sonography: Correlation with age, sex, and habitus in 665 adult volunteers. AJR Am J Roentgenol 160:83–86, 1993.
21. Han DK, Babcock DS: Sonography of kidneys in childhood. AJR Am J Roentgenol 145:611–616, 1985.
22. Dinkel E, Ertel M, Dittrich M, Peters H, Berres M, Schulte-Wissermann H: Kidney size in childhood: Sonographical growth charts for kidney length and volume. Pediatr Radiol 15:38–43, 1985.
23. Erwin BC, Carroll BA, Muller H: A sonographic assessment of neonatal renal parameters. J Ultrasound Med 4:217–229, 1985.
24. Rosenbaum DM, Korngold E, Teele RL: Sonographic assessment of renal length in normal children. AJR Am J Roentgenol 142:467–469, 1984.
25. Schlesinger AE, Hernandez RJ, Zerin JM, Marks TI, Kelsch RC: Interobserver and intraobserver variations in sonographic renal length measurements in children. AJR Am J Roentgenol 156:1029–1032, 1991.
26. Love L, Meyers MA, Churchill RJ, Reynes CJ,

Moncada R, Gibson D: Computed tomography of extraperitoneal spaces. AJR Am J Roentgenol 136:781–789, 1981.

27. Weill FS, Perriguey G, Rohmer P: Sonographic study of the juxtarenal retroperitoneal compartments. J Ultrasound Med 1:307–310, 1982.

28. Raptopoulos V, Kleinman PK, Marks S, Snyder M, Silverman PM: Renal fascial pathway: Posterior extension of pancreatic effusions within the anterior pararenal space. Radiology 158:367–374, 1986.

29. Kneeland JB, Auh YH, Rubenstein WA, Zirinsky K, Morrison H, Whalen JP, Kazam E: Perirenal spaces: CT evidence for communication across the midline. Radiology 164:657–664, 1987.

30. Jequier S, Rousseau O: Sonographic measurements of the normal bladder wall in children. AJR Am J Roentgenol 149:563–566, 1987.

31. Jequier S, Paltiel H, and Lafortune M: Ureterovesical jets in infants and children: Duplex and color Doppler US studies. Radiology 175:349–353, 1990.

32. Burge H, Middleton WD, McClennan BL, Hildebolt CF: Ureteral jets in healthy subjects with unilateral ureteral calculi: Comparison with color Doppler US. Radiology 180:437–442, 1991.

33. Elejalde BR, de Elejalde MM: Ureteral ejaculation of urine visualized by ultrasound. J Clin Ultrasound 11:475–476, 1983.

Chapter 17

Normal Variants and Developmental Anomalies of the Urinary Tract

William J. Zwiebel

NORMAL ANATOMIC VARIANTS

Fetal Lobation

As noted in the preceding chapter, indentations that mark the boundaries of the renal lobes are present on the surfaces of the kidneys during fetal life. These surface indentations impart a lobulated appearance that commonly is described as "fetal lobulation." The proper term, however, is "fetal lobation," since the surface indentations define the renal lobes.

Fetal lobation usually disappears by birth, but the surface indentations may persist into childhood (Fig. 17–1) or even into adult life.[1, 2] Persistent fetal lobation may be mistaken for cortical scarring, but this error can be avoided if the following characteristics of fetal lobation are noted: (1) the interlobar septa are linear, thin, and sharply defined; (2) a small, triangular "notch" is present at the cortical end of each lobar boundary; (3) the septa and notches are spaced regularly *between* the medullary rays; and (4) parenchymal thinning is *not* present. In contrast, cortical scars are thick, broad, poorly defined, and associated with parenchymal thinning.

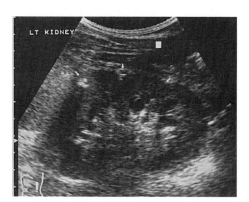

Figure 17–1—Fetal Lobation. Discrete cortical indentations (arrows) are visible at the boundaries of the renal lobes in this 17 year old man.

Junctional Parenchymal Defect

Embryologically, each kidney is formed from upper and lower units of parenchyma that fuse along an oblique line. The junction points of these units may persist as a prominent indentation of the cortical surface, called the "junctional parenchymal defect,"[1, 3, 4] which the unwary may mistake for a cortical scar. Correct identification of this common normal variant (Fig. 17–2) is based on the following observations:

1. The parenchymal defect most often is anterior, at the junction of the upper and middle thirds of the kidney.
2. Less commonly, the junctional defect is posterior, between the middle and lower thirds of the kidney.
3. The junctional defect is visible *only* on longitudinal images.
4. An oblique echogenic band (the junctional line) may connect the junctional defect with the renal sinus.
5. The junctional defect is variably associated with a prominent septum of Bertin, as described next.

Prominent Septum of Bertin

The cortex intervening between adjacent medullary pyramids may be unusually thick in the midportion of the kidney, as illustrated in Figure 17–3. This thick mass of parenchyma is a normal variant called a prominent septum of Bertin, which is important only because it may be mistaken for a renal mass.[1, 5–7] This error can be avoided through the following observations:

1. The prominent septum is located directly opposite the renal sinus.
2. The prominent septum usually is triangular in shape (either on transverse or longitudinal images), as opposed to the spherical shape of a tumor.

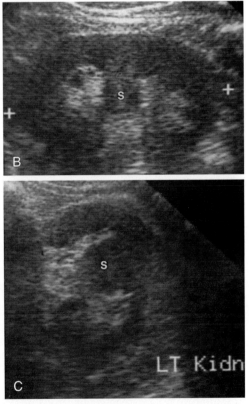

Figure 17-2—Junctional Line. A longitudinal view of a right kidney demonstrates a prominent junctional notch (arrow) in the anterior aspect of the kidney. Note that the notch is sharply defined and is in the characteristic location of a junctional line.

3. Echo characteristics of the septum are identical to other portions of the renal cortex.
4. The septum is variably associated with a bifid renal pelvis and a junctional parenchymal defect, as described earlier.

Most septa of Bertin are less than 3 cm in maximum dimension, but some may be larger and may have a strikingly bulbous, masslike appearance. When it is not possible to differentiate with ultrasound between a prominent septum and a neoplasm, scintigraphy or contrast-enhanced computed tomography may be of value.

Dromedary Hump

Either kidney, but more commonly the left, may exhibit a prominent, laterally directed bump

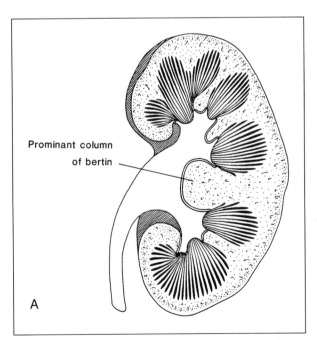

Figure 17-3—Prominent Septum of Bertin. (**A**) Illustration of the anatomy of the septum (column) of Bertin. (**B**) Longitudinal, and (**C**) transverse views of a prominent septum of Bertin (S). Note that the septum points toward the hilum and has a somewhat triangular shape as seen in the transverse plane. The echogenicity of the septum is identical to the remainder of the renal parenchyma.

in its mid portion, called a dromedary hump.[1] This normal variant may be recognized by assessing the internal architecture of the kidney. If the shape of the corticomedullary junction and the renal sinus corresponds to the shape of the hump, then a mass is easily excluded. A dromedary hump commonly is associated with a bifid pelvis or a prominent septum of Bertin.

Extrarenal Pelvis

In most instances, the renal pelvis is largely confined within the renal sinus. Less commonly, a sizeable portion of the renal pelvis extends outside the renal sinus. Such "extrarenal" pelves typically have a distended appearance that may be mistakenly attributed to hydronephrosis. The calyces are not dilated, however, and this finding best differentiates this variant from hydronephrosis.

Ureteropelvic Junction Obstruction

Congenital narrowing at the junction of the ureter and the renal pelvis is a common developmental variant that may impede the flow of urine, causing distention of the renal pelvis as well as the major and minor calyces (hydronephrosis). In many cases, it is difficult to differentiate between this harmless anomaly and significant, pathologic urinary tract obstruction. Congenital ureteropelvic junction (UPJ) obstruction is suggested if calyceal dilatation is minimal, kidney size is normal, and renal parenchymal thickness is normal. Moderate or severe urinary tract distention and parenchymal thinning suggest significant obstructive uropathy and are not features of innocuous UPJ narrowing.

ANOMALIES

A fine etymologic line separates normal variants and anomalies. We clearly have crossed this line, however, when we talk about renal agenesis, hypoplasia, dysplasia, and ectopy, which are the anomalies included in this section. Before proceeding, it is important to define these terms and the related term "atrophy."[8] *Agenesis* refers to failure of development of an organ or body part. *Dysplasia* implies disordered (abnormal) development, either from a primary defect (e.g., chromosomal) or a secondary insult (e.g., urinary tract obstruction); *hypoplasia* implies subnormal size, resulting from a developmental problem; *ectopy* refers to abnormal location; and *atrophy* indicates partial or full development followed by regression in size, usually as a result of a damaging insult. More than one of these terms may be

applicable to a given condition. For example, renal dysplasia (maldevelopment) may result in hypoplasia (small size).

Missing Kidney

When a kidney cannot be located sonographically, renal ectopy, agenesis, hypoplasia, dysplasia, or atrophy all are considerations. The sonographer should do four things to investigate a missing kidney: (1) search carefully for an ectopic kidney; (2) look for a small but normotopic kidney (hypoplasia, dysplasia, or atrophy); (3) look for hypertrophy of the contralateral kidney; and (4) in women, look for associated anomalies of the reproductive organs (Chapter 28). The size of the contralateral kidney is particularly important, since compensatory hypertrophy (enlargement) usually occurs when one kidney is absent or small. The presence of a normal-sized contralateral kidney suggests that the missing kidney is ectopic, rather than absent or small.

Renal agenesis is a primary consideration when one or both kidneys cannot be found.[9–13] The term "agenesis" implies a primary failure of kidney (metanephros) development, but some cases of agenesis clearly are secondary abnormalities; that is, the metanephros forms but then is damaged and disappears during fetal life. A prime example is disappearance of a multicystic dysplastic kidney,[10, 11] as discussed in Chapter 21.

Bilateral renal agenesis is, of course, incompatible with postnatal life, and results in Potter syndrome (Chapter 42). Unilateral renal agenesis generally does not reduce life expectancy, unless other anomalies are present.[10, 11] Unilateral agenesis is about twice as common as bilateral agenesis.

The Small Kidney

An abnormally small kidney represents a diagnostic dilemma. Hypoplasia, dysplasia, or atrophy are all potential causes, and differentiation among these etiologies generally is difficult or impossible,[9] as illustrated in Figure 17–4.

Cystic Dysplasia

Multicystic dysplasia, infantile polycystic kidney disease, and other types of cystic dysplasia are developmental anomalies that are discussed in detail in Chapter 21.

Pelvic Kidney

Ectopia, or displacement, of a kidney is a common renal anomaly. The pelvic kidney, in which cephalad "migration" of the kidney does not occur, is the simplest form of renal ectopy.[14–19] In this genetically random anomaly, the kidney re-

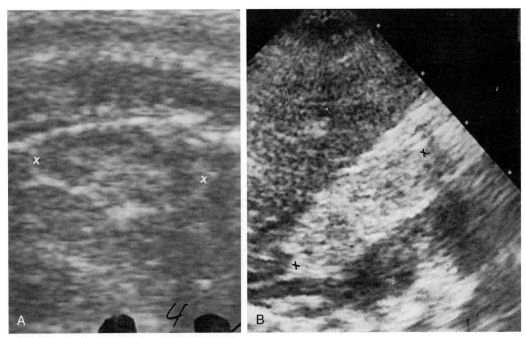

Figure 17-4—Congenital Small Kidneys. (**A**) This neonatal left kidney measures 33 mm in length (cursors), which is substantially smaller than the usual 45 to 50 mm for a term infant. The shape of the kidney is normal, and the renal sinus is well defined. The kidney functioned normally on an intravenous pyelogram (not shown) and apparently was small for embryologic reasons (reduced branching of the nephrogenic bud[9]). (**B**) Longitudinal sonogram of the right kidney in a term neonate thought to have renal agenesis on the basis of prenatal sonograms. Postnatal ultrasound, however, demonstrated small, highly echogenic, dysplastic kidneys, as shown here. The kidney shown measures only 25 mm in length (cursors) and is so echogenic that it blends in with the retroperitoneal fat. The featureless appearance provides no information about the etiology of dysplasia.

mains on the proper side of the body but is positioned lower than normal, either in the iliac fossa or the true pelvis. The displaced kidney may be asymptomatic and detected incidentally on physical examination or an imaging procedure. Alternatively, complications such as infection or hydronephrosis may cause symptoms.

Except for being displaced, most pelvic kidneys are normal developmentally, and these "normal" kidneys are easily recognized with ultrasound (Fig. 17–5A). Occasionally, however, a pelvic kidney is grossly abnormal in appearance because it is affected by dysplasia, duplication anomalies, vesicoureteral reflux, and/or hydronephrosis. These abnormal pelvic kidneys are easily mistaken for cystic or solid masses (Fig. 17–5B) or abnormal segments of bowel.[9, 15, 16] Diagnostic error may be avoided if the ipsilateral renal fossa is examined routinely in patients with pelvic pathology. The empty renal fossa should be a powerful clue as to the nature of the pelvic mass. (Elementary, Watson!)

Horseshoe Kidney

The horseshoe kidney[9, 16, 17] is a genetically random fusion anomaly in which the lower poles of the kidneys are united by a band of tissue that crosses the midline anterior to the aorta and inferior vena cava. The fusion band usually crosses at the level of the fourth or fifth lumbar vertebra and usually consists of functional renal parenchyma. Less commonly, the kidneys are joined only by a fibrous band. About 20% of horseshoe kidneys are low-lying, and some may be located as far inferior as the true pelvis.[16] Discrepancy in the size of the fused kidneys occurs uncommonly and is attributed to hypoplasia of one kidney and compensatory hypertrophy of the other.

The orientation of a horseshoe kidney is always abnormal. The lower renal poles are positioned *medial* to the upper poles, which is opposite to the normal relationship, and the renal pelves are directed anteriorly rather than anteromedially.

Sonographic diagnosis of a horseshoe kidney (Fig. 17–6) depends on the identification of a mass of tissue connecting the lower poles or the appreciation of abnormal renal orientation. The latter is an extremely important diagnostic clue, particularly when the kidneys are joined only by a fibrous band that may be invisible sonographically. The two most common sonographic errors in relation to horseshoe kidneys are to miss the anomaly entirely or to mistake the preaortic parenchymal band for adenopathy.

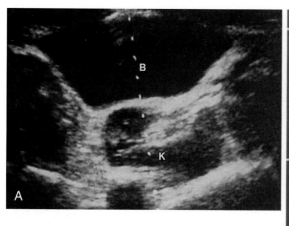

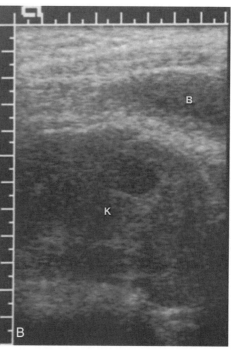

Figure 17-5—Pelvic Kidney. (**A**) An easily recognized kidney (K) is seen posterior to the bladder (B) in this transverse sonogram. (**B**) This hydronephrotic pelvic kidney (K) presents a bizarre appearance that might easily be mistaken for a pelvic mass. B = bladder (virtually empty).

Crossed, Fused Ectopy

Crossed, fused ectopy[9, 18, 19] is a genetically random, complicated form of renal ectopia of unknown embryogenesis. In this anomaly, the upper pole of the ectopic kidney is fused with the lower pole of the contralateral, normotopic kidney. The axis of the fused kidney is more longitudinal (less oblique) than normal. The pelvis of the ectopic kidney is directed anteriorly (rather than anteromedial). The pelvis of the normotopic kidney may be positioned similarly or may have a normal orientation. The ureter from the ectopic kidney crosses the midline to insert on the correct side of the bladder.

Several sonographic findings identify crossed, fused ectopy (Fig. 17–7): (1) the fused kidney is unusually long, but it is normal in transverse dimensions; (2) a notchlike defect is usually present at the fusion point; (3) two separate renal sinuses, pelves and ureters are present; and (4) the contralateral kidney is absent.

It is surprisingly easy to misdiagnose crossed, fused ectopy with ultrasound. First, the ectopic

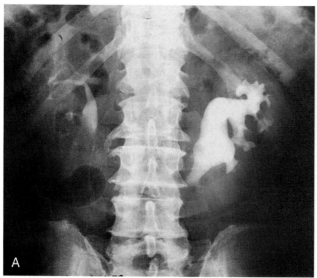

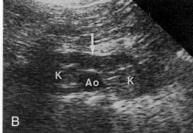

Figure 17-6—Horseshoe Kidney. (**A**) An intravenous pyelogram demonstrates an abnormal renal axis bilaterally. Note that the lower poles of both kidneys are medial to the upper poles and are poorly defined. (**B**) A transverse image of the lower poles of the kidneys (K) demonstrate a bridge of tissue (arrow) that connects the lower poles. Ao = aorta.

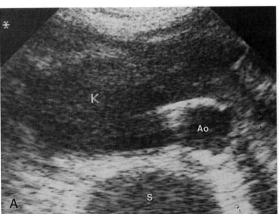

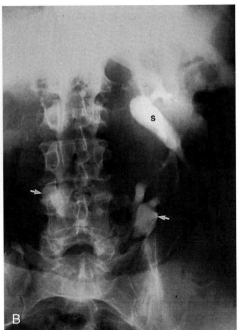

Figure 17-7—Cross-Fused Ectopy. (**A**) An ill-defined, abnormally shaped kidney (K) is seen adjacent to the aorta (Ao) and spine (S). (**B**) Intravenous pyelography demonstrates crossed, fused ectopia. The superior component (S) is the normotopic left kidney. The inferior component (arrows) is the anatomic right kidney, which is attached to the lower pole of the left kidney.

kidney may be overlooked if it is oddly oriented and is not visible in the same image planes as the normotopic kidney. In such instances, absence of the contralateral kidney typically is attributed to agenesis. Second, it may be assumed that the inordinately large, fused kidney is merely hypertrophic (in response to contralateral renal agenesis). Finally, the ectopic kidney may be mistaken for a renal mass arising from the normotopic kidney.

Ureteral Duplication

One of the most important renal anomalies from a clinical perspective is ureteral duplication.[9, 12–15, 20–23] This anomaly is important because it is common and because early recognition (in utero or in infancy) appears to lessen adverse consequences substantially (especially urinary tract infection).

Ureteral duplication results from premature splitting of the ureteric bud, or from the independent development of two ureteric buds (see preceding chapter). Duplication is classified as *incomplete* if the two ureters unite before entering the bladder. With incomplete duplication, the insertion of the united ureter into the bladder usually is normal, and for this reason, incomplete duplication generally has no pathologic consequences. Incomplete duplication is rarely recognized sonographically. With *complete* duplication, two completely separate ureters enter the bladder at distinct locations. Patients with this anom-

aly are subject to significant renal damage from infection, obstruction, or reflux, for reasons discussed later. In cases of complete ureteral duplication, the ureter draining the upper moiety (portion) of the kidney enters the bladder *below* the ureter from the lower moiety. The anatomy and pathologic consequences of complete duplication are summarized as follows:

Upper Moiety Ureter

1. Enters the bladder *below and medial* to the lower moiety ureter.
2. Enters the bladder medial to the normal ureteral insertion site.
3. May insert ectopically at remote locations (e.g., the urethra, the seminal vesicle, the vas deferens, the uterus, or the vagina).
4. Is subject to obstruction and ureterocele development.

Lower Moiety Ureter

1. Enters the bladder *superior* to the upper moiety ureter.
2. Enters the bladder superior and lateral to the normal ureteral insertion site.
3. Has an abnormal course through the bladder wall (relatively acute angle with the bladder wall and short intramuscular distance).
4. Is subject to vesicoureteral reflux (72% to 88% of cases).[21]

Obstruction is the predominant pathologic feature of the upper pole of a duplicated collecting system, and in some cases obstruction may result in massive upper moiety hydronephrosis. The parenchyma surrounding the hydronephrotic collecting system may be atrophic, and in some instances, atrophy may be so severe that no parenchyma is visible. In such cases, the upper pole of the kidney resembles a cyst (Fig. 17–8). If this "cyst" is large, it may alter the renal axis, causing the pyelographic "drooping lily" sign. Infectious or noninfectious debris may produce diffuse or dependent echoes within the dilated collecting system. In addition to the upper pole findings, massive hydroureter may be visible sonographically. Massively distended ureters in children tend to elongate and fold into a serpentine configuration. On ultrasound slices, the folded segments look like a series of round or ovoid cysts, rather than the tubular shape usually associated with ureteral dilatation. A ureterocele (discussed next) is present at the bladder inser-

tion site in about one half the cases of upper moiety ureteral dilatation.

Not all duplicated upper poles suffer the effects of massive dilatation, and some may not be dilated at all.[23] The sonographic appearance in these cases ranges from normal to mild or moderate upper pole hydronephrosis. Uncommonly, the obstructed upper pole may undergo atrophy, and the accumulated fluid within the collecting system may be reabsorbed. The only findings then may be small kidney size (the atrophic upper pole being invisible), a ureterocele, and compensatory hypertrophy of the contralateral kidney.

The principal adverse effect of complete duplication on the lower moiety of the kidney is vesicoureteral reflux. The resultant sonographic findings may include hydronephrosis (usually mild),[21] generalized parenchymal thinning, or focal scarring. In most cases, however, the lower pole moiety is normal sonographically.

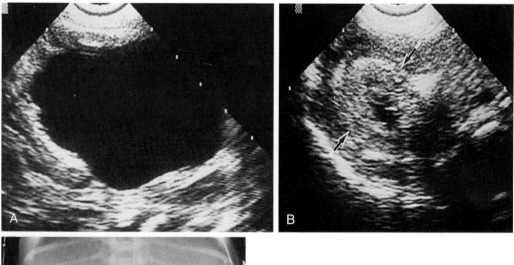

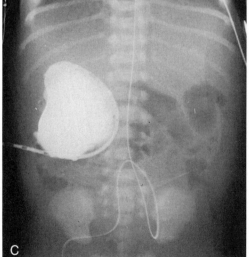

Figure 17-8—Duplicated Collecting System with Obstructed Upper Pole Moiety. (**A**) Coronal scans show a 6-cm diameter fluid collection in the right upper quadrant of this term infant. This fluid collection is a massively dilated upper pole moiety of a duplicated collecting system. (The right upper pole ureter was subsequently found to implant ectopically in the bladder.) (**B**) A transverse scan in the right iliac fossa shows an apparently normal lower component of the duplicated kidney (arrows), which is displaced inferiorly by the massively dilated upper pole. (**C**) Percutaneous nephrostomy demonstrates the dilated upper pole moiety.

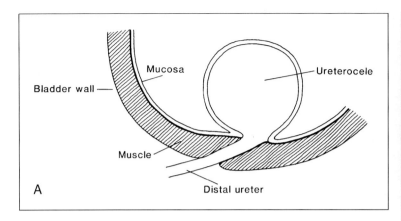

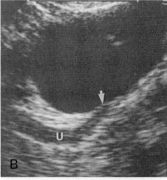

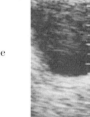

Figure 17-9—Ureterocele. (**A**) Illustration of ureterocele anatomy. (**B**) A longitudinal sonogram demonstrates distal ureteral dilatation (U) extending to the ureterovesical junction (arrow). (**C**) A longitudinal view at the ureterovesical junction shows a ureterocele (arrows) projecting into the bladder lumen. The ureteral insertion was ectopic.

Ureterocele

A ureterocele[13, 20–26] is a focal outpouching of the intramural portion of the ureter, as illustrated in Figure 17–9A. Most ureteroceles project into the lumen of the bladder, but they also may project externally, into the peritoneal space or retroperitoneum. Ureteroceles are usually associated with obstruction (partial or complete) at the ureterovesical junction (Fig. 17–9B). They may occur in normally located ureters, but they are most common in ureters that enter the bladder ectopically. Rarely, a ureterocele may form at the site where an ectopic ureter inserts into another structure, such as the vagina.

When a ureterocele is seen with ultrasound, it usually looks like a "cyst" contained *within* the lumen of the bladder (Fig. 17–9C). Some ureteroceles change size or disappear in response to pressure changes in the ureter or bladder, and these may be overlooked sonographically. A ureterocele also may be overlooked if the bladder is empty and the ureterocele is mistaken for the bladder! Finally, a ureterocele that projects *outside* the bladder may easily be mistaken for a bladder diverticulum, pelvic cysts, or another cystlike pelvic mass. Most, but not all, ureteroceles, are accompanied by ureteral dilatation and hydronephrosis.

Posterior Urethral Valve

The most common cause of urethral (not ureteral) obstruction in a male fetus or infant is a posterior urethral valve,[27–30] which is a diaphragmatic obstruction of the bulbomembranous portion of the urethra. Other causes of urethral obstruction are rare. The most important sonographic finding associated with the posterior urethral valve is dilatation of the prostatic urethra (Fig. 17–10), as seen during voiding or using the Credé method. Ancillary, but nonspecific, findings are a thick walled, distended bladder and upper urinary tract dilatation.

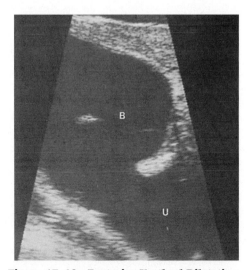

Figure 17-10—Posterior Urethral Dilatation. The posterior urethra (U) is massively enlarged in this male patient with an obstructive urethral anomaly. B = bladder.

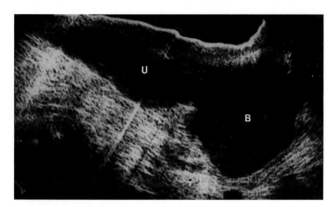

Figure 17-11—Urachal Remnant. A dilated urachal remnant (U) is seen to extend cephalad from the bladder (B) on this longitudinal sonogram. The patient was a 9 year old girl who presented with a tender midline abdominal mass.

Urachal Cyst

The urachus is an embryonic structure that regresses by the time bladder formation is complete, leaving only a small, cordlike remnant that connects the dome of the bladder with the umbilicus (see preceding chapter).[15] Vestiges of the urachal epithelium and lumen persist into adulthood in about one third of individuals,[31] but these do not usually cause problems. Rarely, however, pathology develops in the urachal remnant in one of the following forms:[24, 31-35]

1. A urachal fistula occurs if both the bladder and umbilical ends of the urachus remain patent.
2. A urachal sinus occurs at the umbilicus if the umbilical end remains patent but the bladder end closes normally.
3. A urachal diverticulum develops in the bladder wall if the bladder end remains patent but the umbilical end closes normally.
4. A urachal cyst develops in the abdominal wall if both the umbilical and bladder ends are closed but the lumen persists.

A urachal diverticulum may cause urine stasis and recurrent urinary tract infection. A urachal sinus or cyst may become infected, leading to abscess formation (Fig. 17–11). Finally, the urachal epithelium may undergo adenomatous metaplasia and become a urachal carcinoma.

REFERENCES

1. Marchal G, Verbeken E, Oyen R, et al: Ultrasound of the normal kidney: A sonographic, anatomic and histologic correlation. Ultrasound Med Biol 12:999–1009, 1986.
2. Partiquin H, Lefaivre JF, Lafortune M, et al: Fetal lobation, an anatamo-ultrasonographic correlation. J Ultrasound Med 9:191–197, 1990.
3. Carter AR, Horgan JG, Jennings TA, Rosenfeld AT: The junctional parenchymal defect: A sonographic variant of renal anatomy. Radiology 154:499–502, 1985.
4. Hoffer FA, Hanabergh AM, Teele RL: The interrenicular junction: A mimic of renal scarring on normal pediatric sonograms. AJR Am J Roentgenol 145:1075–1078, 1985.
5. Leekam RN, Matzinger MA, Brunelle M, Gray RR, Grosman H: The sonography of renal columnar hypertrophy. J Clin Ultrasound 11:491–494, 1983.
6. Mahony BS, Jeffrey RB, Laing FC: Septa of Bertin: A sonographic pseudotumor. J Clin Ultrasound 11:317–319, 1983.
7. Prando A, Pereira RM, Marins JLC: Sonographic evaluation of hypertrophy of septum of Bertin. Urology 24:505–510, 1984.
8. Taylor EJ (ed): Dorland's Illustrated Medical Dictionary. 27th ed. Philadelphia, WB Saunders, 1988, pp 37, 165, 519, 528, 797.
9. Jones DB: Kidneys. In Kissane JM (ed): Anderson's Pathology. 8th ed. St Louis, CV Mosby, 1985, pp 765–767.
10. Vinocar L, Slovis TL, Perlmutter AD, et al: Follow-up studies of multicystic dysplastic kidneys. Radiology 167:311–315, 1988.
11. Pedicelli G, Jequier S, Bowen A, Boisvert J: Multicystic dysplastic kidneys: Spontaneous regression demonstrated with US. Radiology 160:23–26, 1986.
12. Elder JS, Duckett JW: Management of the fetus and neonate with hydronephrosis detected by prenatal ultrasonography. Pediatr Ann 17:19–28, 1988.
13. Nusbaum AR, Dorst JP, Jeffs RD, Gearhart JP, Sanders RC: Ectopic ureter and ureterocele: Their varied sonographic manifestations. Radiology 159:227–235, 1986.
14. Warwick R, Williams DL (eds): Gray's Anatomy. 35th British ed. Philadelphia, WB Saunders, 1973, p 183.
15. Tourney TW: The early development of the human nephros. Embryology Carnegie Inst 35:159–197, 1954.
16. Trackler RT, Resnick ML, Leopold GR: Pelvic horseshoe kidney: Ultrasound findings and case report. J Clin Ultrasound 6:51–52, 1978.
17. Grandone CH, Haller JO, Berdon WE, Friedman AP: Asymmetric horseshoe kidney in the infant: Value of renal nuclear scanning. Radiology 154:366, 1985.
18. McCarty S, Rosenfield AT: Ultrasonography in crossed renal ectopia. J Ultrasound Med 3:107–112, 1984.
19. Lubat E, Hernanz-Schulman M, Genieser NB,

Ambrosino MM, Teele RL: Sonography of the simple and complicated ipsilateral fused kidney. J Ultrasound Med 8:109–114, 1989.

20. Bisset GS, Strife JL: The duplex collecting system in girls with urinary tract infection. AJR Am J Roentgenol 148:497–500, 1987.

21. Markle BM, Potter BM: Surgical diseases of the urinary tract. *In* Haller JO, Shkolnik A (eds): Ultrasound in Pediatrics. New York, Churchill Livingstone, 1981.

22. Winters WD, Lebowitz RL: Importance of prenatal detection of hydronephrosis of the upper pole. AJR Am J Roentgenol 155:125–129, 1990.

23. Share JC, Lebowitz RL: Ectopic ureterocele without ureteral and calyceal dilatation (ureterocele disproportion): Findings on urography and sonography. AJR Am J Roentgenol 152:567–571, 1989.

24. Friedman AP, Haller JO, Schulze G, Schaffer R: Sonography of vesical and perivesical abnormalities in children. J Ultrasound Med 2:385–390, 1983.

25. Andrew WK, Thomas RG, Aitken FG: Simple ureteroceles—ultrasonographic recognition and diagnosis of complications. SAMT 67:20–22, 1985.

26. Hantman SS: Sonographic diagnosis of vaginal ectopic ureter. J Ultrasound Med 2:523–524, 1983.

27. Willi UV, Lebowitz RL: The so-called megaureter-megacystis syndrome. AJR Am J Roentgenol 133:409–416, 1979.

28. Gaisie G, Mandell J, Scatliff JH: Congenital stenosis of the male urethra. AJR Am J Roentgenol 142:1269–1271, 1984.

29. McAlister WH: Demonstration of the dilated prostatic urethra in posterior urethral valve patients. J Ultrasound Med 3:189–190, 1984.

30. Gilsanz V, Miller JH, Reid BS: Ultrasonic characteristics of posterior urethral valves. Radiology 145:143–145, 1982.

31. Shubert GE, Pavkovic MB, Bethke-Bedurftig BA: Tubular urachal remnants in adult bladders. J Urol 127:40–42, 1992.

32. Spataro RF, Davis RS, McLachlan MSF, Linke CA, Barbaric ZL: Urachal abnormalities in the adult. Radiology 149:659–663, 1983.

33. Cacciarelli AA, Kass EJ, Yang SS: Urachal remnants: Sonographic demonstration in children. Radiology 174:473–475, 1990.

34. Wan Y-L, Lee T-Y, Tsai C-C, Chen S-MS, Chou F-F: The role of sonography in the diagnosis and management of urachal abscesses. J Clin Ultrasound 19:203–208, 1991.

35. Brick SH, Friedman AC, Pollack HM, Fishman EK, Radecki PD, Siegelbaum MH, Mitchell DG, Lev-Toaff AS, Caroline DF: Urachal carcinoma: CT findings. Radiology 169:377–381, 1988.

Chapter 18

Renal Failure and Renal Vascular Disease

William J. Zwiebel

Renal failure may result from three types of pathology: obstruction of urine outflow, renal parenchymal disease, and vascular occlusion. Because diagnostic ultrasound provides information about all three of these conditions, it is regarded as a valuable method for assessing patients with renal failure. Significant urinary tract abnormalities may be detected with ultrasound in up to 50% of renal failure patients.[1]

URINARY TRACT OBSTRUCTION

The detection of urinary tract obstruction[1–5] is the principal goal of ultrasound in patients with renal failure. Urinary tract obstruction is one of the few forms of renal failure that may be cured; therefore, the liberal use of sonography to detect obstruction in azotemic patients is warranted. The cost effectiveness of ultrasound is enhanced, however, by consideration of clinical factors. Ultrasound detects hydronephrosis in only 1% of azotemic patients in whom the risk for obstruction is low, compared with 29% of patients in whom history, signs, or symptoms suggest an obstructive etiology.[2]

Sonographic Diagnosis

Urinary tract obstruction is diagnosed *by inference* when ultrasound demonstrates dilatation of the intrarenal collection structures (hydronephrosis), ureteral dilatation (ureterectasis), or persistent dilatation of the urinary bladder after attempted voiding. The sensitivity and specificity of ultrasound in diagnosing hydronephrosis both exceed 90%, hence sonography is an accurate diagnostic method.[3–5]

Various schemes for grading hydronephrosis have been devised, but precision in quantifying dilatation has not been achieved. Therefore, I continue to use the traditional subjective categories: minimal, moderate, and severe, as illustrated in Figure 18–1.

Whenever hydronephrosis is detected, the sonographer should always try to determine the *extent* of dilatation. Dilatation limited to a portion of the kidney suggests obstruction of a major calyx or obstruction of one portion of a duplicated collecting system (Chapter 17). Dilatation of the renal pelvis and intrarenal structures, but not of the proximal ureter, suggests ureteropelvic junction obstruction. Ureteral dilatation may be caused by obstruction anywhere along the course of the ureter, as well as at the bladder outlet. The latter etiology is confirmed when postvoiding examination shows massive urine retention or when urinary tract dilatation disappears with bladder decompression.

In addition to determining the extent of obstruction, sonographers should also try to determine the cause of obstruction. Masses, calculi, and bladder-emptying problems are the principal causes of obstruction that are amenable to sonographic diagnosis, but it is an unfortunate fact that the cause of obstruction cannot be determined with ultrasound in many cases. This failing occurs for two reasons. First, the only portions of the ureters that can be seen regularly are a short segment adjacent to the kidney and a short segment behind the bladder. The remaining portions of the ureters are obscured by echogenic bowel contents. Second, many lesions that block the ureters (e.g., uroepithelial tumors and calculi) are quite small and would be difficult to identify even if the ureter could be seen. Urography and computed tomography[6] often are more effective than ultrasound for determining the extent and cause of urinary tract obstruction.

Diagnostic Caveats

We have stated that ultrasound is highly accurate for identifying hydronephrosis, but sonographic misdiagnoses are possible.[7–24] (Remember that the sonologist's motto is "You can always be fooled.") Please note the following caveats (also listed in Table 18–1) that will help avoid errors.

Failure to Look at the Bladder. Bladder outlet obstruction is easily detected, but the sonographer must look at the bladder and obtain

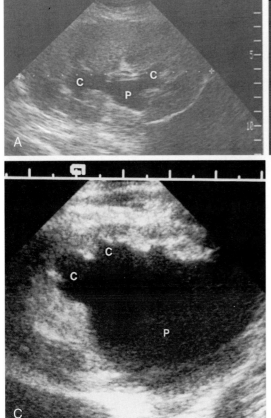
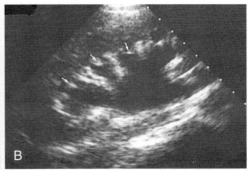

Figure 18-1—Hydronephrosis Grades.
(**A**) Minimal; note that the major calyces (C) and pelvis (P) are visible. (**B**) Moderate; the major and minor calyces are visible. The tips of the pyramids (arrows) are visible in this case. (**C**) Severe; the calyces (C) and pelvis (P) are massively dilated. (Longitudinal view of the upper pole of the left kidney.)

postvoid bladder views! Examine the bladder in *all* patients with renal failure, *even those with Foley catheters in place.* An improperly positioned catheter may drain a few milliliters of urine but will not relieve bladder outlet obstruction!

Failure to Look at the Distal Ureter. Obstructing calculi are readily visible in the retrovesical portions of the ureters (Chapter 22). If you find a distal ureteral calculus, the referring clinician thinks you are a hero! Why miss this opportunity by not looking?

The Problem of Minimal Hydronephrosis. Minimal dilatation of intrarenal collecting structures may be a normal finding in a well-hydrated patient, may be caused by vesicoureteral reflux, or may be the only manifestation of significant obstruction (especially soon after an abrupt obstruction).[7-11] In many cases, it is not possible to determine when minimal hydronephrosis is significant. The incidence of obstructive uropathy is low (6%), however, when minimal hydronephrosis is accompanied by a low index of suspicion for obstruction,[8] but minimal dilatation should be taken seriously in patients who are at risk for obstruction. Remember, obstruction is one of the few treatable causes of renal failure!

Obstruction Without Dilatation. Rarely, abruptly occurring obstruction does not produce hydronephrosis because it results in abrupt "shut down" of urine production.[24-26]

Dilatation Without Obstruction. Collecting system dilatation may occur in the absence of flow-reducing obstruction, as for example in renal allografts and congenital ureteropelvic junction narrowing.[9, 11, 15-19]

Dilatation from Reflux. The only sonographic finding that differentiates between obstruction-induced and reflux-induced hydronephrosis is minute-to-minute variation in the

Table 18-1. Pitfalls in Diagnosing Hydronephrosis

Failure to examine the bladder
Failure to examine the distal ureters
Visualization of prominent but normal calyces
Dilatation without obstruction
Obstruction without dilatation
Dilatation from vesicoureteral reflux
Normal blood vessels mimicking dilated calyces
Peripelvic cysts
Papillary necrosis

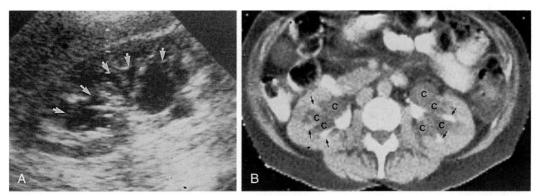

Figure 18-2—Peripelvic Cysts Mistaken for Hydronephrosis. (A) This longitudinal view of the right kidney shows sonolucent renal sinus fluid collections (arrows). The left kidney (not shown) has a similar appearance, leading to a diagnosis of bilateral hydronephrosis. Note, however, that these fluid collections vary in size and that they do not connect with a dilated renal pelvis. (B) A contrast-enhanced computed tomogram performed subsequent to the ultrasound examination demonstrates nondilated renal collecting structures (arrows) bilaterally. Both renal sinuses are filled with peripelvic cysts (C).

degree of dilatation, particularly when the ureters and calyces become larger as the bladder becomes smaller.[18, 19]

Blood Vessels Mimic Dilated Calyces. Normal intrarenal blood vessels (arteries or veins) are visible sonographically and may mimic dilated calyces, particularly in children.[10] Differentiation is possible with color Doppler.

Peripelvic Cysts Mimic Dilated Calyces. Multiple benign cysts, called peripelvic cysts, may be present in the renal sinus of middle-aged and elderly individuals, and these may readily be mistaken for dilated calyces[20, 21] (Fig. 18-2). A simple rule helps prevent this error: diagnose hydronephrosis only when the dilated calyces are *similar in size* and clearly *communicate* with a centrally located, dilated renal pelvis. Dilated collecting structures should resemble a hand, with the fingers representing the major calyces and the palm representing the renal pelvis!*

Papillary Necrosis. Parenchymal cavities resulting from papillary necrosis may be mistaken for hydronephrosis.[22, 23] Two findings in papillary necrosis are diagnostic: (1) *only the calyces are enlarged* (the infundibula and pelvis are not dilated); and (2) the medullary pyramids are blunted, small, or invisible.

Doppler Assessment of Hydronephrosis

Platt and colleagues[11] suggest the use of the resistivity index,† as calculated from Doppler waveforms, for differentiating between obstruc-

tive and nonobstructive dilatation. These investigators have found that the resistive index in parenchymal arteries (e.g., interlobar) exceeds 0.70 with obstructive dilatation and is below 0.70 with nonobstructive dilatation. Although a normal (low) resistive index appears to *exclude* urodynamically significant dilatation, a high resistive index is not specific for obstruction, since high resistance also occurs with diffuse parenchymal disease, including allograft rejection.[12-14]

RENAL PARENCHYMAL DISEASE

The second major cause of renal failure that may be evaluated with ultrasound is renal parenchymal disease.[12-14, 22, 23, 27-54] Renal failure due to parenchymal disease often cannot be cured; nonetheless, ultrasound findings in renal parenchymal disease have relevance from both a diagnostic and therapeutic perspective.

The sonographic findings associated with renal parenchymal disease [12-14, 22, 23, 27-60] are listed in Table 18-2. Generally speaking, the severity of these abnormalities correlates poorly with the severity of renal injury and dysfunction; therefore, the ultrasound findings are poor prognosti-

Table 18-2. Sonographic Findings in Renal Parenchymal Disease

Altered cortical echogenicity
Focal parenchymal sonolucency
Altered size and/or appearance of the medullary pyramids
Diminished renal sinus echogenicity
Altered kidney size
Irregular kidney contours
Papillary necrosis

---

*To a former radiology resident, this appearance was reminiscent of brass knuckles, which may say something about his background.

†The resistive index is the peak systolic frequency, minus the end diastolic frequency, divided by the peak systolic frequency.

Table 18-3. Sonographic Findings in Selected Renal Parenchymal Diseases

Acute Glomerulonephritis

Normal appearance
Variable enlargement
Variable increase in cortical echogenicity

Acute Nephrotic Syndrome

Normal appearance
Enlargement
Increased cortical echogenicity
Variable prominence of pyramids

Acute Toxic Nephritis

Normal appearance
Increased cortical echogenicity (may be very bright)
Variable prominence of pyramids
Variable enlargement

Acute Tubular Necrosis

Normal appearance
Increased cortical echogenicity with prominent, hypoechoic
    pyramids
Markedly increased pyramidal echogenicity (deposition of
    Tamm-Horsfall protein)

Diabetic and Hypertensive Nephropathy

Gradual decrease in kidney size
Gradual increase in echogenicity and decrease of
    corticomedullary contrast (due to fibrosis)

cators. The exception to this rule is the shrunken "end stage" kidney (described later), which always implies severe, irremediable damage.

A glance at Table 18–2 shows that parenchymal disease causes a broad array of echographic changes. To make matters worse, a single parenchymal disorder may produce a variety of sonographic findings, as indicated in Table 18–3.[12, 14, 27-31, 35-60] This lack of specificity occurs because disorders that *primarily* affect one component of the renal parenchyma may *secondarily* affect other components.* For instance, the kidneys remain normal in most cases of acute glomerulonephritis because only the glomeruli are affected. In some cases of glomerulonephritis, however, cortical echogenicity is increased because the inflammatory response "spills over" into the interstitium and visibly increases tissue echogenicity.

The following section reviews briefly the sonographic findings listed in Table 18–2.

Increased Cortical Echogenicity

Cortical echogenicity is considered to be increased when the "brightness" of the cortex *exceeds* that of the adjacent liver parenchyma[27, 32, 33]

*Renal parenchyma is composed of four major tissue components: glomeruli, tubules, the interstitium (the supporting structure of the kidney), and the microvasculature.

(Fig. 18–3). Although this finding is highly specific for renal parenchymal disease (98%), it occurs in only 18% of cases[27, 32]; furthermore, interobserver variability is considerable.[33, 34] The older ultrasound literature states that cortical echogenicity in adults is abnormal if it equals the echogenicity of the liver,[28, 29, 31] but it has been shown that cortical and hepatic echogenicity are equal in 40% of normal adult kidneys.[32, 33] (Remember, however, the renal cortex is normally more echogenic than the liver in infants and small children![27, 32-34])

Increased cortical echogenicity is a manifestation of diseases that prominently affect the renal interstitium, particularly those associated with active cellular infiltration of the interstitium.[27-32, 43] Examples include acute nephrotic syndrome, acute allograft rejection, and acute toxic injury. Interstitial fibrosis also increases cortical echogenicity, but only to a moderate degree.

Decreased Cortical Echogenicity

Cortical echogenicity may be decreased by massive kidney edema[27-29, 35-38, 41, 55-60] or by diffuse neoplastic infiltration (Chapter 20). Reduced echogenicity usually is accompanied by renomegaly. Renal vein thrombosis is an example.

Focal Decreased Cortical Echogenicity

Localized areas of decreased cortical echogenicity (Figure 18–4) may occur with severe inflammatory or edematous processes, and with parenchymal infarction.[35-37] Examples include acute renal transplant rejection, focal bacterial nephritis, and lupus nephritis.

Medullary Pyramidal Changes

In most parenchymal diseases, the medullary pyramids become more conspicuous (Fig. 18–5). Increased conspicuousness is attributed to hyperemia, edema, necrosis at the corticomedullary junction, and tubular distention. Less commonly, the pyramids become less conspicuous, as occurs with medullary fibrosis (seen in elderly patients). Striking *increases* in pyramidal echogenicity occur in nephrocalcinosis and several additional disorders considered in Chapter 22.[27-29, 39, 40]

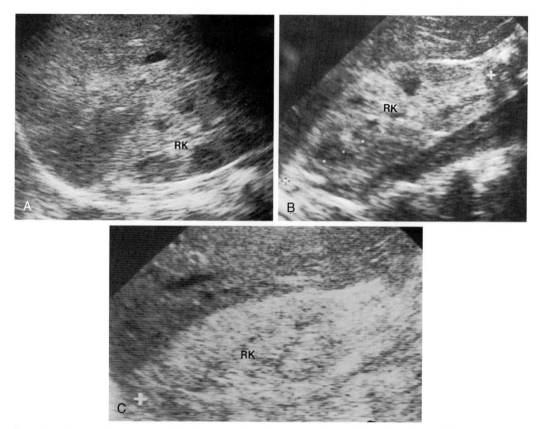

Figure 18-3—Renal Parenchymal Disease. (**A, B**) Longitudinal views of the right kidney (RK) demonstrate moderately increased cortical echogenicity (relative to the liver) in this child with acute glomerulonephritis. Note that the pyramids are not enlarged but are more conspicuous due to enhanced corticomedullary contrast. (**C**) A longitudinal view of the right kidney (RK) in a patient who has ingested toxic alcohol demonstrates markedly increased cortical and medullary echogenicity. Note that the medullary pyramids are not visible.

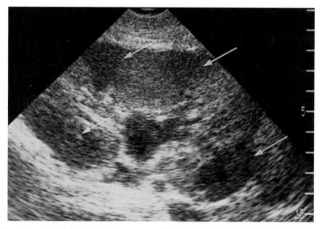

Figure 18-4—Focal Decreased Echogenicity. Areas of decreased echogenicity (arrows) are seen peripherally in this renal allograft during an episode of acute rejection. Note the lack of renal sinus echogenicity surrounding the renal pelvis.

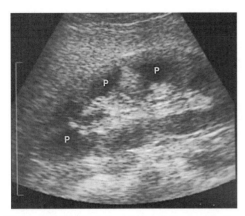

Figure 18-5—Prominent Renal Pyramids. Large and poorly defined renal pyramids (P) stand out against the renal cortex in this 50 year old man with acute interstitial nephritis of undetermined origin.

Diminished Renal Sinus Echogenicity

The normally strong echogenicity of the renal sinus is diminished or lost (Fig. 18–4) in severe inflammatory processes such as pyelonephritis, acute transplant rejection, and neoplastic infiltration. This loss of echogenicity may result from edema, inflammation-induced degeneration of fat cells, or neoplastic infiltration of the sinus fat.[41]

Increased Kidney Size

The kidneys may be enlarged by a host of inflammatory, infiltrative, neoplastic, and metabolic disorders, as listed in Table 18–4.° Bilateral enlargement is the rule with most of these conditions.

Diminished Kidney Size

Shrinkage of the kidneys (Fig. 18–6) implies parenchymal destruction from myriad primary and secondary disorders, invariably leading to parenchymal fibrosis.[27, 42, 43] The end result is the end-stage kidney, which is a featureless, scarred remnant, as shown in Figure 18–7.

Irregular Kidney Contours

Loss of the usual smooth renal outline (Fig. 18–8) implies focal parenchymal destruction and scar formation, usually due to infection or infarction. The kidneys are smoothly marginated in virtually all other forms of renal parenchymal disease.

°References 2, 12–14, 17, 27–30, 41–48, 55–60.

The Confusing Findings in Acute Tubular Necrosis

Acute tubular necrosis (ATN) deserves particular mention, since this condition presents seemingly contradictory ultrasound findings.[12, 27–29, 35–41, 46–48] In most cases of ATN the kidneys remain normal sonographically. This is especially true of ischemic injury associated with renal transplantation. Less commonly, the cortex becomes echogenic and the pyramids become more conspicuous (hypoechoic and/or large), as occurs with toxic injury. Rarely, pyramidal echogenicity is dramatically increased, mimicking the findings of nephrocalcinosis (Chapter 22). This appearance occurs primarily in infants and is due to precipitation of Tamm-Horsfall proteins in the renal tubules.

RENOVASCULAR DISORDERS

The final cause of renal failure that we will consider is circulatory failure, which may result from obstruction of either the renal artery or renal vein.[55–74] Readers who are unfamiliar with the normal features of renal blood flow should review this material in Chapter 16.

Renal Artery Occlusion

Occlusion or hemodynamically significant stenosis of the main renal artery[62, 64–75] causes ischemic damage to all renal tissues. The net results are cellular death, diminished kidney size, and fibrosis, which occur in proportion to the duration and severity of ischemia. Kidneys injured by "global" ischemia retain normal echogenicity and shape until the injury is advanced. If blood flow is not restored, however, fibrosis ensues, ultimately leading to the end stage appearance described earlier.

Failure to detect blood flow in the renal hilum with color Doppler sonography strongly suggests arterial occlusion.[62, 66–73] Before this judgment is reached, however, it is essential to confirm that the Doppler instrument is sufficiently sensitive to detect flow in other abdominal arteries at an equivalent depth, or in the other kidney.

It is logical to assume that the renal artery is patent when arterial flow is present at the renal hilum, but this is not necessarily so. Collateral flow through accessory renal arteries or capsular branches may produce normal-appearing color Doppler images at the renal hilum and even normal-appearing spectral Doppler waveforms.[64, 69, 70, 72, 73] The only way to *confirm* the patency of the renal artery is to trace it in its entirety, from its aortic origin to the renal hilum!

Table 18-4. Causes of Kidney Enlargement

Hydronephrosis
Diabetes mellitus
Acute glomerulonephritis
Acute vasculitis
Lupus nephritis
AIDS-related nephropathy
Acute toxic nephropathy
Neoplastic infiltration (usually lymphoma or leukemia; less
  commonly renal cell carcinoma, transitional cell
  carcinoma, or other neoplasms)
Amyloidosis
Acute renal vein thrombosis
Obesity and large body habitus
Chronic steroid use
Acromegaly
Cystic disorders

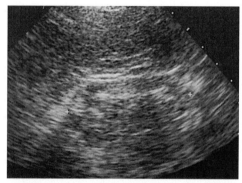

Figure 18-7—End-Stage Kidney. A poorly defined, hyperechoic end-stage kidney (cursors) measuring 6 cm in length is barely detectable in this adult with diabetic nephropathy.

Renal Artery Stenosis

Ultrasound diagnosis of renal artery stenosis [61, 62, 65-70] is based on the detection of increased flow velocity in the stenotic portion of the vessel and turbulence in the immediate poststenotic region. With severe stenosis, arterial signals distal to the stenosis are "damped" (low amplitude and rounded). Renal artery stenosis is considered to be hemodynamically significant (pressure reducing) when the lumen diameter is narrowed by at least 50%. This—or greater levels of narrowing (Fig. 18–9)—is indicated when peak systole (peak systolic velocity) in the stenosis exceeds 180 cm/sec, or when peak systole in the stenosis is 3.5 (or more) times higher than peak systole in the aorta at the level of the renal arteries. (See Figure 18–9 following page 268.)

Two problems have limited the value of color Doppler sonography for detecting renal artery stenosis. First, the renal arteries are difficult to follow throughout their course, even with the best color Doppler systems. Second, stenoses of accessory renal arteries (present in one third of individuals with renovascular hypertension) cannot be identified reliably.

Arterial Embolization

Focal obstruction of arterial branches within the kidney (typically embolic) causes ischemic damage to the portions of the kidney (lobes or segments) served by the occluded branches. The occlusion of multiple segmental or lobar arteries produces a "pruned tree" appearance on color Doppler examination, rather than the normal, uniform distribution of parenchymal vessels. Power Doppler sonography[75] may be of particular value for assessing parenchymal renal vessels.

The net effect of arterial embolization is parenchymal destruction, which is manifested by focal cortical thinning that is broad based, triangular in shape, and centered *between* adjacent pyramids. In theory, this appearance differs from that seen with infectious scarring, in which the cortical defects are directly *over* the pyramids,

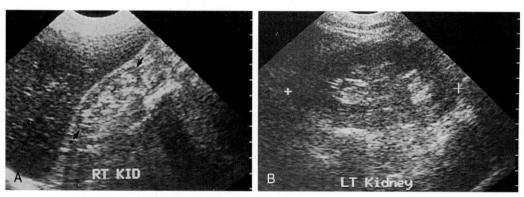

Figure 18-6—Decreased Renal Size. (**A**) The right kidney (arrows) in this patient with renal artery stenosis is considerably smaller (6.8 cm) than the left kidney (**B**), which measured 11 cm (the same scale was used for both pictures). Note that the volume of parenchyma on the right is small in comparison to the volume of the renal sinus fat. Contrast this appearance with the left kidney.

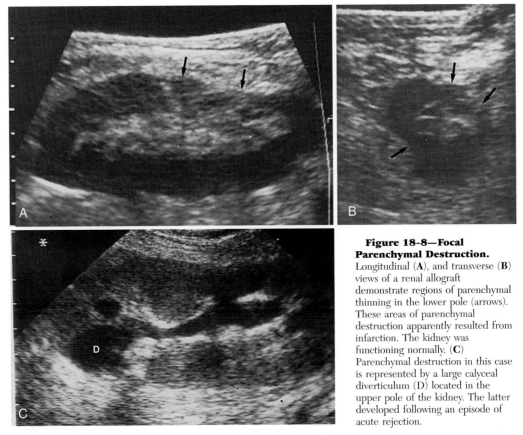

Figure 18-8—Focal Parenchymal Destruction. Longitudinal (**A**), and transverse (**B**) views of a renal allograft demonstrate regions of parenchymal thinning in the lower pole (arrows). These areas of parenchymal destruction apparently resulted from infarction. The kidney was functioning normally. (**C**) Parenchymal destruction in this case is represented by a large calyceal diverticulum (D) located in the upper pole of the kidney. The latter developed following an episode of acute rejection.

but in my opinion this distinction can rarely be appreciated sonographically.

Renal Vein Thrombosis

Renal vein thrombosis also may result in ischemic parenchymal destruction and acute renal failure.[55-61] The potential exists for recanalization of the renal vein or the development of venous collaterals, but renal damage from venous occlusion often is permanent. Acute renal vein occlusion causes parenchymal edema (congestion) and hemorrhage. If severe, these processes may cause renomegaly as well as altered renal echogenicity, including the following: (1) hypoechoic cortex with decreased corticomedullary differentiation; (2) hyperechoic cortex with preservation of corticomedullary differentiation; and (3) mottled heterogeneity accompanied by the loss of normal intrarenal architecture. In some cases, linear echogenic streaks of unknown origin course through the renal parenchyma, and these are thought to be pathognomonic for renal vein thrombosis.[58, 59]

Renal vein thrombosis can be diagnosed with certainty only through direct identification of thrombus in the renal vein. The acutely throm-bosed renal vein invariably is enlarged, and Doppler signals typically are absent. A small "trickle" of flow may be present around the clot, but such flow is low in velocity and continuous (lacks normal phasic variation). Recently formed thrombus is hypoechoic, and in some cases is virtually anechoic. As a result the thrombus may be invisible with gray-scale sonography and detectable only with Doppler ultrasound. Two additional pitfalls are noteworthy. First, venous flow may be evident within the kidney, even though the renal vein is occluded, since large collaterals may develop quickly and restore flow. Second, very sluggish flow may mimic thrombosis since no Doppler signal is detectable at very slow flow rates.

The long-term effects of renal vein thrombosis are varied. In some cases, the kidney returns to a normal sonographic appearance, but if the kidney is severely damaged, chronic changes may include diminished kidney size, increased echogenicity (due to fibrosis), and even the end stage appearance described earlier.

REFERENCES

1. Chang VH, Cunningham JJ: Efficacy of sonography as a screening method in renal insufficiency. J Clin Ultrasound 13:415–417, 1985.

2. Ritchie WW, Vick CW, Glocheski SK, Cook DE: Evaluation of azotemic patients: Diagnostic yield of initial US examination. Radiology 167:245–247, 1988.

3. Denton T, Cochlin DL, Evans C: The value of ultrasound in previously undiagnosed renal failure. Br J Radiol 57:673–675, 1984.

4. Lee JKT, Baron RL, Melson GL, McClennan BL, Weyman PJ: Can real-time ultrasonography replace static B-scanning in the diagnosis of renal obstruction? Radiology 139:161–165, 1981.

5. Malave SR, Neiman HL, Spies SM, Cisternino SJ, Adamo G: Diagnosis of hydronephrosis: Comparison of radionuclide scanning and sonography. AJR Am J Roentgenol 135:1179–1185, 1980.

6. Bosniak MA, Megibow AJ, Ambos MA, Mitnick JS, Lefleur RS, Gordon R: Computed tomography of ureteral obstruction. AJR Am J Roentgenol 138:1107–1113, 1982.

7. Morin ME, Baker DA: The influence of hydration and bladder distension on the sonographic diagnosis of hydronephrosis. J Clin Ultrasound 7:192–194, 1979.

8. Kamholtz RG, Cronan JJ, Dorfman GS: Obstruction and the minimally dilated renal collecting system: US evaluation. Radiology 170:51–53, 1989.

9. Jaffe RB, Middleton AW Jr: Whitaker test: Differentiation of obstructive from nonobstructive uropathy. AJR Am J Roentgenol 134:9–15, 1980.

10. Scola FH, Cronan JJ, Schepps B: Grade I hydronephrosis: Pulsed Doppler US evaluation. Radiology 171:519–520, 1989.

11. Platt JF, Rubin JM, Ellis JH: Distinction between obstructive and nonobstructive pyelocaliectasis with duplex Doppler sonography. AJR Am J Roentgenol 153:997–1000, 1989.

12. Platt JF, Rubin JM, Ellis JH: Acute renal failure: Possible role of duplex Doppler US in distinction between acute perirenal failure and acute tubular necrosis. Radiology 179:419–423, 1991.

13. Platt JF, Ellis JH, Rubin JM, DiPietro MA, Sedman AB: Intrarenal arterial Doppler sonography in patients with nonobstructive renal disease: Correlation of resistive index with biopsy findings. AJR Am J Roentgenol 154:1223–1227, 1990.

14. Mostbeck GH, Kain R, Mallek R, Derfler K, Walter R, Havelec L, Tscholakoff D: Duplex Doppler sonography in renal parenchymal disease: Histopathologic correlation. J Ultrasound Med 10:189–194, 1991.

15. Peake SL, Roxburgh HB, Langlois S: Ultrasonic assessment of hydronephrosis of pregnancy. Radiology 146:167–170, 1983.

16. Fried AM, Woodring JH, Thompson DJ: Hydronephrosis of pregnancy: A prospective sequential study of the course of dilatation. J Ultrasound Med 2:255–259, 1983.

17. Schutz K, Siffring PA, Forrest TS, Hill WC, Frick MP: Serial renal sonographic changes in preeclampsia. J Ultrasound Med 9:415–418, 1990.

18. Lucaya J, Enriquez G, Delgado R, Castellote A: Infundibulopelvic stenosis in children. AJR Am J Roentgenol 142:471–474, 1984.

19. Cronan JJ, Amis ES, Scola FH, Schepps B: Renal obstruction in patients with ileal loops: US evaluation. Radiology 158:647–648, 1986.

20. Rosenfield AT, Taylor KJW, Dembner AG, Jacobson P: Ultrasound of renal sinus: New observations. AJR Am J Roentgenol 133:441–448, 1979.

21. Ralls PW, Esensten ML, Boger D, Halls JM: Severe hydronephrosis and severe renal cystic disease: Ultrasonic differentiation. AJR Am J Roentgenol 134:473–475, 1980.

22. Hoffman JC, Schnur MJ, Koenigsberg M: Demonstration of renal papillary necrosis by sonography. Radiology 145:785–787, 1982.

23. Shapeero LG, Vordermark JS: Papillary necrosis causing hydronephrosis in the renal allograft. J Ultrasound Med 8:579–581, 1989.

24. Curry NS, Gobien RP, Schabel SI: Minimal-dilatation obstructive nephropathy. Radiology 143:531–534, 1982.

25. Maillet PJ, Pelle-Francoz D, Laville M, Gay F, Pinet A: Nondilated obstructive acute renal failure: Diagnostic procedures and therapeutic management. Radiology 160:659–662, 1986.

26. Naidich JB, Rackson ME, Mossey RT, Stein HL: Nondilated obstructive uropathy: Percutaneous nephrostomy performed to reverse renal failure. Radiology 160:653–657, 1986.

27. Huntington DK, Hill SC, Hill MC: Sonographic manifestations of medical renal disease. Semin Ultrasound CT MR 12:290–307, 1991.

28. Rosenfield AT, Siegel NJ: Renal parenchymal disease: Histopathologic-sonographic correlation. AJR Am J Roentgenol 137:793–798, 1981.

29. Hricak H, Cruz C, Romanski R, et al: Renal parenchymal disease: Sonographic-histologic correlation. Radiology 144:141–147, 1982.

30. Walker JT, Keller MS, Katz SM: Computed tomographic and sonographic findings in acute ethylene glycol poisoning. J Ultrasound Med 2:429–431, 1983.

31. Brenbridge AN, Chevalier RL, Kaiser DL: Increased renal cortical echogenicity in pediatric renal disease: Histopathologic correlations. J Clin Ultrasound 14:595–600, 1986.

32. Platt JF, Rubin JM, Bowerman RA, Marn CS: The inability to detect kidney disease on the basis of echogenicity. AJR Am J Roentgenol 151:317–319, 1988.

33. Lamont AC, Graebe AC, Pelmore JM, Thompson JR: Ultrasound assessment of renal cortical brightness in infants: Is naked eye evaluation reliable? Invest Radiol 25:250–253, 1990.

34. Fontaine S, Lafortune M, Breton G, Vallée C: Ascites as a cause of hyperechogenic kidneys. J Clin Ultrasound 13:633–636, 1985.

35. Swobodnik WL, Spohn BE, Wechsler JG, et al: Real-time ultrasound evaluation of renal transport failure during the early postoperative period. Ultrasound Med Biol 12:97–105, 1986.

36. Frick MP, Feinberg SB, Sibley R, Idstrom ME: Ultrasound in acute renal transplant rejection. Radiology 138:657–660, 1981.

37. Singh A, Cohen WN: Renal allograft rejection: Sonography and scintigraphy. AJR Am J Roentgenol 135:73–77, 1980.

38. Hricak H, Cruz C, Eyler WR, Madrazo BL, Romanski R, Sandler MA: Acute post-transplantation renal failure: Differential diagnosis by ultrasound. Radiology 139:441–449, 1981.

39. Hoddick W, Filly RA, Backman U, Callen PW, Vincenti F, Hricak H, Mahony BS, Amend W: Renal allograft rejection: US evaluation. Radiology 161:469–473, 1986.

40. Fried AM, Woodring JH, Loh FK, Lucas BA, Kryscio RJ: The medullary pyramid index: An objective assessment of prominence in renal transplant rejection. Radiology 149:787–791, 1983.

41. Hricak H, Romanski RN, Eyler WR: The renal sinus during allograft rejection: Sonographic and

histopathologic findings. Radiology 142:693–699, 1982.

42. Troell S, Berg U, Johansson J, Wikstad I: Ultrasonographic renal parenchymal volume related to kidney and renal parenchymal area in children with recurrent urinary tract infections and asymptomatic bacteriuria. Acta Radiol Diagn 25:411–416, 1984.

43. Päivänsalo M, Pyhtinen J, Seppänen U: An ultrasonographic renal parenchymal index. Acta Radiol 56:57–61, 1982.

44. Segel MC, Leaky J, Slasky BS: Diabetes mellitus: The predominant cause of bilateral renal enlargement. Radiology 153:341–342, 1984.

45. Chesney RW, O'Regan S, Kaplan BS, Nograde MB: Asymmetric renal enlargement in acute glomerulonephritis. Radiology 122:431–434, 1977.

46. Hricak H, Toledo-Pereyra LH, Eyler WR, Madrazo BL, Sy GS: Evaluation of acute post-transplant renal failure by ultrasound. Radiology 133:443–447, 1979.

47. Rosenfield AT, Zeman RK, Cicchetti DV, Siegel NJ: Experimental acute tubular necrosis: US appearance. Radiology 157:771–774, 1985.

48. Nomura G, Kinoshita E, Yamagata Y, Koga N: Usefulness of renal ultrasonography for assessment of severity and course of acute tubular necrosis. J Clin Ultrasound 12:135–139, 1984.

49. Choyke PL, Grant EG, Hoffer FA, Tina L, Korec S: Cortical echogenicity in the hemolytic uremic syndrome: Clinical correlation. J Ultrasound Med 7:439–442, 1988.

50. Patriquin HB, O'Regan S, Robitaille P, Paltiel H: Hemolytic-uremic syndrome: Intrarenal arterial Doppler patterns as a useful guide to therapy. Radiology 172:625–628, 1989.

51. Stanley JH, Cornella R, Loevinger E, Schabel SI, Curry NS: Sonography of systemic lupus nephritis. AJR Am J Roentgenol 142:1165–1168, 1984.

52. Longmaid HE, Rider E, Tymkiw J: Lupus nephritis: New sonographic findings. J Ultrasound Med 6:75–79, 1987.

53. Hamper UM, Goldblum LE, Hutchins GM, Sheth S, Dahnert WF, Bartlett JG, Sanders RC: Renal involvement in AIDS: Sonographic-pathologic correlation. AJR Am J Roentgenol 150:1321–1325, 1988.

54. Schaffer RM, Schwartz GE, Becker JA, Rao TKS, Shih YH: Renal ultrasound in acquired immune deficiency syndrome. Radiology 153:511–513, 1984.

55. Keating MA, Althausen AF: The clinical spectrum of renal vein thrombosis. J Urol 133:938–945, 1985.

56. Rosenberg ER, Trought WS, Kirks DR, Summer TE, Grossman H: Ultrasonic diagnosis of renal vein thrombosis in neonates. AJR Am J Roentgenol 134:35–38, 1980.

57. Paling MR, Wakefield JA, Watson LR: Sonography of experimental acute renal vein occlusion. J Clin Ultrasound 13:647–653, 1985.

58. Metreweli C, Pearson R: Echographic diagnosis of neonatal renal venous thrombosis. Pediatr Radiol 14:105–108, 1984.

59. Lalmand B, Avni EF, Nasr A, Ketelbant P, Struyven

J: Perinatal renal vein thrombosis. J Ultrasound Med 9:437–442, 1990.

60. Rosenfield AT, Zeman RK, Cronan JJ, Taylor KJW: Ultrasound in experimental and clinical renal vein thrombosis. Radiology 137:735–741, 1980.

61. Taylor KJW, Burns PN: Duplex Doppler scanning in the pelvis and abdomen. Ultrasound Med Biol 11:643–658, 1985.

62. Hillman BJ: Imaging advances in the diagnosis of renovascular hypertension. AJR Am J Roentgenol 153:5–14, 1989.

63. Friedman DM, Schacht RG: Doppler waveforms in the renal arteries of normal children. J Clin Ultrasound 19:387–392, 1991.

64. Yune HY, Klatte EC: Collateral circulation to an ischemic kidney. Radiology 119:539–546, 1976.

65. Greene ER, Venters MD, Avasthi PS, Conn RL, Jahnke RW: Noninvasive characterization of renal artery blood flow. Kidney Int 20:523–529, 1981.

66. Avasthi PS, Voyles WF, Greene ER: Noninvasive diagnosis of renal artery stenosis by echo-Doppler velocimetry. Kidney Int 25:824–829, 1984.

67. Spies JB, Hricak H, Slemmer TM, Zeineh S, Alpers CE, Zayat P, Lue TF, Kerlan RK Jr, Madrazo BL, Sandler MA: Sonographic evaluation of experimental acute renal arterial occlusion in dogs. AJR Am J Roentgenol 142:341–346, 1984.

68. Norris CS, Pfeiffer JS, Rittgers SE, Barnes RW: Noninvasive evaluation of renal artery stenosis and renovascular resistance. J Vasc Surg 1:192–201, 1984.

69. Rittgers SE, Norris CS, Barnes RW: Detection of renal artery stenosis: Experimental and clinical analysis of velocity waveforms. Ultrasound Med Biol 11:523–531, 1985.

70. Kohler TR, Zierler RE, Martin RL, Nicholls SC, Bergelin RO, Kazmers A, Beach KW, Strandness DE Jr: Noninvasive diagnosis of renal artery stenosis by ultrasonic duplex scanning. J Vasc Surg 4:450–456, 1986.

71. Handa N, Fukanaga R, Ogawa S, Matsumoto M, Kimura K, Kamada T: A new, accurate, and non-invasive screening method for renovascular hypertension: The renal artery Doppler technique. J Hypertension 6:S458–S460, 1988.

72. Taylor DC, Kettler MD, Moneta GL, Kohler TR, Kazmers A, Beach KW, Strandness DE Jr: Duplex ultrasound scanning in the diagnosis of renal artery stenosis: A prospective evaluation. J Vasc Surg 7:363–369, 1988.

73. Berland LL, Koslin DB, Routh WD, Keller FS: Renal artery stenosis: Prospective evaluation of diagnosis with color duplex US compared with angiography. Radiology 174:421–423, 1990.

74. Martin RL, Nanra RS, Wlodarczyk J, DeSilva A, Bray AE: Renal hilar Doppler analysis in the detection of renal artery stenosis. J Vasc Tech 15:173–180, 1991.

75. Rubin JM, Bude RO, Carson PL, et al: Power Doppler US: A potentially useful alternative to mean frequency-based color Doppler US. Radiology 190:853–856, 1994.

Chapter 19

Renal Allografts and Hemodialysis

William J. Zwiebel

Practitioners in both referral and community hospitals are likely to be asked to evaluate renal transplant patients, for renal transplantation is a common surgical procedure in Western nations. It is pertinent, therefore, to consider the role of sonography in renal transplantation.

GENERAL CONSIDERATIONS

The term "allograft" refers to any tissue transplanted from one human to another. The proper term for the transplanted kidney, therefore, is "renal allograft." The allograft may be harvested (removed) from a living related donor, or from a brain-dead donor. The term "cadaveric renal allograft" is used in the latter circumstance, even though the donor is alive at the time the kidney is removed.

The renal allograft almost always is placed in the right or left iliac fossa of the recipient. Usually the allograft is extraperitoneal (between the peritoneum and the iliacus muscle). In a child, the allograft may be placed intraperitoneally if it is too large for extraperitoneal transplantation. The allograft ureter is passed through an oblique tunnel in the muscular layer of the bladder, forming a nonrefluxing ureterovesical junction. The allograft artery is attached in one of three ways: (1) the end of the allograft artery to the side of the external iliac artery (end-to-side); (2) the end of the allograft artery to the end of an internal iliac branch (end-to-end); or (3) for multiple renal arteries or for a small renal artery from a child, a patch of the donor aorta containing the arterial orifice(s) (Carrell patch) is attached to an opening made in the external iliac artery. In almost all cases, the cut end of the allograft vein is attached to the side of the external iliac vein (end-to-side).

The native kidneys of the allograft recipient usually are left in place, but they may be removed for a variety of reasons, including chronic or recurrent infection. Native kidneys are subject to the development of cysts and neoplasms in dialysis patients, as discussed later, but these le-

sions do not result from renal transplantation per se.

Renal allografts are subject to a variety of complications, including acute tubular necrosis (ATN) (in the postoperative period), acute rejection, chronic rejection, infection, ureteral obstruction, ureteral reflux, vascular obstruction, and extrarenal fluid collections.[1–54]

TECHNICAL CONSIDERATIONS

Renal allografts usually are quite superficial in location, which necessitates the use of linear array or curved array transducers. These transducers provide a broad field of view and good nearfield image quality.

From an ultrasound perspective, a transplanted kidney looks like a native kidney, with several minor exceptions.[1, 2] First, anatomic detail often is clearer than in native kidneys due to the superficial location of the allograft. Second, the cortex may appear more echogenic than that of a normotopic kidney, due to lack of ultrasound attenuation by overlying structures (Fig. 19–1).

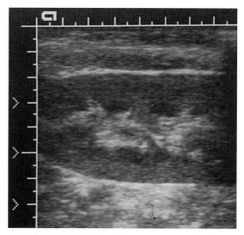

Figure 19-1—Normal Renal Allograft. A long axis view of a renal allograft 1 month postsurgery demonstrates prominent cortical echogenicity and pyramids, which in this case were normal findings.

It may be unclear whether enhanced cortical echogenicity is normal or is related to rejection. Third, the allograft usually enlarges over a period of several months following transplantation, and such enlargement should not be mistakenly attributed to rejection. In adults, the volume of the allograft typically increases up to 30%,[2, 9] but this increase may be as much as 200% if a kidney from a young (and relatively small) donor is transplanted into a much larger recipient (e.g., an adult).[13] Finally, slight dilatation of the allograft collecting system (hydronephrosis) is a common finding, particularly in the postoperative period. In most instances, such dilatation is not of urodynamic importance.

The sonographic diagnosis of allograft pathology is aided by a baseline scan conducted within the first 2 days following surgery. This scan represents an important standard with which later changes may be compared. Typically, a second scan is obtained at 1 to 2 weeks post-transplant, and a third scan is obtained at about 3 months.

ALLOGRAFT REJECTION

Renal allograft rejection may produce a host of sonographic abnormalities, as listed in Table 19–1.[1, 3–19] The most common and important manifestations of allograft rejection (Fig. 19–2) are (1) increased size of the graft (best appreciated through volume measurements); (2) increased cortical echogenicity; and (3) increased size and/or conspicuousness of the renal pyramids.[7, 12, 16, 19] Additional important features of acute rejection are peripheral hypoechoic zones (see Figure 18–5) and diminished sinus echogenicity (Fig. 19–2), but these are seen only in cases of severe rejection.[3, 5, 7, 10, 12, 19] The etiology of these changes is discussed in Chapter 18.

Doppler waveform abnormalities that indicate high peripheral arterial resistance (Fig. 19–3) also occur in renal transplant rejection. These flow abnormalities are evident in the segmental or lobar arteries of the allograft, both in acute and chronic rejection.[20–40] As summarized in Table 19–2, the waveform changes associated with

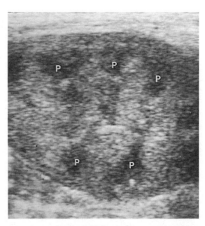

Figure 19-2—Renal Transplant Rejection. Prominent, enlarged medullary pyramids (P) stand out against echogenic renal cortex. The renal sinus is undefined because of decreased echogenicity of the sinus fat. Allograft volume had increased 40% from the preceding study.

rejection include (1) absence of flow throughout diastole; (2) flow reversal in diastole; (3) a resistivity index* that equals or exceeds 0.7; and (4) a pulsatility index† that equals or exceeds 1.8.[20–22, 24–27, 30–37] Specificity for rejection is increased by using a resistivity index of 0.9 or greater as a sign of rejection.

ACUTE TUBULAR NECROSIS

In contrast to allograft rejection, postsurgical ATN, resulting from ischemia, does not generally alter the B-mode appearance of the renal allografts or the Doppler flow characteristics. Uncommonly, however, cortical echogenicity or arterial pulsatility is increased in post-transplant ATN. Please see Chapter 18 for further information about ATN.

Accuracy for Rejection and Acute Tubular Necrosis

Initially it was hoped that ultrasound could be used to diagnose renal allograft rejection noninvasively and differentiate between rejection and ATN in the postoperative period.[4–6, 8, 9, 21, 24, 25] These hopes have faded with time, for experience has shown that ultrasound is neither sensitive nor specific for allograft rejection.[3, 12, 15–20, 22, 25–35, 39] To optimize specificity (to avoid false-positive diagnosis), *rejection should not be diagnosed sonographically unless several rejection-*

Table 19-1. Sonographic Manifestations of Renal Allograft Rejection

Increased allograft size (volume)
Increased cortical echogenicity (cellular infiltration)
Increased prominence of the renal pyramids*
Focal cortical hypoechoic regions (edema, necrosis)
Decreased echogenicity of the renal sinus (edema)
Increased flow resistance in parenchymal arteries

*Increased pyramid size and increased contrast between the hypoechoic pyramids and the echogenic cortex.

*The resistivity index is the peak systolic frequency minus the end diastolic frequency, divided by the peak systolic frequency.
†The pulsatility index is the peak systolic frequency minus the lowest diastolic frequency (including reversed flow), divided by the mean frequency.

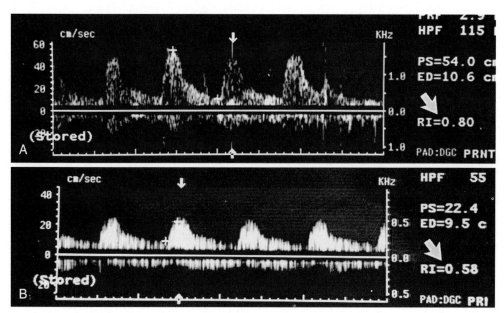

Figure 19-3—Rejection-Related Increase in Pulsatility. (**A**) Abnormal pulsatility. The resistivity index is 0.80 (arrow at right). (**B**) Normal pulsatility for comparison, with resistivity index of 0.58 (arrow at right).

related abnormalities are present.[9, 11, 12, 16, 19] Unfortunately, this requirement reduces the sensitivity for rejection to 70% or less. To make matters worse, sonographic changes seen with cyclosporine toxicity mimic those seen with rejection.[15, 25, 29, 40] (Cyclosporine is a commonly used immunosuppressant drug.)

In my opinion, ultrasound findings are most useful in cases of severe acute rejection. In such instances, the kidney is grossly enlarged, the pyramids are prominent, the renal sinus fat is hypoechoic, arterial flow resistance is elevated, and hypoechoic areas may be present in the renal cortex. I feel that ultrasound findings are not very helpful when acute rejection is mild or moderate in severity. Furthermore, I believe that the primary role of renal transplant ultrasound is not the detection of rejection but the detection of other complications—particularly hydronephrosis and fluid collections.

ALLOGRAFT HYDRONEPHROSIS

As noted previously, mild allograft hydronephrosis may occur normally during the first week

Table 19-2. Doppler Features of Allograft Rejection

High-resistance waveform appearance
Sharp, narrow systolic peaks
Second systolic peak higher than first
Minimal or absent diastolic flow
Flow reversal early in diastole
Pulsatility index ≥ 1.8
Resistivity index ≥ 0.7

or two following renal transplantation and probably results from postoperative edema at the insertion site of the ureter into the bladder. In some cases, mild hydronephrosis persists indefinitely, for no apparent reason. This finding is insignificant as long as urine output is good, renal function is satisfactory, and the degree of dilatation remains constant or regresses. The urodynamic significance of hydronephrosis may be evaluated with the Whitaker test,[41] scintigraphy, or pyelography in patients with abnormal renal function.

Moderate or severe hydronephrosis is a more disturbing finding in a renal allograft patient, particularly if the degree of hydronephrosis increases over time. Functionally significant hydronephrosis occurring in the immediate postoperative period usually results from surgical complications. Hydronephrosis appearing later generally is due to one of the following problems: (1) scarring at the ureterovesical junction; (2) obstructing debris (blood clots or fungal mycelia) within the ureter; (3) ureteral compression by extrinsic fluid collections; (4) bladder-emptying disorders; or (5) vesicoureteral reflux. Sonographic findings cannot differentiate among many of these causes. (See Chapter 18 for additional details.)

PERIGRAFT FLUID

Fluid collections are quite common following renal transplantation.[42–45] In the immediate postoperative period, a small volume of serous fluid

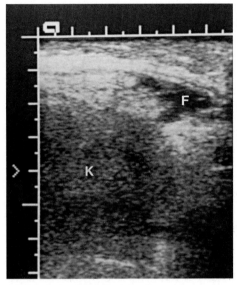

Figure 19-4—Seroma. A baseline postoperative scan shows a small fluid collection (F) in a location corresponding to the surgical incision. K = kidney.

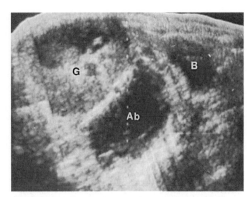

Figure 19-5—Abscess. A large, debris-containing abscess (Ab) is seen posteromedial to the allograft (G) on a transverse scan, at 3 weeks postsurgery. Diagnosis was confirmed surgically. B = bladder.

fluid collections are outlined in Table 19–3 and illustrated in Figures 19–4 through 19–7. Please review this material before proceeding as it is not repeated in the text.

VASCULAR COMPLICATIONS

The final and important role of ultrasound with respect to renal transplantation concerns the diagnosis of vascular problems.[43, 46–54] I believe that color Doppler examination should be a routine component of renal allograft sonography, because such examination is relatively easy and yields valuable information. It is possible, in most cases, to trace the allograft vessels in their entirety, from the iliac anastomoses to the kidney, and this should be the goal of the vascular examination, in addition to the assessment of parenchymal arterial pulsatility, as discussed earlier.

Vascular complications of renal allografts fall into four broad categories: arterial stenosis, vascular occlusion, pseudoaneurysm, and arteriovenous fistula.

(seroma) commonly accumulates adjacent to the transplanted kidney or in the operative wound, and this fluid should not be viewed with alarm as long as it does not increase in volume. Moderate-to-large collections generally are pathologic, regardless of when they appear, and these usually require further investigation with percutaneous aspiration or other means. The differential possibilities for perigraft fluid collections include serous fluid (seroma), blood (hematoma), pus (abscess), urine (urinoma), and lymph (lymphocele). Ultrasound does not accurately differentiate among these collections in all cases, but an educated guess can be made by considering four factors: the time of appearance (following surgery), symptomatology, location, and sonographic appearance. These aspects of allograft-related

Table 19-3. Diagnostic Features of Perigraft Fluid Collections

Collection	Clinical Features	Sonographic Features
Seroma/hematoma	Asymptomatic. Immediate postoperative period	Anechoic or mixed echogenicity. Adjacent to kidney or in wound. Irregular shape. Regresses in days or weeks
Abscess	Fever, leukocytosis, pain. May be relatively asymptomatic due to immunosuppression. Often postoperative, may be later (weeks to months)	May be perinephric, in the renal parenchyma, or in the wound. Usually well defined. Contents anechoic to echogenic
Urinoma	Pain, decreased renal output, fever. Virtually always in immediate postoperative period	Anechoic, often large, sometimes loculated. Location variable. Resembles lymphocele, but too early. Scintigraphy is diagnostic.
Lymphocele	Asymptomatic or pain. May obstruct ureter by extrinsic compression. Typically 1–2 months or later postsurgery, rarely earlier. Attributed to interrupted allograft lymphatics	Classically multilocular, with thin septa and anechoic fluid. May be unilocular. Classically located medially, between the allograft lower pole and the bladder

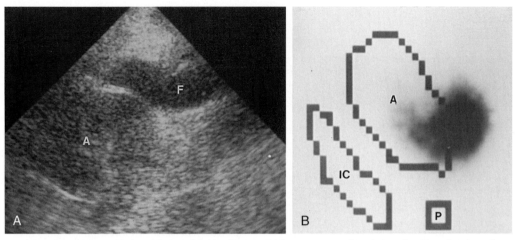

Figure 19-6—Urinoma. (**A**) An elongated fluid collection (F) lies anterior and medial to the allograft (A) on this transverse sonogram in an obese and difficult-to-scan patient with pelvic pain and decreased urine output, 1 month postsurgery. (**B**) The accumulation of radiotracer in an equivalent location is seen on this ⁹⁹ᵐTc scintigram, confirming the diagnosis of urinoma. A = allograft; IC = iliac crest; P = pubis.

Arterial Stenosis

The most common vascular complication of renal transplantation (about 10% of patients) is arterial stenosis.[47] Typically, stenosis occurs within 3 years of transplantation and is heralded by hypertension.* Short-segment stenosis at the allograft artery origin occurs early after transplantation and almost always is a surgical complication. Occasionally such stenoses result from

---

*In about 80% of cases, post-transplantation hypertension is caused by conditions other than renal artery stenosis.[47]

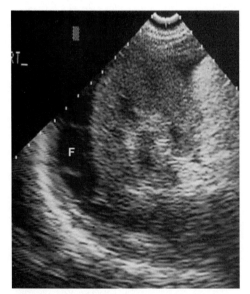

Figure 19-7—Lymphocele. A transverse sonogram demonstrates a loculated fluid collection (F) located between the allograft and the pelvic side wall.

allograft artery rejection. Long-segment, distal allograft artery stenosis is a later complication that results from intimal hyperplasia or scarring. Distal stenoses may be multiple and may be related to rejection. Recipient iliac artery stenosis is uncommon and almost invariably results from surgical injury.

The Doppler hallmarks of renal artery stenosis are increased flow velocity in the stenotic segment, coupled with poststenotic disturbed flow. Arterial waveforms may be damped distal to very severe stenoses. The quantification of allograft stenosis has not been worked out in any detail, but a few diagnostic parameters are available, as listed in Table 19–4.[46–51]

Vascular Occlusion

Occlusion (thrombosis) of the allograft renal artery is an unusual complication (less than 1%

Table 19-4. Diagnostic Criteria for Allograft Renal Arteries

Normal Flow Parameters
  Velocity: 80–118 cm/sec
  Volume flow: 346–422 ml/min

Parameters for Stenosis Exceeding 50% or 60% Decrease in Diameter

  Stenotic zone frequency > 7.5 kHz (+ poststenotic disturbed flow)
  Systolic velocity > 190 cm/sec (+ poststenotic disturbed flow)
  Systolic velocity ratio* > 3 (+ poststenotic disturbed flow)

---

*Ratio of stenotic zone peak systolic velocity–to–external iliac artery peak systolic velocity.
Data from references 48 and 49.

of renal transplants)[47] that typically occurs acutely in the postoperative period and is related to rejection or technical factors. Arterial occlusion is readily detected with duplex sonography, since arterial and venous flow are absent in the allograft.[47, 48]

Occlusion of the allograft vein also is a rare complication (less than 1% of cases) that occurs primarily in the immediate post-transplant period.[47] The affected allograft is enlarged because of congestion and typically has a nonhomogeneous appearance. Flow is absent in the renal vein, and the renal artery waveform exhibits a peculiar pattern characterized by sustained flow reversal in diastole.[47, 52]

Arteriovenous Fistula

Fistula formation between an artery and vein may occur within the renal allograft as a result of biopsy trauma.[47, 53, 54] Many such parenchymal fistulas are asymptomatic, but others are associated with sustained hypertension. Color Doppler sonography readily detects arteriovenous fistulas, since markedly disturbed flow within the fistula stands out like a beacon within the renal parenchyma. Additional findings are high-velocity flow in the artery that feeds the fistula, and a montage of color, called a "visible bruit," in the parenchyma adjacent to the fistula.

Pseudoaneurysm

Most pseudoaneurysms in renal allografts occur within the renal parenchyma and result from arterial laceration during renal biopsy.[47, 54] These false aneurysms are represented on gray scale images as well-defined, focal anechoic areas that are indistinguishable from renal cysts. Color Doppler sonography demonstrates blood flow in the pseudoaneurysm, confirming the diagnosis. In some cases, a characteristic high-velocity jet is visible in the aneurysm neck. Pseudoaneurysms also occur at the renal artery–iliac artery anastomosis, but these are uncommon.[47]

DIALYSIS COMPLICATIONS

Cysts and neoplasms have been identified with remarkable frequency in the end stage kidneys of chronic hemodialysis or peritoneal dialysis patients.[55-61] No satisfactory pathologic explanation is available for this phenomenon. Cysts (Fig. 19–8) generally do not become visible until the patient has completed 3 years of dialysis. Thereafter, they increase rapidly in number to a prevalence level approaching 100%.[58, 59, 61] Renal cysts may be complicated by intracyst hemorrhage (17% of dialysis patients) and the formation of perinephric hematomas.[56, 58, 61] The latter complications result when a hemorrhagic cyst ruptures into the perinephric space.

A more significant problem than cyst formation in long-term hemodialysis patients is the development of renal tumors (Fig. 19–9). Hyperplastic processes are thought to cause such lesions, but the pathogenesis of renal neoplasms in these patients is poorly understood. The majority of native kidney tumors in dialysis patients are adenomas,[58] but carcinomas also occur frequently. Overall, about 8% of long-term dialysis patients develop renal cell carcinoma.[61] This figure represents a prevalence about five to seven times greater than in the general population.[59, 61] As with cysts, renal carcinomas do not generally

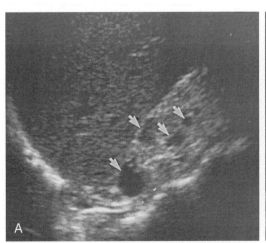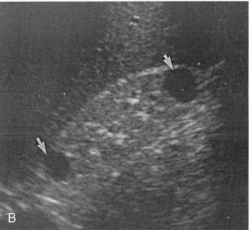

Figure 19-8—Hemodialysis-Related Cysts. (A, B) Two longitudinal views of the right kidney in a chronic hemodialysis patient show several cysts (arrows). This end-stage fibrotic kidney is diffusely echogenic.

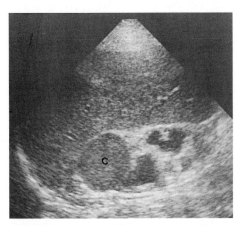

Figure 19-9—Hemodialysis-Related Renal Cell Carcinoma. A well-defined, homogeneous renal cell carcinoma (C) is seen in the right kidney in this chronic hemodialysis patient. Note hydronephrosis and increased renal echogenicity due to fibrosis.

appear until dialysis treatment has continued for 3 or more years.

Owing to the high incidence of renal carcinoma, routine native kidney surveillance, using ultrasound or computed tomography, has been proposed in patients receiving dialysis therapy for 3 or more years.[57, 59, 61] The need for such screening has not been uniformly accepted, and strong arguments have been raised against it. First, routine screening is costly. Second, routine screening is unlikely to increase the already limited life expectancy of many dialysis patients. Finally, most tumors that develop in dialysis patients are small, low-grade malignancies, and are nonmetastatic. Either ultrasound or computed tomography may be employed in those dialysis patients for whom a favorable long-term prognosis warrants native kidney tumor surveillance.

REFERENCES

1. Pozniak MA, Kelcz F, Dodd GD: Renal transplant ultrasound: Imaging and Doppler. Semin Ultrasound CT MR 12:319–334, 1991.
2. Lachance SL, Adamson D, Barry JM: Ultrasonically determined kidney transplant hypertrophy. J Urol 139:497–498, 1988.
3. Hillman BJ, Birnholz JC, Busch GJ: Correlation of echographic and histologic findings in suspected renal allograft rejection. Radiology 132:673–676, 1979.
4. Maklad NF, Wright CH, Rosenthal SJ: Gray scale ultrasonic appearances of renal transplant rejection. Radiology 131:711–717, 1979.
5. Hricak H, Toledo-Pereyra LH, Eyler WR, Madrazo BL, Zammit M: The role of ultrasound in the diagnosis of kidney allograft rejection. Radiology 132:667–672, 1979.
6. Hricak H, Toledo-Pereyra LH, Eyler WR, Madrazo BL, Sy GS: Evaluation of acute post-transplant renal failure by ultrasound. Radiology 133:443–447, 1979.
7. Singh A, Cohen WN: Renal allograft rejection: Sonography and scintigraphy. AJR Am J Roentgenol 135:73–77, 1980.
8. Frick MP, Feinberg SB, Sibley R, Idstrom ME: Ultrasound in acute renal transplant rejection. Radiology 138:657–660, 1981.
9. Hricak H, Cruz C, Eyler WR, Madrazo BL, Romanski R, Sandler MA: Acute post-transplantation renal failure: Differential diagnosis by ultrasound. Radiology 139:441–449, 1981.
10. Hricak H, Romanski RN, Eyler WR: The renal sinus during allograft rejection: Sonographic and histopathologic findings. Radiology 142:693–699, 1982.
11. Fried AM, Woodring JH, Loh FK, Lucas BA, Kryscio RJ: The medullary pyramid index: An objective assessment of prominence in renal transplant rejection. Radiology 149:787–791, 1983.
12. Slovis TL, Babcock DS, Hricak H, Han BK, Rose G, McEnery P, Muz J, Chang C-H, Fleischman LE, Corbett DP: Renal transplant rejection: Sonographic evaluation in children. Radiology 153:659–665, 1984.
13. Babcock DS, Slovis TL, Han BK, McEnery P, McWilliams DR: Renal transplants in children: Long-term follow-up using sonography. Radiology 156:165–167, 1985.
14. Rosenfield AT, Zeman RK, Cicchetti DV, Siegel NJ: Experimental acute tubular necrosis: US appearance. Radiology 157:771–774, 1985.
15. Linkowski GD, Warvariv V, Filly RA, Vincenti F: Sonography in the diagnosis of acute renal allograft rejection and cyclosporine nephrotoxicity. AJR Am J Roentgenol 148:291–295, 1987.
16. Swobodnik WL, Spohn BE, Wechsler JG, Schusdziarra V, Blum S, Franz HE, Ditschuneit H: Real-time ultrasound evaluation of renal transplant failure during the early postoperative period. Ultrasound Med Biol 12:97–105, 1986.
17. Hoddick W, Filly RA, Backman U, Callen PW, Vincenti F, Hricak H, Mahony BS, Amend W: Renal allograft rejection: US evaluation. Radiology 161:469–473, 1986.
18. Hricak H, Terrier F, Marotti M, Engelstad BL, Filly RA, Vincenti F, Duca RM, Bretan PN, Higgins CH, Feduska N: Post-transplant renal rejection: Comparison of quantitative scintigraphy, US, and MR imaging. Radiology 162:685–688, 1987.
19. Cochlin DL, Wake A, Salaman JR, Griffin PJA: Ultrasound changes in the transplant kidney. Clin Radiol 39:373–376, 1988.
20. Rifkin MD, Needleman L, Pasto ME, Kurtz AB, Foy PM, McGlynn E, Canino C, Baltarowich OH, Pennell RG, Goldberg BB: Evaluation of renal transplant rejection by duplex Doppler examination: Value of the resistive index. AJR Am J Roentgenol 148:759–762, 1987.
21. Taylor KJW, Morse SS, Rigsby CM, Bia M, Schiff M: Vascular complications in renal allografts: Detection with duplex Doppler US. Radiology 162:31–38, 1987.
22. Rigsby CM, Burns PN, Weltin GG, Chen B, Bia M, Taylor KJW: Doppler signal quantification in renal allografts: Comparison in normal and rejecting transplants with pathologic correlation. Radiology 162:39–42, 1987.
23. Sternberg HV, Nelson RC, Murphy FB, Chezmar JL, Baumgartner BR, Delaney VB, Whelchel JD, Bernardino ME: Renal allograft rejection: Evaluation by Doppler US and MR imaging. Radiology 162:337–342, 1987.
24. Taylor KJW, Marks WH: Use of Doppler imaging

for evaluation of dysfunction in renal allografts. AJR Am J Roentgenol 155:536–537, 1990.

25. Grant EG, Perrella RR: Wishing won't make it so: Duplex sonography in the evaluation of renal transplant dysfunction. AJR Am J Roentgenol 155:538–539, 1990.

26. Rigsby CM, Burns PN, Weltin GG, Chen B, Bia M, Taylor KJW: Doppler signal quantitation in renal allografts: Comparison in normal and rejecting transplants, with pathologic correlation. Radiology 162:39–42, 1987.

27. Genkins SM, Sanfilippo FP, Carroll BA: Duplex Doppler sonography of renal transplants: Lack of sensitivity and specificity in establishing pathologic diagnosis. AJR Am J Roentgenol 152:535–539, 1989.

28. Waltzer WC, Shabtai M, Anaise D, Rapaport FT: Usefulness and limitations of Doppler ultrasonography in the evaluation of postoperative renal allograft dysfunction. Transplant Proc 21:1901–1902, 1989.

29. Ward RE, Bartlett ST, O'Green Koenig J, Ballenger J, Neylan J, Friend M: The use of duplex scanning in evaluation of the posttransplant kidney. Transplant Proc 21:1912–1916, 1989.

30. Allen KS, Jorkasky DK, Arger PH, Velchik MG, Grumbach K, Coleman BG, Mintz MC, Betsch SE, Perloff LJ: Renal allografts: Prospective analysis of Doppler sonography. Radiology 169:371–376, 1988.

31. Harris DCH, Allen AR, Gruenewald S, Lawrence S, Stewart JH, Chapman JR: Doppler assessment in renal transplantation. Transplant Proc 21:1895–1896, 1989.

32. Townsend RR, Tomlanovich SJ, Goldstein RB, Filly RA: Combined Doppler and morphologic sonographic evaluation of renal transplant rejection. J Ultrasound Med 9:199–206, 1990.

33. Drake DG, Day DL, Letourneau JG, Alford BA, Sibley RK, Mauer SM, Bunchman TE: Doppler evaluation of renal transplants in children: A prospective analysis with histopathologic correlation. AJR Am J Roentgenol 154:785–787, 1990.

34. Perchik JE, Baumgartner BR, Bernardino ME: Renal transplant rejection: Limited value of duplex Doppler sonography. Invest Radiol 26:422–426, 1991.

35. Kelcz F, Pozniak MA, Pirsch JD, Oberly TD: Pyramidal appearance and resistive index: Insensitive and nonspecific sonographic indicators of renal transplant rejection. AJR Am J Roentgenol 155:531–535, 1990.

36. Schwaighofer B, Kainberger F, Fruehwald F, Huebsch P, Gritzmann N, Karnel F, Tscholakoff D: Duplex sonography of normal renal allografts. Acta Radiol 30:53–56, 1989.

37. Don S, Kopechy KK, Filo RS, Leapman SB, Thomalla JV, Jones JA, Klatte EC: Duplex Doppler US of renal allografts: Causes of elevated resistive index. Radiology 171:709–712, 1989.

38. Warshauer DM, Taylor KJW, Bia MJ, Marks WH, Weltin GG, Rigsby CM, True LD, Lorber MI: Unusual causes of increased vascular impedance in renal transplants: Duplex Doppler evaluation. Radiology 169:367–370, 1988.

39. Pozniak MA, Kelcz F, Stratta RJ, Oberley TD: Extraneous factors affecting resistive index. Invest Radiol 23:899–904, 1988.

40. Pozniak MA, Kelcz F, D'Alessandro A, Oberley T, Stratta R: Sonography of renal transplants in dogs: The effect of acute tubular necrosis, cyclosporine nephrotoxicity, and acute rejection on resistive index

and renal length. AJR Am J Roentgenol 158:791–797, 1992.

41. Jaffe RB, Middleton AW Jr: Whitaker test: Differentiation of obstructive from nonobstructive uropathy. AJR Am J Roentgenol 134:9–15, 1980.

42. Siler TM, Campbell D, Wicks JD, Lorber MI, Surace P, Turcotte J: Peritransplant fluid collections. Radiology 138:145–151, 1981.

43. Coyne SS, Walsh JW, Tisnado WH, Sharpe AR, Amendola MA, Mendez-Picon G, Lee HM: Surgically correctable renal transplant complications: An integrated clinical and radiologic approach. AJR Am J Roentgenol 136:1113–1119, 1981.

44. Hildell J, Aspelin P, Nyman U, Husberg B, Molde A: Ultrasonography in complications of renal transplantation. Acta Radiol Diagn 25:299–304, 1984.

45. Surratt JT, Siegel MJ, Middleton WD: Sonography of complications in pediatric renal allografts. RadioGraphics 10:687–699, 1990.

46. McGee GS, Peterson-Kennedy L, Astleford P, Yao JST: Duplex assessment of the renal transplant. Surg Clin North Am 70:133–141, 1990.

47. Dodd GD, Tublin ME, Shah A, Zajko AB: Imaging of vascular complications associated with renal transplants. AJR Am J Roentgenol 157:449–459, 1991.

48. Grenier N, Douws C, Morel D, Ferriére J-M, Le Guillou M, Potaux L, Broussin J: Detection of vascular complications in renal allografts with color Doppler flow imaging. Radiology 178:217–223, 1991.

49. Guzzo JA, Kupinski AM, Stone MP, Lempert N, Shah DM: Evaluation of renal allograft blood flow rates by duplex ultrasonography. J Vasc Technol 14:232–234, 1990.

50. Snider JF, Hunter DW, Moradian GP, Castaneda-Zuniga WR, Letourneau JG: Transplant renal artery stenosis: Evaluation with duplex sonography. Radiology 172:1027–1030, 1989.

51. Stringer DA, O'Halpin D, Daneman A, Liu P, Geary DF: Duplex Doppler sonography for renal artery stenosis in the post-transplant pediatric patient. Pediatr Radiol 19:187–192, 1989.

52. Reuther G, Wanjura D, Bauer H: Acute renal vein thrombosis in renal allografts: Detection with duplex Doppler US. Radiology 170:557–558, 1989.

53. Middleton WD, Kellman GM, Melson GL, Madrazo BL: Postbiopsy renal transplant arteriovenous fistulas: Color Doppler US characteristics. Radiology 171:253–257, 1989.

54. Hübsch PJS, Mostbeck G, Barton PP, Gritzmann N, Fruehwald FXJ, Schurawitzki H, Kovarik J: Evaluation of arteriovenous fistulas and pseudoaneurysms in renal allografts following percutaneous needle biopsy: Color-coded Doppler sonography versus duplex Doppler sonography. J Ultrasound Med 9:95–100, 1990.

55. Scanlon MH, Karasick SR: Acquired renal cystic disease and neoplasia: Complications of chronic hemodialysis. Radiology 147:837–838, 1983.

56. Weissberg DL, Miller RB: Renal cell carcinoma and acquired cystic disease of the kidneys in a chronically dialyzed patient. J Ultrasound Med 2:191–194, 1983.

57. Kutcher R, Amodio JB, Rosenblatt R: Uremic renal cystic disease: Value of sonographic screening. Radiology 147:833–835, 1983.

58. Levine E, Grantham JJ, Slusher SL, Greathouse JL, Krohn BP: CT of acquired cystic kidney disease and

renal tumors in long-term dialysis patients. AJR Am J Roentgenol 142:125–131, 1984.

59. Jabour BA, Ralls PW, Tang WW, Boswell WD, Colletti PM, Feinstein EI, Massry SG: Acquired cystic disease of the kidneys: Computed tomography and ultrasonography appraisal in patients on peritoneal and hemodialysis. Invest Radiol 22:728–732, 1987.

60. Taylor AJ, Cihen EP, Erickson SJ, Olson DL, Foley WD: Renal imaging in long-term dialysis patients: A comparison of CT and sonography. AJR Am J Roentgenol 153:765–767, 1989.

61. Levine E, Slusher SL, Grantham JJ, Wetzel LH: Natural history of acquired renal cystic disease in dialysis patients: A prospective longitudinal CT study. AJR Am J Roentgenol 156:501–506, 1991.

Chapter 20

Solid Renal Masses

William J. Zwiebel

CLASSIFICATION

A comprehensive list of solid-appearing renal masses[1-5] is presented in Table 20–1. It should be noted that a few of these lesions are not, in fact, solid masses, but only *appear* solid by sonographic criteria. Conversely, certain solid renal masses may undergo degeneration, cyst formation, or hemorrhage, making them *appear* cystlike (Chapter 21).

The most important tumor of the kidney, by far, is renal cell carcinoma,[1-51] which constitutes approximately 80% to 83% of clinically identified renal neoplasms.[1] Uroepithelial tumors account for 7% to 10% of renal neoplasms, Wilms tumor for 5% to 6%, and miscellaneous other tumors constitute 3% to 4%. Although Wilms tumor is relatively uncommon overall, it is the most important renal neoplasm in children.

Renal cell carcinoma and Wilms tumor are emphasized in this text because of their importance in adult and childhood patient populations. Other solid renal neoplasms are treated less extensively.

INTRARENAL OR EXTRARENAL

Sonography is an excellent medium for confirming or excluding the renal origin of a mass (Fig. 20–1). The ultrasound features used to differentiate between intra- and extrarenal masses are analogous to those used to differentiate between intra- and extrahepatic masses (Chapter 8). Among these, the demonstration of a fat plane between the mass and the lesion is perhaps the most useful sign of extrarenal origin. Conversely, intrarenal origin is most clearly indicated by continuity of the mass with the renal parenchyma (absence of a fat plane or other boundary). Intrarenal origin also is indicated by the sonographic equivalent of the radiographic "beak sign," as illustrated in Figure 20–1B.

RENAL CELL CARCINOMA

Renal cell carcinoma,[1] or hypernephroma, is thought to originate from renal tubular epithelial cells. The peak incidence of this tumor is the 6th decade, but the tumor can occur at virtually any age, including childhood. Hematuria, back or flank pain, and a palpable mass are the most frequent presenting signs and symptoms. Weight loss, malaise, and hypertension also may herald the presence of this tumor. Most renal cell carcinomas are diagnosed at a late stage, as indicated by an average tumor size of 9 cm at the time of discovery![1] In the last 10 to 15 years, however, the incidental diagnosis of renal cell carcinoma has increased substantially (as much as fivefold), due to the widespread use of ultrasound and computed tomography.[5, 10, 20] Early diagnosis is important, because renal cell carcinoma seems to be a slow-growing (300-day doubling time), late-metastasizing neoplasm.[10, 13] Patients with small renal cell carcinomas (less than 3 cm) have a 5-year survival rate of 70%, which represents a decidedly better prognosis than in larger lesions. The improved chance of survival with small tumors is attributed to a lower incidence of metastasis and local recurrence. A nearly linear relationship exists, furthermore, between tumor size and renal vein invasion, which negatively affects survival.[1, 5, 9, 12, 13, 16, 17, 19, 20, 22] It is unfortunate that the diagnosis rate for small, asymptomatic renal cell carcinomas remains low in comparison with the rate for symptomatic tumors.[1, 19] As a result, the overall survival statistics for this tumor remain poor (30% to 50% at 5 years; 17% to 28% at 10 years).[1, 5, 10-22]

Table 20–1. Differential Considerations for Solid-Appearing Renal Masses

Neoplasms
  Renal cell carcinoma
  Uroepithelial tumors
  Metastasis
  Lymphoma
  Leukemia
  Wilms tumor
  Nephroblastoma
  Angiomyolipoma
  Oncocytoma
  Other rare neoplasms (e.g., fibroma)
Focal severe bacterial nephritis°
Abscess°
Echogenic Cyst†

°See Chapter 22.
†See Chapter 21.

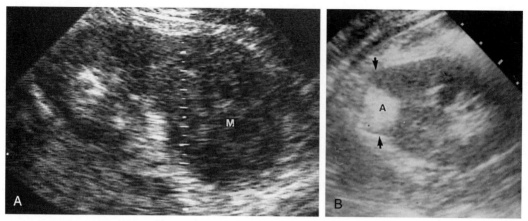

Figure 20-1—Localization of Mass Lesions. (**A**) This left flank mass (renal cell carcinoma) clearly arises from the kidney. The mass (M) is continuous with the renal parenchyma, without a plane of demarcation intervening between the mass and the kidney. (**B**) The renal origin of this incidentally discovered angiomyolipoma (A) is indicated by two findings. First, the locus of the mass is within the boundaries of the kidney. Second, beaklike projections of renal parenchyma (arrows) are seen at the margins of the mass.

Sonographic Findings

The sonographic appearance of renal cell carcinoma is variable, as illustrated in Figures 20–2 and 20–3. Most renal cell carcinomas are hypoechoic or isoechoic relative to normal renal parenchyma. Ten percent, however, are more echogenic than normal parenchyma.[4, 23–40] The existence of these hyperechoic lesions is noteworthy, since they may be mistaken for benign, hyperechoic cysts or fat-containing tumors. Renal cell carcinoma is not an encapsulated tumor; therefore, the borders of the mass sometimes are poorly defined. The borders of small tumors tend to be sharp, however, and these well-defined tumors may be mistaken for benign lesions such as cysts. The internal architecture of renal cell carcinoma may be homogeneous or heteroge-

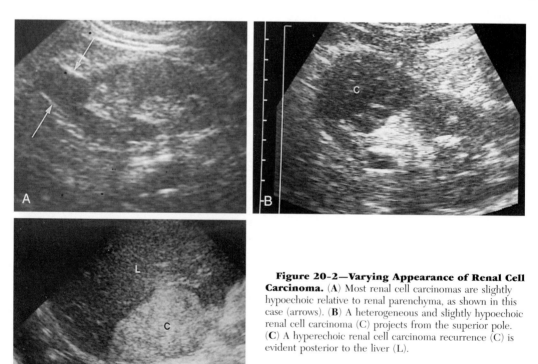

Figure 20-2—Varying Appearance of Renal Cell Carcinoma. (**A**) Most renal cell carcinomas are slightly hypoechoic relative to renal parenchyma, as shown in this case (arrows). (**B**) A heterogeneous and slightly hypoechoic renal cell carcinoma (C) projects from the superior pole. (**C**) A hyperechoic renal cell carcinoma recurrence (C) is evident posterior to the liver (L).

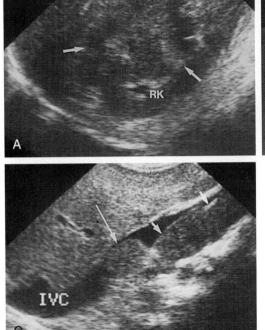

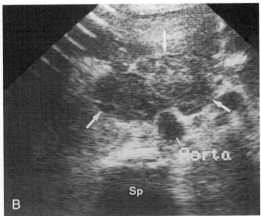

Figure 20-3—Renal Carcinoma with Local Metastases. (**A**) A large, ill-defined mass (arrows) arises from the right kidney (RK). This mass has invaded locally into the liver (L) and adjacent structures. Note the heterogeneity of this lesion, which relates to necrosis and the presence of small calcifications (documented with computed tomography). (**B**) A transverse image demonstrates periaortic adenopathy (arrows) medial to the tumor. Sp = spine. (**C**) Tumor is seen to extend into the inferior vena cava (IVC) (long arrow). The IVC also is compressed by extrinsic tumor metastases (short arrows).

neous, with a tendency for small tumors to be homogeneous and for larger ones to be heterogeneous. Heterogeneity results from necrosis, hemorrhage, or calcification, all of which are common histologic features of larger renal cell carcinomas. Necrotic areas may be anechoic, sonolucent, or even hyperechoic compared with the rest of the tumor or normal renal parenchyma. Massive necrosis and hemorrhage may cause "cystic" degeneration (discussed later), in which the bulk of the tumor is converted to hypoechoic or anechoic fluid.

In rare instances, renal cell carcinoma may infiltrate the renal parenchyma along the existing structural framework of the kidney.[38] This mode of growth causes enlargement of either a portion or all of the kidney, without a focal mass. The sonographic features of infiltrating carcinoma are indistinguishable from those of transitional cell carcinoma, lymphoma, and other infiltrating neoplasms.

Calcification is common in renal cell carcinoma[39, 40] and may be peripheral or central in location. Calcification sometimes produces discrete strong reflections and acoustic shadowing; alternatively, it may simply contribute to sonographic inhomogeneity. Generally speaking, tumor calcification is more easily identified radiographically than sonographically.

Doppler assessment of renal neoplasms is in an investigational state. High-velocity Doppler signals (exceeding 4 kHz) have been detected within or at the periphery of 81% (22 of 29) of renal cell carcinomas.[41, 42] In contrast, such signals appear to be uncommon in a variety of other benign and malignant renal masses. Thus, Doppler may be of some value in differentiating between renal cell carcinoma and other mass lesions, but this hypothesis is not firmly proved.

Metastasis

Ultrasound may identify local metastasis of renal cell carcinoma, as well as metastasis to regional lymph nodes and the liver (Fig. 20–3). The usual locations for nodal metastasis are along the renal vessels, at the junction of the renal vessels with the aorta and inferior vena cava (IVC), and along the para-aortocaval area cephalad to the renal vessels. Hepatic metastasis may be hematogenous or by direct extension.

Renal cell carcinoma has a great propensity for metastasis (or extension) into the renal vein and the IVC (up to 20% and 10% of cases, respectively).[1] Though it may seem improbable, venous extension does not preclude surgical cure, as it often is possible to "shell out" the tumor from the venous system.

As seen with ultrasound, intravenous tumor[47–49] (Fig. 20–3C) typically is homogeneous, and of low or intermediate echogenicity. The tumor-containing renal vein almost always is distended to a distinctly abnormal size, and even the IVC may be distended when tumor is present. Doppler signals are absent within the tumor itself, but flow may be present around the tumor.

Ultrasound has received mixed reviews as a modality for detecting venous extension.[42, 45, 47–49] If the renal vein and IVC are well visualized, sonographic accuracy is good (96% sensitivity, 100% specificity), but renal vein visualization is inadequate in 34% to 54% of patients, and the IVC is inadequately seen in 4% to 21% of cases.[45, 49] Thus, the overall sensitivity for venous tumor extension may be as low as 18% for the renal veins and 33% for the IVC.[45]

Cystic Renal Cell Carcinoma

The term "cystic" renal cell carcinoma should be reserved for tumors that principally consist of a circumscribed collection of fluid. The mechanism by which a cystic renal cell carcinoma forms is unclear. Four potential mechanisms have been cited: (1) the tumor may develop within the wall of a cyst, (2) a solid tumor may excavate as a result of liquefactive necrosis, (3) the tumor may develop adjacent to a cyst, and (4) the tumor may somehow induce cyst development.[29–34]

The sonographic findings in cystic renal cell carcinoma include the following: (1) a focal nodule or thickening in an otherwise typical renal cyst; (2) diffuse, irregular wall thickening in a distinctly "atypical" cyst; (3) a multilocular cyst (Fig. 20–4); and (4) a cyst with diffuse or dependent echogenicity, with or without other atypical cyst findings.[4, 29–37] A focal tumor nodule or focal wall thickening is particularly problematic, since these subtle features may easily be overlooked with ultrasound if the cyst is otherwise unremarkable. Although this type of tumor development seems to be rare,[32] the need for close ultrasound scrutiny of cystic renal masses cannot be overemphasized. Any deviation from the classic cyst appearance described in the chapter that follows deserves further diagnostic evaluation, and possible biopsy.

Surveillance for Small Renal Cell Carcinomas

Individuals who are at higher-than-normal risk for renal cell carcinoma fall into two categories: (1) those with a hereditary predisposition—e.g., hereditary telangiectasia (Osler-Weber-Rendu disease) or retinocerebral angiomatosis (von Hippel–Lindau disease), and (2) patients with hematuria.[1, 5, 7–9, 15] Hereditary disorders are rare, but the prevalence of renal cell carcinoma in these conditions is as high as 35% (with a 75% rate of bilaterality).[1, 7, 8, 15] In contrast, asymptomatic (microscopic) hematuria[5, 9] is a common problem (1% to 13% of adults) but is associated with a low incidence of renal cell carcinoma (3%–6%). Hematuria may result from multiple conditions in addition to tumors, including inflammatory processes and calculi.

The following is a summary of the comparative accuracy of imaging techniques used to detect renal neoplasms in high-risk patients.

1. Intravenous urography (IVU)[2, 11, 12, 14–16, 20–22] is excellent for detecting uroepithelial tumors. IVU is fairly good for detecting renal masses

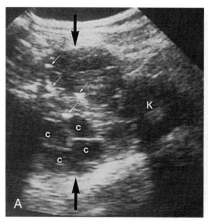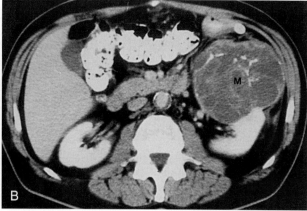

Figure 20-4—Cystic Renal Cell Carcinoma. (**A**) A large mass (dark arrows) is seen in intimate association with the left kidney (K). The mass contains solid elements and calcifications (white arrows), in addition to the cystic spaces (c). (**B**) A contrast-enhanced computed tomogram demonstrates more clearly the cystic character of the mass (M) as well as linear calcification.

larger than 3 cm (85% sensitivity), but it is poor for tumors 3 cm or smaller (range, 33% to 67%). Furthermore, the detection rate for small tumors drops off rapidly as tumor size decreases. In one study, IVU detected only 52% of 2- to 3-cm masses seen with computed tomography (CT), and only 13% of 1- to 2-cm masses.[21]

2. Sonography is superior to IVU for detection of small renal masses,[2, 5, 13–16, 20–22] but the performance of this modality is less than ideal. In one study,[16] sonography detected only 79% of tumors 3 cm or smaller. In another study, sonography identified 82% of 2- to 3-cm masses seen with CT, 60% of 1- to 2-cm masses, and only 20% of masses smaller than 1 cm.[21]

3. CT detects 94% of renal cell carcinomas 3 cm in diameter or smaller and 98% of renal neoplasms of any size.[5, 7, 8, 14, 16, 20–22]

4. The performance of magnetic resonance imaging (MRI) probably is as good as that of CT, but information on this subject is limited.[5, 8, 20]

From these data, it is clear that a negative urographic examination is insufficient for excluding small, occult renal neoplasms, and that patients at risk for such lesions generally should be evaluated with CT rather than with ultrasound. In small children, however, ultrasound may be the preferred method for tumor surveillance, since ultrasound tolerates patient motion better than CT, and ionizing radiation is avoided. Urography continues to be the most sensitive method for detection of uroepithelial tumors[9]; therefore, a combination of urography and CT appears to be the preferred approach to adults with persistent hematuria. MRI also is valuable for renal tumor surveillance, but its use probably should be restricted to patients who cannot receive intravenous contrast, since it is more costly than CT.[8]

UROEPITHELIAL CARCINOMA

More than 85% to 95% of uroepithelial cancers[1, 3, 38, 52–54] are transitional cell carcinomas, and approximately 10% are squamous cell tumors. The squamous lesions are almost always associated with calculi and chronic infection. Most uroepithelial malignancies develop in the renal pelvis or major calyces and produce mass lesions within the renal sinus. Occasionally, however, transitional cell carcinoma may infiltrate the renal parenchyma focally or diffusely, causing enlargement of the kidney (and loss of function) in the absence of a discrete mass. Gross or microscopic hematuria are the presenting findings in 75% of patients with transitional cell carcinoma, and flank pain is present in about 25% of patients, as a result of ureteral obstruction.

Sonographic Findings

In most cases of uroepithelial carcinoma, the sonographic findings[38, 52–54] consist of a discrete, solid-appearing mass centered within the renal sinus (Fig. 20–5). Cystic degeneration is uncommon, and the tumor usually is homogeneous, with echogenicity equal to or slightly greater than that of normal renal parenchyma. Differentiation from other renal neoplasms is not possible in most cases; nonetheless, the sonologist should think of a uroepithelial carcinoma when a mass is localized to the renal sinus and is associated

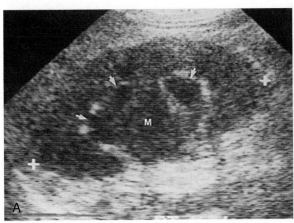 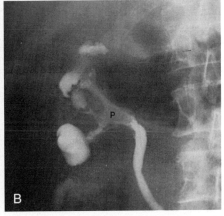

Figure 20-5—Uroepithelial Carcinoma. (A) An isoechoic mass (M) fills the renal sinus of the right kidney in this elderly man with hematuria. Dilated calyces (arrows) are evident. (B) A retrograde pyelogram shows extensive narrowing and irregularity of the renal pelvis (P) and the major calyces. The minor calyces are dilated.

with hydronephrosis. Uroepithelial tumors commonly obstruct the urinary tract because they originate in the wall of the collecting structures.

The following additional sonographic findings may be seen in cases of uroepithelial carcinoma: (1) hydronephrosis without a visible tumor; (2) a focal mass projecting into a dilated collecting structure (Fig. 20–6); (3) obliteration of the usual bright echogenicity of the renal sinus; (4) evidence of calculi (bright reflections and acoustic shadowing) in conjunction with a central renal mass (especially with squamous tumors); (5) renal vein invasion (less common than with renal cell carcinoma); and (6) focal or diffuse parenchymal thickening, renal enlargement, and perhaps loss of corticomedullary differentiation (caused by an infiltrating form of transitional cell carcinoma).

RENAL METASTASES

The widespread use of CT for tumor staging has increased our awareness of metastasis to the kidneys from distant sources.[1, 4, 38, 55, 56] Lung carcinoma is the most frequent source of renal metastases, but various additional tumors commonly metastasize to the kidneys, including renal cell carcinoma arising in the contralateral kidney.

The sonographic appearance of renal metastases is nonspecific. Most are hypo- or isoechoic relative to normal renal parenchyma, and the tumors may be homogeneous or heterogeneous in texture. The presence of multiple renal tumors is particularly suggestive of metastasis.

LYMPHOMA AND LEUKEMIA

Renal parenchymal involvement is common in pediatric patients with acute leukemia and in adults with lymphoma (particularly non-Hodgkin lymphoma).[38, 57–65] The detection of renal involvement in these tumors has important ramifications concerning therapeutic approaches and remission status.

Lymphoma and leukemia have a predilection for infiltration of the renal parenchyma and often cause focal or diffuse (Fig. 20–7) renal enlargement. Parenchymal infiltration also is manifested by diminution or loss of corticomedullary differentiation. The affected renal parenchyma tends to be iso- or hypoechoic relative to the normal renal cortex, but diffusely increased echogenicity has been reported in rare cases. Lymphoma also may infiltrate the renal sinus, and thereby reduce sinus echogenicity or generate a discrete sinus mass (Fig. 20–7).

Both lymphoma and leukemia also may generate discrete renal parenchymal masses. These masses are homogeneous and characteristically are strikingly hypoechoic. The latter finding is a useful diagnostic feature, but it enables these lesions to be mistaken for renal cysts. Scrutiny of the echogenicity within and distal to such masses is the key to avoidance of this pitfall (Chapter 21). Occasionally, lymphomatous or leukemic masses may be isoechoic with normal renal parenchyma.

WILMS TUMOR AND NEUROBLASTOMA

Sonography is the primary method for assessment of abdominal masses that present in infants (under 2 years of age) and young children.[66–70] The origin and nature of the mass may be ascertained quickly and painlessly with ultrasound,

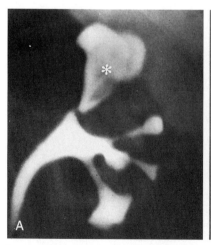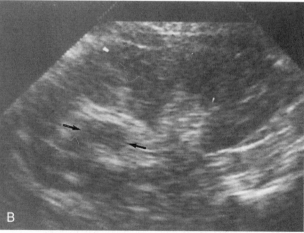

Figure 20-6—Calyceal Tumor Mass. (**A**) A radiolucent filling defect (asterisk) is seen in the upper pole calyx of the right kidney in a patient with hematuria. (**B**) A soft tissue mass (arrows) is seen on this coronal sonogram. Retrograde pyelography and brush biopsy were performed, confirming the diagnosis of uroepithelial carcinoma.

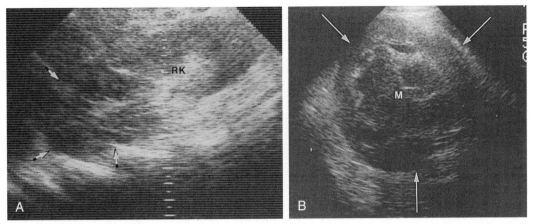

Figure 20-7—Renal Lymphoma. Two cases of renal involvement with lymphoma are shown. (**A**) This longitudinal sonogram demonstrates diffuse, decreased echogenicity and enlargement of the upper pole (arrows) of the right kidney (RK), due to infiltration by non-Hodgkin lymphoma. (**B**) A transverse sonogram in another patient with non-Hodgkin lymphoma demonstrates a lymphomatous mass (M) that fills the renal sinus of the right kidney (arrows).

and this vital information may then be used to plan for additional diagnostic studies. Wilms tumor and neuroblastoma[66–83] are the most common abdominal tumors of infancy and early childhood. Although neuroblastoma is not a renal neoplasm, it is included in this chapter because it often involves the kidneys and because imaging procedures are the primary means for differential diagnosis between Wilms tumor and neuroblastoma.

Age of Presentation

The age of presentation of Wilms tumor and neuroblastoma overlap, as indicated in Table 20–2.[72] It is noteworthy, however, that Wilms tumor only rarely presents at birth. A renal neoplasm detected at birth most likely is a mesoblastic nephroma or other variant of nephroblastomatosis, as discussed later.[72, 78, 79] A *perinephric* tumor presenting at birth is likely to be a neuroblastoma.[69]

Wilms Tumor

Wilms tumor, or nephroblastoma,[72–79] is a malignant tumor of renal origin that arises from

Table 20-2. Age of Presentation of Wilms Tumor and Neuroblastoma

Wilms tumor
Does not present at birth
⅓ present within 1st year of life
¾ present before age 4 years
Neuroblastoma
May present at birth (or in utero)
⅓ present within 1st year of life
80% present by age 5 years

rests of the embryonic metanephric blastoma. The renal origin generally is evident on imaging studies (Fig. 20–8), but it may be obscured by massive tumor extension into adjacent viscera, or by encapsulation of the tumor. In the latter instance, the capsule may give a false impression that the tumor is separate from the kidney. Wilms tumor tends to be smooth in shape, with regular, well-defined margins or a well-defined capsule. The tumor rarely is calcified, rarely crosses the midline, and rarely envelops major blood vessels, such as the aorta or IVC. A distinctive and frequently seen feature is growth of Wilms tumor *within* the lumen of the renal vein or IVC.[75] Necrotic degeneration and hemorrhage occur commonly within Wilms tumor, but the necrotic areas are relatively small and give the appearance of localized, well-defined anechoic areas within an otherwise solid mass.[76] Large, irregular necrotic spaces suggest neuroblastoma, as discussed later.

The objectives for sonographic examination in Wilms tumor are to document the origin and solid nature of the mass (e.g., as opposed to a benign cyst), to detect invasion of surrounding viscera, to detect venous extension, and to search for lesions in the opposite kidney. The latter objective is particularly important, since Wilms tumor occurs bilaterally in 5% to 10% of cases.[72]

Nephroblastomatosis

Normally, all blastic tissue disappears from the kidneys by 36 weeks' gestation. The persistence of blastic tissue after 36 weeks is termed "nephroblastomatosis."[78, 79] The residual blastic tissue may evolve into a variety of renal neoplasms, including Wilms tumor, that range from

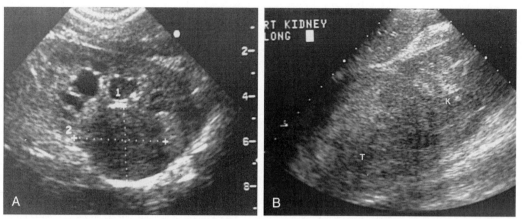

Figure 20-8—Wilms Tumor. (**A**) A longitudinal scan shows a 4-cm diameter, hypoechoic, well-encapsulated Wilms tumor (cursors 1 and 2) that clearly arises from the kidney. (**B**) This 6-cm diameter Wilms tumor (T) appears to arise from the superior pole of the kidney (K), but differentiation from a neuroblastoma of adrenal origin is difficult. Note the difference in the echogenicity between this tumor and that shown in **A.** (Both courtesy of Paula Shultz, MD, Primary Children's Hospital, Salt Lake City. Reproduced with permission.)

benign to malignant. Blastic rests per se are not visible with any imaging modality, but those that evolve into tumors may be visualized with ultrasound, CT, or MRI. On ultrasound studies, nephroblastic tumors present as hypoechoic, rounded, peripheral masses of various sizes that typically distort the renal contours. Bilaterality and multiplicity of the masses are common. These masses are visualized more clearly with CT than with ultrasound, and for this reason CT is recommended for confirming the diagnosis of nephroblastomatosis and for determining the number and size of lesions. Both ultrasound and CT may have a surveillance role in individuals who have a genetic predisposition for nephroblastomatosis. For a review of this subject, see the paper by White and colleagues.[79]

Neuroblastoma

Neuroblastoma[66, 67, 71, 77–85] is a highly malignant neoplasm of neural crest origin. Approximately two thirds of neuroblastomas arise in the adrenal medulla. The remainder may originate at any location along the neural crest, including the chest, abdomen, and pelvis. The imaging characteristics of neuroblastoma (Fig. 20–9) include irregular shape and margins, lack of encapsulation, large size, and a tendency to cross the midline and envelop major abdominal vessels. Since neuroblastoma is *not* a renal tumor, the kidneys tend to be displaced rather than invaded, and intraluminal vascular extension does not occur. (Note the differences between this growth pattern and that of Wilms tumor, as presented earlier.)

Although some neuroblastomas are uniformly

solid and homogeneous, sonographic heterogeneity is the rule, due to the formation of large necrotic/hemorrhagic areas.[69, 71, 83] In rare cases, necrosis may be so extensive that the neuroblastoma presents as a multilocular cystic mass, as shown in Figure 20–9. Tumor calcification is common in neuroblastoma, and it may be massive. Calcification is identified through typical sonographic features—bright reflections and acoustic shadows. Massive necrosis and massive calcification are important differential findings, since they are common in neuroblastoma but uncommon in Wilms tumor.

The adrenal origin of smaller neuroblastomas

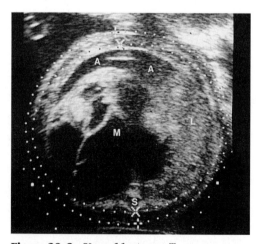

Figure 20-9—Neuroblastoma. Transverse sonogram at the inferior margin of the liver (L) in a fetus at 32 weeks' menstrual age. A huge mass (M) with cystic and solid elements crosses the midline. Ascites (A) is present. S = spine; cursors = inner and outer margins of the abdominal wall. The fetus died in utero from hydrops.

may be suggested by suprarenal tumor location, replacement of the adrenal gland, and inferior displacement of the ipsilateral kidney. Tumor origin is obscure, however, in most cases of neuroblastoma, due to large tumor size and extensive invasion.

TWO DISTINCTIVE RENAL TUMORS

Considerable attention has been devoted in the medical literature to two benign renal tumors, seen principally in adults, that have fairly distinctive sonographic features: angiomyolipomas and oncocytomas. Although these are uncommon renal lesions, sonologists should be aware of their diagnostic features, for open renal biopsy or nephrectomy may be avoided when these distinctive features can be demonstrated.

Angiomyolipoma. Renal neoplasms composed primarily or completely of fat[86–92] have a fairly characteristic appearance, since their echogenicity equals or exceeds that of the renal sinus and perinephric fat (Figs. 20–1B, 20–10). The most common fatty tumor with this sonographic presentation is an angiomyolipoma, which is composed of blood vessels, muscle, and fat, as its name infers. Angiomyolipoma should be a primary consideration for a highly echogenic renal mass, but it is noteworthy that other renal masses also may be highly echogenic, including liposarcoma, renal cell carcinoma, hemangioma, hemorrhagic cyst, milk of calcium cyst, and parenchymal scar.[23–29, 86–88, 91, 92] When a hyperechoic mass is detected, therefore, CT should be performed to document the fatty nature of the lesion. Even if the mass proves to be fatty, biopsy or close follow-up may be advisable. It should be noted that all angiomyolipomas are *not* highly echogenic, since echogenicity varies in relation to the quantity and type of fat present in the tumor.

Most angiomyolipomas are large at the time of discovery (mean diameter, 9.4 cm) but tumor size ranges widely from 1 or 2 cm to more than 20 cm.[86] Large tumors tend to be exophytic and often contain anechoic or hypoechoic areas caused by hemorrhage and necrosis. Angiomyolipomas are strongly associated with tuberous sclerosis, and multiple tumors may be present in tuberous sclerosis patients. Renal vein invasion has been reported rarely with angiomyolipomas.[90]

Oncocytoma. A great deal has been made of oncocytomas recently in the radiology literature, and I feel that this is much ado about a very rare tumor. Oncocytomas[93–95] are benign renal neoplasms composed primarily of cells called oncocytes, which are uniform and large and contain a great number of mitochondria. These tumors usually present in the 6th or 7th decade, as an incidentally found (asymptomatic), typically solitary renal lesion. These tumors are important from an imaging perspective because a characteristic central band of fibrosis (thought to be a "healed" region of necrosis) is seen with ultrasound or CT in about 25% of cases (and only in lesions greater than 3 cm in diameter). The branching (stellate) central "scar" is hyperechoic on ultrasound examination and hypodense (relative to the rest of the tumor) on CT images. The remainder of the tumor is homogeneous and medium in echogeneity.

Although the central scar is virtually diagnostic of oncocytoma *in lesions larger than 3 cm in diameter,*[94] there are two significant diagnostic limitations of the scar sign. First, a central scar may be seen in some renal cell carcinomas

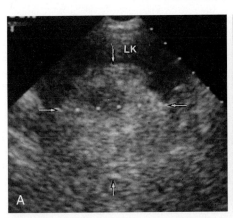
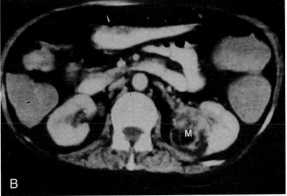

Figure 20-10—Angiomyolipoma, Incidentally Discovered in a 62 Year Old Woman. (**A**) A highly echogenic mass (arrows) is visualized at the medial border of the left kidney (LK) on this coronal image. Angiomyolipoma was suggested on the basis of the strong echogenicity of this tumor. (**B**) The diagnosis was confirmed with this contrast-enhanced CT scan that demonstrates a large, left renal mass (M) with extensive fat-density components.

smaller than 3 cm in diameter; hence the finding can be applied only to tumors larger than 3 cm. Second, small foci of renal cell carcinoma may be embedded in bona fide oncocytomas, necessitating the removal of the tumor in most cases.[94] There is a redeeming value of the scar sign, however, for a kidney-sparing operation may be employed if the diagnosis of oncocytoma is suggested preoperatively.

REFERENCES

1. Jones DB: Kidneys. *In* Kissane JM (ed): Anderson's Pathology. 8th ed. St Louis, CV Mosby, 1985, pp 765–768.
2. Pollack HM, Goldberg BB, Morales JO, Bogash M: A systematized approach to the differential diagnosis of renal masses. Diagn Radiol 113:653–659, 1974.
3. Abrams HL: Mass lesions: A diagnostic approach to renal vascular tumors and cysts. J Cont Educ Radiol 1:11–51, 1979.
4. Charboneau JW, Hattery RR, Ernst EC, James EM, Williamson B, Hartman GW: Spectrum of sonographic findings in 125 renal masses other than benign simple cysts. AJR Am J Roentgenol 140:87–94, 1983.
5. Bosniak MA: The small (≤3.0 cm) renal parenchymal tumor: Detection, diagnosis and controversies. Radiology 179:307–317, 1991.
6. Bosniak MA: The management of the small (≤1.5 cm) renal parenchymal tumor. Radiology 179:288–294, 1991.
7. Malek RS, Omess PJ, Benson RC, Zincke H: Renal cell carcinoma in von Hippel–Lindau syndrome. Am J Med 82:236–238, 1987.
8. Choyke PL, Filling-Katz MR, Shawker TH, Gorin MB, Travis WD, Chang R, Seizinger BR, Dwyer AJ, Lineham WM: Von Hippel–Lindau disease: Radiologic screening for visceral manifestations. Radiology 174:815–820, 1990.
9. Corwin HL, Silverstein MD: The diagnosis of neoplasia in patients with asymptomatic microscopic hematuria: A decision analysis. J Urol 139:1002–1006, 1988.
10. Birnbaum BA, Bosniak MA, Megibow AJ, Lubat E, Gordon RB: Observations on the growth of renal neoplasms. Radiology 176:695–701, 1990.
11. Kass DA, Hricak H, Davidson AJ: Renal malignancies with normal excretory urograms. AJR Am J Roentgenol 141:731–734, 1983.
12. Rinsho K, Ishikawa S, Uchida K, Koiso K: The value of ultrasonography in early detection of renal cell carcinoma. Jpn J Clin Oncol 14:329–334, 1984.
13. Clayman RV, Surya V, Miller RP, Reinke DB, Fraley EE: Pursuit of the renal mass. Am J Med 77:218–223, 1984.
14. Curry NS, Reinig J, Schabel SI, et al: An evaluation of the effectiveness of CT vs. other imaging modalities in the diagnosis of atypical renal masses. Invest Radiol 19:447–452, 1984.
15. Curry NS, Schabel SI, Betsill WL: Small renal neoplasms: Diagnostic imaging, pathologic features, and clinical course. Radiology 158:113–117, 1986.
16. Amendola MA, Bree BL, Pollak HM, et al: Small renal cell carcinomas: Resolving a diagnostic dilemma. Radiology 166:637–641, 1988.
17. Hijdu SI, Thomas AG: Renal cell carcinoma at autopsy. J Urol 97:978–982, 1967.
18. Talmo TS, Shonnard JW: Small renal adenocarcinoma with metastases. J Urol 124:132–134, 1980.
19. Skinner DG, Colvin RB, Vermillion CD, et al: Diagnosis and management of renal cell carcinoma: A clinical and pathological study of 309 cases. Cancer 28:1165–1177, 1971.
20. Smith SJ, Bosniak MA, Megibow AJ, Hulnick DH, Horii SC, Raghavendra BN: Renal cell carcinoma: Earlier discovery and increased detection. Radiology 170:699–703, 1989.
21. Warshauer DM, McCarthy SM, Street L, Bookbinder MJ, Glickman MG, Richter J, Hammers L, Taylor C, Rosenfield AT: Detection of renal masses: Sensitivities and specificities of excretory urography/linear tomography, US, and CT. Radiology 169:363–365, 1988.
22. Levine E, Huntrakoon M, Wetzel LH: Small renal neoplasms: Clinical, pathologic, and imaging features. AJR Am J Roentgenol 153:69–73, 1989.
23. Coleman BG, Arger PH, Mintz MC, Pollack HM, Banner MP: Hyperdense renal masses: A computed tomographic dilemma. AJR Am J Roentgenol 143:291–294, 1984.
24. Sussman S, Cochran ST, Pagani JJ, McArdle C, Wong W, Austin R, Curry N, Kelly KM: Hyperdense renal masses: A CT manifestation of hemorrhagic renal cysts. Radiology 150:207–211, 1984.
25. Zirinsky K, Auh YH, Rubenstein WA, Williams JJ, Pasmantier MW, Kazam E: CT of the hyperdense renal cysts: Sonographic correlation. AJR Am J Roentgenol 143:151–156, 1984.
26. Balfe DM, McClennan BL, Stanley RJ, Weyman PJ, Sagel SS: Evaluation of renal masses considered indeterminate on computed tomography. Radiology 142:421–428, 1982.
27. Japerrière J, Ethier S, Boisjoly A: Cholesterol crystals as the source of diffuse echoes in a benign renal cyst. J Clin Ultrasound 12:183–185, 1984.
28. Gooding GAW: Sonography of hemorrhagic cysts with computed tomographic correlation. J Ultrasound Med 5:699–702, 1986.
29. Rosenberg ER, Korobkin M, Foster W, Silverman PM, Bowie JD, Dunnick NR: The significance of septations in a renal cyst. AJR Am J Roentgenol 144:593–595, 1985.
30. Dery R, Lewandowski B, Richard L: Real-time sonographic diagnosis of a carcinoma in a renal cyst. J Can Assoc Radiol 35:392–394, 1984.
31. Parienty RA, Pradel J, Parienty I: Cystic renal cancers: CT characteristics. Radiology 157:741–744, 1985.
32. Foster WL, Vollmer RT, Halvorsen RA, Williford ME: Ultrasonographic findings of small hypernephroma associated with renal cyst. J Clin Ultrasound 11:463–466, 1983.
33. Pollack HM, Banner MP, Arger PH, Peters J, Mulhern CB, Coleman BG: The accuracy of gray-scale renal ultrasonography in differentiating cystic neoplasms from benign cysts. Radiology 143:741–745, 1982.
34. Green WM, King DL, Casarella WJ: A reappraisal of sonolucent renal masses. Radiology 121:163–171, 1976.
35. Coleman BG, Arger PH, Mulhern CB, Pollack HM, Banner MP, Arenson RL: Gray-scale sonographic spectrum of hypernephromas. Radiology 137:757–765, 1980.
36. Pamilo M, Suramo I, Päivänsalo M: Characteristics of hypernephromas as seen with ultrasound and

computed tomography. J Clin Ultrasound 11:245–249, 1983.

37. Sugimoto S, Tsujimoto F, Kato Y, Tada S, Onishi T, Masuda F, Machida T: Sonographic patterns of renal cell carcinoma with emphasis on relation to tumor size. J Clin Ultrasound 12:247–250, 1984.

38. Hartman DS, Davidson AJ, Davis CJ, Goldman SM: Infiltrative renal lesions: CT-sonographic-pathologic correlation. AJR Am J Roentgenol 150:1061–1064, 1988.

39. Sniderman KW, Krieger JN, Seligson GR, Sos TA: The radiologic and clinical aspects of calcified hypernephroma. Radiology 131:31–35, 1979.

40. Weyman PJ, McClennan BL, Lee JKT, Stanley RJ: CT of calcified renal masses. AJR Am J Roentgenol 138:1095–1099, 1982.

41. Kuijpers D, Jaspers R: Renal masses: Differential diagnosis with pulsed Doppler US. Radiology 170:59–60, 1989.

42. Dubbins PA, Wells I: Renal carcinoma: Duplex Doppler evaluation. Br J Radiol 59:231–236, 1986.

43. Bassil B, Dosoretz D, Prout GR: Classification and staging of renal cell carcinoma. CA Cancer J Clin 35:152–163, 1985.

44. Johnson CD, Dunnick NR, Cohan RH, Illescas FF: Renal adenocarcinoma: CT staging of 100 tumors. AJR Am J Roentgenol 148:59–63, 1987.

45. London NJM, Messios N, Kinder RB, Smart JG, Osborn DE, Watkin EM, Flynn JT: A prospective study of the value of conventional CT, dynamic CT, ultrasonography, and arteriography for staging renal carcinoma. Br J Urol 64:209–217, 1989.

46. Weyman PJ, McClennan BL, Stanley RJ, Levitt RG, Sagel SS: Comparison of computed tomography and angiography in the evaluation of renal cell carcinoma. Radiology 137:417–424, 1980.

47. Roubidoux MA, Dunnick NR, Sostman HD, Leder RA: Renal carcinoma: Detection of venous extension with gradient-echo MR imaging. Radiology 182:269–272, 1992.

48. Thomas JL, Bernardino ME: Neoplastic-induced renal vein enlargement: Sonographic detection. AJR Am J Roentgenol 136:75–79, 1981.

49. Schwerk WB, Schwerk WN, Rodeck G: Venous renal tumor extension: A prospective US evaluation. Radiology 156:491–495, 1985.

50. Bernardino ME, Green B, Goldstein HM: Ultrasonography in the evaluation of post-nephrectomy renal cancer patients. Radiology 128:455–458, 1978.

51. Alter AJ, Uehling DT, Zwiebel WJ: Computed tomography of the retroperitoneum post nephrectomy. Radiology 133:663–668, 1979.

52. Graeb DA, Uhrich P: Diffuse renal transitional cell carcinoma and hydronephrosis. AJR Am J Roentgenol 135:620–621, 1980.

53. Dalla-Palma L, Bazzocchi M, Pozzi-Mucelli RS, Rossi M, Stacul F, Agostini R, Maffessanti M: The role of ultrasonography in the diagnosis of tumours of the renal pelvis. Eur J Radiol 4:156–160, 1984.

54. Leder RA, Dunnick NR: Transitional cell carcinoma of the pelvicalices and ureter. AJR Am J Roentgenol 155:713–722, 1990.

55. Mitnick JS, Bosniak MA, Rothberg M, Megibow AJ, Raghavendra BN, Subramanyam BA: Metastasis neoplasm to the kidney studied by computed tomography and sonography. J Comp Assist Tomogr 9:43–49, 1985.

56. Choyke PL, White EM, Zeman RK, Jaffe MH, Clark LR: Renal metastases: Clinicopathologic and radiologic correlation. Radiology 162:359–363, 1987.

57. Kumari-Subaiya S, Lee WJ, Festa R, Phillips G, Pochaczevsky R: Sonographic findings in leukemic renal disease. J Clin Ultrasound 12:465–472, 1984.

58. Heiberg E, Wolverson MK, Sundaram M, Shields JB: CT findings in leukemia. AJR Am J Roentgenol 143:1317–1323, 1984.

59. Jayagopal S, Cohen HL, Bhagat J, Eaton DH: Hyperechoic renal cortical masses: An unusual sonographic presentation of acute lymphoblastic leukemia in a child. J Clin Ultrasound 19:425–429, 1991.

60. Hahn FJ, Peterson N: Renal lymphoma simulating adult polycystic disease. Radiology 122:655–656, 1977.

61. Shirkhoda A, Staab EV, Mittelstaedt CA: Renal lymphoma imaged by ultrasound and gallium-67. Radiology 137:175–180, 1980.

62. Gregory A, Behan M: Lymphoma of the kidneys: Unusual ultrasound appearance due to infiltration of the renal sinus. J Clin Ultrasound 9:343–345, 1981.

63. Jafri SZH, Bree RL, Amendola MA, Glazer GM, Schwab RE, Francis IR, Borlaza G: CT of renal and perirenal non-Hodgkin lymphoma. AJR Am J Roentgenol 138:1101–1105, 1982.

64. Bruneton JN, Drouillard J, Caramella E, Manzino JJ: Lymphomes du rein: Intérêt de l'échographie et de la scanographie. J Radiol 65:755–760, 1984.

65. Weinberger E, Rosenbaum DM, Pendergrass TW: Renal involvement in children with lymphoma: Comparison of CT with sonography. AJR Am J Roentgenol 155:347–349, 1990.

66. Crist WM, Kun LE: Common solid tumors of childhood. N Engl J Med 324:461–471, 1991.

67. Kohler JA, Metreweli C, Pritchard J: How useful is ultrasound in the management of abdominal malignancy? Arch Dis Child 59:1000–1002, 1984.

68. Chevalier RL, Campbell F, Brenbridge ANAG: Nephrosonography and renal scintigraphy in evaluation of newborns with renomegaly. Urology 24:96–103, 1984.

69. Shkolnik A: Applications of ultrasound in the neonatal abdomen. Radiol Clin North Am 23:141–156, 1985.

70. Hammou A, Montague JP, Cordier MD, Neuenschwander S: "Gros rein" unilatéral néonatal approche echotomographique du diagnostic. Ann Radiol 28:56–60, 1985.

71. Sommers S: Adrenal glands. *In* Kissane JM (ed): Anderson's Pathology. 8th ed. St Louis, CV Mosby, 1985, pp 1429–1450.

72. Marble B, Pater B: Surgical diseases of the urinary tract. *In* Halter JO, Shkolnik A: Ultrasound in Pediatrics (Clinics in Diagnostic Ultrasound #8). New York, Churchill Livingstone, 1981, pp 135–164.

73. Belt TG, Cohen MD, Smith JA, Cory DA, McKenna S, Weetman R: MRI of Wilms' tumor: Promise as the primary imaging method. AJR Am J Roentgenol 146:955–961, 1986.

74. Jaffe MH, White SJ, Silver TM, Heidelberger KP: Wilms tumor: Ultrasonic features, pathologic correlation, and diagnostic pitfalls. Radiology 140:147–152, 1981.

75. Reiman TAH, Siegel MJ, Shackelford GD: Wilms tumor in children: Abdominal CT and US evaluation. Radiology 160:501–505, 1986.

76. Hartman DS, Sanders RC: Wilms' tumor versus neuroblastoma: Usefulness of ultrasound in differentiation. J Ultrasound Med 1:117–122, 1982.

77. Lowe RE, Cohen MD: Computed tomographic evaluation of Wilms tumor and neuroblastoma. RadioGraphics 4:915–928, 1984.

78. Fernbach SK, Feinstein KA, Donaldson JS, Baum ES: Nephroblastomatosis: Comparison of CT with US and urography. Radiology 166:153–156, 1988.

79. White KS, Kirks DR, Bove KE: Imaging of nephroblastomatosis: An overview. Radiology 182:1–5, 1992.

80. White SJ, Stuck KJ, Blane CE, Silver TM: Sonography of neuroblastoma. AJR Am J Roentgenol 141:465–468, 1983.

81. Stark DD, Moss AA, Brasch RC, deLorimier AA, Albin AR, London DA, Gooding CA: Neuroblastoma: Diagnostic imaging and staging. Radiology 148:101–105, 1983.

82. Atkinson GO, Zaatari GS, Lorenzo RL, Gay BB, Garvin AJ: Cystic neuroblastoma in infants: Radiographic and pathologic features. AJR Am J Roentgenol 146:113–117, 1986.

83. Forman HP, Leonidas JC, Berdon WE, Slovis TL, Wood BP, Samudrala R: Congenital neuroblastoma: Evaluation with multimodality imaging. Radiology 175:365–368, 1990.

84. Brasch RC, Randel SB, Gould RG: Follow-up of Wilms tumor: Comparison of CT with other imaging procedures. AJR Am J Roentgenol 137:1005–1009, 1981.

85. Stark DD, Brasch RC, Moss AA, deLorimier AA, Albin AR, London DA, Gooding CA: Recurrent neuroblastoma: The role of CT and alternative imaging tests. Radiology 148:107–112, 1983.

86. Hartman DS, Goldman SM, Friedman AC, Davis CJ, Madewell JE, Sherman JL: Angiomyolipoma: Ultrasonic-pathologic correlation. Radiology 139:451–458, 1981.

87. Sherman JL, Hartman DS, Friedman AC, Madewell JE, Davis CJ, Goldman SM: Angiomyolipoma: Computed tomographic-pathologic correlation of 17 cases. AJR Am J Roentgenol 137:1221–1226, 1981.

88. Raghavendra BN, Bosniak MA, Megibow AJ: Small angiomyolipoma of the kidney: Sonographic-CT evaluation. AJR Am J Roentgenol 141:575–578, 1983.

89. Bret PM, Bretagnolle M, Gaillard D, Plauchu H, Labadie M, Lapray J-F, Roullaud Y, Cooperberg P: Small, asymptomatic angiomyolipomas of the kidney. Radiology 154:7–10, 1985.

90. Kutcher R, Rosenblatt R, Mitsudo SM, Goldman M, Kogan S: Renal angiomyolipoma with sonographic demonstration of extension into the inferior vena cava. Radiology 143:755–756, 1982.

91. Shirkhoda A, Lewis E: Renal sarcoma and sarcomatoid renal cell carcinoma: CT and angiographic features. Radiology 162:353–357, 1987.

92. Khan AN, Gould DA, Shah SM, Mouasher YK: Primary renal liposarcoma mimicking angiomyolipoma on ultrasonography and conventional radiology. J Clin Ultrasound 13:58–59, 1985.

93. Levine E, Huntrakoon M: Computed tomography of renal oncocytoma. AJR Am J Roentgenol 141:741–746, 1983.

94. Quinn MJ, Hartman DS, Friedman AC, Sherman JL, Lautin EM, Pyatt RS, Ho CK, Csere R, Fromowitz FB: Renal oncocytoma: New observations. Radiology 153:49–53, 1984.

95. Goiney RC, Goldenberg L, Cooperberg PL, Charboneau JW, Rosenfield AT, Russin LD, McCarthy S, Zeman RK, Gordon PB, Rowley BA: Renal oncocytoma: Sonographic analysis of 14 cases. AJR Am J Roentgenol 143:1001–1004, 1984.

Chapter 21

Cysts and Cystic Diseases of the Kidneys

William J. Zwiebel

A broad spectrum of "cystic" disorders may affect the kidneys, ranging from harmless, benign serous cysts to potentially fatal cystic dysplasia. Renal cystic disorders are a confusing subject for several reasons. First, cystic diseases with widely different pathologic roots may have identical sonographic features. Second, several cystic diseases that are classified by age of presentation (e.g., infantile, juvenile, or adult) actually present over a much wider age range than their names imply. Third, several classification schemes have been published over the years, using inconsistent terminology.

Our task in this chapter is to simplify and clarify this subject. To this end, we begin with Table 21–1, which is my classification of cystic renal diseases. Cystic disorders are divided into four primary categories: (1) benign serous cysts, (2) sporadic dysplasia, (3) hereditary dysplasia, and (4) cystic masses of diverse etiologies. Please review this table before proceeding.

Table 21–1. Classification of Cystic Renal Diseases

Benign Serous Cysts

Sporadic Cystic Dysplasia
  Multicystic dysplasia
  Glomerulocystic disease

Hereditary Cystic Dysplasia
  Recessive
    Infantile polycystic kidney disease
    Juvenile polycystic kidney disease
  Dominant
    Adult polycystic kidney disease, PKD1 locus
    Adult polycystic kidney disease, undefined locus
  Undefined inheritance pattern
    Medullary cystic disease

Cystic Masses and Cyst-Mimicking Masses
  Multilocular cystic nephroma
  Cystic renal cell carcinoma
  Arteriovenous malformation
  Hematoma
  Parenchymal abscess
  Segmental xanthogranulomatous pyelonephritis
  Echinococcal cyst

BENIGN SEROUS CYSTS

Nonhereditary, idiopathic, benign serous cysts[1–36] may occur at any age but are particularly common in elderly people. These cysts also are called "simple cysts," which is an appropriate pathologic term, but I prefer the term "benign serous cyst" or "benign cyst." Fifty percent of persons older than 50 years have one or more benign serous renal cysts.[2] These cysts range widely in size from less than 1 cm to over 10 cm, and the number of cysts also ranges widely. Benign serous cysts also occur uncommonly in children (incidence, 0.22%; equal male/female distribution).[5, 15]

Benign serous cysts are epithelium-lined and are thought to arise from obstructed tubular elements. The exact etiology, however, is unknown. These cysts may develop at any location within the renal parenchyma. If they arise near the cortex, they project exophytically from the kidney. Alternatively, they may be imbedded within the parenchyma, or they may project into the renal sinus as so-called "parapelvic cysts."

Benign serous cysts assume a spherical shape if their growth is unrestricted, but an irregular configuration may be imposed by surrounding structures, particularly in the case of parapelvic cysts. The cysts have extremely thin walls. Incomplete septation and minor loculation occur infrequently. A multilocular appearance, however, is atypical and suggests other conditions such as neoplasms. Most benign renal cysts are asymptomatic, but symptoms may develop when large cysts compress adjacent viscera, when cysts become infected, or when hemorrhage into a cyst occurs.

Classic Cyst Features

Benign serous cysts (Fig. 21–1) have three classic features: (1) a thin (invisible) and smooth wall, (2) absence of internal echoes, and (3) enhanced through-transmission of ultrasound, relative to adjacent solid tissue.[3–15] *All three of these features must be observed before the diagnosis of*

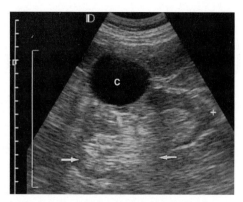

Figure 21-1—Benign Renal Cyst. The classic features of a benign renal cyst (C) are illustrated in this transverse sonogram of the right kidney. The cyst is anechoic (except for artifacts in the nearfield), the interior surface is smooth, the wall is invisible, and enhanced through-transmission (arrows) is evident.

renal cyst is made. If all these characteristics are documented, benignity is assured with 98% to 100% probability.[7-11]

Atypical Cysts

Cysts that do not exhibit the three classic features just described are considered atypical.[16-36] The principal atypical findings are calcification, septation, wall abnormalities, and echoes within the cyst contents. These atypical features are problematic, for they can be seen in benign renal cysts, cystic neoplasms, and abscesses, and sonographic findings do not differentiate among these etiologies. The following atypical cyst features are noteworthy.

- **Wall Calcification.** Calcification occurs in the walls of approximately 1% to 3% of benign renal cysts.[16-19, 35, 36] It produces strong reflections and acoustic shadows (if sufficiently large). Calcification also occurs in cystic or solid renal cell carcinomas; hence, the detection of calcification is cause for close scrutiny. Calcified cysts should be considered benign only under the following circumstances: (1) the calcification is punctate or arcuate; (2) the calcification is clearly located in the wall (Fig. 21–2); (3) the cyst wall is exquisitely thin (usually invisible); and (4) no other atypical features are present.
- **Milk of Calcium.** A second form of calcification, called milk of calcium, occurs very rarely in benign serous cysts. Milk of calcium is crystalline calcium salt that precipitates within the cyst fluid and generates high-level echogenicity. If the salts are "stirred up," the echogenicity is diffuse, but classically, milk of calcium

produces dependent echogenicity of high intensity. The echogenic fluid may cast an acoustic shadow.
- **Atypical Walls and Septation.** Cyst wall thickening, wall irregularity, mural nodules (Fig. 21–3), and multiple internal septa (Fig. 21–4) are atypical features of particular concern. These features may occur in benign cysts, but they also occur in cystic renal cell carcinoma or other malignant renal masses,[20, 21, 25-34] as considered in the preceding chapter.
- **Echogenic Contents.** The contents of benign serous renal cysts normally are anechoic, but the cyst contents occasionally exhibit diffuse, low-to-medium echogenicity (Fig. 21–5). In such cases, the echogenic material may be hemorrhage debris, cellular debris from infection, or crystalline material (calcium salts or cholesterol).[20-22, 27]

Classification of Atypical Cysts

It is noteworthy that about 20% of atypical renal cysts are benign on follow-up studies, which, unfortunately, may be invasive and expensive.[8] Bosniak[27] has proposed the following classification scheme, which relies on both ultrasound and computed tomographic (CT) features, to define more precisely which cystic renal lesions require extended evaluation, and which can be ignored or followed conservatively.

- **Class I—benign, no follow-up needed.** Classic ultrasound features of a benign cyst are present, as described earlier; on CT, the cyst contents are less than 20 Hounsfield (density) units, and no enhancement of the wall or contents is seen.

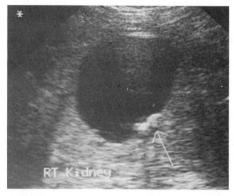

Figure 21-2—Cyst Wall Calcification. Punctate calcification (arrow) is seen in this renal cyst in a patient in the 8th decade of life. Note that there is no evidence of a soft tissue mass or wall thickening in association with this calcification.

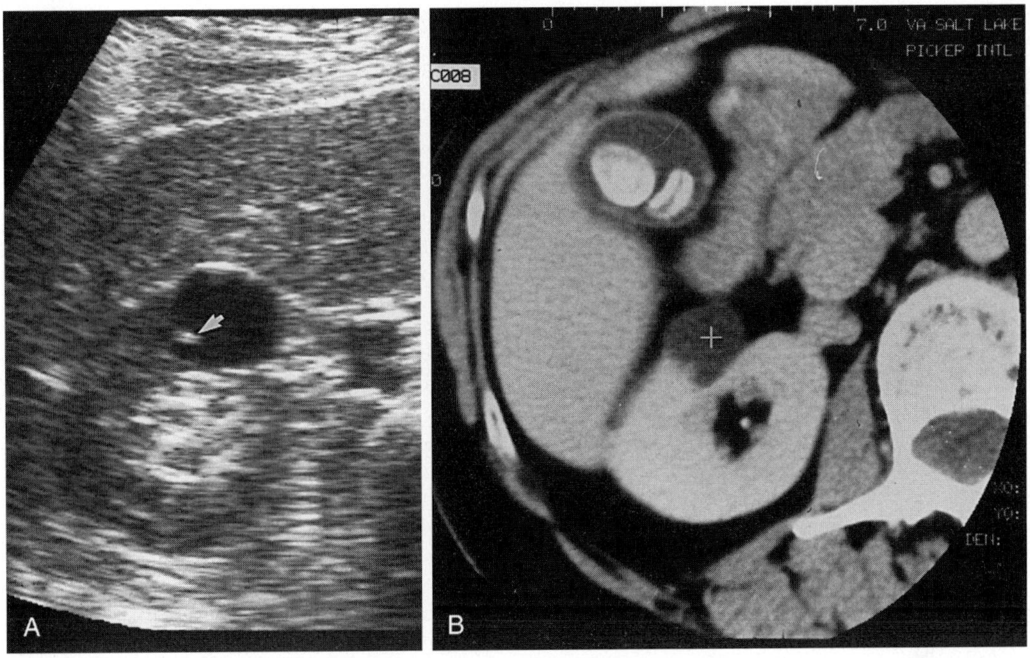

Figure 21-3—Cyst Wall Abnormality. (**A**) A nonshadowing mural nodule (arrow) is evident in this atypical cyst. (**B**) Corresponding CT scan shows the cyst (cursor) and mural nodule. No change has been seen during 12 months of follow-up.

- **Class II—benign, no follow-up needed.** The same features as listed for class I, except for thin septa, or calcification that is focal, thin, and peripheral.
- **Class III—indeterminate, needing follow-up or additional diagnostic studies.** All the benignity criteria for categories I and II are not met, but the overall impression is one of benignity.
- **Class IV—highly suspicious for malignancy, biopsy needed.** Thick, irregular walls; thick septa; solid components; enhancement of the cyst walls or septa; central calcification; cyst contents of intermediate or high CT density.

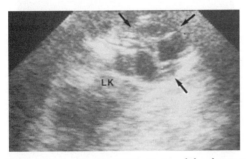

Figure 21-4—Loculated Cyst. A multilocular cystic mass (arrows) is seen in the lower pole of the left kidney (LK) on this longitudinal view. This was thought to be a cystic carcinoma or a multilocular cystic nephroma, and a partial nephrectomy was performed. It was merely a multilocular benign cyst on pathologic examination.

The Problem of the Hyperdense Cyst

Hemorrhage into benign renal cysts may make the fluid hyperdense on CT examination (about 50 to 90 Hounsfield units).[20, 21, 23–27] Bosniak[27] considers these cysts to be benign (Class II) if the following criteria are met: 3 cm or less in diameter, round shape, sharply marginated, peripheral location (so that the cyst wall can be evaluated), and no enhancement of the wall. About 50% of hyperdense cysts have classic benign features on ultrasound examination, supporting their inclusion in Class II.[27] If benignity cannot be demonstrated conclusively with CT and ultrasound, a hyperdense cyst is placed in class IV (biopsy required).

MULTICYSTIC DYSPLASIA

Pathologic and Clinical Features

Multicystic dysplasia[1–5, 37–51] is a sporadic form of renal dysplasia that usually presents in fetal life or infancy and is thought to result from obstruction or atresia of the embryonic ureter or renal pelvis. This failure of ureteric development disrupts metanephros induction and maturation, and the metanephros degenerates into a collection of cysts. The great majority of multicystic dysplastic kidneys are nonfunctioning. Rarely,

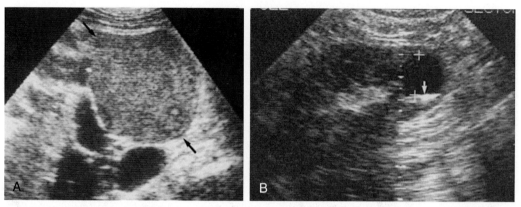

Figure 21-5—Echogenic Cysts. (A) Uniform, medium-level echogenicity is seen in a renal cyst (arrows) in a patient with dominant polycystic kidney disease who presented with acute left flank pain. High density on CT (not shown) suggested cyst hemorrhage. Note that the sonographic findings are indistinguishable from a solid mass. (B) A layer of echogenic material (arrow) is present in the dependent portion of this cyst (cursors). The layer changed position with patient motion (not shown).

however, renal function may be present at a markedly subnormal level. The presence or absence of renal function appears to depend on the degree of ureteral obstruction and the age at which ureteral development fails. The nonfunctioning form of polycystic dysplasia seems to be caused by *complete* ureteric bud obstruction before the 10th week of life, whereas the functioning form is caused by incomplete ureteral obstruction occurring after the 10th week.[40–42]

Multicystic dysplasia is bilateral in up to 21% of cases, and in these instances the disease usually is fatal in the neonatal period.[1, 2, 4, 38, 39, 41–43] Patients with the rare "functional" variant may survive for several years, however, without dialysis or transplantation. In cases of unilateral multicystic dysplasia, the opposite kidney is abnormal in an estimated 20% to 45% of cases.[43] Contralateral abnormalities include agenesis, hypoplasia, hydronephrosis, and ureteropelvic junction (UPJ) obstruction.[43] Historically, UPJ obstruction was thought to be the most common contralateral anomaly (up to 27% of cases), but a recent report suggests that UPJ obstruction is relatively uncommon, occurring in only about 7% of cases.[43] The most significant contralateral abnormality is renal agenesis (2.6% to 11% of cases), which usually results in neonatal death.[43]

In the past, surgical excision was routine for a unilateral multicystic dysplastic kidney discovered in infancy or childhood. Sonographic follow-up has shown, however, that many of these kidneys regress substantially in size or disappear by 3 years of age.[44, 45] It now is common practice to follow a multicystic dysplastic kidney with the expectation that it will disappear spontaneously. If the kidney does not regress, or increases in size, then surgery is considered. A multicystic

dysplastic kidney may persist into adult life as a collection of calcified cysts. Fortunately, the incidence of neoplastic transformation and other complications in these remnants appears to be negligible.[46, 47]

Sonographic Findings

The sonographic findings in multicystic dysplasia (Fig. 21–6, Table 21–2) are diagnostic in most cases. The kidney consists of relatively large (over 1 cm), randomly arranged cysts of various sizes.[3–5, 37–39, 43–45] The cysts exhibit benign features, as described earlier for serous cysts. No renal parenchyma is visible, and the renal pelvis is not evident. The cystic kidney has a roughly

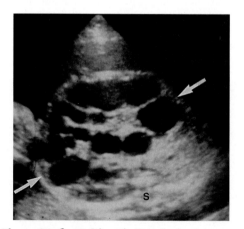

Figure 21-6—Multicystic Dysplasia. A transverse sonogram in a 26-week fetus demonstrates a large, multicystic left renal mass (arrows) that occupies much of the fetal abdomen. Various-sized cysts are present. No normal kidney components could be identified. S = fetal spine.

Table 21-2. Differential Features of Renal Cystic Dysplasias

Dysplasia	Age Range	Findings
Multicystic	Fetus, infancy	Collection of cysts of various sizes. Roughly reniform shape
Autosomal recessive	Usually fetus or infancy; also later in childhood (juvenile variety)	Large, highly echogenic kidneys, visible small cysts up to 1 cm in diameter. Corticomedullary differentiation absent. Bilateral
Autosomal dominant	Usually adulthood; wide range, down to childhood	Early: small (1–3 cm) cysts, large kidneys with irregular margins, some parenchyma visible. Late: massive kidney enlargement, innumerable cysts of various sizes, some large (≥5 cm). Bilateral

reniform shape and usually is quite large at the time of diagnosis—in keeping with the usual clinical presentation as a palpable abdominal mass. It should be noted that the size of the kidney varies widely in relation to the degree of spontaneous regression.

In some cases, differentiation between multicystic dysplasia and hydronephrosis is difficult, and in such instances the following ultrasound findings are helpful: (1) in multicystic dysplasia, the cysts are arranged *randomly* and *vary* in size; (2) in hydronephrosis, the dilated calyces are fairly similar in size and are uniformly positioned around a large, *centrally located* renal pelvis; and (3) in hydronephrosis, the dilated calyces are connected with the renal pelvis, like the fingers and palm of a glove.

AUTOSOMAL RECESSIVE POLYCYSTIC KIDNEY DISEASE

Pathologic and Clinical Features

Recessively inherited polycystic kidney disease[1, 3–5, 37, 38, 48–51] usually is discovered in utero in association with oligohydramnios, or is discovered in infancy in the setting of azotemia and kidney enlargement. The term "infantile" polycystic kidney disease is applicable in these cases. A second form of this recessive disorder exists, however, called juvenile polycystic kidney disease, and this form presents later in childhood. The infantile and juvenile varieties share two pathologic features: (1) renal cyst formation associated with renal dysfunction and (2) hepatic fibrosis (see Chapters 9 and 15).[1–5, 38, 48, 49] If renal cyst formation is predominant, the disorder presents in infancy with renal failure. If the renal component is less severe, the disorder presents later in childhood, either with renal failure or systemic hypertension. If the renal component is mild and hepatic fibrosis is predominant, the

disorder presents late in childhood as hepatic failure, portal hypertension, or both.

The renal pathology in recessive polycystic kidney disease (infantile and juvenile) is characteristic: myriad tiny cysts are present in the medulla and cortex of *both* kidneys. These cysts originate as tubular dilatation, but they gradually "round out" in a "string-of-beads" fashion to form cysts. Renal function is present to varying degrees, and when function is sufficient for pyelographic visualization, the dilated tubules produce characteristic linear striations that radiate outward from the renal hilum.

Sonographic Findings

The sonographic findings in recessive polycystic kidney disease are characteristic. The principal features (Fig. 21–7, Table 21–2) are *bilateral* kidney enlargement, markedly increased parenchymal echogenicity, and loss of corticomedullary differentiation.[3–5, 38, 48–51] Renal enlargement is caused by the combined volume of innumerable tiny cysts; increased echogenicity is attributed to the myriad echogenic interfaces that the cysts create; and corticomedullary differentiation is lost because cysts are present both in the medulla and the cortex. Although this is a cystic condition, cysts per se are not the predominant sonographic finding, because the great majority of the cysts are too small for sonographic resolution. The preservation of a thin rim of *hypoechoic* cortex at the periphery of an otherwise echogenic kidney appears to be pathognomonic, but this finding is rare.[4, 49] Another apparently pathognomonic (but uncommon) finding is the presence of tiny, dilated tubules in the medullary rays.[4]

Differential Considerations

Not all kidneys affected by recessive polycystic kidney disease have the classic appearance shown in Figure 21–7A. Variations occur (Fig. 21–7B), including visualization of innumerable tiny cysts,

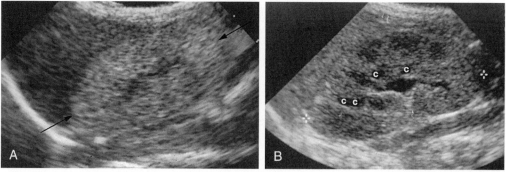

Figure 21-7—Recessive (Infantile) Polycystic Kidney Disease. Two cases are illustrated. (**A**) A longitudinal sonogram shortly after birth in a 31-week premature infant demonstrates increased echogenicity. Innumerable tiny cysts are barely visible throughout the renal parenchyma. The kidney (arrows) is enlarged (48 mm, or 40-weeks size), and corticomedullary differentiation is absent. The other kidney had a similar appearance. The infant died within a week. (**B**) Slight variation of findings is seen in another neonate with recessive polycystic kidney disease. The kidney is markedly enlarged (8.6 cm at term) and hyperechoic, but the echotexture is more heterogeneous than in **A**. Innumerable barely resolved, small cysts are present, as well as several larger (macroscopic) cysts (c).

and the presence of some larger cysts. These seldom exceed 1 cm in diameter, are few in number, and are not the predominant finding. The latter points are important for sonographic differentiation of recessive and dominant polycystic kidney disease in children. *In the recessive form, the predominant finding is increased echogenicity caused by myriad tiny cysts, whereas in the dominant form the predominant findings are cysts per se, which generally are moderate to large in size.* These differences notwithstanding, recessive and dominant polycystic kidney disease may sometimes be indistinguishable sonographically. Furthermore, both these conditions can be mistaken for a rare cystic dysplasia, called glomerulocystic disease, that presents in late childhood or early adulthood.[1–5, 38, 51]

AUTOSOMAL DOMINANT POLYCYSTIC KIDNEY DISEASE

Clinical and Pathologic Features

The dominant form of polycystic kidney disease[1–5, 38, 40, 48, 52–61] frequently is called "adult polycystic kidney disease" since this disorder most often presents clinically in adulthood. "Dominant polycystic kidney disease" (DPKD) is the preferred term since this is not an exclusively adult condition, and DPKD may present in childhood or even in infancy.[38, 48, 58, 59]

DPKD is one of the most common genetic disorders of humans.[52, 55] In North America and Europe, about 1 in 1000 persons carries a mutant gene for DPKD; furthermore, this disease accounts for 6% to 9% of end-stage renal failure cases.[52, 54–56] The marked prevalence of DPKD is explained by two factors. First, the dominant inheritance pattern ensures that 50% of offspring are affected (penetrance varies, however). Second, renal failure usually does not occur until the fourth or fifth decade, well within or beyond the reproductive years.

In the great majority of cases, DPKD is caused by a gene mutation at a specific locus called PKD1, but in about 4% of families the gene mutation is elsewhere, at a second location, called PKD2.[52–55] This is important, as renal cysts, hypertension, and renal failure occur earlier, and with greater severity, with the PKD1 disease (mean survival, 57 years) than with PKD2 disease (mean survival, 69 years). A third genetic mutation at an unidentified locus accounts for a small number of DPKD cases.

As of this writing (January, 1997), genetic markers remain under development for the identification of DPKD family members who have received a gene mutation. Thus, the fate of potential recipients is uncertain since the disease often is clinically silent well into adult life. Genetic uncertainty is worsened by the occurrence of a variety of genetic defects at a given locus, widely variable penetrance of the polycystic trait, and uncertainty as to whether the patient has PKD1 disease or the less severe PKD2 disease.[52–55]

DPKD is a systemic disorder,[54, 55] as suggested by the occurrence, in some individuals, of cysts in organs other than the kidneys, valvular heart disease, and cerebral aneurysms. Liver cysts occur in about 30% of affected individuals, and cysts are present less commonly in the pancreas, ovaries, uterus, and seminal vesicles.[53–55] Complications of DPKD (in addition to renal failure) are frequent, and include hypertension, pain, hematuria, cyst hemorrhage, cyst rupture, cyst infection, and urinary tract obstruction.[3–5, 57, 60, 61]

Sonographic Features

The sonographic findings in DPKD[3–5, 38, 48, 57–61] vary in direct relationship to the degree of cyst development (Fig. 21–8). Early in the course of the disease, the kidneys may appear normal, or only a few cysts may be present (see diagnostic criteria later). In addition, cyst development may be greater in one kidney than the other in the early stages. With time, however, the cysts become larger, more numerous, and more sonographically apparent. By the time renal dysfunction is apparent clinically, sonographic diagnosis usually is straightforward. The kidneys are grossly enlarged and irregular, innumerable cysts of various sizes are readily seen, the borders of the kidney are difficult to define, and little or no renal parenchyma is visible.

Note that although cyst formation may be more apparent in one kidney or the other in the early stages of this disease, cysts inevitably develop bilaterally. Older medical articles refer to a condition called segmental or unilateral polycystic kidney disease. This is actually an unrelated, rare disorder currently called multilocular cystic nephroma.[62–66]

The Role of Sonography

Ultrasound serves two purposes in patients with DPKD: early detection of cysts for genetic counseling, and assessment of complications of the disorder. With respect to genetic counseling, the detection of two cysts on one kidney, or one cyst on both kidneys, constitutes a positive sonographic examination in potentially affected individuals aged 30 years or less.[59] The presence of a single cyst is nondiagnostic, because isolated, benign serous cysts may occur sporadically in children and young adults. The number of cysts, as well as the age at which the cysts become visible, predicts the severity of the disease.[48, 52, 53, 58, 59] For a person in the second decade (ages 10 to 19 years) with numerous cysts, the probability of clinically significant renal failure exceeds 90%; furthermore, such an individual is likely to suffer from renal failure before his or her children are mature.[52, 53, 59] In contrast, the *absence* of cysts during the second decade reduces the probability of significant renal disease to about 60%, and the absence of cysts during the third decade (ages 20 to 29 years) reduces the probability further, to about 14%.[52, 53, 59] An individual without cysts after age 30 years very likely does not have the PKD1 mutation, and, if affected by DPKD, probably will not suffer from renal failure until late in life, or not at all.[52]

The second function of sonography is assessment for complications of DPKD, especially cyst hemorrhage, cyst infection, calculus formation, and urinary tract obstruction. These complications should be sought with vigor in patients who present with pain, hematuria, or signs of infection. Unfortunately, most of these complications occur in advanced DPKD patients, in whom adequate sonographic examination is not possible due to the massive size of the kidneys. On occasion, sonography may demonstrate a calculus, hydronephrosis, or echogenic cyst fluid that indicates hemorrhage or infection, but in most cases sonographic examination is futile. CT is the preferred imaging modality for seeking complications of DPKD, as this modality provides a comprehensive view of the massively enlarged kidneys.

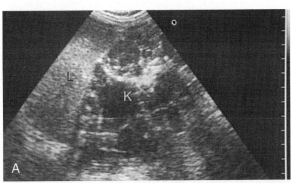
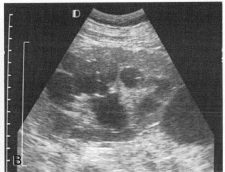

Figure 21-8—Dominant (Adult) Polycystic Kidney Disease. Two cases of dominant polycystic kidney disease are shown. (**A**) A longitudinal view demonstrates massive enlargement of the right kidney (K) in comparison with the adjacent liver (L). Innumerable cysts of varying size are seen, and no renal parenchyma is visible. (**B**) In a less severely affected individual, a longitudinal view of the right kidney demonstrates cysts of different sizes. Note that some parenchyma is visible in this patient.

Sonographic Differential Diagnosis

The differential diagnosis of adult polycystic kidney disease includes hydronephrosis, certain cystic dysplasias, cystic neoplasms, xanthogranulomatous pyelonephritis, and multiple nonhereditary renal cysts. The latter condition is noteworthy, since elderly individuals occasionally have numerous benign renal cysts. If the patient is elderly, if the cysts are few enough to be counted, and if normal-appearing renal parenchyma is seen among the cysts, then the diagnosis of polycystic kidney disease should be withheld. If the cysts are too numerous to count and normal renal parenchyma cannot be detected, then the diagnosis of adult polycystic kidney disease should be considered.

REFERENCES

1. Jones DB: Kidneys. *In* Kissane JM (ed): Anderson's Pathology. 8th ed. St Louis, CV Mosby, 1985, pp 765–767.
2. Kissane JM: Congenital malformations. *In* Hepinstall RH (ed): Pathology of the Kidneys. Boston, Little, Brown, 1974, pp 69–119.
3. Grossman H, Rosenberg ER, Bowie JD, Ram P, Merten DF: Sonographic diagnosis of renal cystic diseases. AJR Am J Roentgenol 140:81–85, 1983.
4. Hayden CK, Swischuk LE: Renal cystic disease. Semin Ultrasound CT MR 12:361–373, 1991.
5. Hayden CK, Swischuk LE, Smith TH, Armstrong EA: Renal cystic disease in childhood. RadioGraphics 6:97–116, 1986.
6. Leopold GR, Talner LB, Asher WM, et al: Renal ultrasonography: An updated approach to the diagnosis of renal cysts. Radiology 109:671–678, 1973.
7. Pollack HM, Goldberg BB, Morales JO, Bogash M: A systematized approach to the differential diagnosis of renal masses. Radiology 113:653–659, 1974.
8. Pollack HM, Banner MP, Arger PH, Peters J, Mulhern CB, Coleman BG: The accuracy of gray-scale renal ultrasonography in differentiating cystic neoplasms from benign cysts. Radiology 143:741–745, 1982.
9. Lingard DA, Lawson TL: Accuracy of ultrasound in predicting the nature of renal masses. J Urol 122:724–727, 1979.
10. Chan SL, Cooperberg P, McLoughlin MG, Ewart B: Grey-scale ultrasonography: A refined tool for differentiating renal mass lesions. Can Med Assoc J 122:321–322, 1980.
11. McClennan BL, Stanley RJ, Melson GL, Levitt RG, Sagel SS: CT of the renal cyst: Is cyst aspiration necessary? AJR Am J Roentgenol 133:671–675, 1979.
12. Hidalgo H, Dunnick NR, Rosenberg ER, Ram PC, Korobkin M: Parapelvic cysts: Appearance on CT and sonography. AJR Am J Roentgenol 138:667–671, 1982.
13. Patel K, Caro PA, Chatten J: Parapelvic renal cyst causing UPJ obstruction. Pediatr Radiol 19:2–5, 1988.
14. Gordon RL, Pollack HM, Popky GL, Duckett JW: Simple serous cysts of the kidney in children. Radiology 131:357–361, 1979.
15. McHugh K, Stringer DA, Hebert D, Babiak CA: Simple renal cysts in children: Diagnosis and follow-up with US. Radiology 178:383–385, 1991.
16. Cho KJ, Thornbury JR, Berkstein J, et al: Localized cystic disease of the kidneys: Angiographic, pathologic correlation. AJR Am J Roentgenol 132:891–895, 1979.
17. Love L, Yedlicka J: Computed tomography of internally calcified renal cysts. AJR Am J Roentgenol 145:1225–1227, 1985.
18. Weyman PJ, McClennan BL, Lee JKT, Stanley RJ: CT of calcified renal masses. AJR Am J Roentgenol 138:1095–1099, 1982.
19. Sniderman KW, Krieger JN, Seligson GR, Sos TA: The radiologic and clinical aspects of calcified hypernephroma. Radiology 131:31–35, 1979.
20. Gooding GAW: Sonography of hemorrhagic cysts with computed tomographic correlation. J Ultrasound Med 5:699–702, 1986.
21. Sussman S, Cochran ST, Pagani JJ, McArdle C, Wong W, Austin R, Curry N, Kelly KM: Hyperdense renal masses: A CT manifestation of hemorrhagic renal cysts. Radiology 150:207–211, 1984.
22. Japerrière J, Ethier S, Boisjoly A: Cholesterol crystals as the source of diffuse echoes in a benign renal cyst. J Clin Ultrasound 12:183–185, 1984.
23. Coleman BG, Arger PH, Mintz MC, Pollack HM, Banner MP: Hyperdense renal masses: A computed tomographic dilemma. AJR Am J Roentgenol 143:291–294, 1984.
24. Zirinsky K, Auh YH, Rubenstein WA, Williams JJ, Pasmantier MW, Kazam E: CT of the hyperdense renal cyst: Sonographic correlation. AJR Am J Roentgenol 143:151–156, 1984.
25. Balfe DM, McClennan BL, Stanley RJ, Weyman PJ, Sagel SS: Evaluation of renal masses considered indeterminate on computed tomography. Radiology 142:421–428, 1982.
26. Green WM, King DL, Casarella WJ: A reappraisal of sonolucent renal masses. Radiology 121:163–171, 1976.
27. Bosniak MA: The small (≤3.0 cm) renal parenchymal tumor: Detection, diagnosis, and controversies. Radiology 179:307–317, 1991.
28. Charboneau JW, Hattery RR, Ernst EC, James EM, Williamson B, Hartman GW: Spectrum of sonographic findings in 125 renal masses other than benign simple cysts. AJR Am J Roentgenol 140:87–94, 1983.
29. Risenberg ER, Korobkin M, Foster W, Silverman PM, Bowie JD, Dunnick NR: The significance of septations in a renal cyst. AJR Am J Roentgenol 144:593–595, 1985.
30. Coleman BG, Arger PH, Mulhern CB, Pollack HM, Banner MP, Arenson RL: Gray-scale sonographic spectrum of hypernephromas. Radiology 137:757–765, 1980.
31. Parienty RA, Pradel J, Parienty I: Cystic renal cancers: CT characteristics. Radiology 157:741–744, 1985.
32. Dery R, Lewandowski B, Richard L: Real-time sonographic diagnosis of a carcinoma in a renal cyst. J Can Assoc Radiol 35:392–394, 1984.
33. Foster WL, Vollmer RT, Halvorsen RA, Williford ME: Ultrasonographic findings of small hypernephroma associated with renal cyst. J Clin Ultrasound 11:463–466, 1983.
34. Amis ES, Cronan JJ, Pfister RC: Needle puncture

of cystic renal masses: A survey of the Society of Uroradiology. AJR Am J Roentgenol 148:297–299, 1987.

35. Daniel WW Jr, Hartman GW, Witten DM, et al: Calcified renal masses: A review of 10 years' experience at the Mayo Clinic. Radiology 103:501–508, 1972.

36. Phillips TL, Chin FG, Palubinskas AJ: Calcification in renal masses: An eleven-year survey. Radiology 80:786–794, 1963.

37. Tourey TW: The early development of the human nephros. Embryol Carnegie Inst 35:159–197, 1954.

38. Worthington JL, Shackelford GD, Cole BR, Tack ED, Kissane JM: Sonographically detectable cysts in polycystic kidney disease in newborn and young infants. Pediatr Radiol 18:287, 1988.

39. Stuck KJ, Koff SA, Silver TM: Ultrasonic features of multicystic dysplastic kidney: Expanded diagnostic criteria. Radiology 143:217–221, 1982.

40. Osathanondh V, Potter EL: Pathogenesis of polycystic kidneys. Arch Pathol 77:459–512, 1964.

41. Felson B, Cussen LJ: The hydronephrotic type of unilateral congenital multicystic disease of the kidney. Semin Roentgenol 10:113–123, 1975.

42. Griscom MT, Vawter GF, Fellers FX: Pelvoinfundibular atresia; The usual form of multicystic kidney: 44 unilateral and 22 bilateral cases. Semin Roentgenol 10:125–131, 1975.

43. Kleiner B, Filly RA, Mack K, Callen PW: Multicystic dysplastic kidney: Observations of contralateral disease in the fetal population. Radiology 161:27–29, 1986.

44. Pedicelli G, Jequier S, Bowen A'D, Boisvert J: Multicystic dysplastic kidneys: Spontaneous regression demonstrated with US. Radiology 160:23–26, 1986.

45. Vinocur L, Slovis TL, Perlmutter AD, Watts FB, Chang C-H: Follow-up studies of multicystic dysplastic kidneys. Radiology 167:311–315, 1988.

46. Barrett DM, Wineland RS: Renal cell carcinoma in a multicystic dysplastic kidney. Urology 15:152–154, 1980.

47. Ambrose SS, Jould RA, Turlock TS, Parrott TS: Unilateral multicystic renal disease in adults. J Urol 128:366–369, 1982.

48. Kääriäinen H, Jääskeläinen L, Kivisaari L, Koskimies O, Norio R: Dominant and recessive polycystic kidney disease in children: Classification by intravenous pyelography, ultrasound, and computed tomography. Pediatr Radiol 18:45–50, 1988.

49. Melson GL, Shackelford GD, Cole BR, and McClennan BL: The spectrum of sonographic findings in infantile polycystic kidney disease with urographic and clinical correlation. J Clin Ultrasound 13:113–119, 1985.

50. Boal DK, Teele RL: Sonography of infantile polycystic kidney disease. AJR Am J Roentgenol 135:575–580, 1980.

51. Rego JD, Laing FC, Jeffrey RB: Ultrasonographic diagnosis of medullary cystic disease. J Ultrasound Med 2:433–436, 1983.

52. Parfrey PS, Bear JC, Morgan J, Cramer BC, McManamon PJ, Gault MH, Churchill DN, Singh M, Hewitt R, Somlo S, Reeders ST: The diagnosis and prognosis of autosomal dominant polycystic kidney disease. N Engl J Med 323:1085–1090, 1990.

53. Grantham JJ: Polycystic kidney disease—an old problem in a new context. N Engl J Med 319:944–946, 1988.

54. European Polycystic Kidney Disease Consortium (Harris PC): The polycystic kidney disease 1 gene encodes a 14 kb transcript and lies within a duplicated region on chromosome 16. Cell 77:881–894, 1994.

55. Grantham JJ: Polycystic kidney disease—there goes the neighborhood. N Engl J Med 333:36–37, 1995.

56. Lowrie EG, Hampers CL: The success of Medicare's end-stage renal disease program: The case for profits and the private marketplace. N Engl J Med 305:434–438, 1981.

57. Kelsey JA, Bowie JD: Gray-scale ultrasonography in the diagnosis of polycystic kidney disease. Radiology 122:791–795, 1977.

58. Walker FC, Loney LC, Root ER, Melson GL, McAlister WH, Cole BR: Diagnostic evaluation of adult polycystic kidney disease in childhood. AJR Am J Roentgenol 142:1273–1277, 1984.

59. Bear JC, McManamon P, Morgan J, Payne RH, Lewis H, Gault MH, Churchill DN: Age at clinical onset and at ultrasonographic detection of adult polycystic kidney disease: Data for genetic counselling. Am J Med Genet 18:45–53, 1984.

60. Barbaric ZL, Spataro RF, Segal AJ: Urinary tract obstruction in polycystic renal disease. Radiology 125:627–629, 1977.

61. Levine E, Grantham JJ: High-density renal cysts in autosomal dominant polycystic kidney disease demonstrated by CT. Radiology 154:477–482, 1985.

62. Banner MP, Pollack HM, Chatten J, Witzleben C: Multilocular renal cysts: Radiologic-pathologic correlation. AJR Am J Roentgenol 136:239–247, 1981.

63. Beckwith JB, Kiviat NB: Multilocular renal cysts and cystic renal tumors. AJR Am J Roentgenol 136:435–436, 1981.

64. Hantman SS: Unilateral adult polycystic kidney. J Ultrasound Med 1:371–374, 1982.

65. Madewell JE, Goldman SM, Davis CJ, Hartman DS, Feigin DS, Lichtenstein JE: Multilocular cystic nephroma: A radiographic-pathologic correlation of 58 patients. Radiology 146:309–321, 1983.

66. Hartman DS, Davis CJ, Sanders RC, Johns TT, Smirniotopoulos J, Goldman SM: The multiloculated renal mass: Considerations and differential features. RadioGraphics 7:29–52, 1987.

Chapter 22

Urinary Tract Infection and Calculi

William J. Zwiebel

URINARY TRACT INFECTION

Sonography does not generally have a role in the management of uncomplicated urinary tract infections (cystitis or pyelonephritis) that respond promptly to antibiotic therapy. The value of sonography is realized in cases of persistent, recurrent, or chronic infection and in urosepsis. In these settings, ultrasound serves three functions.[1–16] First, ultrasound can identify urinary tract dilatation, calculi, or congenital anomalies that may contribute to acute or chronic infection. Second, ultrasound can differentiate between uncomplicated pyelonephritis and so-called "complicated" pyelonephritis (e.g., abscess and pyonephrosis) that may require radiologic or surgical intervention. Finally, sonography can identify unusual consequences of chronic infection, such as xanthogranulomatous pyelonephritis.

Routes of Infection

The great majority of urinary tract infections[1–45] are caused by bacteria, particularly gram-negative intestinal flora. Fungal infections occur uncommonly and are usually restricted to immunocompromised or otherwise debilitated individuals. The risk factors for urinary tract infections are diabetes mellitus, immunosuppression, chronic calculus disease, and urine stasis (due to obstruction, vesicoureteral reflux, paralysis, or collecting system anomalies).

Most urinary tract infections begin in the bladder and "ascend" via the ureters to the renal pelvis and calyces. The bacteria then enter the renal parenchyma, possibly via lymphatics within the walls of the collecting channels, and spread within the interstitium to the periphery of the kidney. The infection then may "seed" the perinephric space. Hematogenous infection of the kidneys also occurs, but this route of infection is uncommon and usually occurs in immunocompromised individuals, intravenous drug users, or in cases of tuberculosis (discussed later).

Pyelonephritis

The term "pyelonephritis" refers to infection of the renal pelvis, calyces, and parenchyma. The most significant site of infection is the parenchyma, since irreparable damage may occur if parenchymal infection is severe. One or both kidneys may be involved in acute pyelonephritis. The clinical manifestations include flank pain, fever, chills, leukocytosis, dysuria, and bacteriuria.

The sonographic findings in *uncomplicated* acute pyelonephritis[1–10] are renomegaly, decreased parenchymal echogenicity, and loss of corticomedullary differentiation (Fig. 22–1). In addition, the wall of the renal pelvis or major calyces may be thickened and may have a "tram track" or halo appearance (Fig. 22–2).* All of these abnormalities result from infection-induced inflammation and accompanying edema. Sonography is relatively insensitive for detection of acute pyelonephritis (31% to 64%)[3, 13]; therefore, many infected kidneys may appear normal on ultrasound examination.

Acute, Focal Bacterial Nephritis

Studies of pyelonephritic kidneys[5] suggest that each lobe is infected as a unit and that the severity of the infection may vary considerably from one renal lobe to another. The term "acute, focal bacterial nephritis" is applied to disproportionately severe infection of one or more lobes.[1, 2, 4, 5, 7, 11–16] The severity of lobar infections in such cases falls somewhere between the usual form of pyelonephritis and renal abscess. Microscopic abscesses may in fact be present in the highly infected area, and tissue destruction may result, even if antibiotic therapy is prompt and effective. Follow-up studies have demonstrated, however, that most cases of acute focal bacterial nephritis resolve without appreciable loss of renal parenchyma.[5, 14, 15]

The sonographic manifestations of acute, focal bacterial nephritis are enlargement and altered

---

*Thickening of collecting structures (pelvis or calyces) was originally thought to be specific for acute pyelonephritis, but this finding is nonspecific and also may occur in uncomplicated urinary tract obstruction, vesicoureteral reflux, and renal transplant rejection.[9, 10]

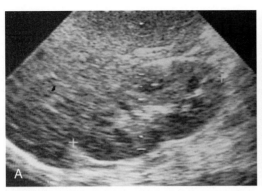 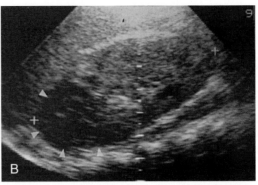

Figure 22-1—Acute Pyelonephritis. (13 year old male with fever and *Pseudomonas* pyuria). (**A**) Longitudinal sonogram of the unaffected (normal) right kidney; length: 6.5 cm. Note that the pyramids are clearly visible. (**B**) The pyelonephritic left kidney is diffusely hypoechoic. The kidney also is markedly enlarged (9 cm) but this is not obvious due to differences in scale. Corticomedullary differentiation is absent, and the renal sinus is poorly defined. All these changes are related to inflammatory edema. The superior pole (arrowheads) is less echogenic than the rest of the kidney, representing a focal region of severe nephritis.

echogenicity confined to a localized portion (or portions) of the kidney (Figs. 22–1*B*, 22–3). These findings usually are accompanied by more generalized changes of acute pyelonephritis. The echogenicity of the affected area(s) usually is diminished, owing to the intensity of the inflammatory reaction, and corticomedullary differentiation typically is lost. In some cases, however, the affected area(s) may contain scattered, more intense reflections or may be diffusely hyperechoic. The latter finding may be related to hemorrhage or microabscess formation, but its cause

is unknown. The presence of a large, discrete, anechoic area is reason for concern, as such an area probably represents frank tissue breakdown with abscess formation.

In acute, focal bacterial nephritis, the enlarged, highly inflamed portion of the kidney may resemble a neoplastic mass (Fig. 22–3). To avoid significant diagnostic error, it is important to think of this condition when a masslike lesion is found in a patient with acute pyelonephritis.

Close follow-up of focal, acute bacterial nephritis is desirable for two reasons. First, percutaneous or surgical drainage may be necessary if an abscess forms. Second, it may be useful to know the extent of parenchymal damage, as sub-

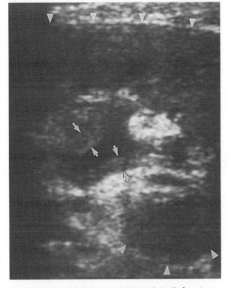

Figure 22-2—Thickened Renal Pelvis. A transverse scan of a renal allograft shows thickening of the renal pelvis walls (arrows) due to acute pyelonephritis. Arrowheads mark the borders of the kidney. (Courtesy of Paula Woodward, MD, University of Utah Medical Center, Salt Lake City.)

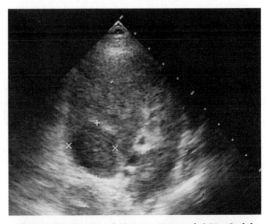

Figure 22-3—Focal, Severe Bacterial Nephritis. A masslike, focal hypoechoic zone (cursors) is seen in this transverse view of the left kidney in a 27 year old woman with acute pyelonephritis examined at 36 weeks of pregnancy. Other changes of acute perinephritis were evident sonographically but are not illustrated here. This finding resolved without apparent tissue destruction.

sequently revealed by parenchymal scar formation.

Renal Abscess

Vasospasm is a prominent feature of severe acute pyelonephritis,[4] and vasospasm-induced ischemia, combined with severe infection, may lead to tissue necrosis, liquefaction, and parenchymal abscess formation. An abscess also may develop adjacent to a pyelonephritic kidney, within the perinephric space. Both parenchymal and perinephric abscesses[1, 4, 5, 7, 8, 11–13, 17, 18] are significant complications of pyelonephritis since they may be associated with massive tissue destruction and sepsis. Small abscesses confined to the parenchyma may resolve with antibiotic therapy, but large parenchymal abscesses require surgical or percutaneous drainage. Perinephric abscesses are resistant to antibiotic therapy; therefore, drainage is required in most cases.[12, 17, 18]

Parenchymal renal abscesses (Figs. 22–4, 22–5) are represented sonographically as well-defined, rounded areas that either are anechoic or strikingly hypoechogenic relative to normal renal parenchyma. The abscess fluid may contain

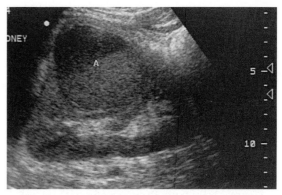

Figure 22-5—Renal Carbuncle. A large, debris-laden abscess (A) is present in the midportion of the left kidney in this 45 year old man with acute pyelonephritis who was examined because of failure to respond to routine antibiotic therapy. The abscess projects externally, consistent with the term "carbuncle."

diffuse or dependent low-level echoes generated by debris. Enhanced through-transmission is the rule, but distal enhancement may be absent if the abscess contents are echogenic. The margins of renal abscesses typically are somewhat "shaggy," and a discrete wall or capsule is not

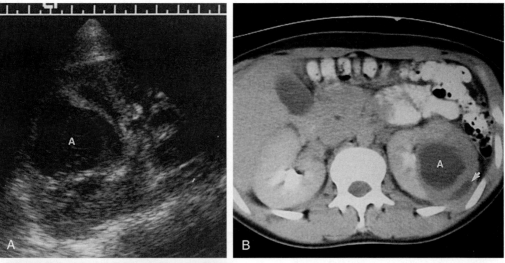

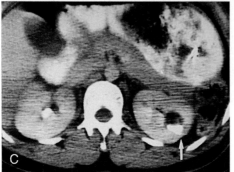

Figure 22-4—Parenchymal Renal Abscess. (A) This longitudinal sonogram demonstrates a large, intraparenchymal abscess (A) in the superior pole of the left kidney. Note the presence of debris within the abscess and the mass effect on surrounding kidney structures. (**B**) Contrast-enhanced computed tomography performed on the same day as the sonogram demonstrates the abscess cavity (A) surrounded by edema, as well as a small perinephric abscess (arrow). (**C**) A contrast-enhanced computed tomogram 18 months later demonstrates parenchymal thinning and a large calyceal diverticulum (arrow) at the former abscess site. Contrast is present in the dependent portion of the diverticulum. (Technically limited scan performed in relation to acute trauma.)

evident. Occasionally, however, abscesses may have smooth walls and anechoic contents, and these lesions may be indistinguishable from benign serous cysts. In rare instances, gas accumulation within the abscess cavity may produce focal strong reflections and acoustic shadows. These findings may be attributed mistakenly to renal calculi.

Perinephric abscesses are represented sonographically as well-defined anechoic or hypoechoic collections that surround part or all of the kidney (Fig. 22–6). Debris within the abscess fluid may generate dependent or diffuse low-level echoes. Abscesses may spread extensively within the confines of the perinephric space and achieve massive proportions (Fig. 22–6B). Differentiation between perinephric abscess and hematoma generally is not possible sonographically.

Emphysematous Pyelonephritis and Pyelitis

If a gas-forming organism infects the renal parenchyma, gas may accumulate within affected portions of the renal tissue. The term "emphysematous pyelonephritis"[1, 19–21] is applied to this uncommon but highly dangerous condition, which usually occurs in diabetic patients. The sonographic findings in emphysematous pyelonephritis are striking, for strong reflections (Fig. 22–7), possibly accompanied by acoustic shadows, emanate from the parenchymal gas bubbles. Other manifestations of acute pyelonephritis also may be seen, as described earlier.

It is important to differentiate between emphysematous pyelonephritis and emphysematous *pyelitis* in which infection-related gas accumulates within the renal pelvis and calyces. Emphysematous pyelitis may not represent a clinically dangerous situation, whereas emphysematous pyelonephritis is a serious condition that in some cases is curable only with nephrectomy.

Pyonephrosis

Gross purulence within the collecting system of the kidney is termed "pyonephrosis."[23–26] In essence, pyonephrosis is an intra–collecting system abscess and as such may be associated with sepsis as well as significant morbidity and mortality. Pyonephrosis occurs only in hydronephrotic (and usually obstructed) kidneys. Predisposing factors include diabetes, large calculi, and collecting system anomalies.

Pyonephrosis is characterized sonographically by diffuse or dependent low-level echogenicity within distended renal collecting structures (Fig. 22–8). The walls of the collecting system may be thickened, and other changes of pyelonephritis may be evident, as described previously. An obstructing calculus also may be present. *Echogenic fluid within a hydronephrotic kidney should not be passed over as artifactual or inconsequential,* for if this finding is due to pyonephrosis, prompt drainage may be required to avoid significant complications.

Echogenic collecting system fluid is not specific for pyonephrosis. Fungal mycelia, blood, and crystalline material also may generate echoes within the renal collecting system. Furthermore, the spectrum of findings in renal tuberculosis and xanthogranulomatosis pyelonephritis (discussed later) may mimic pyonephrosis.

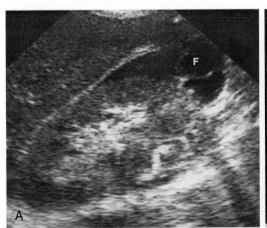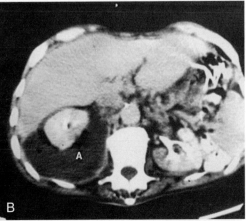

Figure 22-6—Perinephric Abscess. (A) A longitudinal sonogram shows a loculated fluid collection (F) adjacent to the inferior pole of the right kidney. An inexperienced sonologist misinterpreted this as fluid-filled bowel. (B) A contrast-enhanced CT scan five days later demonstrates a massive perinephric abscess (A) surrounding the right kidney. The abscess was drained successfully with a percutaneous catheter.

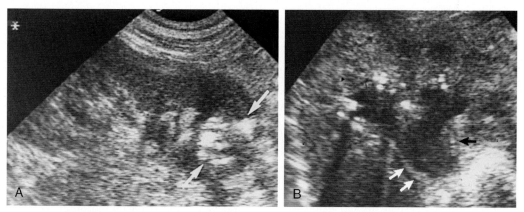

Figure 22-7—Emphysematous Pyelonephritis. (**A**) A longitudinal sonogram in an elderly diabetic patient demonstrates poorly defined, highly echoic areas (arrows) in the lower pole of the left kidney. These represent areas of gas accumulation in infected parenchyma. (**B**) In another patient, a longitudinal scan of the right kidney demonstrates focal gas bubbles (bright dots) in the parenchyma *adjacent* to dilated renal collecting structures. These gas bubbles could not be displaced with changes in patient position, indicating that they were in the parenchyma, rather than the collecting structures. Note the "tram track" appearance of the walls of the renal pelvis (arrows), caused by edema in this patient with acute pyelonephritis.

Sonography Versus Computed Tomography for Pyelonephritis Complications

The relative diagnostic value of sonography and computed tomography (CT) for detecting abscess and other complications of acute pyelonephritis has been the subject of considerable debate in the radiologic literature.[1, 3–5, 7, 8, 11, 15, 16, 26] CT is more sensitive than sonography for renal abscesses, particularly for collections 2 cm or smaller in diameter. CT also appears to differentiate better between acute focal bacterial nephritis and renal abscess. Ultrasound, on the other hand, offers safety (no ionizing radiation), ease of examination, portability, and low cost. In my opinion, sonography should be used first in cases of complicated pyelonephritis, because it readily detects hydronephrosis and large abscesses that require drainage. CT should be reserved for cases in which sonography fails.

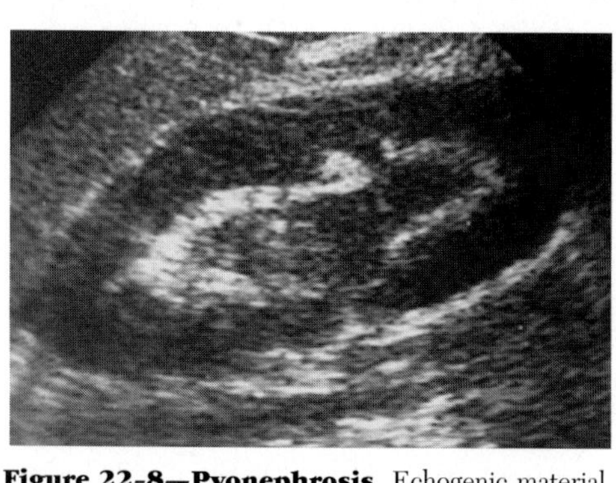

CHRONIC RENAL INFECTION

The sonographic manifestations of chronic renal infection, regardless of cause, include diminished kidney size and cortical irregularity (scarring), both of which result from parenchymal destruction[26] (see Figure 22–4C). Focal zones of parenchymal destruction are represented by triangular parenchymal defects centered over the renal pyramids. Undamaged portions of the kidney may undergo compensatory hypertrophy, and the resultant distortion of kidney anatomy can mimic a neoplastic mass.

CHILDHOOD URINARY TRACT INFECTION

Infection of the urinary tract in children[27–37] is harmless as long as such infection is confined to the bladder and is treated effectively. If, however, the infecting agent ascends to the kidneys and infects the renal parenchyma, significant renal damage may result, particularly if the infection is chronic or recurrent.[27] To prevent or limit infection-induced renal damage, urinary tract examination is recommended in children with urinary tract infection, particularly before the age of 5 years.[27–29, 34] The principal goals of sonography in such children[28–34] are to detect the following: (1) structural abnormalities of the kidneys, ureters, and urinary bladder; (2) hydronephrosis related to anomalies or reflux; (3) calculi; and

Figure 22-8—Pyonephrosis. Echogenic material related to bacterial infection is seen within the dilated collecting structures of this right kidney. The patient was immunosuppressed due to cancer chemotherapy.

(4) complications of acute pyelonephritis, such as abscess.

The main shortcomings of sonography are inability to diagnose vesicoureteral reflux reliably, and a general lack of urodynamic information.[30] Because of these shortcomings, scintigraphy and voiding cystourethrography (VCUG) are used in conjunction with sonography for assessment of pediatric urinary tract infection. Jequier and associates[29] feel that in children over 5 years of age with only one episode of urinary tract infection, additional imaging studies are not required if a comprehensive ultrasound examination is normal. All investigators agree that additional evaluation, at least with radionuclide imaging, is indicated in children younger than 5 years and in older children with recurrent infection.[28–34, 37]

FUNGAL INFECTION

Candida albicans is the most common fungus to infect the urinary tract.[38–41] The infection usually is confined to the major collecting structures, including the bladder, ureters, and renal pelvis, but renal parenchymal infection also may occur. Most fungal infections occur in immunocompromised individuals.

The sonographic hallmark of urinary fungal infection is the visualization of fungal elements within the collecting system. Fungal organisms grow as branching structures, called mycelia, that form interwoven masses. In early stages of infection, the mycelial aggregates are small and are represented only by low-level, dependent echogenicity. With time, larger aggregates form that are visible as discrete intraluminal masses with medium-to-high echogenicity. Within the bladder, fungal masses usually are spherical, but within the kidney, they may conform to the shape of the collecting system and even form "casts" that distend the collecting structures.

Renal parenchymal fungal infection results in parenchymal thickening and *increased* echogenicity of the cortex and medulla. These findings may be diffuse or localized, in accordance with the distribution of the infection.

URINARY TRACT TUBERCULOSIS

The tuberculous bacillus spreads to the urinary tract via the blood stream very early following the initial pulmonary infection. If the pulmonary infection is confined and heals, chest radiographs may remain normal. Only 30% of patients with urinary tract tuberculosis (TB) have an abnormal chest radiograph, and only 50% have a history of tuberculous infection.[1, 26, 44, 45]

Tuberculous infection of the kidney begins in the renal cortex, spreads to the medulla, and flourishes in the papilla, where it causes papillary necrosis. Necrosis of the papilla usually is the earliest manifestation of TB that can be detected with imaging studies. Pyelography can detect early changes of papillary necrosis, but sonography can detect only advanced destructive changes that occur when the infection spreads from the medullary tip to the rest of the medullary ray. The tuberculous infection also may spread to the cortex where it can cause cortical defects or diffuse parenchymal thinning, depending on the extent of parenchymal involvement.

The papillary/medullary infection seeds the urine with bacteria, spreading the infection into the collecting system. Favorite secondary sites of infection are the infundibula (major calyces), the ureters (particularly at the ureteropelvic junction), and the bladder. Scarring, which is a prominent feature of mucosal infection, results in calycectasis or more generalized hydronephrosis, depending on the location of obstructive scars. Dystrophic calcification forms commonly in areas of mucosal scarring, or elsewhere in infected renal parenchyma.

Urinary tract TB may present sonographically with any of the following findings, seen in isolation or in combination[1, 26, 44, 45]: (1) calycectasis, pyelocalyectasis, or ureterectasis (depending on the site of scarring/obstruction); (2) papillary or medullary cavitation; (3) cortical scarring; (4) generalized parenchymal thinning (advanced disease); (5) calcification (strong reflections with acoustic shadowing); and (6) a thick-walled, contracted bladder (from scarring). Obviously, these findings are diverse and nonspecific, but TB should be a particular consideration when hydronephrosis and papillary or medullary cavitation are confined to one or a few major calyces (due to infundibular scarring), or when the calyces are diffusely dilated but the renal pelvis is not seen (due to scarring).

Although calcification is a prominent radiographic feature of TB, it is not as easily detected sonographically and usually is not a prominent diagnostic feature. Uncommonly, the granulomatous reaction replaces the renal parenchyma, generating a nonfunctioning "putty" kidney that may appear relatively normal sonographically.

URINARY TRACT CALCULI

Urinary tract calculi are macroscopic aggregates of crystalline material that are precipitated within the major collecting structures (calyces, pelvis, ureter). Fifty to seventy percent of such aggregates contain calcium salts, and the calcium content is sufficient for radiographic visualization in about 85% of cases.[46] Most urinary tract calculi develop in healthy individuals without identifiable precipitating causes. Calculus formation is enhanced, however, by prolonged ingestion of stone-forming substances, diminished urine output (e.g., in hot climates), urine stasis, chronic urinary tract infection, and certain systemic diseases.

Sonographic Findings

Calculi within the urinary tract generate strong ultrasonic reflections and acoustic shadows[47-67] (Fig. 22–9). Shadowing from smaller calculi may be difficult to demonstrate, however[48, 49, 59] (Fig. 22–10). The sonographic properties of renal calculi are unrelated to composition; hence, all calculi are visible sonographically, including those that are not calcified. Ancillary sonographic findings are a hypoechoic halo around the calculus (of undetermined origin), and movement of the calculus if it is contained within a capacious portion of the urinary tract such as the bladder.[59]

Diagnostic Accuracy

Sonographic detection of urinary tract calculi is affected by image quality, calculus size, and echo contrast with surrounding tissues.[47-60] Ultrasound detects 80% to 90% of calculi located in the kidney and virtually 100% of calculi in the distal ureter (behind or in the wall of the bladder).[52, 57] These excellent detection rates are attributed to good visualization and excellent echo contrast between the calculus and its surroundings. The sonographic detection rate is only about 65%, however, for calculi located *anywhere* in the urinary tract (kidney, renal pelvis,

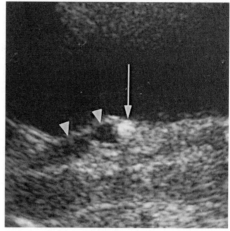

Figure 22-10—Distal Ureteral Calculus. A longitudinal sonogram in a patient with acute renal colic shows dilatation of the intramural portion of the ureter (arrowheads), caused by an obstructing calculus (arrow) at the ureterovesical junction. An acoustic shadow is only minimally visible distal to the calculus, due to the small size of the calculus and its location.

or ureter), and it is as low as 40% for calculi *anywhere* in the ureters.[53-57]

False-positive sonographic diagnoses of calculi are said to occur in about 10% of urinary tract examinations.[59-67] These occur when various structures are mistaken for calculi, including arterial calcifications, gas bubbles, small echogenic masses, milk of calcium, and papillary necrosis. With respect to papillary necrosis, note that the papillae may be highly echogenic during the initial ischemic stage of papillary necrosis. Later, the sloughed papillae may again be quite echogenic when surrounded by urine within the dilated medullary cavity.

Clinical Applications

It has been suggested that ultrasound and an abdominal radiograph are sufficient for assessment of patients with acute renal colic,[68, 69] but this is not a universally held opinion. In my opinion, there are four principal situations in which ultrasound may be useful for the diagnosis of urinary tract calculi: (1) as a means for detecting *distal* ureteral calculi in patients with acute renal colic (Fig. 22–10); (2) for assistance during or following shock wave lithotripsy; (3) for differentiating between nonopaque calculi and soft tissue masses; and (4) to search for renal calculi in nonfunctioning kidneys and when urography is contraindicated (e.g., renal failure, history of contrast reaction, or in pregnancy).

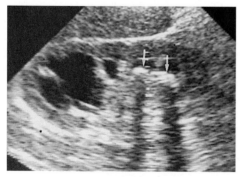

Figure 22-9—Renal Calculi. A longitudinal view of this right kidney demonstrates several large calculi (arrows) within collecting structures. Note that these are strongly echogenic and cast prominent acoustic shadows. The kidney is hydronephrotic.

NEPHROCALCINOSIS

Nephrocalcinosis[70-84] refers to the deposition of calcium salts within the renal tissues, usually in the form of microscopic aggregates. Nephrocalcinosis most commonly occurs in the medullary pyramids, but calcium salts also may be deposited in the renal cortex—either exclusive of, or in conjunction with, medullary calcification. A host of diseases (e.g., hypervitaminosis D, hypercalcemia, hypercalciuria, renal tubular acidosis, and medullary sponge kidney) may cause nephrocalcinosis on a primary or secondary basis. One condition, however, has become particularly common in recent years: furosemide-induced nephrocalcinosis in premature infants receiving intensive care.

Nephrocalcinosis most commonly affects the renal medulla; therefore, the classic sonographic finding is *striking echogenicity of the medullary pyramids* in an otherwise normal kidney (Fig. 22–11). In rare instances, the cortex may be affected and the pyramids spared, or both the cortex and medulla may be strongly echogenic (according to the distribution of calcification). Acoustic shadowing is not a prominent finding, since the individual calcifications are extremely small (often microscopic) and are interspersed among soft tissue elements that transmit ultrasound. Sonography is the primary means for detecting nephrocalcinosis as it is vastly more sensitive to microscopic calcification than is radiography.

Disorders other than nephrocalcinosis may cause "bright" pyramids. These include renal tubular urate deposition (hyperuricemia), protein deposition (e.g., Tamm-Horsfall protein in acute renal failure), vascular congestion (e.g., sickle cell disease), acute papillary necrosis, and medullary fibrosis. The sonographic findings in these conditions may be indistinguishable from those of nephrocalcinosis.

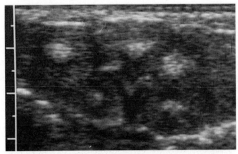

Figure 22-11—Nephrocalcinosis (26 week gestational age infant in a neonatal intensive care patient). A longitudinal sonogram of the left kidney demonstrates strongly echogenic but nonshadowing renal pyramids. The right kidney had a similar appearance.

REFERENCES

1. Goldman SM, Fishman EK: Upper urinary tract infection: The current role of CT, ultrasound, and MRI. Semin Ultrasound CT MR 12:335–361, 1991.
2. Dinkel E, Orth S, Dittrich M, Schulte-Wissermann H: Renal sonography in the differentiation of upper from lower urinary tract infection. AJR Am J Roentgenol 146:775–780, 1986.
3. Sty JR, Wells RG, Starshak RJ, Schroeder BA: Imaging in acute renal infection in children. AJR Am J Roentgenol 148:471–477, 1987.
4. Morehouse HT, Weiner SN, Hoffman JC: Imaging in inflammatory disease of the kidney. AJR Am J Roentgenol 143:135–141, 1984.
5. Gold RP, McClennan BL, Rottenberg RR: CT appearance of acute inflammatory disease of the renal interstitium. AJR Am J Roentgenol 141:343–349, 1983.
6. Edell SL, Bonavita JA: The sonographic appearance of acute pyelonephritis. Radiology 132:683–685, 1979.
7. Björgvinsson E, Massoud M, Eggli KD: Diagnosis of acute pyelonephritis in children: Comparison of sonography and ^{99m}Tc-DMSA scintigraphy. AJR Am J Roentgenol 157:539–543, 1991.
8. Soulen MC, Fishman EK, Goldman SM, Gatewood OMB: Bacterial renal infection: Role of CT. Radiology 171:703–707, 1989.
9. Nicolet V, Carignan L, Dubuc G, Hébert G, Bourdon F, Paquin F: Thickening of the renal collecting system: A nonspecific finding at US. Radiology 168:411–413, 1988.
10. Avni EF, Van Gansbeke D, Thoua Y, Matos C, Marconi V, Lemaitre L, Schulman CC: US demonstration of pyelitis and ureteritis in children. Pediatr Radiol 18:134–139, 1988.
11. Hoddick W, Jeffrey RB, Goldbert HI, Federle MP, Laing FC: CT and sonography of severe renal and perirenal infections. AJR Am J Roentgenol 140:517–520, 1983.
12. Kuligowska E, Newman B, White SJ, Caldarone A: Interventional ultrasound in detection and treatment of renal inflammatory disease. Radiology 147:521–526, 1983.
13. June CH, Browning MD, Smith LP, Wenzel DJ, Pyatt RS, Checchio LM, Amis ES: Ultrasonography and computed tomography in severe urinary tract infection. Arch Intern Med 145:841–845, 1985.
14. Rosenfield AT, Glickman MG, Taylor KJW, Crade M, Hodson J: Acute focal bacterial nephritis (acute lobar nephronia). Radiology 132:553–561, 1979.
15. Lee JKT, McClennan BL, Melson GL, Stanley RJ: Acute focal bacterial nephritis: Emphasis on gray scale sonography and computed tomography. AJR Am J Roentgenol 135:87–92, 1980.
16. Rigsby CM, Rosenfield AT, Glickman MG, Hodson J: Hemorrhagic focal bacterial nephritis: Findings on gray-scale sonography and CT. AJR Am J Roentgenol 146:1173–1177, 1986.
17. Lang EK: Renal, perirenal, and pararenal abscesses: Percutaneous drainage. Radiology 174:109–113, 1990.
18. Deyoe LA, Cronan JJ, Lambiase RE, Dorfman GS: Percutaneous drainage of renal and perirenal abscesses: Results in 30 patients. AJR Am J Roentgenol 155:81–83, 1990.
19. Allen HA, Walsh JW, Brewer WH, Vick CW, Haynes JW: Sonography of emphysematous pyelonephritis. J Ultrasound Med 3:533–537, 1984.

20. Balsara VJ, Raval B, Maklad NF: Emphysematous pyelonephritis in a renal transplant: Sonographic and computed tomographic features. J Ultrasound Med 4:97–99, 1985.

21. Cook DJ, Achong MR, Dobranowski J: Emphysematous pyelonephritis complicates urinary tract infection in diabetes. Diabetes Care 12:229–232, 1989.

22. Coleman BG, Arger PH, Mulhern CB, Pollack HM, Banner MP: Pyonephrosis: Sonography in the diagnosis and management. AJR Am J Roentgenol 137:939–943, 1981.

23. Yoder IC, Pfister RC, Lindfors KK, Newhouse JH: Pyonephrosis: Imaging and intervention. AJR Am J Roentgenol 141:735–740, 1983.

24. Subramanyam BR, Raghavendra BN, Bosniak MA, Lefleur RS, Rosen RJ, Horii SC: Sonography of pyonephrosis: A prospective study. AJR Am J Roentgenol 140:991–993, 1983.

25. Jeffrey RB, Laing FC, Wing VW, Hoddick W: Sensitivity of sonography in pyonephrosis: A reevaluation. AJR Am J Roentgenol 144:71–73, 1985.

26. Kenney PJ: Imaging of chronic renal infections. AJR Am J Roentgenol 155:485–494, 1990.

27. Hodson CJ: Reflux nephropathy: A personal historical review. AJR Am J Roentgenol 137:451–462, 1981.

28. Hayden CK, Swischuk LE, Fawcett HD, Rytting JE, McCord G: Urinary tract infections in childhood: A current imaging approach. RadioGraphics 6:1023–1038, 1986.

29. Jequier S, Forbes PA, Nogrady MB: The value of ultrasonography as a screening procedure in a first-documented urinary tract infection in children. J Ultrasound Med 4:393–400, 1985.

30. Kessler RM, Altman DH: Real-time sonographic detection of vesicoureteral reflux in children. AJR Am J Roentgenol 138:1033–1036, 1982.

31. Mason WG: Urinary tract infections in children: Renal ultrasound evaluation. Radiology 153:109–111, 1984.

32. Leonidas JC, McCauley RGK, Klauber GC, Fretzayas AM: Sonography as a substitute for excretory urography in children with urinary tract infection. AJR Am J Roentgenol 144:815–819, 1985.

33. Kangarloo H, Gold RH, Fine RN, Diament MJ, Boechat MI: Urinary tract infection in infants and children evaluated by ultrasound. Radiology 154:367–373, 1985.

34. Strife JL, Bisset GS, Kirks DR, Schlueter FJ, Gelfand MJ, Babcock DS, Han BK: Nuclear cystography and renal sonography: Findings in girls with urinary tract infection. AJR Am J Roentgenol 153:115–119, 1989.

35. Bisset GS, Strife JL, Dunbar JS: The voiding cystourethrogram—is it necessary in the evaluation of the female child with urinary tract infection? Presented at the 28th Annual Meeting of the Society for Pediatric Radiology, Boston, April 1985.

36. Lebowitz RL: The detection of vesicoureteral reflux in the child. Invest Radiol 21:519–531, 1986.

37. Zerin ML: Hydronephrosis in the neonate and young infant: Current concepts. Semin Ultrasound CT MR 15:306–316, 1994.

38. Stuck KJ, Silver TM, Jaffe MH, Bowerman RA: Sonographic demonstration of renal fungus balls. Radiology 142:473–474, 1981.

39. Schmitt GH, Hsu AS: Renal fungus balls: Diagnosis by ultrasound and percutaneous antegrade pyelography and brush biopsy in a premature infant. J Ultrasound Med 4:155–156, 1985.

40. Kintanar C, Cramer BC, Reid WD, Andrews WL: Neonatal renal candidiasis: Sonographic diagnosis. AJR Am J Roentgenol 147:801–805, 1986.

41. Berman LH, Stringer DA, St Onge O, Daneman A, Whyte H: An assessment of sonography in the diagnosis and management of neonatal renal candidiasis. Clin Radiol 40:577–581, 1989.

42. Van Kirk OC, Go RT, Wedel VJ: Sonographic features of xanthogranulomatous pyelonephritis. AJR Am J Roentgenol 134:1035–1039, 1980.

43. Hartman DS, Davis CJ, Goldman SM, Isbister SS, Sanders RC: Xanthogranulomatous pyelonephritis: Sonographic-pathologic correlation of 16 cases. J Ultrasound Med 3:481–488, 1984.

44. Premkumar A, Lattimer J, Newhouse JH: CT and sonography of advanced urinary tract tuberculosis. AJR Am J Roentgenol 148:65–69, 1987.

45. Scott F, Engelbrecht HE: Ultrasonography of the advanced tuberculous kidney. S Afr Med J 75:371–372, 1989.

46. Jones DB: Kidneys. In Kissane JM (ed): Anderson's Pathology. 8th ed. St Louis, CV Mosby, 1985, pp 765–767.

47. Stafford SJ, Jenkins JM, Staab EV, Boyce I, Fried FA: Ultrasonic detection of renal calculi: Accuracy tested in an in vitro porcine kidney model. J Clin Ultrasound 9:359–363, 1981.

48. King W, Kimme-Smith C, Winter J: Renal stone shadowing: An investigation of contributing factors. Radiology 154:191–196, 1985.

49. Kimme-Smith C, Perrella RR, Kaveggia LP, Cochran S, Grant EG: Detection of renal stones with real-time sonography: Effect of transducers and scanning parameters. AJR Am J Roentgenol 157:975–980, 1991.

50. Pollack HM, Arger PH, Goldberg BB, Mulholland SG: Ultrasonic detection of nonopaque renal calculi. Radiology 127:233–237, 1978.

51. Brennan RE, Curtis JA, Kurtz AB, Dalton JR: Use of tomography and ultrasound in the diagnosis of nonopaque renal calculi. JAMA 244:594–596, 1980.

52. Middleton WD, Dodds WJ, Lawson TL, Foley WD: Renal calculi: Sensitivity for detection with US. Radiology 167:239–244, 1988.

53. Erwin BC, Carroll BA, Sommer FG: Renal colic: The role of ultrasound in initial evaluation. Radiology 152:147–150, 1984.

54. Hill MC, Rich JI, Mardiat JG, Finder CA: Sonography vs. excretory urography in acute flank pain. AJR Am J Roentgenol 144:1235–1238, 1985.

55. Lerner RM, Rubens D: Distal ureteral calculi: Diagnosis by transrectal sonography. AJR Am J Roentgenol 147:1189–1191, 1986.

56. Omnishi K, Watanabe H, Ohe H, Saitoh M: Ultrasound findings in urolithiasis in the lower ureter. Ultrasound Med Biol 12:577–579, 1986.

57. Baumgartner BR, Steinberg HV, Ambrose SS, Walton KN, Bernardino ME: Sonographic evaluation of renal stones treated by extracorporeal shock-wave lithotripsy. AJR Am J Roentgenol 149:131–135, 1987.

58. Kaude JV, Williams JL, Wright PG, Bush D, Derau C, Newman RC: Sonographic evaluation of the kidney following extracorporeal shock wave lithotripsy. J Ultrasound Med 6:299–306, 1987.

59. Neisius D, Moll V: Renal ultrasonography in the management of calculus disease. Urol Clin North Am 16:829–840, 1989.

60. Watson LR, Abbitt PL, Jenkins AD: Adjunctive use

of ultrasonography in the management of kidney stones treated by ESWL. Appl Radiol April:19–23, 1990.

61. Gould RJ, Rochester D, Panella JS: Sonographic demonstration of renal arterial calcification simulating multiple renal calculi. Urology 25:330–331, 1985.

62. Kane RA, Manco LG: Renal arterial calcification simulating nephrolithiasis on sonography. AJR Am J Roentgenol 140:101–104, 1983.

63. Jacobs RP, Kane RA: Sonographic appearance of calculi in renal calyceal diverticula. J Clin Ultrasound 12:289–291, 1984.

64. Patriquin H, Lafortune M, Filiatrault D: Urinary milk of calcium in children and adults: Use of gravity-dependent sonography. AJR Am J Roentgenol 144:407–413, 1985.

65. Hernanz-Schulman M: Hyperechoic renal medullary pyramids in infants and children. Radiology 181:9–11, 1991.

66. Braden GL, Kozinn DR, Hampf FE, Parker TH, Germain MJ: Ultrasound diagnosis of early renal papillary necrosis. J Ultrasound Med 10:401–403, 1991.

67. Dillard JP, Tainer LB, Pinckney L: Normal renal papillae simulating caliceal filling defects on sonography. AJR Am J Roentgenol 148:895–896, 1987.

68. Haddad MC, Sharif HS, Shahed MS, et al: Renal colic: Diagnosis and outcome. Radiology 184:83–88, 1992.

69. Choyke PL: The urogram: Are rumors of its death premature? Radiology 184:33–36, 1992.

70. Cacciarelli AA, Young N, Levine AJ: Gray-scale ultrasonic demonstration of nephrocalcinosis. Radiology 128:459–460, 1978.

71. Shuman WP, Mack LA, Rogers JV: Diffuse nephrocalcinosis: Hyperechoic sonographic appearance. AJR Am J Roentgenol 136:830–832, 1981.

72. Glazer GM, Callen PW, Filly RA: Medullary nephrocalcinosis: Sonographic evaluation. AJR Am J Roentgenol 138:55–57, 1982.

73. Brennan JN, Diwan RV, Makker SP, Cromer BA, Bellon EM: Ultrasonic diagnosis of primary hyperoxaluria in infancy. Radiology 145:147–148, 1982.

74. Pearse DM, Kaude JV, Williams JL, Bush D, Wright PG: Sonographic diagnosis of furosemide-induced nephrocalcinosis in newborn infants. J Ultrasound Med 3:553–556, 1984.

75. Martino CR, Pakter RL, Schultz CL, Andriole J, Ling A: Small, dense kidneys in a 7-year-old. Presented at the 16th Annual Symposium of the Association of Academic Radiologists and Chief Radiology Residents, Newport Beach, California, May 8, 1984.

76. Gilsanz V, Fernal W, Reid BS, Stanley P, Ramos A: Nephrolithiasis in premature infants. Radiology 154:107–110, 1985.

77. Patriquin HB, O'Reagan S: Medullary sponge kidney in childhood. AJR Am J Roentgenol 145:315–319, 1985.

78. Schumacher R, Klingmüller V, Reither M: Stellenwert der Sonographie gegenuber Röntgen und Computertomographie bei der Diagnose von Nephrokalzinosen. Röfo Fortschr Geb Rontgenstr Neuen Bildgeb Verfahr 141:75–79, 1984.

79. Weber M, Braun B, Köhler H: Ultrasonic findings in analgesic nephropathy. Nephron 39:216–222, 1985.

80. Falkoff GE, Rigsby CM, Rosenfield AT: Partial, combined cortical and medullary nephrocalcinosis: US and CT patterns in AIDS-associated MAI infection. Radiology 162:343–344, 1987.

81. Ginalski JM, Portmann L, Jaeger P: Does medullary sponge kidney cause nephrolithiasis? AJR Am J Roentgenol 155:299–302, 1990.

82. Kraus RA, Gaisie G, Young LW: Increased renal parenchymal echogenicity: Causes in pediatric patients. RadioGraphics 10:1009–1018, 1990.

83. Jequier S, Kaplan BS: Echogenic renal pyramids in children. J Clin Ultrasound 19:85–92, 1991.

84. Shultz PK, Strife JL, Strife CF, McDaniel JD: Hyperechoic renal medullary pyramids in infants and children. Radiology 181:163–167, 1991.

Chapter 23

Bladder Pathology

William J. Zwiebel

Ultrasound provides valuable information about urinary bladder pathology, because the urinary bladder is readily visualized sonographically. The normal features of the urinary bladder are presented in Chapter 16.

URINE RETENTION

The retention of an abnormally large volume of urine after attempted voiding may result from bladder outlet obstruction or neurologic dysfunction. Imaging studies generally do not differentiate well between these causes of urine retention, and ultrasound is no exception. Nonetheless, ultrasound is an excellent method for *detecting* urine retention and *quantifying* the severity of the problem. Several calculations have been proposed for estimating the volume of (retained) urine within the bladder,[1, 2] but the following calculation, which is relatively simple, is accurate to within 15% of catheter-measured volume:[1]

$$\text{Volume} = (\text{length} \times \text{width} \times \text{height}) / 0.5$$

This formula is a commonly used method for estimating the volume of an ellipsoid. The measurement points are illustrated in Figure 16–14.

DIFFUSE WALL THICKENING

Diffuse thickening of the bladder wall may be caused by inflammation, muscular hypertrophy, or neoplasia. In most cases, sonographic findings do not effectively differentiate among these causes, however. The bladder wall is considered to be abnormally thick (Fig. 23–1) when it measures more than 3 mm from the lumen to the adventitia (the bright outer layer). The mucosa and muscular layers tend to blend together; hence, it may not be possible to differentiate between mucosal and muscular abnormalities with ultrasound. The wall of an empty bladder always appears thick, so the bladder must be reasonably well distended for assessing wall thickness.

Hypertrophy of the muscular layer is caused by attempted emptying against an obstructed bladder outlet.[3] Muscular hypertrophy commonly produces localized bandlike thickening, in addition to more generalized thickening. The localized bands, which are called trabeculae, are visible sonographically as longitudinal ridges in the bladder wall. Alternatively, if the image plane cuts across a trabecular ridge, the ultrasound appearance may mimic a focal mass, as shown in Figure 23–2.

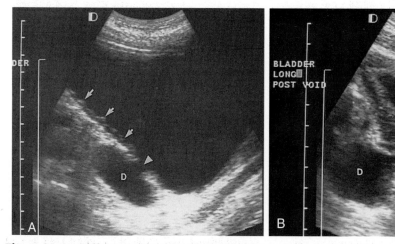

Figure 23-1—Diffuse Bladder Wall Thickening (34 year old man with bladder outlet obstruction). **(A)** The bladder wall (arrows) is visibly thickened (5 mm), even though the bladder is well distended. A diverticulum (D) is visible on this longitudinal view. The arrowhead marks the communication between the diverticulum and the bladder. **(B)** Wall thickening is very striking on this postvoid film in the same patient (calculated residual volume: 150 ml). The diverticulum (D) does not empty with voiding.

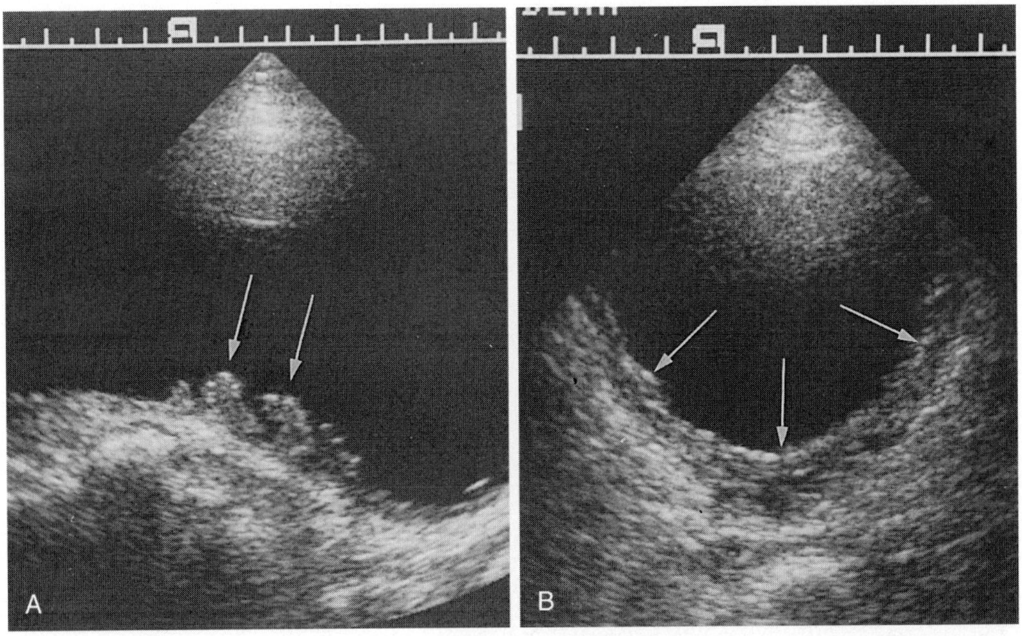

Figure 23-2—Trabeculation. (A) This view shows a series of frondlike excrescences projecting into the bladder lumen (arrows), suggesting inflammation or neoplasia. (B) A scan 90 degrees to **A** shows that the fronds are in fact a series of ridges (only one is shown here, arrows). These muscular ridges (trabeculae) resulted from bladder outlet obstruction.

Inflammation of the bladder wall, or cystitis, is usually caused by infection. In most patients with acute cystitis the bladder wall is normal sonographically. Visible abnormality is much more common with chronic inflammation and usually consists of nonspecific, diffuse wall thickening.

FOCAL WALL THICKENING

Focal thickening of the bladder wall may result from inflammation, from neoplasia, or, uncommonly, from endometriosis. In general, these conditions are indistinguishable sonographically, which is problematic since focal inflammatory masses may be regarded as tumors out of hand, without consideration of inflammation as a cause.

Focal inflammation may produce localized wall thickening or a polypoid mass that projects into the bladder lumen (Fig. 23–3). The surface of the mass often is irregular, further mimicking the appearance of an epithelial neoplasm. The mass may be homogeneous sonographically, or it may have a "cystic" appearance. The latter finding suggests bullous cystitis, a chronic form of bladder inflammation associated with the formation of fluid-filled bullae within the wall. Focal inflammatory thickening may be accompanied by generalized (but less severe) wall thickening as well as intraluminal inflammatory debris.[3–8]

Ectopic endometrial tissue implanted on the serosal surface of the bladder in patients with endometriosis (Chapter 31) occasionally penetrates the bladder wall and protrudes into the bladder lumen.[3, 13, 14] Alternatively, the endometrial tissue may incite the formation of a focal inflammatory mass, as illustrated in Figure 23–3.

Transitional cell carcinoma is by far the most common neoplasm[3, 9–12, 15] that originates in the bladder wall. Other bladder neoplasms are almost invariably metastatic and usually enter the bladder by direct extension (e.g., rectal, prostate,

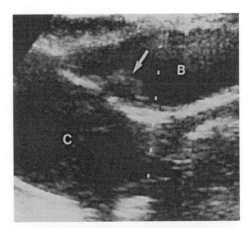

Figure 23-3—Focal Inflammatory Mass. A longitudinal scan shows a mass of tissue (arrow) projecting into the bladder lumen (B). A large, endometriosis-related chocolate cyst (C) is seen adjacent to the bladder. The initial diagnosis was endometriosis invading the bladder wall, but an inflammatory process called cystitis cystica was diagnosed via cystoscopic biopsy.

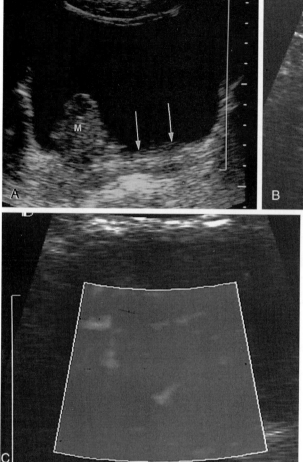

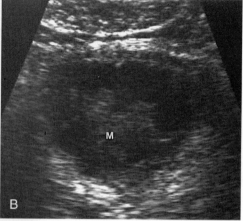

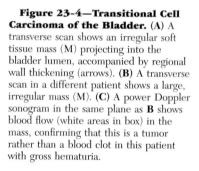

Figure 23-4—Transitional Cell Carcinoma of the Bladder. (A) A transverse scan shows an irregular soft tissue mass (M) projecting into the bladder lumen, accompanied by regional wall thickening (arrows). **(B)** A transverse scan in a different patient shows a large, irregular mass (M). **(C)** A power Doppler sonogram in the same plane as **B** shows blood flow (white areas in box) in the mass, confirming that this is a tumor rather than a blood clot in this patient with gross hematuria.

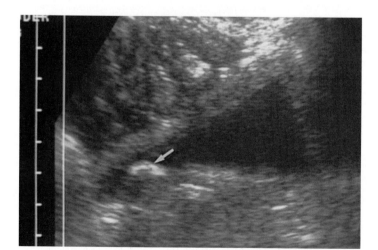

Figure 23-5—Bladder Calculus. A longitudinal sonogram shows a large calculus (arrow) in the dependent portion of the bladder.

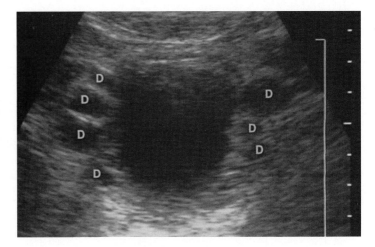

Figure 23-6—Diverticula. Multiple diverticula (D) are seen on this transverse scan in a patient with chronic bladder outlet obstruction.

uterine, and ovarian carcinomas). Transitional cell carcinoma may cause regional thickening of the bladder wall or a polypoid mass that projects into the bladder lumen (Fig. 23–4). Tumor echogenicity and "texture" are variable. Bulky bladder tumors commonly have an irregular, poorly marginated intraluminal border. Color Doppler demonstration of blood flow in the mass differentiates between tumor and intraluminal thrombi, which are indistinguishable otherwise.

Tumor extension to the bladder wall from an adjacent pelvic organ typically is quite apparent as the bladder wall findings are accompanied by a mass outside the bladder. With large masses, it may be impossible to tell whether the tumor originated outside the bladder and spread in, or vice versa.

EMPHYSEMATOUS CYSTITIS

Emphysematous cystitis refers to infection of the bladder with a gas-forming organism, causing gas bubbles to form within the bladder wall or lumen. The result, from a sonographic perspective, is unusually strong echogenicity of the bladder wall, typically accompanied by wall thickening. Acoustic shadows may be present if the gas bubbles are sufficiently large, but shadows are absent when the bubbles are microscopic. Calcium within the bladder wall may mimic the appearance of emphysematous cystitis, but calcium and gas are easily differentiated radiographically. Gas that accumulates *within* the bladder lumen produces strong reflections in a *supernatant* location, accompanied by distal acoustic shadows. Intraluminal gas is very uncommon in patients with cystitis; therefore, when gas is seen in the bladder lumen, think first of other causes such as bowel fistulization, vaginal fistulization, and especially catheterization or other types of instrumentation.

BLADDER CALCULI

Bladder calculi[3, 7, 16, 17] generally occur in the presence of urine stasis, chronic infection, or chronic use of an indwelling catheter. Symptomatic bladder calculi are usually quite large (2 cm or more) and have characteristic ultrasound features: strong, arcuate surface reflections, prominent acoustic shadows, and movement with altered patient position (Fig. 23–5). Small, gravel-like calculi are less obvious and may produce dependent echoes resembling other debris.

BLADDER DIVERTICULA

Bladder diverticula are thin-walled mucosal sacs that protrude through the muscular wall of the bladder into the peritoneal space. Although congenital diverticula occur, they are uncommon, and most bladder diverticula result from recurrent contraction of the bladder against an obstructed outlet. Bladder diverticula present sonographically as intramural or extravesicular fluid collections (Figs. 23–2, 23–6). If the "neck" that connects the diverticulum with the bladder lumen is visible, then the diagnosis is obvious. If the neck is not visible, an extravesicular diverticulum is indistinguishable from a pelvic cyst, abscess, or other pelvic fluid collections.[3]

REFERENCES

1. Kiely EA, Hartnell GG, Gibson RN, Williams G: Measurement of bladder volume by real-time ultrasound. Br J Urol 60:33–35, 1987.
2. Griffiths CJ, Murray A, Ramsden PD: Accuracy and repeatability of bladder volume measurement using ultrasound imaging. J Urol 136:808–812, 1986.
3. Bree RL, Silver TM: Sonography of bladder and perivesical abnormalities. Am J Roentgenol 136:1101–1104, 1981.
4. Gooding GAW: Varied sonographic manifestations of cystitis. J Ultrasound Med 5:61–63, 1986.

5. Rifkin MD, Kurtz AB, Pasto ME, Goldberg BB: Unusual presentations of cystitis. J Ultrasound Med 2:25–28, 1983.

6. Morley P: The bladder. *In* Rosenfield RT (ed): Genitourinary Ultrasonography. New York, Churchill Livingstone, 1979, p 139.

7. Kauzlaric D, Barmeir E: Sonography of emphysematous cystitis. J Ultrasound Med 4:3189–3200, 1985.

8. Gooding GAW: Sonography of *Candida albicans* cystitis. J Ultrasound Med 8:121–124, 1989.

9. Abu-Yousef MM, Narayana AS, Franken EA, Brown RC: Urinary bladder tumors studied by cystosonography. Part I: Detection. Radiology 153:223–226, 1984.

10. Abu-Yousef MM, Narayana AS, Brown RC, Franken EA: Urinary bladder tumors studied by cystosonography. Part II: Staging. Radiology 153:227–231, 1984.

11. Brun B, Gammelgaard J, Christoffersen J: Transabdominal dynamic ultrasonography in detection of bladder tumors. J Urol 132:19–20, 1984.

12. Fornage BD, Rifkin MD, Lemaire AD, Touche DH: Bladder metastasis of gastric carcinoma: Diagnosis by sonography. J Clin Ultrasound 12:578–580, 1984.

13. Goodman JD, Macchia RJ, Macasaet MA, Schneider M: Endometriosis of the urinary bladder: Sonographic findings. Am J Roentgenol 135:625–626, 1980.

14. Kumar R, Haque AK, Cohen MS: Endometriosis of the urinary bladder: Demonstration by sonography. J Clin Ultrasound 12:363–365, 1984.

15. Bornstein I, Charboneau JW, Hartman GW: Leiomyoma of the bladder: Sonographic and urographic findings. J Ultrasound Med 5:407–408, 1986.

16. Lebowitz RL, Vargas B: Stones in the urinary bladder in children and young adults. Am J Roentgenol 148:491–495, 1987.

17. Pollack HM, Banner MP, Martinez LO, Hodson CJ: Diagnostic considerations in urinary bladder wall calcification. Am J Roentgenol 136:791–797, 1981.

Miscellaneous Abdominal Topics

INTRODUCTION

The preceding chapters have covered the major abdominal applications of diagnostic ultrasound on an organ-by-organ basis. A number of other applications exist that are grouped here as miscellaneous abdominal subjects. The fact that these ultrasound applications are collected under the term "miscellaneous" does not imply that they are unimportant. Included herein are several applications for which ultrasound is the primary diagnostic modality, such as examination of the abdominal wall and aorta, and the diagnosis of appendicitis and pyloric stenosis.

This section is divided into four chapters that cover the following topics: (1) the abdominal survey examination; (2) the abdominal wall; (3) bowel pathology; (4) the peritoneal space, including abscesses and masses; (5) The aorta and iliac arteries; and (6) the adrenal glands.

Chapter 24

The Abdominal Wall, Peritoneal Space, and Adrenal Glands

William J. Zwiebel

THE ABDOMINAL WALL

Ultrasound is an excellent tool for detecting hernias and other lesions of the abdominal wall[1-7] and for determining whether pathologic processes are located in the wall or in the peritoneal space. Accurate diagnosis of abdominal wall disorders requires knowledge of abdominal wall anatomy and a consistent, effective scanning technique.

Anatomy

The structure of the abdominal wall[1-4] is illustrated in Figure 24–1. The appearance of the abdominal wall varies somewhat with the degree of muscular development and the amount of subcutaneous fat, but the major wall components are visible in most individuals. The most crucial wall structure, from a sonographic perspective, is the transversalis fascia, which lies adjacent to the peritoneum (Figs. 24–1, 24–2). This strongly echogenic layer is important, for it serves as an easily recognized marker for the peritoneum. Pathology that is deep to the transversalis fascia is intraperitoneal, and that which is superficial to this fascial layer lies within the abdominal wall. Since the transversalis fascia marks the peritoneum, it is key to the diagnosis of herniation, as discussed later.

The peritoneum also is marked by motion of intraperitoneal contents. With respiration, the abdominal contents move caudad and cephalad, while the abdominal wall remains stationary. Likewise, peristaltic motion is evident in the peritoneal space but not in the abdominal wall.

Examination Technique

Linear or gently curved array transducers are ideal for examining the abdominal wall since they have a large field of view and clearly define structures located close to the skin. The first step in the examination is to get oriented. Transverse scans generally work best for the orienting process, as they effectively display abdominal wall anatomy. Wall anatomy should be scrutinized to the extent that the transversalis/peritoneal interface is clearly identified. If the anatomy of the wall is distorted by pathology, get oriented in another area where the wall is normal, and then move back to the area of pathology. Take advantage of the normal symmetry of the wall to detect pathology!

Abscesses and Hematomas

Ultrasound is a useful means for diagnosis of abdominal wall abscess and for differentiating between abscess and cellulitis. Abdominal wall abscesses[1, 5] vary in appearance. They may be circumscribed and well defined, or they may have irregular borders. The abscess contents may be anechoic, or echogenic debris may be present. Strong reflections and acoustic shadows may be seen in gas-containing collections. Abscesses sometimes originate in the abdominal wall, but they also may spread to the wall from the peritoneal space. It is important, therefore, to define the relationship between the abscess and the transversalis/peritoneal interface. It also is important to look for intraperitoneal pathology associated with a wall abscess, especially bowel wall thickening resulting from Crohn's disease, diverticulitis, or tumors.

Abdominal wall hematomas[1, 6] usually occur in the rectus muscles (Fig. 24–3), but they also may occur elsewhere in the abdominal wall. They may develop "spontaneously" in elderly people, in athletes, in anticoagulated patients, or in any person following an unusual abdominal wall strain. They typically present with acute abdominal pain that may be attributed clinically to intra-abdominal pathology. Very recently formed hematomas are mildly echogenic. With time, thrombus retracts and the hematoma becomes heterogeneous, with highly echogenic thrombus surrounded by anechoic fluid. Eventually the entire collection becomes anechoic as the clot lyses (Chapter 7). Hematomas and abscesses cannot be distinguished sonographically, but clinical differentiation usually is possible. Furthermore, the shape of the collection may suggest one diagnosis

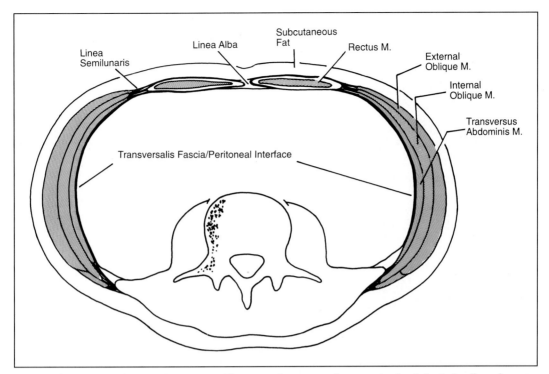

Figure 24-1—Abdominal Wall Anatomy. The principal structures that comprise the abdominal wall are the rectus muscles, the lateral musculature (oblique and transverse muscles), and intervening fascial bands (linea alba and linea semilunaris). The juxtaposed transversalis fascia and peritoneum mark the boundary between the abdominal wall and the peritoneal cavity.

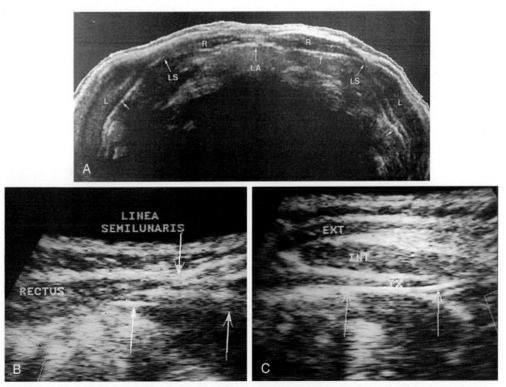

Figure 24-2—Sonographic Anatomy of the Abdominal Wall. (A) A transverse static ultrasound scan shows the rectus muscles (R), the lateral abdominal musculature (L), the linea alba (LA), and the linea semilunaris (LS). The transversalis/peritoneal interface (small arrows) is clearly seen. **(B)** A transverse image shows the lateral border of the rectus muscle and the area of the linea semilunaris. Upward arrows depict the transversalis/peritoneal interface. **(C)** The three layers of the lateral abdominal musculature are clearly visible (EXT = external oblique; INT = internal oblique; TX = transversus abdominis). Arrows depict the location of the transversalis/peritoneal interface.

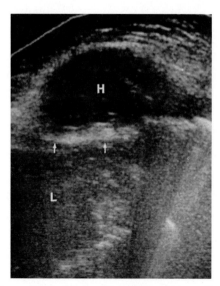

Figure 24-3—Rectus Hematoma (66 year old woman with thrombocytopenia and sudden onset of right upper quadrant abdominal pain 6 hours before examination). This longitudinal sonogram shows a sharply marginated hematoma (H) in the anterior abdominal wall. The hematoma measures 6 cm (maximum) and is lens shaped. Arrows mark the transversalis/peritoneal interface. L, liver.

or another. Blood tends to spread throughout a muscle group until confined by fascial boundaries, and, as a result, hematomas tend to have an elongated or lentiform shape. Abscesses, on the other hand, tend to form as rounded collections.

Neoplasms

Neoplastic masses[1, 7] occur uncommonly in the abdominal wall, with the exception of lipomas (Fig. 24–4). Abdominal wall neoplasms may be primary tumors, hematogenous metastases, or direct metastases from the intra-abdominal tumor. Owing to the latter possibility, it is important to determine whether the mass is localized to the wall or communicates with deeper structures.

Abdominal wall neoplasms generally are hypoechoic relative to other wall structures, but they vary in echogenicity. They also range from sharply delineated to poorly delineated, and from focal to more diffuse. Differentiation among neoplastic masses, inflammatory masses, and scar is not possible sonographically.

Hernia

Bowel or omentum may herniate through defects in the musculofascial layers of the abdominal wall and come to lie between the muscular layers, within the subcutaneous fat, or within inguinal structures.[1-4] Hernias commonly are classified as reducible, incarcerated, or strangulated. A hernia is said to be reducible when its contents return to the peritoneal space in response to manual pressure, altered patient position, or changes in intra-abdominal pressure. If the hernia cannot be reduced, the contents are described as incarcerated. The contents of an incarcerated hernia may suffer "strangulation" if the vessels are entrapped or undergo torsion. The result may be ischemia or infarction of the hernia contents.

The clinical diagnosis of abdominal wall herniation usually is an easy matter, and, in such cases, sonography does not have a diagnostic role. In some instances, however, the clinical diagnosis may be uncertain. For example, a "bulge" at the site of a surgical incision may be caused by weakening of the wall or frank herniation through a musculofascial defect. The former usually is innocuous, but the latter could lead to strangulation of bowel. A second example is an obese patient with unexplained abdominal pain. Sonography can determine whether or not the pain is related to occult herniation.

Herniation in the inguinal area is very common and is usually diagnosed clinically. Occasionally, however, ultrasound is useful for differentiating between a hernia and other pathology, such as a solid mass, and for confirming that scrotal enlargement is due to herniation. In such cases, echogenic omentum or peristaltic bowel is present in the hernia contents. Differential problems can occur if the herniated bowel is strangulated

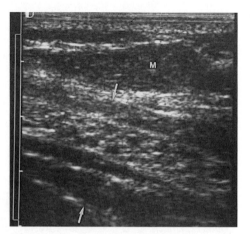

Figure 24-4—Abdominal Wall Lipoma. A 3-cm long, hypoechoic mass (M) is evident in the abdominal wall in this patient with an asymptomatic palpable mass. The echogenicity of the mass is identical to that of adjacent subcutaneous fat. The mass clearly is outside the wall musculature (between arrows).

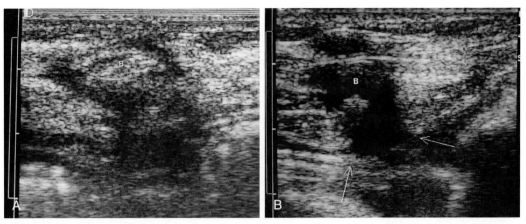

Figure 24-5—Bowel Herniation (30 year old man 5 years after renal allograft with pain superior to the graft and a vague, palpable fullness). **(A)** Bowel (B) is present in the abdominal wall. **(B)** An adjacent image shows a defect (arrows) in the transversalis/peritoneal interface through which the bowel (B) herniated. The location of the defect corresponded with the renal transplantation incision.

and aperistaltic, in which case the dilated bowel loops may appear as nonspecific fluid collections.

Inguinal hernias that extend well into the scrotal sac (following the spermatic cord) are usually so-called "direct" hernias, but "indirect" inguinal hernias may have a similar appearance. Femoral hernias, furthermore, may be confused with either type of inguinal hernia. Differentiation is based on the relationship of the hernia neck to the inferior epigastric vessels and the femoral vessels. Ultrasound does not function well for classifying inguinal hernias; computed tomography is the preferred diagnostic method.[2]

Abdominal wall herniation outside the inguinal area is readily evaluated sonographically (Figs. 24–5, 24–6), but two diagnostic findings are key to accurate diagnosis: (1) the demonstration of bowel or omentum *extrinsic* to the peritoneal cavity, and (2) the detection of an actual *defect* in the transversalis/peritoneal layer. A "bulge" in a weakened portion of the abdominal wall may

mimic herniation, since the abdominal contents seem to project outside of the peritoneal cavity. Herniation, however, implies that the abdominal contents have in fact left the abdominal cavity and are *extraperitoneal,* within the wall. This distinction can be made only through demonstration of a gap in the transversalis layer, and such a gap must be carefully documented.

Herniation of abdominal contents often is intermittent and commonly occurs only with straining, lifting, or other maneuvers that increase abdominal pressure. It is imperative, therefore, to reproduce the conditions that cause signs or symptoms of herniation. For example, if lifting causes symptoms, then have the patient attempt to lift the ultrasound machine!

Urachal Abnormalities

The urachus is a vestigial, midline structure that persists in the anterior abdominal wall in some individuals. Cysts, abscesses, sinuses, and fistulas may develop from a persistent urachus, as described in Chapter 17.

THE PERITONEAL SPACES

Note that the term "spaces" is used in the above subtitle. There are, in fact, several peritoneal spaces, all of which communicate with one another.* In this chapter, we consider only the lesser and greater peritoneal spaces.[8–12] The lesser peritoneal space, which also is called the lesser sac, lies roughly posterior to the body of the stomach and anterior to the pancreas (Fig.

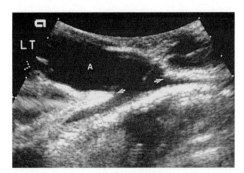

Figure 24-6—Hernia Containing Ascites. A defect (arrows) is clearly visible in the abdominal wall at the incision site of this postoperative patient. Ascites (A) is present in the incision as well as in the abdominal cavity.

---

*For further information, see the excellent articles by Weill et al[8] and Dodds et al.[9]

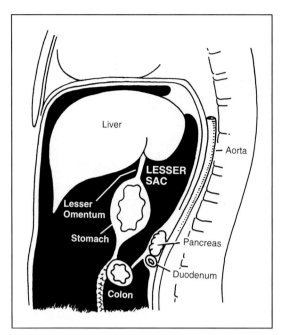

Figure 24-7—Lesser Peritoneal Space. The location of the lesser peritoneal space (lesser sac) is illustrated on this sagittal section of the abdomen.

24–7). This space is "lesser" because it is relatively small and contains no viscera, compared with the "major" peritoneal space, which is much larger and contains the bowel and other abdominal organs. The only communication between the lesser and greater peritoneal spaces is an opening a fingerwidth in diameter, called the foramen of Winslow, that lies adjacent to the second portion of the duodenum.

The most noteworthy aspect of the lesser sac is that it usually is empty, or nearly so, even when ascites is present in the greater peritoneal space. The presence of lesser sac fluid should bring to mind two forms of pathology. The first is *significant nearby disease,* particularly pancreatitis, or complications of gastric ulcer, such as abscess. The second is peritoneal carcinomatosis, which causes malignant ascites. The ordinary transudative form of ascites (e.g., from hepatocellular disease) does not usually enter the lesser sac unless the quantity of ascites is massive.[10–12]

Ascites

Pathologic fluid *dispersed* within the peritoneal space is called ascites.[10–23] This fluid may be a transudate (acellular and low in protein), as in hepatocellular disease, renal failure, or "third space" fluid disorders; or an exudate, as in peritonitis or peritoneal carcinomatosis. A second important type of fluid may be found in the perito-

neal space: blood. Blood may accumulate and move freely in the peritoneal space in trauma patients with ruptured viscera, in patients with ectopic pregnancy, and less commonly in other conditions leading to visceral rupture.[19, 20]

Sonography is quite sensitive to the presence of peritoneal fluid. As little as 100 ml may be detected in adults,[14] but a more realistic minimum volume probably lies between 100 and 300 ml.[15, 16] Because of its sensitivity, ultrasound is an excellent modality for detecting intraperitoneal hemorrhage, and it is used increasingly for detecting free peritoneal blood in trauma patients.[20] Ultrasound is also an excellent medium for differentiating between ascites and other causes of abdominal distention, such as dilated bowel.

Large volumes of intraperitoneal fluid are easily seen with ultrasound (Fig. 24–8), but smaller amounts may be detected only if the sonographer knows where to look (i.e., knows where fluid is likely to collect).[13, 17, 18] The most dependent part of the peritoneal space, with the patient supine, is the pelvic cavity; hence, the pelvis is a good location to look for ascites. The next most likely location is along the lateral or anterior aspect of the liver. (Don't forget to look anterior to the left lobe as well as the right.) The next most common locations are Morison's pouch (between the kidney and the right lobe of the liver) and the right paracolic gutter.

Transudative ascites is echo-free (Fig. 24–8), but exudative ascites, containing cells or proteinaceous debris, may be echogenic. In the latter case, the echoes may be fine grained or coarse, depending on the amount of material suspended in the fluid.[21–23] Fine fibrinous strands sometimes form in ascites (Fig. 24–9). On ultrasound exami-

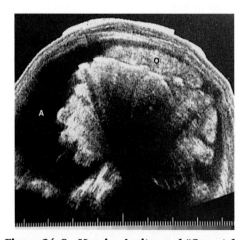

Figure 24-8—Massive Ascites and "Omental Cake." A transverse static scan shows massive ascites (A), with bowel "floating" centrally, in this patient with anaplastic lung cancer. Extensive tumor infiltration of the omentum (O) (omental cake) also is visible.

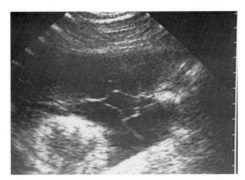

Figure 24-9—Strands Within Ascites. Delicate membranous strands traverse malignant ascites (image of left upper quadrant of the abdomen).

nation, these thin, echogenic bands wave back and forth with respiration or other movement. Fibrinous bands *suggest* that the fluid is exudative, but this is not a specific finding. Blood in the peritoneal cavity is faintly echogenic, due to the reflectivity of red blood cells. One should always think of hemorrhage when echogenic pelvic fluid is seen in a patient with pelvic pain (Chapter 36 [OB ectopic]).

Free Versus Loculated Peritoneal Fluid

Four features differentiate between free fluid, such as ascites (Fig. 24–8), and loculated fluid, such as an abscess (Fig. 24–10): (1) free fluid "insinuates itself" among bowel loops and other abdominal viscera; (2) it can be displaced with pressure; (3) its location changes when the pa-

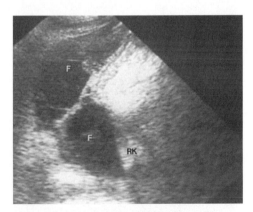

Figure 24-10—Peritoneal Abscess (postcholecystectomy). A walled-off, loculated fluid collection (F) is present in the right paracolic gutter, adjacent to the right kidney (RK). This collection somewhat resembles loculated ascites, as shown in Figure 24–9; however, the septa are thick and irregular, and the fluid is echogenic. Most important, this collection was localized, displaced surrounding viscera, and could not be displaced by changing the patient's position.

tient moves; and (4) it has no "mass effect." Loculated fluid, on the other hand, is confined, cannot be displaced with patient motion, and may exhibit mass effect if the collection is large. The differential possibilities are broad for loculated peritoneal fluid collections,[17–31] as indicated in Table 24–1. Unfortunately, sonographic findings help only to cull this list in a general way. The sonographic diagnosis of localized intraperitoneal fluid collections can be made only in the context of clinical information.

Peritoneal Carcinomatosis

The term "peritoneal carcinomatosis" refers to the diffuse spread of tumor within the peritoneal space, with resultant "seeding" or "studding" of the peritoneum. Peritoneal carcinomatosis usually originates from tumors of the abdominal or pelvic viscera.[20–34] Ovarian tumors are the most likely source in women.[34] In men, the likely source is a gastrointestinal neoplasm (particularly pancreas, stomach, and colon carcinoma).[34] Malignant neoplasms such as breast carcinoma, malignant melanoma, and lung carcinoma also can spread to the peritoneum hematogenously.

Ascites usually is the only sonographic finding in patients with peritoneal carcinomatosis, as the peritoneal implants generally are too small for visualization.[32, 33] Ascites almost invariably accompanies peritoneal carcinomatosis, and in some cases it facilitates sonographic visualization of peritoneal tumor implants by displacing bowel loops from the peritoneal surfaces. Peritoneal metastases (Figs. 24–8, 24–11) have a variety of sonographic appearances, including (1) focal nodules (or masses); (2) focal plaquelike thickening; (3) diffuse peritoneal thickening; and (4) bowel wall thickening.[32–37] The natural progression is from nodules to plaques to diffuse involvement. A dramatic manifestation of diffuse implantation is gross thickening of the greater omentum, described pathologically as an "omen-

Table 24-1. Loculated Peritoneal Fluid: Differential Diagnosis

Type of Collection	Examples
Developmental cysts	GI duplication cyst, urachal cyst
Lymphatic cysts	Cystic hygroma, lymphocele
Inclusion cyst	Postsurgical adhesions
Cystic neoplasm	Cystadenoma, cystadenocarcinoma, mucocele
Necrotic neoplasms	Sarcomas, carcinomas
Extravasated fluid	Hematoma, urinoma, biloma
Parasitic cysts	Ameboma, echinococcal cyst
Abscess	Numerous sources
Pseudocyst	Acute pancreatitis

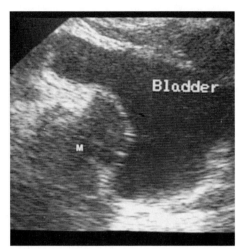

Figure 24-11—Peritoneal Carcinomatosis
(Anaplastic Lung Carcinoma). Longitudinal scan showing a tumor mass (M) adjacent to the bladder. Although this could be a primary pelvic tumor, the presence of tumor implants elsewhere and omental cake (not shown) indicated peritoneal carcinomatosis.

tal cake." The thickened omentum is seen as a medium-echogenicity tissue mass that extends across the anterior aspect of the abdominal cavity (Fig. 24–8).

Pseudomyxoma peritonei[30, 31] is a special form of carcinomatosis that occurs when a mucin-containing cystic tumor ruptures and "seeds" the peritoneal surfaces with malignant cells. These cells produce mucoid ascites that fills the interstices of the peritoneal space. The name "pseudomyxoma" describes the gelatin-like consistency of the mucoid ascites that resembles the contents of mucinous tumors. In addition to mucinous ascites, cellular implants may generate daughter cysts, either focally or diffusely, within the peritoneal space. Both benign and malignant mucinous tumors may cause pseudomyxoma peritonei, but the outcome is likely to be disastrous in either case. The origin of the mucinous tumor may be the appendix (benign or malignant mucocele) or the ovary (mucinous cystadenoma or cystadenocarcinoma).

Ascites is the most common sonographic finding in patients with pseudomyxoma peritonei, and the mucoid material may generate diffuse low-level echoes throughout the fluid. These findings are nonspecific, however. The only specific finding is the presence of "mucin balls" suspended in an ascitic matrix, as illustrated in Figure 24–12. Other manifestations of pseudomyxoma peritonei include multicystic masses, solid-appearing masses, matting of the bowel, and bowel distention (due to obstruction).

Recognition of Adenopathy

The presence of enlarged abdominal lymph nodes can be recognized by the location of the resultant mass and in some cases by the appearance of the nodal mass. Massive lymph node enlargement usually occurs along the course of the aorta, inferior vena cava, and iliac vessels as well as in the mesentery and the porta hepatis. Enlarged nodes almost invariably are hypoechoic, and initially the borders of individual nodes are visible sonographically, as seen in Figure 24–13. With progression of disease, however, the borders fade, and the nodes merge into featureless masses that are suggestive of adenopathy only by their location.

THE ADRENAL GLANDS

In adults, computed tomography is the preferred method for imaging the adrenal glands, for this method is technically simple and accurate.[38–43] Magnetic resonance imaging holds promise as an adjunctive method for adrenal imaging.[44, 45] Ultrasound is not a primary method for adrenal examination in adults, principally because the normal adrenal glands are difficult to identify, and adrenal hyperplasia is not readily detected.[38–40, 42, 43, 46] Adrenal masses, on the other hand, are fairly easy to visualize (sensitivity 77% to 97% in adults) and are accurately portrayed (specificity 75% to 97%).[38, 40, 47, 48]

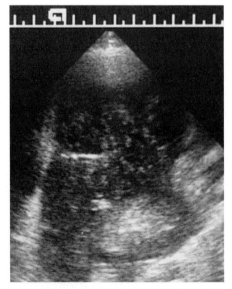

Figure 24-12—Pseudomyxoma Peritonei (origin: mucinous adenocarcinoma of the ovary). A transverse view of the left upper quadrant shows innumerable moderately echogenic globules of mucin suspended within peritoneal fluid. The peritoneal space was filled with multiloculated cysts and solid tumor masses.

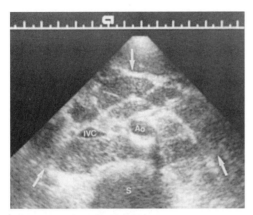

Figure 24-13—Adenopathy. A transverse scan shows multiple enlarged lymph nodes (arrows) surrounding the inferior vena cava (IVC) and aorta (Ao) in a patient with Hodgkin lymphoma. Note that the cava and aorta are displaced from their usual position adjacent to the spine (S).

In contrast to the situation in adults, sonography is the primary method for adrenal examination in children, in whom diagnostic accuracy approaches 100%.[49] The difference in sonographic efficacy is due to the small size and lean body habitus of most children.

Sonographic Anatomy

The adrenal glands[38, 42, 43, 46–52] are located anteromedial to the superior poles of the kidneys, as shown in Figure 24–14. Because of this position, large adrenal masses tend to displace the kidney inferiorly. The right gland lies posterior to the inferior vena cava (IVC), and masses in this gland displace the IVC *anteriorly.* Adrenal origin is likely for a suprarenal mass that displaces the IVC anteriorly.

The adrenal glands are complex in shape, and roughly resemble an inverted Y or V (Fig. 24–15). Because of this complex shape, the sonographic appearance varies greatly with different planes of section. A normal gland may be V- or Y-shaped, or it may be linear. Two adjacent limbs may be mistaken for hyperplasia or a mass.

The adrenal cortex is relatively sonolucent compared with the echogenic adrenal medulla. This difference is most apparent in the neonatal period (Fig. 24–16), when the cortex is quite thick. Because fetal or neonatal adrenal glands are relatively large and have a hypoechoic periphery and echogenic center, they may be mistaken for the kidneys, particularly in cases of renal agenesis.[51, 53, 54] In older children and adults, the cortex and medulla can sometimes be differentiated sonographically, but in most cases they blend together, and the adrenal glands have a uniform, hypoechoic appearance (relative to surrounding fat) (Fig. 24–17).

The maximum length of the right adrenal gland in adults is 3 cm.[46] The left gland invariably is smaller, since it has shorter limbs. The maximum normal thickness of any limb in adults is 7.1 mm.[46, 47] The adrenal glands are disproportionately large in neonates; the right gland may be up to 3.5 cm in length.[49, 51] Adrenal size decreases rapidly in infants, and by 12 months the adrenal glands have an adult appearance.[49]

Examination Technique

Visualization rates for the normal adrenal glands in adults range from 79% to 92% on

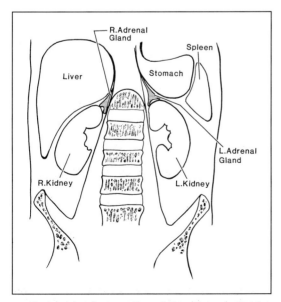

Figure 24-14—Location of the adrenal glands.

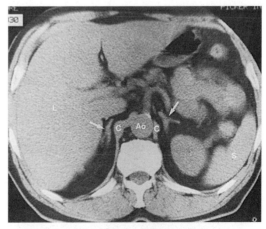

Figure 24-15—Adrenal Gland Location. Computed tomographic image shows the location of the adrenal glands (arrows). L = liver; S = spleen; Ao = aorta; C = crus of diaphragm.

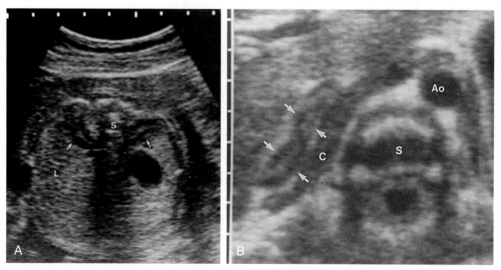

Figure 24-16—Normal Adrenal Glands. Fetal **(A)** and neonatal **(B)** adrenal glands (arrows) are shown. S = spine; L = liver; C = crus of diaphragm; Ao = aorta. The hypoechoic adrenal cortex surrounds the more echogenic medulla.

the right and 38% to 71% on the left.[46, 47, 52] Sonographic examination is best accomplished from a posterolateral transducer position through the ninth or tenth intercostal space. Coronal planes are best, but transverse planes also may be helpful. The right adrenal gland also may be seen from an anterior approach, using the liver as a window.

The kidneys serve as the primary orienting structures in the search for the adrenal glands. To find an adrenal, first visualize the upper pole of the ipsilateral kidney and then look slightly superior and medial to the kidney.

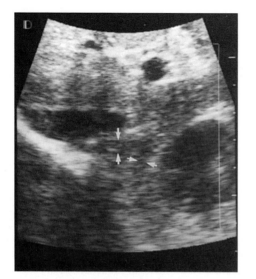

Figure 24-17—Normal Adrenal Gland (arrows). Outside of the fetal or neonatal period, the adrenal medulla and cortex cannot be differentiated.

Clinical and Pathologic Features

A detailed discussion of adrenal pathology is beyond the scope of this work. From a pathologic perspective, adrenal disorders are categorized on the basis of anatomic origin and hormonal function, as summarized in Tables 24-2 and 24-3.[39] Please review these tables before proceeding, as their contents are not repeated in the text.

Sonographic Features of Adrenal Pathology

Hyperplasia. Hyperplastic adrenal glands[40, 42, 43, 52] generally are easier to visualize sonographically than normal glands. They are characterized by greater-than-normal limb thickness and clear differentiation between the adrenal cortex and medulla. Both of these features result from abnormal thickness of the adrenal cortex, which is relatively sonolucent. The medulla is unaffected.

Hematoma. Adrenal hematomas[55–58] generally are hypoechoic relative to surrounding structures

Table 24-2. Categories of Adrenal Pathology

Cortical hyperplasia
Adrenocortical adenoma
Adrenocortical carcinoma
Cyst
Pheochromocytoma
Metastasis
Lymphoma
Hematoma
Infection

Table 24-3. Adrenal Pathology in Relation to Endocrine Function

Excess cortisol production°	Adrenal insufficiency
Cortical hyperplasia (70%)	Tuberculous infection (most common cause)
Cortical adenoma (20%)	Metastasis (uncommon cause)
Cortical carcinoma (10%)	Adrenal hemorrhage (uncommon cause)
Excess aldosterone production°	**Normal adrenal function**
Cortical hyperplasia (20%)	Cortical adenoma
Cortical adenoma (80%)	Cortical carcinoma
Cortical carcinoma (rare)	Cyst
Excess catecholamine production	Hematoma†
	Metastasis†
Pheochromocytoma	Lymphoma

°Other hormones may be produced, but these are most common.
†Adrenal insufficiency occurs rarely with these lesions.

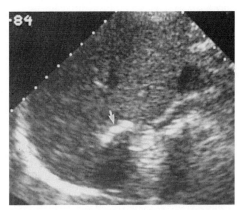

Figure 24-19—Calcified Adrenal. A longitudinal sonogram in a 54 year old woman shows bright reflections and shadowing at the posterior aspect of the liver. Similar findings were seen in an equivalent location in the left upper quadrant. A radiograph (not shown) confirmed the presence of bilateral adrenal calcification that was idiopathic.

(Fig. 24–18), and some may be anechoic. The echogenicity varies, however, in relation to the age of the collection (Chapter 7). Heterogeneity is a common finding, with echogenic components imbedded in a hypoechoic background. Hematomas are more commonly unilateral than bilateral. The sonographic features do not differentiate between adrenal hematomas and neoplastic masses. However, the correct diagnosis usually is suggested by the clinical circumstances, which may include trauma or overwhelming intercurrent illness.

Neonatal adrenal hematomas tend to be large relative to the size of the neonate (Fig. 24–18), and they may exceed the size of the adjacent kidney. Adrenal hematomas are relatively small in adults, and in reported cases do not seem to exceed 3 to 4 cm in size.

Calcification. Adrenal calcification occurs most commonly following adrenal hemorrhage, tuberculosis infection, and occasionally fungal infection. As such, calcification may be an incidental finding (Fig. 24–19).

Neoplasms. The sonographic features of adrenal neoplasms (Fig. 24–20) are nonspecific and do not permit reliable differential diagnosis. The differential list can be culled, however, by considering imaging findings in lieu of clinical information. Sonographic features of adrenal neoplasms

Table 24-4. Ultrasound Features of Common Adrenal Masses

Hematoma	Anechoic, hypoechoic, clumps of echoes in anechoic matrix. May be very large in neonates. Not exceeding 3–4 cm in adults
Adenoma	Homogeneous, hypoechoic,° well-defined, roughly sperical, *6 cm or less* in size and usually under 3 cm. Less often heterogeneous due to necrosis or calcification
Carcinoma	Usually *exceeds* 6 cm in diameter, hypoechoic,° and almost always heterogeneous due to large areas of necrosis or calcification. May also resemble a cyst.
Pheochromocytoma	Tends to be large, but ranges from 2–9.5 cm. Sharply marginated by fibrous capsule. Small tumors homogeneous, low-to-medium echoes.° Large tumors heterogeneous due to hemorrhages that vary in age. May be cystlike.
Metastases	Three cm or less in size, hypoechoic, and usually homogeneous

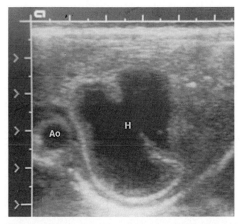

Figure 24-18—Massive Adrenal Hematoma. A transverse scan in a neonate who had suffered interpartum distress shows a large left adrenal hematoma (H). Ao = aorta.

°Relative to surrounding structures.

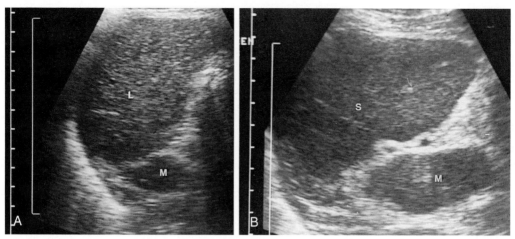

Figure 24-20—Bilateral Adrenal Metastases (bronchogenic carcinoma). (A) A longitudinal scan of the right upper quadrant shows a hypoechoic mass (M) posterior to the right lobe of the liver (L) and just above the right kidney (not shown). (B) A coronal scan of the left upper quadrant shows a similar mass (M) medial to the spleen (S). Both locations are consistent with the adrenal glands, and the findings were confirmed in the course of chest computed tomography.

are listed in Table 24–4.[38, 39, 41, 42, 47, 50, 59–65] Neuroblastoma is an important adrenal tumor of infancy and childhood. This neoplasm is discussed in Chapter 20.

REFERENCES

1. Miller EI, Rogers A: Sonography of the anterior abdominal wall. Semin Ultrasound 4:278–287, 1982.
2. Wechsler RJ, Kurtz AB, Needleman L, et al: Cross-sectional imaging of abdominal wall hernias. Am J Roentgenol 153:517–521, 1989.
3. Miller PA, Mezwa DG, Feczko PJ, Jafri ZH, Madrazo BL: Imaging of abdominal hernias. RadioGraphics 15:333–347, 1995.
4. Harrison LA, Keesling CA, Martin NL, Lee KR, Wetzel LH: Abdominal wall hernias: Review of herniography and correlation with cross-sectional imaging. RadioGraphics 15:315–332, 1995.
5. Yeh H-C, Rabinowitz JG: Ultrasonography and computed tomography of inflammatory abdominal wall lesions. Radiology 144:859–863, 1982.
6. Kuligowska E, Mueller PR, Simeone JF, Fine C: Ultrasound in upper abdominal trauma. Semin Roentgenol 4:281–295, 1984.
7. Hanson RD, Hunter TB, Haber K: Ultrasonographic appearance of anterior abdominal wall desmoid tumors. J Ultrasound Med 2:141–142, 1983.
8. Weill F, Watrin J, Rohmer P, Weiler S, Coche G: Ultrasound and CT of peritoneal recesses and ligaments: A pictorial essay. Ultrasound Med Biol 12:977–989, 1986.
9. Dodds WJ, Foley WD, Lawson TL, Stewart ET, Taylor A: Anatomy and imaging of the lesser peritoneal sac. Am J Roentgenol 144:567–575, 1985.
10. Vincent LM, Mauro MA, Mittelstaedt CA: The lesser sac and gastrohepatic recess: Sonographic appearance and differentiation of fluid collections. Radiology 150:515–519, 1984.
11. Weill FS, Rohmer P, Beloir A, Bagni P: The butterfly sign: An indicator of fluid within both the

12. Gore RM, Callen PW, Filly RA: Lesser sac fluid in predicting the etiology of ascites: CT findings. Am J Roentgenol 139:71–74, 1982.
13. Dinkel E, Lehnart R, Tröger J, Peters H, Dittrich M: Sonographic evidence of intraperitoneal fluid: An experimental study and its clinical implications. Pediatr Radiol 14:299–303, 1984.
14. Goldberg BB, Goodman GA, Clearfield HR: Evaluation of ascites by ultrasound. Radiology 96:15–22, 1970.
15. Meyers MA: Dynamic Radiology of the Abdomen: Normal and Pathologic Anatomy. 2nd ed. New York, Springer Verlag, 1982.
16. Proto AV, Lane EJ, Marangola JP: A new concept of ascitic fluid distribution. Am J Roentgenol 126:974, 1976.
17. Yeh H-C, Wold BS: Ultrasonography in ascites. Radiology 124:783–790, 1977.
18. Gooding GA, Cummings SR: Sonographic detection of ascites in liver disease. J Ultrasound Med 3:169–172, 1984.
19. Sivit CJ: Significance of peritoneal fluid identified by ultrasonographic examination in children with acute abdominal pain. J Ultrasound Med 12:743–746, 1993.
20. Levine CD, Patel UJ, Wachsberg RH, Simmons MZ, Baker SR, Cho KC: CT in patients with blunt abdominal trauma: Clinical significance of intraperitoneal fluid detected on a scan with otherwise normal findings. Am J Roentgenol 164:1381–1385, 1995.
21. Edell SL, Gefter WB: Ultrasonic differentiation of types of ascitic fluid. Am J Roentgenol 133:111–114, 1979.
22. Franklin JT, Azose AA: Sonographic appearance of chylous ascites. J Clin Ultrasound 12:239–240, 1984.
23. Hanson RD, Hunter TB: Tuberculous peritonitis: CT appearance. Am J Roentgenol 144:931–932, 1985.
24. Leonidas JC, Brill PW, Bhan I, Smith TH: Cystic retroperitoneal lymphangioma in infants and children. Radiology 127:203–208, 1978.

25. Sheth S, Nussbaum AR, Hutchins GM, Sanders RC: Cystic hygromas in children: Sonographic-pathologic correlation. Radiology 162:821–824, 1987.

26. Geer LL, Mittelstaedt CA, Staab EV, Gaisie G: Mesenteric cyst: Sonographic appearance with CT correlation. Pediatr Radiol 14:102–104, 1984.

27. Teele RL, Henschke CI, Tapper D: The radiographic and ultrasonographic evaluation of enteric duplication cysts. Pediatr Radiol 10:9–14, 1980.

28. Doust BD, Quiroz F, Stewart JM: Ultrasonic distinction of abscesses from other intra-abdominal fluid collections. Radiology 125:213–218, 1977.

29. Voegeli E, Ayer G, Hofer B: Sonographie und computertomographie bei postoperativen, abdominellen Abszedierungen. Radiologe 24:90–94, 1984.

30. Athey PA, Hacken JB, Estrada R: Sonographic appearance of mucocele of the appendix. J Clin Ultrasound 12:333–337, 1984.

31. Yeh H-C, Shafir MK, Slater G, Meyer RJ, Cohen BA, Geller SA: Ultrasonography and computed tomography in pseudomyxoma peritonei. Radiology 153:507–510, 1984.

32. Mitchell DG, Hill MC, Hill S, Zaloudek C: Serous carcinoma of the ovary: CT identification of metastatic calcified implants. Radiology 158:649–652, 1986.

33. Jeffrey RB: CT demonstration of peritoneal implants. Am J Roentgenol 135:323–326, 1980.

34. Meyers MA: Distribution of intra-abdominal malignant seeding: Depending on dynamics of flow of ascitic fluid. Am J Roentgenol 119:198–203, 1973.

35. Yeh H-C, Chachinian AP: Ultrasonography and computed tomography of peritoneal mesothelioma. Radiology 135:705–712, 1980.

36. Yaghoobian J, Demeter E, Colucci J: Ultrasonic demonstration of lymphomatous infiltration of the greater omentum. Med Ultrasound 8:65–66, 1984.

37. Carroll BA, Ta HN: The ultrasonic appearance of extranodal abdominal lymphoma. Radiology 136:419–425, 1980.

38. Sample WF, Sarti DA: Computed tomography and gray scale ultrasonography of the adrenal gland: A comparative study. Radiology 128:377–383, 1978.

39. Dunnick NR: Adrenal imaging: Current status. Am J Roentgenol 154:927–936, 1990.

40. Abrams HL, Siegelman SS, Adams DF, Sanders R, Finberg HJ: Computed tomography versus ultrasound of the adrenal gland: A prospective study. Radiology 143:121–128, 1982.

41. Adams JE, Johnson RJ, Rickards D, Isherwood I: Computed tomography in adrenal disease. Clin Radiol 34:39–49, 1983.

42. Yamakita N, Yasuda K, Goshima E, Murayama M, Murase H, et al: Comparative assessment of ultrasonography and computed tomography in adrenal disorders. Ultrasound Med Biol 12:23–29, 1986.

43. Georgi VM, Hofbauer J, Weiss H, Keller W, Wunschik F: Wertigkeit von Sonographie, Computertomographie und Angiographie in der Nebennierendiagnostik. Fortschr Röntgenstr 140:373–379, 1984.

44. Schultz CL, Haaga JR, Fletcher BD, Alfidi RJ, Schultz MA: Magnetic resonance imaging of the adrenal glands: A comparison with computed tomography. Am J Roentgenol 143:1235–1240, 1984.

45. Glazer GM, Woolsey EJ, Borrello J, Francis IR, Aisen AM: Adrenal tissue characterization using MR imaging. Radiology 158:73–79, 1986.

46. Yamakita N, Yasuda K, Miura K: Delineation of adrenal in controls and nontumorous adrenal disorders by real-time ultrasonic-scanner. Ultrasound Med Biol 12:107–114, 1986.

47. Yeh HC: Sonography of the adrenal glands: Normal glands and small masses. Am J Roentgenol 135:1167–1177, 1980.

48. Günther RW, Kelbel C, Lenner V: Real-time ultrasound of normal adrenal glands and small tumors. J Clin Ultrasound 12:211–217, 1984.

49. Kangarloo H, Diament MJ, Gold RH, Barrett C, Lippe B: Sonography of adrenal glands in neonates and children: Changes in appearance with age. J Clin Ultrasound 14:43–47, 1986.

50. Sample WF: A new technique for the evaluation of the adrenal gland with gray scale ultrasonography. Radiology 124:463–469, 1977.

51. Oppenheimer DA, Carroll BA, Yousem S: Sonography of the normal neonatal adrenal gland. Radiology 146:157–160, 1983.

52. Marchal G, Gelin J, Verbeken E, Baert A, Lauwerijns J: High-resolution real-time sonography of the adrenal glands: A routine examination? J Ultrasound Med 5:65–68, 1986.

53. Silverman PM, Carroll BA, Moskowitz PS: Adrenal sonography in renal agenesis and dysplasia. Am J Roentgenol 134:600–602, 1980.

54. McGahan JP, Myracle MR: Adrenal hypertrophy: Possible pitfall in the sonographic diagnosis of renal agenesis. J Ultrasound Med 5:265–268, 1986.

55. Mittelstaedt CA, Volberg FM, Merten DF, Brill PW: The sonographic diagnosis of neonatal adrenal hemorrhage. Radiology 131:453–457, 1979.

56. Pery M, Kaftori JK, Bar-Maor JA: Sonography for diagnosis and follow-up of neonatal adrenal hemorrhage. J Clin Ultrasound 9:397–401, 1981.

57. Wolverson MK, Kannegiesser H: CT of bilateral adrenal hemorrhage with acute adrenal insufficiency in the adult. Am J Roentgenol 142:311–314, 1984.

58. Murphy BJ, Casillas J, Yrizarry JM: Traumatic adrenal hemorrhage: Radiologic findings. Radiology 169:701–703, 1988.

59. Fishman EK, Deutch BM, Hartman DS, Goldman SM, Zerhouni EA, Siegelman SS: Primary adrenocortical carcinoma: CT evaluation with clinical correlation. Am J Roentgenol 148:531–535, 1987.

60. Cunningham JJ: Ultrasonic findings in "primary" lymphoma of the adrenal area. J Ultrasound Med 2:467–469, 1983.

61. Hamper UM, Fishman EK, Hartman DS, Roberts JL, Sanders RC: Primary adrenocortical carcinoma: Sonographic evaluation with clinical and pathologic correlation in 26 patients. Am J Roentgenol 148:915–919, 1987.

62. Mitnick JS, Bosniak MA, Megibow AJ, Naidich DP: Non-functioning adrenal adenomas discovered incidentally on computed tomography. Radiology 148:495–499, 1983.

63. Davies RP, Lam AH: Adrenocortical neoplasm in children: Ultrasound appearance. J Ultrasound Med 6:325–328, 1987.

64. Bowerman RA, Silver TM, Jaffe MH, Stuck KJ, Hinerman DL: Sonography of adrenal pheochromocytomas. Am J Roentgenol 137:1227–1231, 1981.

65. Antoniou A, Spetseropoulos J, Vlahos L, Pontifex GR, Papavasiliou C: The sonographic appearance of adrenal involvement in non-Hodgkin's lymphoma. J Ultrasound Med 2:235–236, 1983.

Chapter 25
The Bowel

William J. Zwiebel

Sonography is not widely used to diagnose bowel pathology except in a few specific conditions, such as infantile pyloric stenosis and appendicitis. But other important types of bowel pathology may be identified sonographically, either incidentally or when specifically sought. It is important, therefore, for sonologists and sonographers to be familiar with the normal and pathologic appearances of bowel.

NORMAL BOWEL

The component layers of the normal bowel wall (adventitia, muscularis, and mucosa) can sometimes be seen sonographically with close scrutiny (Fig. 25–1),[1-4] but, in my experience, this level of detail is not achieved in most instances. The maximal wall thickness (all layers) of normal bowel in adults is 5 mm for the gastric body, 2 to 3 mm for the small bowel, and 9 mm for the colon. Normal small bowel loops are "crumpled" together in close proximity; therefore, only small segments of individual loops are visible on ultrasound images, and these segments have angular, cut-off borders.[5] When a long segment of small bowel is visible, the possibility of mechanical obstruction or adynamic ileus should be entertained.

Peristalsis is a noteworthy feature of normal small bowel. Peristalsis is manifested by movement of liquid bowel content, changes in bowel loop caliber and shape, and the rapid appearance and disappearance of bowel loops during real-time observation. Peristalsis is considerably more conspicuous in the small bowel than in the large bowel. The absence of peristalsis, therefore, may be pathologic with respect to small bowel but is nondiagnostic with respect to large bowel.

If the bowel is fluid filled, a mucosal pattern is visible that may permit the identification of the distended segment,[1, 6] but in my experience, this is not possible in all cases. The jejunum contains prominent valvulae conniventes, represented by narrow, closely spaced striations oriented transverse to the bowel axis. The valvulae are less prominent or absent in the ilium, which has a largely featureless mucosal pattern. The colon contains large, widely spaced haustral folds oriented transverse to the bowel axis that cause partial segmentation of the lumen.

DISTENTION

Bowel loops are visible as tubular structures only in the distended state (Fig. 25–2). Bowel distention[1, 5–7] may result either from obstruction or from diminished peristalsis, but sonography often cannot differentiate between these etiologies. Sonographic assessment of the mucosal pattern, as just described, may identify the segment(s) of bowel that are dilated. If the bowel is filled principally with fluid and contains little gas,

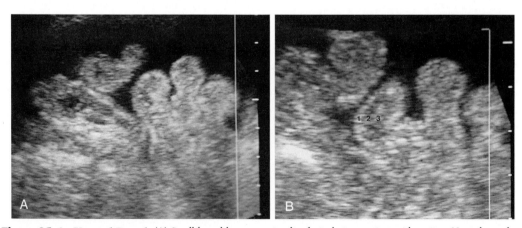

Figure 25-1—Normal Bowel. (A) Small bowel loops are visualized nicely in a patient with ascites. Note that only short segments of bowel are visible. **(B)** On closer inspection, the adventitia (1), muscularis (2) and lumen (3) are visible.

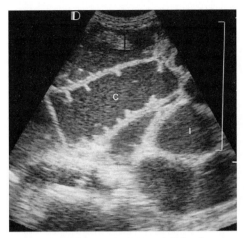

Figure 25-2—Distended Bowel. Dilated portions of the colon (C) and ileum (I) are seen in this 92 year old man with obstructing colon cancer. Note the thick haustral folds in the colon and the featureless appearance of adjacent ileal loops.

distention may be more apparent sonographically than radiographically.

WALL THICKENING

Edema, inflammation, or neoplastic infiltration may visibly increase the thickness of the bowel wall.[1, 4, 7-18] In addition, these processes tend to decrease the echogenicity of the bowel wall and *may* obliterate the aforementioned, normally visible wall layers. The thickened, hypoechoic bowel wall stands out in contrast to the echogenic mucosa and bowel contents, producing a characteristic "doughnut" or "pseudokidney" appearance, which is illustrated in Figure 25–3. The importance of this finding cannot be overstated, for it strongly suggests pathologic bowel wall thickening.[8, 9] Mesenteric thickening in lymphoma and nonbowel pathology occasionally can mimic the doughnut or pseudokidney appearance[9]; nonetheless, bowel pathology should come to mind when findings like those shown in Figure 25–3 are encountered. The causes of bowel wall thickening are multiple and include Crohn disease, lymphoma, primary and secondary neoplasms, and myriad inflammatory processes (e.g., diverticulitis, neutropenic typhlitis, peptic disease, and appendicitis).[1, 4, 7-18] In some cases, tumors or inflammatory processes may produce bulky masses, and it may not be possible to confirm bowel origin with ultrasound (Fig. 25–4).

INCREASED BLOOD FLOW

Little or no flow is evident in normal bowel with color Doppler flow imaging. Bowel that is thickened by inflammatory or neoplastic processes may exhibit increased blood flow, as indicated by enhanced detection of flow with color Doppler.[19-21] The presence of increased flow is nonspecific but suggests pathology since flow is not readily detected in normal bowel.

PNEUMATOSIS

Pneumatosis intestinalis, or the presence of gas in the bowel wall, is manifested by linear or focal bright reflections *within the bowel wall,* which may be accompanied by distal acoustic shadows or comet-tail artifacts.[22-27] These findings are caused by gas bubbles trapped between the component layers of the wall. Gas bubbles also may be seen in the portal venous system or in the hepatic parenchyma (Chapter 7).

In preterm infants, pneumatosis intestinalis is diagnostic of necrotizing enterocolitis, which is a severe form of mucosal ulceration ultimately leading to bowel necrosis and perforation.[22-25] This condition has traditionally been diagnosed radiographically, but ultrasound may provide for earlier diagnosis in some cases. The visualization of a focal fluid collection, an inflammatory mass, or diffuse peritoneal fluid, in association with pneumatosis, is a poor prognostic sign in neonates. These findings suggest frank bowel necrosis or perforation.[24, 25]

In adults, pneumatosis intestinalis also calls to mind serious and potentially life-threatening bowel infection or infarction, but pneumatosis also may occur in the absence of intrinsic bowel pathology, as in patients with bowel dilatation or emphysema.[26, 27]

APPENDICITIS

Sonography has emerged as an important imaging modality for the diagnosis of appendicitis;[20, 22, 23, 28-43] nonetheless, the accuracy and clinical role of sonography continues to be a somewhat controversial subject. The specificity of ultrasound for diagnosis of acute appendicitis is excellent (94% to 100%), but sensitivity ranges more widely, from 76% to 93%.[28-33, 35-38, 40] It appears, therefore, that sonography is more useful for confirming than for excluding the diagnosis of acute appendicitis. Stated differently, a negative ultrasound examination does not definitely exclude acute appendicitis.

Sonographic Technique

A linear array transducer of 5 to 10 MHz is used, depending on the size of the patient. The transducer is placed on the right lower quadrant of the abdomen, in the area of tenderness, and

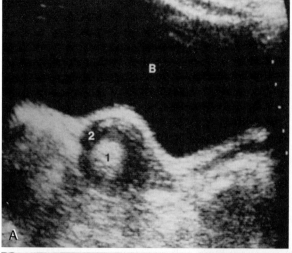

Figure 25-3—Thickened Bowel. (A) The doughnut sign is illustrated in the sigmoid colon in a patient with acute diverticulitis. 1 = lumen; 2 = muscularis; B = bladder. **(B)** The pseudokidney sign is illustrated in the sigmoid colon in a patient with metastatic breast carcinoma. 1 = lumen; 2 = muscularis; B = bladder. **(C)** Marked duodenal wall thickening is apparent in this patient with a duodenal ulcer. 1 = lumen; 2 = muscularis; L = liver; PV = portal vein.

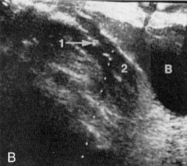

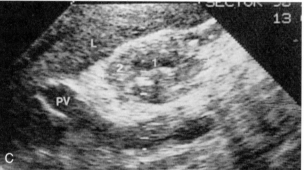

oriented transversely. Graded pressure[28, 30–32, 35–37] is then applied to the transducer, meaning that very light pressure is applied initially, but the pressure subsequently is increased until the transducer indents the abdominal wall. Pressure on the transducer compresses the cecum and gas-containing small bowel that otherwise would obscure the appendix. With graded pressure, it is possible to penetrate deeply into the abdomen with only mild pain, whereas abrupt pressure would cause severe pain that would preclude examination.

If no abnormalities are identified, the pressure is increased until structures delimiting the posterior wall of the abdominal cavity are seen, including the iliacus and psoas muscles, and the iliac artery and vein. When pathology is not identified in the area examined initially, gentle cephalad or caudad movement of the transducer permits the examination of other areas. It sometimes is possible, with graded compression, to move from the iliac fossa inferiorly into the true pelvis to search for gynecologic pathology, even if the bladder is poorly distended.

Normal and Abnormal Findings

If the appendix is normal, then it frequently is not identified.[32, 38, 39] When the normal appendix is seen (Fig. 25–5), its wall is 2 mm or less in thickness, its overall diameter (outer-to-outer) is

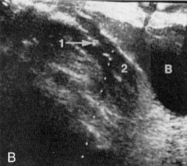

Figure 25-4—Tumor Mass. Eccentric, massive thickening of the bowel wall is present in this patient with gastric adenocarcinoma. LU = lumen.

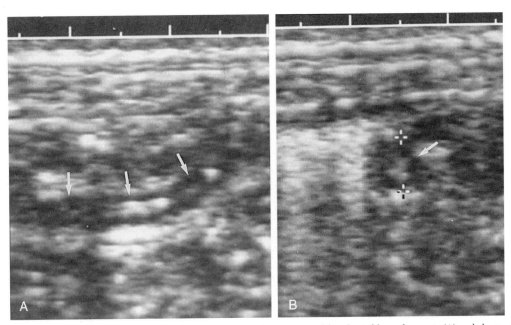

Figure 25-5—Normal Appendix. The appendix (arrows) is empty and barely visible on long axis **(A)** and short axis **(B)** views. The maximum diameter (cursors) is 5 mm.

5 mm or less, the wall is well defined, an echogenic submucosal layer is visible, its lumen is empty, and peristalsis usually is present.[29, 41]

The inflamed appendix[22, 23, 28–43] (Fig. 25–6) is distended with fluid and much easier to identify, therefore, than the normal appendix. The most important diagnostic findings in acute appendicitis are an outer-to-outer diameter of 6 mm or greater,° point tenderness clearly localized to the appendix, and an appendicolith (calculus) within the lumen (or adjacent to the appendix in cases of rupture). The first two of these findings should always be present before a diagnosis of acute

---

°Jeffrey et al[41] regard 6 mm as equivocal and 7 mm or greater as definitely abnormal. They argue that the false-positive rate is excessive, with a cut-off of 6 mm.

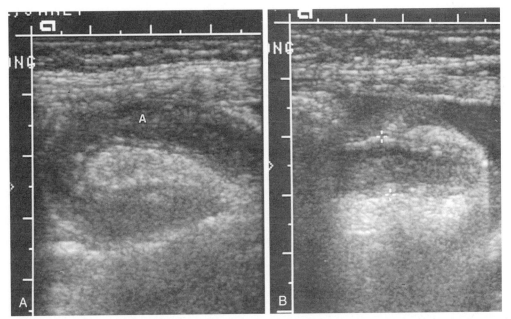

Figure 25-6—Acute Appendicitis. (A) An overview shows a fluid-distended appendix (A) with poor definition of the mucosa. **(B)** Maximum diameter measurement (cursors) near the tip is 12 mm.

appendicitis is made. The third finding (appendicolith) is seen infrequently but is highly specific diagnostically. An appendicolith produces strong focal or arcuate reflections accompanied by acoustic shadows (similar to gallstones or renal calculi).

Numerous ancillary findings may be seen in acute appendicitis, including (1) a sausage-like appearance on long axis images; (2) lack of compressibility; (3) absence of peristalsis; (4) absence or interruption of the echogenic submucosal layer; (5) poor definition of the exterior surface of the appendix because of periappendicitis; (6) periappendiceal fluid; (7) bowel wall thickening near the appendix in the cecum or ileum; and (8) inflammatory nodes of up to 3 cm in nearby mesenteric structures (especially in children).[22, 23, 28–43] The sonographic findings of acute appendicitis are summarized in Table 25–1.

It appears that the most tender appendices represent the acute suppurative state, in which the lumen is distended with fluid. Some investigators[28–30, 32, 37, 43] feel that the absence of severe tenderness is a sign of rupture—the tenderness having been relieved by decompression. Periappendiceal fluid is common with appendiceal rupture, but it is not specific, as the inflammatory process per se can generate fluid. Large fluid collections, however, should be regarded as abscesses related to rupture. Periappendiceal abscesses[32, 34, 39, 42, 43] generally are sonolucent but occasionally may be echogenic and may present a masslike appearance. Appendiceal abscesses should be located adjacent to the appendix and may partially or completely surround the appendix (Fig. 25–7). Inflammatory wall thickening of nearby bowel loops also suggests appendiceal rupture, especially when seen in association with a periappendiceal fluid collection.

False-Negative Diagnoses

The primary source of a false-negative ultrasound examination in acute appendicitis is poor

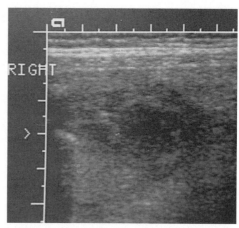

Figure 25–7—Appendiceal Abscess. A transverse scan in the right iliac fossa shows a poorly defined, lucent inflammatory mass about 5 cm in size that corresponded to the point of maximum tenderness. The appendix was not seen. Appendiceal rupture with abscess formation was confirmed surgically.

visualization of the appendiceal region. Lack of visualization results from nondisplaceable echogenic bowel contents, usually associated with excessive pain that prevents effective compression.[32, 37] The nonvisualized appendix, in such cases, is assumed to be normal. False-negative results also are thought to occur early in acute appendicitis when the appendix is inflamed but not distended, and when the appendix has perforated and therefore is decompressed.[32, 37, 43] The decompressed appendix is difficult to identify and less tender than when in the acute, distended state.

INTUSSUSCEPTION

In the condition called intussusception,[21–23, 44–52] one portion of the bowel "telescopes" into another, as illustrated in Figure 25–8. The great majority of intussusceptions occur in children, and, in most of these cases, the ilium intussuscepts into the colon. There usually is no pathologic cause for intussusception in children, but in adults, intussusception is precipitated by a bowel neoplasm (benign or malignant) in about 75% to 85% of cases.[44–46] In these cases, the tumor mass is propelled forward by peristalsis, drawing one portion of the bowel into an adjacent portion.

The classic ultrasound appearance of intussusception is a masslike lesion that resembles a target. The mass is comprised of concentric echogenic and sonolucent rings that represent the concentric layers of the telescoped bowel walls.[48, 49] Although this multiring appearance is

Table 25–1. Sonographic Manifestations of Appendicitis

Primary findings
  The appendix is easily seen
  Distended lumen
  Overall diameter (outer-to-outer) ≥ 6 mm
  Focal tenderness
  Appendicolith
Ancillary findings
  Lack of compressibility
  Interrupted submucosal layer
  Fuzzy exterior wall (periappendicitis)
  Fluid collections adjacent to appendix (periappendicitis or abscess)
  Adjacent bowel wall thickening
  Nearby enlarged lymph nodes

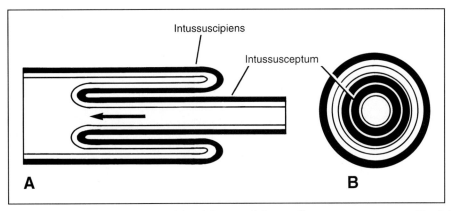

Figure 25-8—Intussusception. Long axis (**A**) and short axis (**B**) views illustrating intussusception. The dark black line is the adventitia, and the light black line is the mucosa.

highly suggestive of intussusception in the right clinical setting, other conditions, particularly tumor infiltration and bowel wall hematoma, may also generate a target appearance.[1, 23, 52] Furthermore, all cases of intussusception are not manifested as concentric rings;[22, 23, 47, 48, 50] some present as nonspecific bowel wall thickening. These problems notwithstanding, ultrasound is an important means for diagnosis of intussusception and may be followed directly by attempts at hydrostatic or pneumatic reduction when findings are typical.[22] Nonsurgical reduction should not be attempted when there are clinical or imaging findings suggesting bowel infarction or perforation.[22, 23]

The presence or absence of blood flow in the wall of the intussusceptum (the "interior" bowel segment) may be an indication of the severity of edema, as well as of the prospect for successful nonsurgical reduction. Blood flow tends to be present in cases that can be reduced nonsurgically and absent in those requiring surgery.[21]

INFANTILE HYPERTROPHIC PYLORIC STENOSIS

Hypertrophic pyloric stenosis of infancy[22, 23, 53–64] is an idiopathic condition characterized pathologically by massive hypertrophy and persistent spasm of the muscularis of the pylorus. The resultant obstruction of the stomach outlet causes gastric distention, vomiting, dehydration, and metabolic acidosis. The condition typically presents at 6 weeks of age in a previously healthy child, but the age of onset ranges from birth to 5 months.[58] The only therapy for hypertrophic pyloric stenosis is surgical myotomy; therefore, accurate differentiation from nonsurgical conditions is of great importance. In many cases, however, differentiation among hypertrophic pyloric

stenosis and other conditions, particularly gastroesophageal reflux, pylorospasm, and peptic disease, is difficult.[58, 65–67] In recent years, sonography has replaced fluoroscopy as the diagnostic procedure of choice for pyloric stenosis. Ultrasound is 91% to 100% sensitive and 80% to 100% specific for diagnosis of this condition,[53–57, 59, 61, 62] but accuracy requires close attention to imaging details.[58, 59]

Sonographic Technique

The technical approach of Haller and Cohen[58] is recommended. Fasting for approximately 2 hours prior to the examination is suggested but is not essential. The pylorus first is localized and then it is examined in detail on images obtained perpendicular and parallel to its axis. If there is unequivocal evidence of pyloric stenosis, then no further evaluation is necessary. If the findings are equivocal or normal, then further examination is recommended using the following technique: A No. 8 French nasogastric tube is inserted and its tip placed in the gastric antrum. The gastric contents are aspirated and 60 to 120 ml of water are instilled, using sonography to monitor gastric filling and to guard against the aspiration of gastric contents. The tube is then removed. The infant then is tipped about 45 degrees toward the right side and the antropyloric area is re-examined for evidence of pyloric stenosis or peptic disease. Finally, the child is turned to a right decubitus position to dump fluid into the duodenum. Gastric emptying may then be assessed through observation of duodenal filling and changes in the size of the pyloric channel.

The Normal and Abnormal Pylorus

The maximum thickness of the normal antropyloric musculature is generally regarded as 2 to

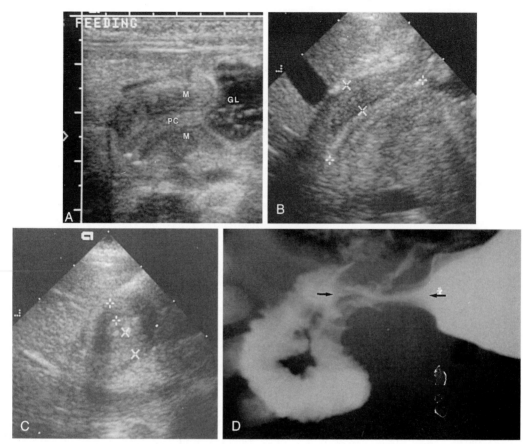

Figure 25-9—Pyloric Stenosis. (**A**) Fluid within the gastric lumen (GL) outlines the gastric end of the pylorus. The hypertrophied pyloric muscularis (M) is clearly visible on either side of the pyloric channel (PC). (**B**) Long axis view showing the entire length of the pylorus (+), which measured 25 mm. The muscularis (X) measured 6 mm. (**C**) A short axis view of the pylorus shows muscularis measurement points (cursors). Outer-to-outer diameter in this case was 16 mm. (**D**) Radiographic demonstration of the elongated, thickened pylorus (arrows) in the same patient.

3 mm.[55, 59, 63] Muscular thickness exceeding 3 mm (Fig. 25–9) is generally considered abnormal and diagnostic of hypertrophic pyloric stenosis in the proper clinical setting[57, 58, 60, 63] (Table 25–2). The maximum anteroposterior (AP) dimension of the normal pylorus (outside-to-outside) is 10 to 15 mm, and a measurement exceeding 15 mm is regarded as abnormal.[53, 54, 58] The overall AP dimension is considered less reliable than muscular thickness and pyloric length, however.[59] The nor-

mal pylorus is 10 to 15 mm long, and a length of 17 mm or greater is a reliable indicator of pyloric stenosis.[57, 59]

Ancillary findings in pyloric stenosis are numerous (Table 25–2) and include gastric distention, prominent peristaltic waves in the stomach, a "nipple" of pyloric mucosa projecting into the gastric lumen, and a tram track appearance of the pyloric mucosa on scans parallel to the pylorus.[56, 58–60, 62, 64] The latter finding, which also is seen radiographically, is caused by infolding of the mucosa under the pressure of the hypertrophied muscle.

Table 25-2. Sonographic Manifestations of Pyloric Stenosis

Primary findings
    Pyloric musculature ≥ 4 mm
    Pyloric outer-to-outer diameter > 15 mm
    Pyloric length ≥ 17 mm
Ancillary findings
    Gastric distention
    Peristaltic waves in gastric body
    Tram-track appearance of pylorus
    Antral nipple

Diagnostic Caveats

The diagnosis of infantile hypertrophic pyloric stenosis is fairly straightforward in the proper clinical setting, but false-positive diagnoses may be made, and other conditions, especially peptic disease, can mimic the findings seen in this condition. Several diagnostic caveats appear to enhance sonographic accuracy.[55, 58, 60] First, the pylorus *must* be assessed both parallel and perpendicular to its axis. Muscular hypertrophy should be diagnosed only when thickening seen in one plane can be confirmed in the orthogonal plane. Second, longitudinal images must fall precisely along the axis of the pylorus, since off-axis images may spuriously thicken the muscularis. Third, overdistention of the stomach should be avoided as this may artifactually shorten the pylorus or result in failure of pyloric visualization. Finally, the sonographer should be alert for other abnormalities, such as mucosal thickening in peptic disease[60, 65] and gastroesophageal reflux.[65, 66]

REFERENCES

1. Pozniak MA, Scanlan K, Yandow D: Ultrasound in the evaluation of bowel disorders. Semin Ultrasound CT MRI 8:366–384, 1987.
2. Bolondi L, Casanova P, Santi V, et al: The sonographic appearance of the normal gastric wall: An in vitro study. Ultrasound Med Biol 12:991–998, 1986.
3. Stringer DA, Daneman A, Brunelle F, et al: Sonography of the normal and abnormal stomach (excluding hypertrophic pyloric stenosis) in children. J Ultrasound Med 5:183–188, 1986.
4. Fleischer AC, Muhletaler CA, James AE: Sonographic assessment of the bowel wall. Am J Roentgenol 136:887–891, 1981.
5. Miller JH, Kemberling CR: Ultrasound of the pediatric gastrointestinal tract. Semin Ultrasound CT MR 8:349–365, 1987.
6. Fleischer AC, Dowling AD, Weinstein ML, James AE: Sonographic patterns of distended, fluid-filled bowel. Radiology 133:681–685, 1979.
7. Morgan CL, Trought WS, Oddson TA, Clark WM, Rice RP: Ultrasound patterns of disorders affecting the gastrointestinal tract. Radiology 135:129–135, 1980.
8. Fakhry JR, Berk RN: The "target" pattern: Characteristic sonographic feature of stomach and bowel abnormalities. Am J Roentgenol 137:969–972, 1981.
9. Chisholm HL, Raptopoulos V, Fabian TM: The sonographic target pattern in nongastrointestinal abnormalities. J Clin Ultrasound 13:42–44, 1985.
10. Mueller PR, Ferrucci JT, Harbin WP, et al: Appearance of lymphomatous involvement of the mesentery by ultrasonography and body computed tomography: The "sandwich sign." Radiology 134:467–473, 1980.
11. Bozkurt T, Richter F, Lux G: Ultrasonography as a primary diagnostic tool in patients with inflammatory disease and tumors of the small intestine and large bowel. J Clin Ultrasound 22:85–91, 1994.
12. Wilson SR, Toi A: The value of sonography in the diagnosis of acute diverticulitis of the colon. Am J Roentgenol 154:1199–1202, 1990.
13. Teefey SA, Montana MA, Goldfogel GA, Shuman WP: Sonographic diagnosis of neutropenic typhlitis. Am J Roentgenol 149:731–733, 1987.
14. Dubbins PA: Ultrasound demonstration of bowel wall thickness in inflammatory bowel disease. Clin Radiol 35:227–231, 1984.
15. Yeh HC, Rabinowitz JG: Ultrasonography and computed tomography of gastric wall lesions. Radiology 141:147–155, 1981.
16. DiCandio G, Mosca F, Campatelli A, et al: Sonographic detection of postsurgical recurrence of Crohn disease. Am J Roentgenol 146:523–526, 1986.
17. Miller JH, Hindman BW, Lam AHK: Ultrasound in the evaluation of small bowel lymphoma in children. Radiology 135:409–414, 1980.
18. Shirahama M, Koga T, Ishibashi H, Uchida S, Ohta Y: Sonographic features of colon carcinoma seen with high-frequency transabdominal ultrasound. J Clin Ultrasound 22:359–365, 1994.
19. Quillin SP, Siegel MJ: Gastrointestinal inflammation in children: Color Doppler ultrasonography. J Ultrasound Med 13:751–756, 1994.
20. Quillin SP, Siegel MJ: Appendicitis: Efficacy of color Doppler sonography. Radiology 191:557–560, 1994.
21. Lim HK, Bae SH, Lee KH, Seo GS, Yoon GS: Assessment of reducibility of ileocolic intussusception in children: Usefulness of color Doppler sonography. Radiology 191:781–785, 1994.
22. Franken EA, Kao SCS, Smith WL, Sato Y: Imaging of the acute abdomen in infants and children. Am J Roentgenol 153:921–928, 1989.
23. Barr LL: Sonography in the infant with acute abdominal symptoms. Semin Ultrasound CT MRI 15:275–289, 1994.
24. Kodroff MB, Hartenberg MA, Goldschmidt RA: Ultrasonographic diagnosis of gangrenous bowel in neonatal necrotizing enterocolitis. Pediatr Radiol 14:168–170, 1984.
25. Miller SF, Seibert JJ, Kinder DL, Wilson AR: Use of ultrasound in the detection of occult bowel perforation in neonates. J Ultrasound Med 12:531–535, 1993.
26. Vernacchia FS, Jeffrey RB, Laing FC, Wing VW: Sonographic recognition of pneumatosis intestinalis. Am J Roentgenol 145:51–52, 1985.
27. Siegel B, Machi J, Ramos JR, Serota AL, Robertson AL: Ultrasonic features of pneumatosis intestinalis. J Clin Ultrasound 13:675–678, 1985.
28. Puylaert JBCM: Acute appendicitis: US evaluation using graded compression. Radiology 158:355–360, 1986.
29. Abu-Yousef MM, Bleicher JJ, Maher JW, et al: High-resolution sonography of acute appendicitis. Am J Roentgenol 149:53–58, 1987.
30. Puylaert JBCM, Rutgers PH, Lalisang RI, et al: A prospective study of ultrasonography in the diagnosis of appendicitis. N Engl J Med 317:666–669, 1987.
31. Jeffrey RB, Laing FC, Lewis FR: Acute appendicitis: High-resolution real-time US findings. Radiology 163:11–14, 1987.
32. Abu-Yosef MM, Franken EA: An overview of graded compression sonography in the diagnosis of acute appendicitis. Semin Ultrasound CT MR 10:352–363, 1989.
33. Larson JM, Peirce JC, Ellinger DM, et al: The validity and utility of sonography in the diagnosis of appendicitis in the community setting. Am J Roentgenol 153:687–691, 1989.
34. Kao SCS, Smith WL, Abu-Yosef MM, et al: Acute appendicitis in children: Sonographic findings. Am J Roentgenol 153:375–379, 1989.
35. Vignault F, Filiatrault D, Brandt ML, et al: Acute appendicitis in children; Evaluation with US. Radiology 176:501–504, 1990.

36. Worrell JA, Drolshagen LE, Kely TC, et al: Graded compression ultrasound in the diagnosis of appendicitis; A comparison of diagnostic criteria. J Ultrasound Med 9:145–150, 1990.

37. Brown JJ: Acute appendicitis: The radiologist's role. Radiology 180:13–14, 1991.

38. Rioux M: Sonographic detection of the normal and abnormal appendix. Am J Roentgenol 158:773–778, 1992.

39. Sivit CJ: Diagnosis of acute appendicitis in children: Spectrum of sonographic findings. Am J Roentgenol 161:147–152, 1993.

40. Balthazar EJ, Birnbaum BA, Yee J, et al: Acute appendicitis: CT and US correlation in 100 patients. Radiology 190:31–55, 1994.

41. Jeffrey RB, Jain KA, Nghiem HV: Sonographic diagnosis of acute appendicitis: Interpretive pitfalls. Am J Roentgenol 162:55–59, 1994.

42. Parulekar SG: Ultrasonographic findings in diseases of the appendix. J Ultrasound Med 2:59–64, 1983.

43. Borushok KF, Jeffrey RB, Laing FC, Townsend RR: Sonographic diagnosis of perforation in patients with acute appendicitis. Am J Roentgenol 154:275–278, 1990.

44. Quillin SP, Siegel MJ: Diagnosis of appendiceal abscess in children with acute appendicitis: Value of color Doppler sonography. Am J Roentgenol 164:1251–1254, 1995.

45. Aston SJ, Machlfeder HL: Intussusception in the adult. Am Surg 41:576–580, 1975.

46. Donhauser JL, Kelly EC: Intussusception in the adult. Am J Surg 79:673–677, 1950.

47. Stubenbord WT, Thorbjarnarson B: Intussusception in adults. Ann Surg 172:306–310, 1970.

48. Morin ME, Blumenthal DH, Tan A, Li YP: The ultrasonic appearance of ileocolic intussusception. J Clin Ultrasound 9:516–518, 1981.

49. Pandher D, Sauerbrei EE: Neonatal ileocolic intussusception with enterogenous cyst: Ultrasonic diagnosis. J Assoc Can Radiol 34:328–330, 1983.

50. Bowerman RA, Silver TM, Jaffe MH: Real-time ultrasound diagnosis of intussusception in children. Radiology 143:527–529, 1982.

51. Lutz HT, Petzold R: Ultrasonic patterns of space-occupying lesions of the stomach and the intestine. Ultrasound Med Biol 2:129–132, 1976.

52. Lee TG, Brickman FE, Avecilia LS: Ultrasound diagnosis of intramural intestinal hematoma. J Clin Ultrasound 5:423–424, 1978.

53. Struck E, Urbanek R: Sonography in the diagnosis of hypertrophic pyloric stenosis. Monatssch Kinderheilkd 130:840–843, 1982.

54. Khamapirad T, Athey PA: Ultrasound diagnosis of hypertrophic pyloric stenosis. J Pediatr 102:23–26, 1983.

55. Blumhagen JD, Noble HGS: Muscle thickness in hypertrophic pyloric stenosis: Sonographic determination. Am J Roentgenol 140:221–223, 1983.

56. Ball TI, Atkinson GO, Gay BB: Ultrasound diagnosis of hypertrophic pyloric stenosis: Real-time application and the demonstration of a new sonographic sign. Radiology 147:499–502, 1983.

57. Wilson DA, Vanhoutte JJ: The reliable sonographic diagnosis of hypertrophic pyloric stenosis. J Clin Ultrasound 12:201–204, 1984.

58. Haller JO, Cohen HL: Hypertrophic pyloric stenosis: Diagnosis using US. Radiology 161:335–339, 1986.

59. Stunden RJ, Lequesne GW, Little KET: The improved ultrasound diagnosis of hypertrophic pyloric stenosis. Pediatr Radiol 16:200–205, 1986.

60. Swischuk LE, Hayden CK, Stansberry SD: Sonographic pitfalls in imaging of the antropyloric region in infants. RadioGraphics 9:437–447, 1989.

61. Strauss S, Itzchak Y, Manor A, Heyman Z, Graif M: Sonography of hypertrophic pyloric stenosis. Am J Roentgenol 136:1057–1058, 1981.

62. Cohen HL, Schechter S, Mestel AL, Eaton DH, Haller JO: Ultrasonic "double track" sign in hypertrophic pyloric stenosis. J Ultrasound Med 6:139–143, 1987.

63. O'Keeffe FN, Stansberry SD, Swischuk LE, Hayden CK: Antropyloric muscle thickness at US in infants: What is normal? Radiology 178:827–830, 1991.

64. Hernanz-Schulman M, Dinauer P, Ambrosino MM, Polk DB, Neblett WW: The antral nipple sign of pyloric mucosal prolapse: Endoscopic correlation of a new sonographic observation in patients with pyloric stenosis. J Ultrasound Med 14:283–287, 1995.

65. Hayden CK, Swischuk LE, Rytting JE: Gastric ulcer disease in infants: US findings. Radiology 164:131–134, 1987.

66. Naik DR, Moore DJ: Ultrasound diagnosis of gastro-oesophageal reflux. Arch Dis Child 59:366–379, 1984.

67. Swischuk LE, Hayden CK, Fawcett HD, Isenberg JN: Gastroesophageal reflux: How much imaging is required? RadioGraphics 8:1137–1145, 1988.

Chapter 26

Abdominal Arterial Aneurysms

William J. Zwiebel

Aneurysms of the aorta and other abdominal vessels are potentially lethal, yet often they are silent clinically. Ultrasound plays an important role in the diagnosis and management of abdominal aneurysms by detecting clinically silent aneurysms, by following aneurysm enlargement over time, and by detecting complications resulting from aneurysm surgery. In this chapter, the clinical and pathologic features of abdominal arterial aneurysms are reviewed, and ultrasound techniques are described that ensure optimum diagnostic results.

NORMAL ANATOMY

The normal abdominal aorta[1-4] (Figs. 26–1, 26–2) has smooth margins and a well-defined wall; it tapers slightly below the level of the renal arteries. The maximum normal diameter of the aorta has traditionally been set at 3 cm,[3, 4] but this value is excessive, based on recent studies showing a maximum normal diameter of only 2 cm in adults.[4] The aorta is located slightly to the left of midline and lies adjacent to the spine throughout its intra-abdominal course. In contrast, the inferior vena cava lies to the right of the midline and gradually moves away from the spine as it passes through the liver and diaphragm. It is possible, therefore, to differentiate between the aorta and the inferior vena cava at a glance.

The normal iliac arteries (see Color Figure 26–3 following page 268) are smoothly marginated and uniform in caliber. The maximum diameter of the common iliac artery (outer-to-outer) generally is about 1 cm, and the external iliac artery is slightly smaller.

TERMINOLOGY

The aorta is considered aneurysmal when the dilated segment is 1.5 times greater in diameter than an adjacent normal segment. Aneurysmal dilatation often is localized, but some aneurysms may extend over long segments of an artery. Certain modifiers are used to describe the extent and shape of aneurysms, including focal aneurysm, diffuse aneurysm, saccular aneurysm, and fusiform aneurysm. The meanings of these terms are self-evident. Other modifiers describe the pathologic causes of aneurysms, including true aneurysm, false aneurysm, arterial dissection, and mycotic aneurysm. It is useful to review these terms as their meanings are *not* self-evident.

True Aneurysm

The composite layers of the vessel wall are intact, but stretched, in a true aneurysm (Fig. 26–4A). The great majority of aortic and iliac aneurysms are true aneurysms. The precise pathogenic mechanism for aortic and iliac aneurysm formation is unknown; after all, atherosclerosis is a ubiquitous condition, yet aneurysms occur in relatively few individuals, and usually they are localized to the infrarenal portion of the aorta. Furthermore, aortoiliac aneurysms occur predominately (76%) in men even though atherosclerosis occurs in both men and women.[5] The tendency for aortic aneurysms to occur infrarenally is of great importance, because the surgeon may conveniently maintain perfusion of the kidneys during surgical repair by cross-clamping the aorta below the renal arteries. Surgical repair is complex for aneurysms that extend cephalad to the renal arteries, and it may involve reimplantation of the renal arteries or mesenteric vessels.

False Aneurysm

A false aneurysm occurs when a hole in the arterial wall permits the escape of blood, which subsequently is confined by surrounding tissues (Fig. 26–4B). The extravasated blood forms a hematoma, into the center of which blood continues to circulate. The aneurysm is "false" since it is not confined by an arterial wall. Most false aneurysms result from iatrogenic arterial puncture followed by inadequate hemostasis, but false aneurysms also may result from violent trauma or localized destruction of the arterial wall by an infectious agent. The term "mycotic aneurysm" is used for infection-related lesions. False aneurysms also may occur at graft anastomoses.

Arterial Dissection

The term "dissecting aneurysm" is a misnomer, for the artery affected by dissection is not always

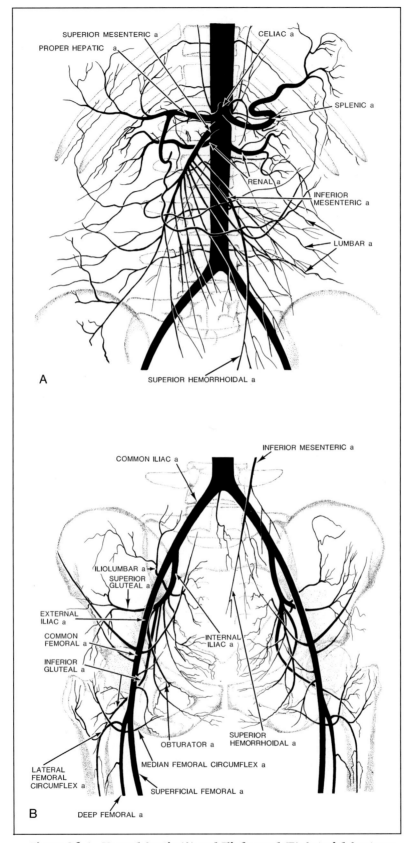

Figure 26-1—Normal Aortic (A) and Iliofemoral (B) Arterial Anatomy.

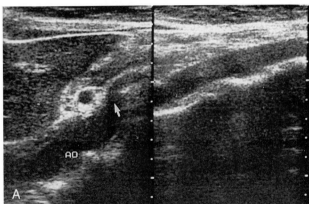

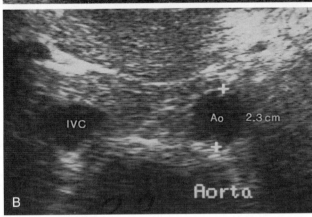

Figure 26-2—Sonography of the Normal Aorta. (A) A longitudinal view demonstrates the entire aorta (AO) from the diaphragmatic hiatus on the left to just proximal to the iliac arteries. Note that the aorta tapers slightly below the level of the superior mesenteric artery (arrow). **(B)** Transverse view of the aorta (Ao, cursors) and the inferior vena cava (IVC), near the diaphragm. The aorta measures 2.3 cm in this individual. The curved white line at the bottom of the image is produced by the spine.

aneurysmal (dilated). The preferred term, therefore, is "arterial dissection."[6] This condition occurs when blood enters the media of the vessel through a rent in the intima and then dissects along the length of the artery (Fig. 26–4C). The intima, and in some cases part of the media, are stripped away and a new lumen, called the false lumen, is formed. Blood may flow freely through both the false lumen and the original (true) lumen, to supply branch vessels. Arterial dissection requires two processes: weakening of the media of the vessel, and the development of a rent in the intima through which blood gains access to the media. Certain uncommon conditions such as Marfan syndrome weaken the arterial media and predispose individuals to arterial dissection, but the great majority of arterial dissections are idiopathic. Although arterial dissection occurs commonly in atherosclerotic vessels, it is not clear that atherosclerosis is a causative factor. Arterial dissection almost invariably begins in the chest and extends into the abdomen.

AORTIC ANEURYSM PRESENTATION

Patients with aortic aneurysms may present with abdominal, back, or leg pain, but 30% to

Figure 26-4—Types of Aneurysms. Normal arterial wall components are shown at the left. In a true aneurysm, the components of the arterial wall are "stretched." In a false aneurysm, a hole is present in the arterial wall. In arterial dissection, a hematoma forms between components of the wall.

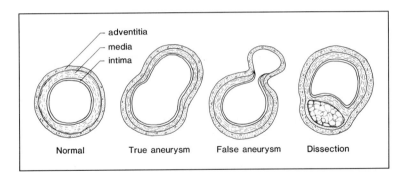

Normal   True aneurysm   False aneurysm   Dissection

60% of them are asymptomatic. In the latter patients, aneurysms are discovered incidentally on physical examination or imaging studies.[5] It is a good practice to check for silent aortic aneurysms in all elderly patients (especially men) who present for abdominal ultrasound examination.

Aortic aneurysms also may present following acute leakage or frank rupture. The signs and symptoms, in such cases, may include pain, prostration, or shock. Aortic aneurysm rupture usually is a catastrophic event and carries a mortality rate of approximately 50%.[6-8]

RISK VERSUS SIZE

The risk of rupture increases with aortic aneurysm size. If the diameter of the aneurysm remains less than 5 cm, the rupture rate is only 5% over a 10-year period. In contrast, if the aneurysm is 5 cm or larger, the rupture rate is 25% over an 8-year period. The risk of rupture increases substantially for aneurysms with a diameter of 6 or more cm,[9, 10] and for this reason surgical repair generally is recommended for aneurysms of this size.

On average, the diameter of an aortic aneurysm "grows" 2 mm to 5 mm per year.[11-13] Average expansion rates are not very meaningful, however, because there is considerable individual variation. When an aneurysm is discovered, therefore, serial ultrasound measurements are usually made at 6-month intervals to determine the rate of expansion. If the aneurysm is small and slow to enlarge, the follow-up interval may be increased to 1 year, but the usual interval for follow-up is 6 months.

Most iliac artery aneurysms occur in association with distal aortic aneurysms, and in such cases the aortic aneurysm generally is the source of clinical concern. Isolated iliac artery aneurysms* are uncommon but may be deadly for two reasons. First, they often cannot be palpated even when they are large. Second, rupture of an iliac artery aneurysm generates nonspecific symptoms of abdominal or pelvic pain, the cause of which may not be recognized until the patient becomes hypotensive or dies. Iliac artery aneurysms 3 cm or larger in diameter generally are felt to pose considerable risk of rupture, and surgical repair or percutaneous stenting are recommended for iliac aneurysms of this size. Iliac artery aneurysms usually are located in the proximal or distal portion of the common iliac arteries. It is useful, therefore to visualize both areas in the course of aneurysm evaluation.

*Not associated with aortic aneurysm.

SONOGRAPHIC APPEARANCE

The primary criterion for the sonographic diagnosis of an arterial aneurysm[13, 14] is a focal increase in the caliber of the artery, with the diameter of the dilated segment measuring at least 1.5 to 2 times greater than adjacent unaffected segment(s) (Fig. 26–5). For aortic aneurysms, an additional feature is the absence of tapering of the vessel below the mesenteric and renal vessels.

Aortic aneurysms have various gross configurations. Some are bulbous, with a sharp junction, or neck, between the normal and aneurysmal portions. Others are fusiform, with a gradual transition between the normal and aneurysmal portions. Many aneurysmal aortas are tortuous, for the aorta typically elongates as well as dilates. Tortuous aortas usually deviate to the left of the spine, as shown in Figure 26–6, but some may deviate anteriorly, creating a prominent kink at the aneurysm neck.

Concentric layers of thrombus usually line the wall of large aortic or iliac aneurysms (Fig. 26–7), and this thrombus may generate emboli that occlude distal arteries. The thrombus in an aneurysm usually is not organized and neither provides structural support nor reduces the risk of rupture.[7] Because of the presence of thrombus, the outer dimensions of an aneurysm often are much greater than the dimensions of the lumen. Arteriography, therefore, usually underestimates the size of an aortic aneurysm.[15, 16]

EXAMINATION PROTOCOL

I recommend the examination protocol presented in Table 26–1 for assessment of aortic and iliac aneurysms. To attain the best results, the following caveats should be noted with respect to this protocol.

1. Always measure an aneurysm the way a surgeon does in the operating room: from the outer surfaces of the vessel (outer-to-outer) (Fig. 26–5).
2. Sagittal and coronal planes are recommended for aneurysm measurement, as shown in Figure 26–5. These planes clearly show the point of maximum dilatation and they avoid error resulting from oblique measurement (Fig. 26–6).
3. Coronal views generally are easier to obtain from the left side of the aorta (Fig. 26–5) than from the right.
4. The maximum interobserver variability for aortic measurement is approximately 5 mm (95% confidence limits), and the mean vari-

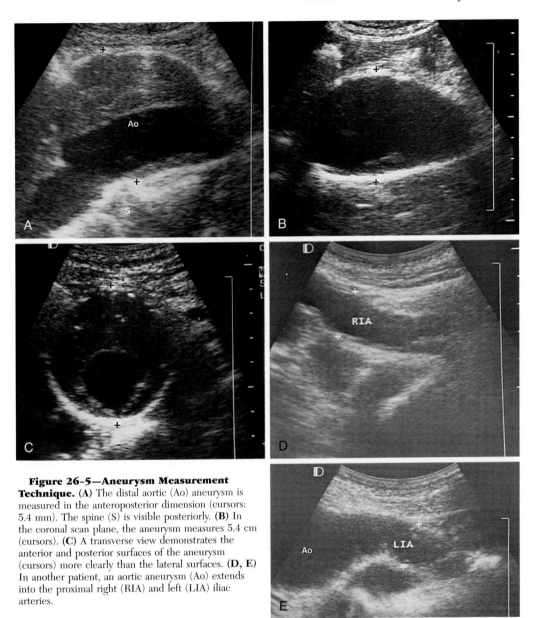

Figure 26-5—Aneurysm Measurement Technique. (A) The distal aortic (Ao) aneurysm is measured in the anteroposterior dimension (cursors: 5.4 mm). The spine (S) is visible posteriorly. (B) In the coronal scan plane, the aneurysm measures 5.4 cm (cursors). (C) A transverse view demonstrates the anterior and posterior surfaces of the aneurysm (cursors) more clearly than the lateral surfaces. (D, E) In another patient, an aortic aneurysm (Ao) extends into the proximal right (RIA) and left (LIA) iliac arteries.

ability is about 2.5 mm.[17] Therefore, an increase in size of less than 5 mm from one examination to another may not be significant.

5. Remember, aneurysms do not decrease in size! To avoid looking foolish, be aware of the measurements reported previously before giving current measurements.

6. Always determine whether or not an aneurysm extends to or above the renal arteries. This is done best by directly visualizing the renal artery origins and measuring the distance from these vessels to the aneurysm. If the renal arteries cannot be visualized directly, their location may be *inferred* by measuring the distance from the superior mesenteric artery (SMA) to the aneurysm (Fig. 26–8). The

renal arteries arise no more than 1.5 cm below the SMA; therefore, the renal arteries should be unaffected if the aneurysm begins 2 cm or more below the SMA.

7. The entire abdominal aorta must be examined to insure that suprarenal aneurysms are not overlooked.

8. Aneurysms at the iliac bifurcations can easily be overlooked (Fig. 26–9) because this area is difficult to visualize. A transducer position lateral to the rectus muscles (Fig. 26–10) is an aid to iliac artery visualization.

COMPLICATIONS

Potential complications of aortic aneurysms are atherosclerotic renal artery obstruction, hy-

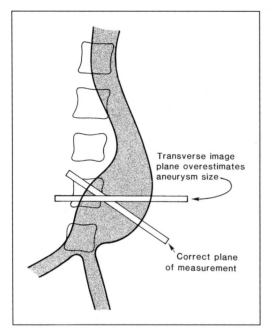

Figure 26-6—Measurement Difficulties Caused by Aortic Tortuosity. Note that the transverse diameter of this tortuous aorta is exaggerated with a true transverse view and is correctly measured only in an oblique view. Coronal images eliminate this problem.

Table 26-1. Examination Protocol for Aortic and Iliac Aneurysms

A. **Longitudinal**
  1. Examine aorta, diaphragm to bifurcation
  2. Determine location and longitudinal extent of aortic aneurysm
  3. Measure aortic aneurysm, anteroposterior (AP), outer-to-outer
  4. Examine iliac arteries to iliac bifurcation
  5. Measure iliac artery aneurysm(s), if present, outer-to-outer
B. **Transverse**
  1. Document the maximum diameter of the aorta at the diaphragm, superior mesenteric artery, and distally
  2. Measure aneurysm, AP and transverse, outer-to-outer
  3. Visualize the iliac arteries
  4. Measure iliac artery aneurysm(s), if present, outer-to-outer
C. **Coronal**
  1. Measure aortic aneurysm, *transverse* dimension, outer-to-outer
  2. Examine iliac arteries and measure aneurysm(s), if present
D. **Color Doppler examination**
  1. Confirm patency of superior mesenteric, celiac, and renal arteries, and examine for flow disturbances associated with stenosis
  2. Measure distance from renal arteries to aneurysm neck
  3. Alternatively, measure distance from superior mesenteric artery to aneurysm neck
E. **Kidneys, longitudinal and transverse**
  1. Document kidney length and normal features
  2. Document hydronephrosis, if present

dronephrosis (due to aneurysm compression of a ureter), retroperitoneal fibrosis, and aneurysm rupture.

Renal artery obstruction, if severe, results in shrinkage of the affected kidney. This finding, as well as hydronephrosis, is easily identified with ultrasound, and for this reason, the kidneys are always evaluated in the course of aortic examination.

Retroperitoneal fibrosis[18, 19] is a rare complication of unknown etiology. Fibrosis is manifested as a hypoechoic soft tissue mantle that partially or completely surrounds the aorta and may ex-

tend bilaterally into the retroperitoneum.[18, 19] The ureters may be entrapped in the fibrotic mass, leading to hydronephrosis.

The most disastrous complication of aortic or iliac aneurysm is rupture.[7, 8, 20, 21] Sonography is only rarely used when aneurysm rupture is suspected, because immediate surgery often is required to maintain life. In some cases, however,

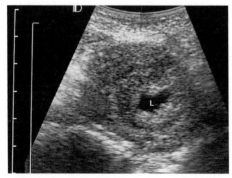

Figure 26-7—Thrombus Within Aneurysm. Concentric layers of thrombus surround the atrial lumen (L) in this 5-cm distal aortic aneurysm.

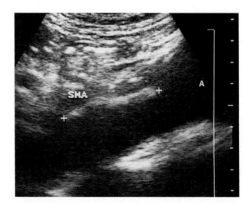

Figure 26-8. Measurement of the distance (cursors) between the SMA and the aneurysm (A) neck (sagittal view). The distance in this case is 4.6 cm, clearly indicating that the aneurysm is infrarenal.

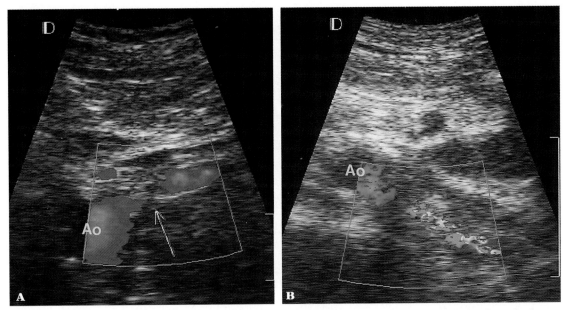

Figure 18-9—Renal Artery Stenosis (in a 68 year old man with diabetes, hypertension, and peripheral vascular disease, confirmed angiographically). **(A)** A transverse power Doppler image through the aorta (Ao) shows a stenosis (arrow) at the origin of the left renal artery. **(B)** A color Doppler image in a slightly different orientation shows the aorta (Ao) and severely disturbed flow (mixture of colors) distal to the left renal artery stenosis. Blood flow could not be detected in the stenosis with power Doppler or conventional color Doppler imaging, but spectral Doppler (not shown) demonstrated an extremely high peak systolic velocity of 665 cm/sec in the stenosis.

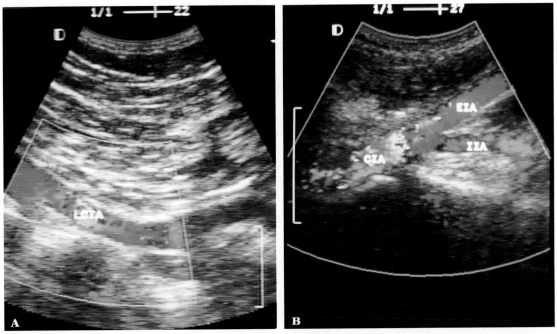

Figure 26-3—Iliac Arteries. **(A)** A longitudinal view shows the left common iliac artery (LCIA) origin from the aorta (left side of image). **(B)** The common iliac artery (CIA) is seen to divide into the external (EIA) and internal (IIA) iliac arteries.

PLATE V

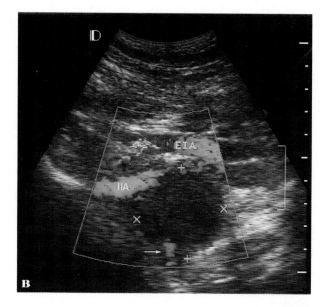

Figure 26-9B. Isolated internal iliac artery (IIA) aneurysm (cursors). Outflow point (arrow) is barely visible. The external iliac artery (EIA) is seen anterior to the aneurysm.

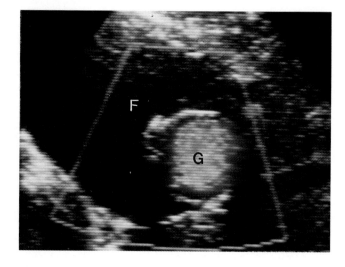

Figure 26-16—Perigraft Fluid. A large fluid collection (F) partially surrounds the graft (G) as seen in this transverse section.

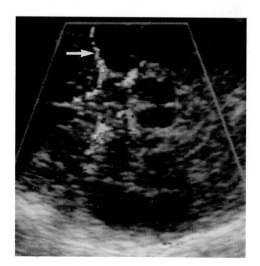

Figure 35-7—Color Doppler of the Circle of Willis. Transverse view at the skull base shows the circle of Willis; the middle cerebral artery is easily seen (arrow) and can be investigated with pulsed Doppler technique.

PLATE VI

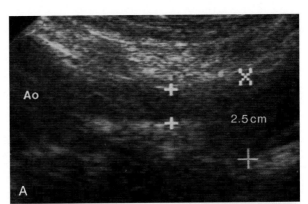

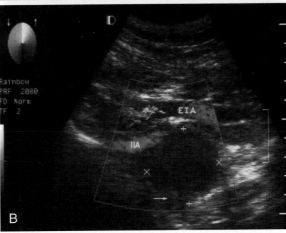

Figure 26-9—Aneurysms at the Iliac Bifurcation. (**A**) A 2.5-cm aneurysm (X and + cursors) is visible at the iliac bifurcation. An aortic aneurysm (Ao) is visible at the left. (**B**) Isolated internal iliac artery (IIA) aneurysm (cursors). Outflow point (arrow) is barely visible posteriorly. The external iliac artery (EIA) is seen anterior to the aneurysm. See Color Figure 26–9*B* following page 268.

leakage of blood is contained by surrounding tissues, lessening the acuteness of the clinical situation. In such instances, computed tomography (CT) is the preferred method for confirming that a leaking aneurysm is the cause of the patient's symptoms[20] (Fig. 26–11*A*). As an expedient, sonography sometimes is used to confirm the presence of an aneurysm, implying that aneurysm rupture is the cause of symptomatology.

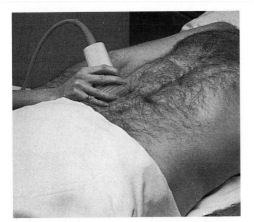

Figure 26-10. Transducer position lateral to the rectus muscle, for visualization of the iliac arteries.

The demonstration of a retroperitoneal hematoma provides direct evidence of aortic rupture (Fig. 26–11*B*). The hematoma is hypoechoic and usually is unilateral or asymmetric. It typically displaces the ipsilateral kidney. Peritoneal fluid also may be present if the aneurysm has leaked into the peritoneal space.

ARTERIAL DISSECTION

CT and magnetic resonance imaging are the primary imaging methods used for detecting and evaluating arterial dissection in the thorax and abdomen. Arterial dissection may be encountered incidentally, however, during sonographic examination. The distinguishing ultrasound finding is a thin membrane that divides the arterial lumen into two compartments (Fig. 26–12). This membrane consists of the intima and in some cases a portion of the media. The membrane moves freely with arterial pulsations if it is thin and if both the true and false lumens are patent. If the membrane is thick or if one lumen is thrombosed, however, the membrane may move little or not at all. Duplex examination may demonstrate flow in both lumina, but different flow

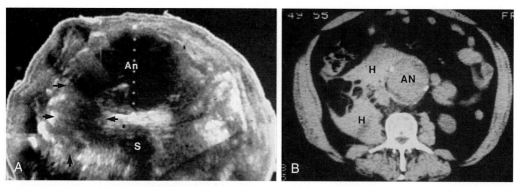

Figure 26-11—Aneurysm Rupture. (A) A transverse abdominal sonogram demonstrates a large hematoma (arrows) that has dissected posterolaterally from an 8-cm aortic aneurysm (An). S = spine. **(B)** Computed tomography demonstrates the hematoma (H) more clearly. AN = aneurysm.

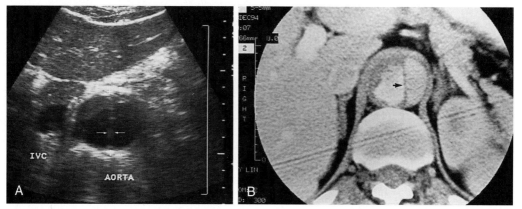

Figure 26-12—Aortic Dissection. (A) A transverse sonogram shows a faintly echogenic intimal flap (arrows) dividing the aortic lumen. The intimal flap is blurred by motion. **(B)** A CT image in the same location more precisely depicts the intimal flap (arrow).

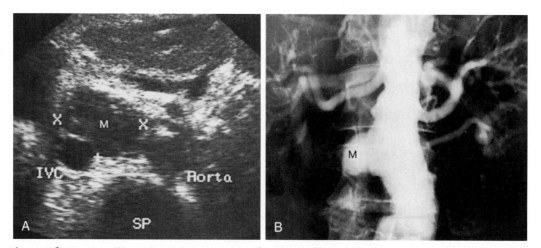

Figure 26-13—Masslike Epigastric Aneurysm. This 75 year old man, who presented with upper abdominal pain, had undergone aortic aneurysm repair approximately 15 years previously, but he had not received regular follow-up. **(A)** Sonography demonstrated a hypoechoic mass (M) located slightly to the right of the aorta, in the vicinity of the pancreatic head. The mass did not pulsate, and Doppler examination was not done. Initially, the mass was thought to be a pancreatic pseudocyst or a necrotic tumor in or near the pancreatic head. IVC = inferior vena cava; SP = spine. **(B)** An arteriogram showed that the mass (M) communicated with the aortic lumen, confirming the diagnosis of pseudoaneurysm.

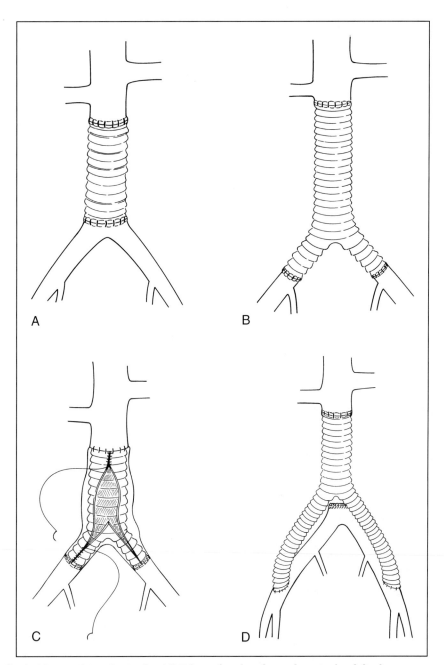

Figure 26-14—Types of Aortic Grafts. **(A)** Tube graft with end-to-end proximal and distal anastomoses. **(B)** Aortoiliac graft with end-to-end distal anastomoses. **(C)** The native aorta is wrapped around the graft and sewn closed. **(D)** Aortobifemoral graft with end-to-side distal anastomoses.

rates may be present, and in some cases flow in the false lumen may be too slow to be detected.

The diameter of the aorta generally is increased by dissection, but not as dramatically as with true aneurysms. In addition, the proximal and distal ends of the dissection may not be as sharply defined as with true aneurysms. Aortic dissection virtually always originates in the chest and extends into the abdominal aorta. Dissection also may extend into the iliac arteries or into other aortic branches. The sonographer should determine the extent of dissection within the abdomen and should look for extension into major aortic branches. Stenosis or occlusion of branch vessels commonly accompanies dissection, and duplex sonography can provide valuable information about these complications.

ANEURYSMS OF EPIGASTRIC AORTIC BRANCHES

Aneurysms form uncommonly in aortic branch arteries, including the superior mesenteric artery, the splenic artery, the hepatic artery, and the renal arteries.[22, 23] Although these aneurysms are uncommon, they are of considerable importance,

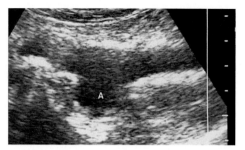

Figure 26–17—Anastomotic Aneurysm. Focal aneurysmal dilatation (A) is evident at the femoral anastomosis of an aortofemoral graft.

for they may be mistaken for abdominal masses arising from the pancreas, liver, or other epigastric structures. This error is particularly apt to occur if the aneurysm does not pulsate because of surrounding fibrosis or intraluminal thrombus. The correct diagnosis, in such cases, can be made only if "aneurysm" comes to the sonographer's mind and Doppler is used to detect flow within the lesion. An example is shown in Figure 26–13.

POSTOPERATIVE ASSESSMENT

Three types of graft procedures are used commonly for aortic aneurysm repair, as illustrated in Figure 26–14. Note from this figure that the aneurysmal aorta sometimes is opened longitudinally and wrapped around the graft. This is done to isolate the graft and the duodenum, lessening the chance of graft infection. The "wrapping" procedure creates a potential space that normally contains fluid during the immediate postoperative period.[24, 25]

Normal Graft Appearance

The objectives of postoperative sonographic examination are to examine the full length of the graft and to evaluate blood flow. The graft material used for aortic bypass has a textured appearance and is quite echogenic (Fig. 26–15). The graft usually can be identified easily. Slight puckering of the graft and native artery occurs at the suture lines, causing visible thickening of the artery wall at the anastomosis. A small layer of fluid normally is present around the graft during the postoperative period. This fluid may be focal or diffuse and may persist for more than a week.

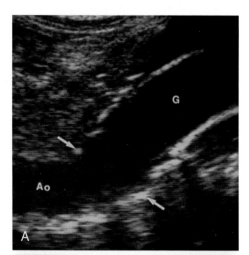

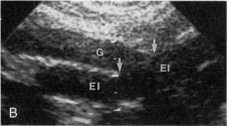

Figure 26-15—Sonogram of an Aortoiliac Graft. **(A)** Proximal end-to-end anastomosis (arrows) of the aorta (Ao) and the graft (G). Note that the weave of the graft is visible. **(B)** End-to-side anastomosis (arrows) of the graft (G) with the external iliac artery (EI).

Complications

The primary complications of aortic graft surgery are hematoma, infection, pseudoaneurysm, true aneurysm, stenosis, and occlusion. All these complications most commonly occur at the anastomoses; therefore, it is imperative to examine the proximal and distal anastomoses carefully. Further discussion of arterial graft complications is beyond the scope of this text, but several graft complications are illustrated in Figure 26–16 following page 268 and Figure 26–17.

REFERENCES

1. Bluth EI: Ultrasound of the abdominal aorta. Arch Intern Med 144:377–380, 1984.
2. Steiner E, Rubens D, Weiss SL, et al: Sonographic examination of the abdominal aorta through the left flank: A prospective study. J Ultrasound Med 5:499–502, 1986.
3. Scott RAP, Ashton HA, Kay DN: Abdominal aortic aneurysm in 4237 screened patients: Prevalence, development and management over 6 years. Br J Surg 78:1122–1124, 1991.
4. Ricci A, Kleeman M, Case T, Pilcher DB: Normal aortic diameter by ultrasound. J Vasc Technol 19:17–19, 1995.
5. Blau SA, Kerstein MD, Deterling RA: Abdominal aortic aneurysm. *In* Kerstein MD, Moulder MD, Webb WR (eds): Aneurysms. Baltimore, Williams & Wilkins, 1983, pp 127–196.
6. DeSanctis RW, Doroghazi RM, Austen G, et al: Aortic dissection. N Engl J Med 317:1060–1067, 1987.
7. Garrett HE, Ilabaca PA: The ruptured abdominal aortic aneurysm. *In* Bergan JJ, Yao JST (eds): Aneurysms: Diagnosis and Treatment. New York, Grune & Stratton, 1982, pp 302–326.
8. Cronenwett JL, Murphy TF, Zelenock GB, et al: Actuarial analysis of variables associated with rupture of small abdominal aortic aneurysms. Surgery 98:462–483, 1985.
9. Bergan JJ, Yao JST: Atherosclerotic aneurysms. *In* Bergan JJ, Yao JST (eds): Aneurysms: Diagnosis and Treatment. New York, Grune & Stratton, 1982, pp 287–301.
10. Nevitt MP, Ballard DJ, Hallett JW: Prognosis of abdominal aortic aneurysms. N Engl J Med 321:1009–1014, 1989.
11. Bernstein EF, Chan EL: Abdominal aortic aneurysm in high-risk patients: Outcome of selective management based on size and expansion rate. Ann Surg 200:255–263, 1984.
12. Sterpetti AV, Shultz RD, Feldhaus RJ, et al: Abdominal aortic aneurysms in elderly patients: Selective management based on clinical status and aneurysmal expansion rate. Am J Surg 150:772–776, 1985.
13. LaRoy LL, Cormier PJ, Matalon TAS, et al: Imaging of abdominal aortic aneurysms. Am J Roentgenol 152:785–792, 1989.
14. Paivansao M, Lahde S, Myllyla V, et al: Ultrasonography in the diagnosis of abdominal aortic aneurysms. Fortschr Röntgenstr 140(6):683–685, 1984.
15. Harter LP, Gross BH, Callen PW, et al: Ultrasonic evaluation of abdominal aortic thrombus. J Ultrasound Med 1:315, 1982.
16. King PS, Copperberg PL, Madigan SM: The anechoic crescent in abdominal aortic aneurysms: Not a sign of dissection. Am J Roentgenol 146:345–348, 1986.
17. Yucel EK, Fillmore DJ, Knox TA, Waltman AC: Sonographic measurement of abdominal aortic diameter: Interobserver variability. J Ultrasound Med 10:681–683, 1991.
18. Bundy AL, Ritchie WGM: Inflammatory aneurysm of the abdominal aorta. J Clin Ultrasound 12:102–104, 1984.
19. Cullenward MJ, Scanlan KA, Pozniak MA, et al: Inflammatory aortic aneurysm (periaortic fibrosis): Radiologic imaging. Radiology 159:75–82, 1986.
20. Clayton MJ, Walsh JW, Brewer WH: Contained rupture of abdominal aortic aneurysms: Sonographic and CT diagnosis. Am J Roentgenol 138:154–156, 1982.
21. Rosen A, Korobkin M, Silverman PM, et al: CT diagnosis of ruptured abdominal aortic aneurysm. Am J Roentgenol 143:265–268, 1984.
22. Falkoff GE, Taylor KJW, Morse S: Hepatic artery pseudoaneurysm: Diagnosis with real-time and pulsed Doppler US. Radiology 158:55–56, 1986.
23. Huey H, Cooperberg PL, Bogoch A: Diagnosis of giant varix of the coronary vein by pulsed-Doppler sonography. Am J Roentgenol 143:77–78, 1984.
24. Mark A, Moss A, Lusby R, et al: CT evaluation of complications of abdominal aortic surgery. Radiology 145:409–414, 1982.
25. Hilton S, Megibow AJ, Naidich DP, et al: Computed tomography of the postoperative abdominal aorta. Radiology 145:403–407, 1982.

Section 7

The Female Pelvis

INTRODUCTION

Sonography is a very effective method for examining the female pelvis. The technique is essentially risk free, and it provides excellent visualization of the pelvic viscera, either through the distended bladder or via a transvaginal approach.

Until recently, sonography was the principal means for imaging the female pelvis; it was the only technique available with sufficient soft tissue discrimination for effective examination of the female reproductive organs. Magnetic resonance imaging (MRI)[1-3] now is challenging the supremacy of diagnostic ultrasound, since this technique also delineates soft tissue clearly. MRI offers a comprehensive view of the female pelvis that can define pathologic conditions in a way that is difficult sonographically. Finally, MRI can delineate the extraperitoneal and musculoskeletal structures of the pelvis far more clearly than ultrasound. In spite of these advantages, however, sonography will continue to be the principal modality used for examining the female pelvis, for it is relatively inexpensive, widely available, and easily performed. Furthermore, in the great majority of patients, sonographic information is adequate for clinical management. MRI undoubtedly will assume an increasingly important role for clarifying pathology that is difficult to assess sonographically, for tumor staging, and for specific indications, such as the assessment of congenital anomalies.

Although sonography is a proven method for pelvic diagnosis, many sonologists are uncomfortable with the interpretation of pelvic sonograms because findings often are nonspecific. The referring clinician also may be unhappy with pelvic sonography because of unrealistic expectations. Pelvic sonography should be viewed not as a definitive diagnostic procedure but as *an adjunct to physical examination*. When the technique is viewed in this context, sonography functions admirably to confirm normality of the pelvic viscera, to detect pathology, to define and clarify physical findings, to follow changes in pelvic lesions, and to provide specific information about genital tract structure and physiologic responses. Let us briefly consider each of these functions.

1. Is the pelvis normal or abnormal? Transabdominal sonography is reported to be 83% to 94% sensitive, and 96% to 97% specific, overall, for detecting or excluding female pelvic pathology.°[4-8] It appears that accuracy for detecting pathology is improved when transvaginal sonography is combined with transabdominal imaging (100% sensitivity and specificity have been reported for detecting and excluding pathology[7]), but only limited data are available about the accuracy of this technique as of this writing. It is clear, nonetheless, that sonography is an excellent method for confirming that the female pelvis either is normal or abnormal. This capability is of particular value when pelvic physical examination is compromised by obesity, anxiety, or other problems.

2. What is the origin of a mass detected by physical examination? In many cases, sonography precisely localizes pelvic pathology to the uterus, the ovary, the adnexal areas, or the posterior pelvic compartment. Such information is extremely useful for directing further diagnostic efforts and for developing a clinical management plan. Unfortunately, sonography cannot always determine the origin of pelvic pathology, or it may be able only to localize pathology in a general way, e.g., "extrauterine." Furthermore, pathology arising in one organ at times may mimic that originating from another structure, as is the case when a pedunculated leiomyoma simulates a solid

---

°Ectopic pregnancy is excluded from this listing (see Chapter 36). Sensitivity specifically for leiomyoma is as low as 63%; see Chapter 29.

ovarian neoplasm. When the origin of pelvic pathology cannot be ascertained clearly with ultrasound, MRI may provide additional localizing information.

3. What are the gross characteristics of a pelvic lesion? Although sonography cannot provide a tissue-specific diagnosis, it serves quite well, in most cases, for assessing gross pathologic characteristics. For instance, sonography may confirm the "cystic" nature of a mass and may differentiate between cysts with benign and malignant appearances. In some cases, however, sonographic characteristics are non-specific and do not provide useful information for guiding patient management. In these instances, the limitation of the procedure should be reported clearly by the sonologist, but without apologies. MRI may be suggested as an additional procedure for characterizing the pathology in selected cases.

4. Does the sonographic appearance of a pelvic lesion match the clinical impression? Sonographic findings are most valuable when correlated with clinical information and the "train of thought" of the referring clinician. For example, in a young woman who is assumed to have a functional ovarian cyst, sonographic characteristics of the mass must be closely scrutinized to exclude more serious pathology. If the sonographic appearance departs significantly from that of a benign cyst, the clinician may have to think again about the clinical impression and the management plan. In some cases, surgical examination of the mass may be chosen rather than clinical observation.

5. Is a pelvic lesion regressing or enlarging? Sonography is extremely accurate in assessing changes in size or appearance of pelvic lesions. This capability is particularly useful in monitoring cysts that are assumed to be functional in origin.

6. What is the status of the female reproductive organs in patients with delayed menarche, precocious puberty, infertility, or congenital anomalies? Sonography provides extremely valuable information about the structure and physiologic response of the reproductive organs in patients with these conditions. Such information is particularly useful in the management of infertile patients and in children, in whom adequate physical examination often is not possible. MRI also can contribute structural information in these conditions and is a valuable adjunctive procedure.

Essential anatomic, technical, and diagnostic information about pelvic sonography is provided in the chapters that follow. In keeping with the approach used elsewhere in this text, pelvic pathology is discussed in the context of sonographic findings rather than anatomic or histologic diagnoses. Thus, different chapters deal with broad sonographic categories, such as vaginal and uterine fluid collections; solid nonuterine masses; and cystic nonuterine masses. This format was chosen because it matches the diagnostic approach used in the course of most sonographic examinations. Pelvic pathology first is defined as uterine or extrauterine; then as ovarian, nonovarian, or tubal; and then in more specific terms, such as cystic or solid.

REFERENCES

1. Hricak H: MRI of the female pelvis: A review. AJR Am J Roentgenol 146:1115–1122, 1986.
2. Chang YCF, Arrive L, Hricak H: Gynecologic tumor imaging. Semin Ultrasound 10:29–42, 1989.
3. Riccio TJ, Adams HG, Munzing DE, Mattrey RF: Magnetic resonance imaging as an adjunct to sonography in the evaluation of the female pelvis. Magn Reson Imaging 8:699–704, 1990.
4. Sanders RC, McNeil BJ, Finberg HJ, et al: A prospective study of computed tomography and ultrasound in detection and staging of pelvic masses. Radiology 146:439–442, 1983.
5. El-Minawi M, El-Halfaway A, Abdel Hadi M, et al: Laparoscopic, synecographic and ultrasonographic vs. clinical evaluation of a pelvic mass. J Reprod Med 29:197–199, 1984.
6. Kurjak A, Jurkovic D: The value of ultrasound in the initial assessment of gynecological patients. Ultrasound Med Biol 13:401–419, 1987.
7. Andolf E, Jörgensen C: A prospective comparison of clinical ultrasound and operative examination of the female pelvis. J Ultrasound Med 7:617–620, 1988.
8. Buy JN, Ghossain MA, Sciot C, et al: Epithelial Tumors of the Ovary: CT Findings and Correlation with US. Radiology 178:811–818, 1991.

Chapter 27
Anatomy and Technique for Female Pelvic Sonography

William J. Zwiebel

THE TRUE AND FALSE PELVIS

The pelvis is divided anatomically into the "true pelvis," which is the bowl-shaped cavity within the bony pelvis, and the "false pelvis," or iliac fossa,[1] as illustrated in Figure 27–1. Clinicians commonly fail to distinguish between the true and false pelves, and as a result, patients often are referred for pelvic sonography when symptoms or findings point instead to the iliac fossa. The sonographer must be cognizant of the location of the patient's signs and symptoms and examine the correct areas. It does no good, for example, to examine the true pelvis in detail while failing to detect abnormalities related to appendicitis that are located in the iliac fossa!

PERITONEAL AND EXTRAPERITONEAL SPACES

The peritoneum envelops the pelvic viscera, as shown in Figure 27–2. Note that the perito-

neum is "draped over" the pelvic viscera and that pathologic processes may be either intra- or extraperitoneal. Although intraperitoneal pelvic pathology is more common than extraperitoneal pathology, significant abnormality may occur in either location.[1-3] The prevesical space (Fig. 27–2) is a particularly noteworthy extraperitoneal space, as hematoma formation is common here following pelvic surgery employing a low transverse ("bikini") incision.[3] Prevesical collections can be overlooked easily if the ultrasound examination is focused on deeper structures.

THE VAGINA

Disorders of the vagina are only rarely the subject of ultrasound examination, but the vagina is an important orienting landmark that "points the way" to the uterus, particularly when pathology distorts pelvic anatomy. The vagina is depicted sonographically as a linear structure extending inferiorly from the cervix, with a distinctive tram track appearance (Fig. 27–3A). In some instances, the anterior and posterior fornices of the vagina are clearly seen, surrounding the anterior and posterior lips of the cervix (Fig. 27–3B). The vagina generally is excluded from the ultrasound field of view on transvaginal scans, since the transducer is positioned at the upper end of the vagina.

THE UTERUS
Childhood Configuration

The shape of the prepubertal uterus[4-12] is much different from the well-recognized, pear-shaped configuration of adulthood. In the normal prepubertal girl, the uterus has either a tubular or a teardrop shape (Fig. 27–4). The uterine body is about equal in size to the cervix, or it may be somewhat smaller than the cervix. Uterine size changes little from 2 to 7 years of age. Between 7 and 12 years of age uterine size increases somewhat, but somatic growth remains greater, proportionally, than uterine growth. Rapid growth of the uterus begins at puberty

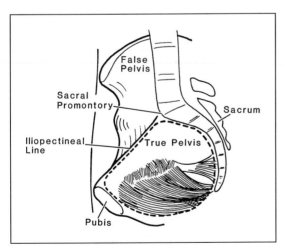

Figure 27-1—Pelvic Anatomy. In this illustration, the true pelvis is outlined by a dotted line. The false pelvis, or iliac fossa, is cephalad to the true pelvis. Note the boundaries of the true pelvis: (1) the sacral promontory; (2) the pubis; (3) the anterior abdominal wall; and (4) the sacrum and associated musculature.

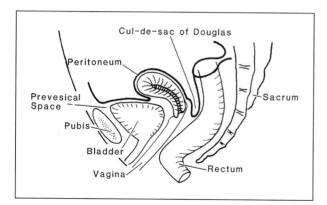

Figure 27-2—Pelvic Peritoneal Reflections. The dark line denotes the location of the peritoneum, which envelopes the pelvic viscera. Note the location of the prevesical space and the cul-de-sac of Douglas.

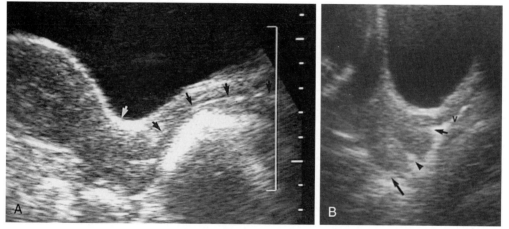

Figure 27-3—Sonographic Anatomy of the Vagina. (A) Longitudinal view showing the "tram track" appearance of the vagina. The central echogenic line is the vaginal lumen (black arrows). The hypoechoic tissue on either side of the lumen represents the vaginal wall. The approximate level of the internal cervical os is shown by the white arrow. **(B)** Longitudinal image showing the anterior (short arrow) and posterior (long arrow) fornices of the vagina. The external cervical os (arrowhead) is flanked by the anterior and posterior lips of the cervix. V = upper portion of vagina.

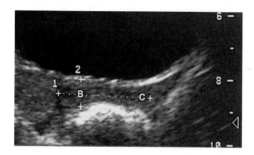

Figure 27-4—Normal Prepubertal Uterus (longitudinal view in a 5 year old girl). Note that the size of the uterine body (B) is similar to that of the cervix (C). The length of the uterus (cursor set 1) is 3.3 cm, corresponding to the normal range for 5 years of age. (Images kindly contributed by Mary Murray, MD, Baystate Medical Center, Springfield, MA.)

Table 27-1. Pediatric Uterine and Ovarian Growth

Age (Years)	Uterine Length (mm)°	Ovarian Volume (cm³)†
2	33.1 ± 4.4	0.75 ± 0.41
4	32.9 ± 3.3	0.82 ± 0.36
6	33.2 ± 4.1	1.19 ± 0.36
8	35.8 ± 7.3	1.05 ± 0.50
10	40.3 ± 6.4	2.22 ± 0.69
12	54.3 ± 8.4	3.80 ± 1.40
13	53.8 ± 11.4	4.18 ± 2.74

°Total uterine length (fundus to cervix); mean, ± 2 SD.
†Mean, ± 2 SD.
From the study of 114 normal females by Orsini LF, Salardi S, Pilu G, et al: Pelvic organs in premenarchal girls: Real-time ultrasonography. Radiology 153:113, 1984.

(about 10 to 12 years). Within a few years after the onset of puberty, uterine size increases five- to sixfold, and the uterus achieves an adult, pear-shaped configuration in which the uterine body is substantially larger than the cervix.[4, 5, 7, 9, 10, 12] The transformation of the uterus to the adult configuration is a valuable landmark for the onset of puberty. Standards for uterine size in children are given in Table 27-1.

Configuration in Menstruating Women

The uterus in adult, menstruating women is a pear-shaped structure that typically is 8 cm long (external cervical os to fundus), 5 cm in the transverse dimension (at its widest point), and 4 cm anteroposterior.[2, 4, 13, 14] Uterine size is slightly greater in parous than in nulliparous women. The adult uterus is divided anatomically into three parts: the cervix, body, and fundus.

The cervix in nonpregnant, menstruating women is approximately 2.5 cm long.[13] The external cervical os often is visible on transabdominal scans, as shown in Figure 27-3B. The internal os can be seen directly in some nonpregnant patients, and even when it cannot be seen directly, its location may be approximated from a distinct angulation of both the anterior uterine surface and the uterine cavity, as shown in Figure 27-5A. The endocervical canal is visible on longitudinal images as a central echogenic line flanked by hypoechoic muscle. On transverse images, the cervix exhibits a "target" configuration (Fig. 27-5B), consisting of a central echogenic canal surrounded by less echogenic myometrium.

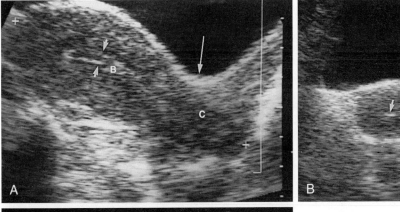

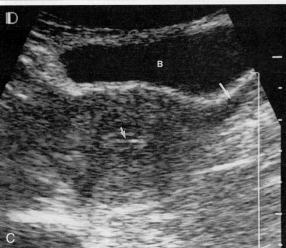

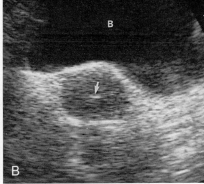

Figure 27-5—Sonographic Anatomy of the Adult Uterus. (A) A long axis view demonstrates the uterine body (B) and cervix (C). Cursors indicate the proper locations from which to measure the uterine length. The notch (large arrow) at the junction of the body and cervix indicates the approximate level of the internal cervical os. The endometrium (small arrows) is echogenic, due to the presence of mucoid material. **(B)** Transverse view of the cervix. Note that the cervix and the cervical canal (arrow) are round in cross section. B = bladder. **(C)** Transverse view of the upper uterine body. Note the ovoid shape of the uterus and the linear endometrial canal (small arrow). The attachment of the round ligament/fallopian tubes complex is visible on the left (large arrow). B = bladder.

The body of the uterus is the portion extending from the internal cervical os to the attachment of the fallopian tubes, and the fundus is the rounded portion cephalad to the tubal insertions (Fig. 27–5A). The body/fundus junction is not denoted sonographically. On transverse sonograms, the body of the uterus has an ovoid configuration, and the uterine cavity is represented by a transverse line (Fig. 27–5B). Laterally directed, triangular projections are apparent in the upper portion of the uterine body, at the attachments of the uterine ligaments and the fallopian tubes (Fig. 27–5C).

The uterus typically is flexed anteriorly at the body/cervix junction, as illustrated in Figure 27–5A. Retroflexion and retroversion (Fig. 27–6A, B) are variations of uterine shape that may produce a bizarre sonographic appearance that can be mistaken for a pelvic mass (Fig. 27–6C). These configurations have no clinical consequences, except on rare occasions during pregnancy, but severe retropositioning may significantly limit sonographic diagnosis.

Serosa, Myometrium, and Endometrium

The serosa, or outer uterine covering, is not visualized sonographically per se, but it is noteworthy that the outer uterine surface is smooth and well defined. The myometrium, or muscular layer of the uterus, produces uniform, medium-level echoes (Figs. 27–3, 27–5). Small lucencies may be visualized occasionally in the periphery of the myometrium (Fig. 27–7). These are normal arcuate arteries and veins that should not be

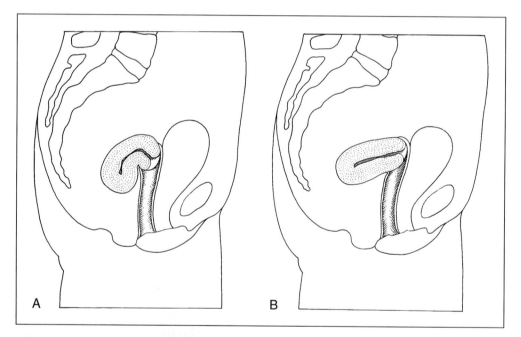

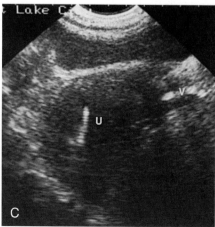

Figure 27-6—Uterine Retroflection and Retroversion. Anatomic drawings illustrate uterine retroflection (**A**), which is common, and retroversion (**B**), which is rare. (**C**) This retroflexed but otherwise normal uterus (U) has a bizarre, masslike shape as seen on this longitudinal scan. The bright reflections are from an intrauterine contraceptive device. V = vagina.

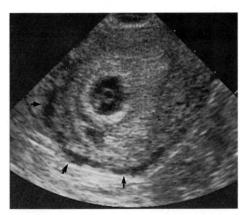

Figure 27-7—Arcuate Uterine Vessels. A coronal, transvaginal sonogram demonstrates prominent arcuate vessels (arrows) in the periphery of a uterus that contains a 6-week gestation.

mistaken for pathology.[15] Color Doppler sonography can provide unequivocal identification of these vessels. The endometrium[4, 16–24] is readily identified in menstrual-aged women as an echogenic structure located centrally within the uterine body (Figs. 27–3, 27–5). The endometrial cavity generally is visible as a thin line centrally located within the uterus (Fig. 27–8). This line may be sonolucent or echogenic, depending on the contents of the uterine cavity. During the late secretory phase of the menstrual cycle, the endometrial cavity is not visible, and in such cases the anterior and posterior portions of the endometrium blend imperceptibly.

The junction of the endometrium and myometrium is marked by a thin sonolucent line called the junctional zone (Fig. 27–8), which is a highly

vascular part of the myometrium. Since *this line is part of the myometrium*, not the endometrium, it should be excluded from sonographic measurements of endometrial thickness.

Endometrial Measurement

There are two ways to measure endometrial thickness. The anterior or posterior components may be measured separately, or the entire endometrial thickness may be measured as a unit, from myometrium to myometrium. I prefer the latter method, because the sonographic landmarks are clear in virtually all cases. It is of utmost importance that the method of measurement is clearly indicated in the sonographic report, lest a false impression of pathologic thickening results. In menstruating, adult women, the myometrium-to-myometrium thickness ranges from 6.2 to 13 mm (5th and 95th percentiles) during the secretory phase of the menstrual cycle.[19–24] The endometrium is less thick during the proliferative phase than during the secretory phase.

Cyclical Endometrial Changes

The hormonal milieu changes dramatically during the menstrual cycle, and these cyclical hormonal changes alter the appearance of the endometrium. The menstrual-related interactions between the ovary and the hypothalamus are illustrated in Figure 27–9. Readers who are unfamiliar with these cyclical interactions should review this figure before proceeding with the text.

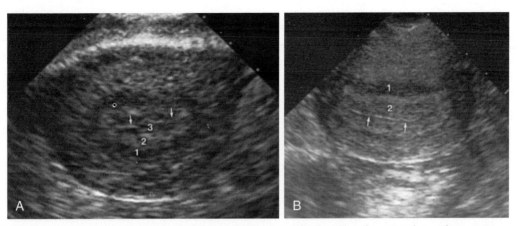

Figure 27-8—Normal Endometrium (Transvaginal). (A) Midcycle—the endometrium has a "three ring" appearance. The outermost dark ring (1) is the junctional zone (hypervascular portion of the myometrium). The outer endometrium (2) is mucus-laden and echogenic. The inner endometrium (3) is sonolucent. The faint white line in the center (arrow) is the endometrial canal. **(B)** Late secretory—the endometrium has a two ring appearance. The junctional zone (1) remains visible, but the endometrium (2) now is uniform in echogenicity. The endometrial cavity (arrows) is clearly seen, but in some cases it may be invisible at this stage (see text).

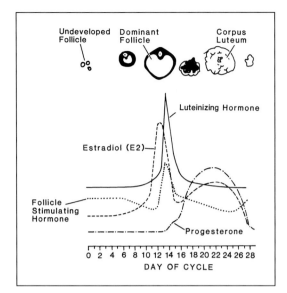

Figure 27-9—Schematic of Menstrual Cycle Changes. The cycle is assumed to be 28 days, but cycle length is variable and may be up to 36 days. The cycle begins on the first day of the menses (day 0 at left), when estrogen and progesterone levels are low and ovarian follicles are small (primordial). The release of follicle-stimulating hormone (FSH) by the anterior pituitary stimulates follicle growth, and the follicles in turn secrete estrogen, raising the serum estrogen (estradiol) level. Via a feedback mechanism, the rising estrogen level suppresses FSH production while promoting luteinizing hormone (LH) secretion in the anterior pituitary. Thus begins the "proliferative" phase of the menstrual cycle, during which the endometrium increases in thickness, and the endometrial glands begin to accumulate mucus.

Near midcycle, follicle growth and estrogen production surge, and typically one follicle increases rapidly in size, becoming the "dominant" follicle. The estrogen surge is followed by a large LH surge, and a smaller FSH surge. These abrupt changes in the hormonal milieu rapidly mature the follicle and ovum, and ovulation (from the dominant follicle) occurs shortly thereafter. The high level of LH stimulates growth of theca-lutein cells, converting the ruptured follicle into a corpus luteum (literally "yellow body"), which secretes progesterone and estrogen. Progesterone stimulates the endometrial glands to secrete mucus, and that is why the postovulatory phase is called the "secretory" phase.

If pregnancy ensues, the gestation secretes human chorionic gonadotropin, which "keeps the corpus luteum going" and in turn maintains the endometrium. If pregnancy does not occur (as shown here), the FSH level drops, followed by a rapid decline of the corpus luteum and decrease in estrogen and progesterone production. The result is sloughing of the endometrium (menstruation), and the start of a new cycle.

Immediately following the menses, the endometrium is very thin (4 mm, myometrium to myometrium[19–24]), and it may be difficult to identify the endometrium sonographically. Endometrial thickness increases throughout the menstrual cycle in normal women. The increase in thickness in the proliferative phase is attributed to estrogen-induced cellular growth. (The graafian follicle is the estrogen source.) Continued thickening in the secretory phase (following ovulation) is attributed to progesterone-induced glandular hyperplasia and mucus accumulation. (The corpus luteum is the progesterone source.)

During the proliferative phase, the endometrium has a three-ring appearance in cross-section. With mucus accumulation in the endometrial glands, however, endometrial echogenicity increases, and by the late secretory phase, the endometrium is uniformly echoic and the endometrium has a two-ring appearance. These changes are illustrated in Figures 27–8 and 27–10. In the late secretory phase, the uterine cavity may disappear from view, because the mucus-laden endometrium is as echogenic as the endometrial cavity.[16, 19, 21–23]

Postmenopausal Appearance

The uterus in elderly, postmenopausal women is smaller than in menstruating women (the mean length is 6.4 cm at or beyond age 60 years).[13] The endometrium also is considerably thinner, and it may be difficult to resolve sonographically. Estrogen replacement therapy, however, may stimulate endometrial growth, causing the endometrium to be visualized easily. Endometrial thickness should not exceed 8 mm in postmenopausal women, including women receiving replacement estrogen therapy.[20, 21, 24]

THE FALLOPIAN TUBES

The ligamentous attachments of the uterus and fallopian tubes are illustrated in Figure 27–11.[2] As shown in this figure, each fallopian tube has a long "tubular" component and a funnel-shaped fimbriated portion that partially surrounds the ovary. The tubular portion is only 1 to 4 mm in diameter.[25–29] The normal fallopian tubes and the broad ligaments are not often resolved with ultrasound as distinct entities, but they may be seen as vague linear structures extending between the uterus and ovary (Fig. 27–12).

THE OVARIES

The ovaries are suspended between the uterus and the pelvic side walls by a slinglike apparatus illustrated in Figure 27–13.[2] This anatomic arrangement allows for considerable mobility of the ovaries; hence, an extended sonographic search may be required before both ovaries are found. Favorite resting places of the ovaries are high along the pelvic side walls, near the iliac

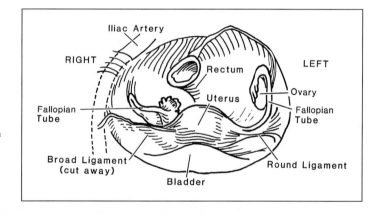

Figure 27-10—Endometrial Changes During the Menstrual Cycle. Early in the cycle (shortly after menstruation), the endometrium is thin and indistinct, but with cellular proliferation and mucus secretion, a three ring appearance develops and becomes increasingly visible (left half of figure). The three rings are the junctional zone, the mucus-laden outer endometrium, and the central endometrium. During the secretory phase, the endometrium develops a two ring appearance consisting of the junctional zone and the endometrium, which at this point is uniformly mucus-laden. The endometrial cavity often is less visible in the secretory phase because it blends in with the echogenic endometrium.

Figure 27-11—Broad Ligament and Fallopian Tube Anatomy. A schematic view looking into the true pelvis shows the broad ligaments extending right and left from the lateral surfaces of the uterus to the pelvic side walls. The fallopian tubes run in the free edge of each broad ligament, as shown on the left side of the subject. The right broad ligament is cut away to illustrate the fallopian tube and ovary.

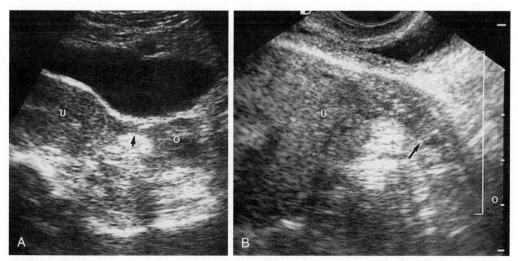

Figure 27-12—Fallopian Tube/Ligament Complex. Transabdominal (**A**) and transvaginal (**B**) images show a bridge of tissue (arrow) representing the fallopian tube and the uterine ligaments (broad and round) that connect the uterus (U) and ovary (O).

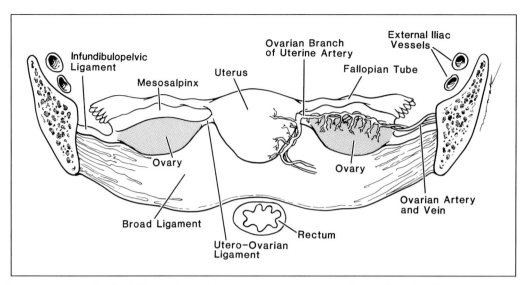

Figure 27-13—Fallopian Tube and Ovarian Anatomy. A cross-section drawing shows that the ovaries are suspended between the uterus and the pelvic side wall by a slinglike apparatus consisting of the broad ligament, utero-ovarian ligament, and infundibulopelvic ligament. The mesosalpinx connects the ovary with the fallopian tube. Note the dual blood supply of the ovary, as illustrated on the right side of the drawing.

vessels and posterolateral to the uterus, within the cul-de-sac of Douglas.

The ovaries (Fig. 27–14) have a fairly distinctive sonographic appearance in older girls and menstruating women.[4–8, 10, 11, 30–33] They are ovoid, well defined, and slightly less echogenic than surrounding structures. A distinctive identifying feature is the presence of follicles, which are anechoic rounded cysts usually seen at the periphery of the ovary.

The ovoid shape of the ovary is an important

indicator of normality that should be documented during every sonographic examination. Departure from an ovoid shape may indicate neoplasia or other pathologic condition (especially when the ovaries are enlarged). Remember: if ovaries were round they would be called roundries, not ovaries!*

Ovarian size[4–8, 10, 12, 30, 32–43] is evaluated most

---

*Observation offered by Diane Engleby, R.D.M.S., Department of Radiology, University of Utah Hospital, Salt Lake City, Utah.

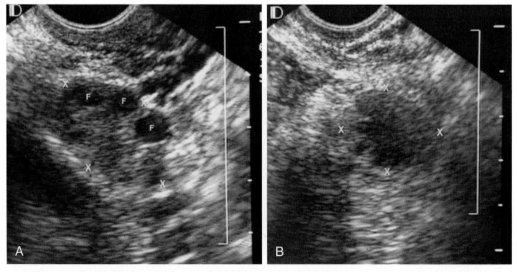

Figure 27-14—Normal Ovary. (A) Long and (B) short axis transvaginal views demonstrate the normal, hypoechoic appearance of the ovaries (cursors). Follicles (F) are illustrated, as well as the points for measuring the long and short axes (cursors).

simply with long-axis measurements, but a more precise way of assessing ovarian size is a volume estimate based on long- and short-axis measurements (Fig. 27–15). Ovarian volume is calculated using the following formula:[4, 30, 32, 40]

$$\text{Ovarian volume} = \text{Long axis} \times \text{short axis A} \times \text{short axis B} \times 0.5$$

In practice, only one short-axis measurement is taken, and this value is used twice for the calculation. Sonographic measurements of ovarian volume correlate well with surgical measurements.[30, 40] Normal values for ovarian size and volume are given in the following sections.

The Ovary in Childhood

Before 7 years of age, normal ovaries are difficult to visualize sonographically, and when they are seen they usually have a solid, homogeneous appearance. Small ovarian cysts representing nonovulatory, "primordial" follicles may be seen occasionally in girls under 6 years of age. From age 6 years to approximately age 12 years, these cysts are seen in increasing numbers but normally are less than 10 mm in diameter (Fig. 27–15). At puberty (approximately age 12 years), larger cysts appear, measuring 10 mm or more in diameter, that are similar histologically to adult follicles. The appearance of these larger cysts heralds the onset of cyclical hormonal changes, as well as the potential for ovulation.[4–8, 10, 11, 35]

During childhood, the ovaries grow slowly until pubertal changes become apparent. Ovarian growth then progresses rapidly, and by menarche the ovaries have an average volume of 3.3 cm[3.6, 10] Standards for ovary size in childhood are given in Table 27–1.

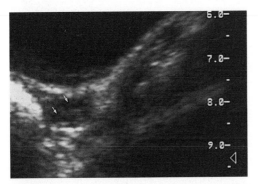

Figure 27-15—Normal Prepubertal Ovary (long axis view in a 5 year old girl). Note that small cysts (arrows) of under 5 mm in diameter are barely visible. The calculated ovarian volume was 0.6 ml, corresponding to that expected for a 5 year old (Table 27–1). (Images kindly contributed by Mary Murray, MD, Baystate Medical Center, Springfield, MA.)

The Ovary in Menstruating Women

Transabdominal sonography visualizes 71% to 92% of normal ovaries in menstruating women. The visualization rate for transvaginal imaging is about 95%.[38, 39, 41] Four centimeters is the generally accepted upper limit of normal for ovarian length (long axis) in adult menstruating women, and 14 cm[3] is the generally accepted upper limit of normal for ovarian volume. The range of reported normal values is broad, however (2.5 to 5.0 cm for ovarian length and 2.2 cm[3] to 21.9 cm[3] for ovarian volume).[*] Until the higher values in these ranges are verified by additional studies, I recommend using the generally accepted size and volume limits given above. Ovaries that exceed these size parameters may be pathologic.

Normal graafian follicles are represented sonographically as anechoic, smoothly marginated cysts imbedded within or on the surface of the ovaries. Normal follicles may be as large as 27 mm, but most do not exceed 20 mm in maximum dimension.[4, 19, 30–33, 44–50]

Cyclical Ovarian Changes

In normal menstruating women, 1 to 11 (mean, 5) graafian follicles may be seen during any phase of the menstrual cycle.[4, 19, 30–33, 44–50] During the proliferative phase, only one follicle is present in 32% of women, but several follicles are present in the remaining 68% of women.[19] Either the solitary follicle or one of the multiple follicles enlarges rapidly during the 5 days that precede ovulation. The rapidly enlarging, or "dominant," follicle reaches a mean size of 21 mm to 23 mm (range, 17 to 27 mm) on the day that the luteinizing hormone "peak" triggers ovulation (Fig. 27–9).[44, 48, 49] It is assumed that ovulation occurs from the dominant follicle.[44–46, 48, 49]

Several investigators report that the cumulus oophorus, which is a ring of cells surrounding the ovum, can be seen sonographically within a day or so before ovulation. The cumulus is visualized as a ringlike structure of 4 to 9 mm (mean, 5.5 mm) attached to the inner surface of the dominant follicle.[44, 46, 47, 49, 50] It seems that the cumulus is quite difficult to identify, however, as some investigators can find it and others cannot.[48]

In the days that follow ovulation, the dominant follicle is converted into the corpus luteum by the effects of luteinizing hormone. As this process occurs, the dominant follicle usually disappears from an ultrasound perspective and leaves

---

[*]Refs. 4, 32, 33, 35, 36, 38, 39, 41, and 42.

no trace. Alternatively, the dominant follicle may persist as a smaller and perhaps crenelated cyst, or as an echogenic area.[44–46, 48] If pregnancy ensues, the corpus luteum may evolve, during the first trimester of pregnancy, into a cyst 3 cm or larger in diameter.

The Postmenopausal Ovary

The ovaries shrink in the postmenopausal period. Most of the shrinkage occurs within the first 4 years after menopause, and thereafter the size decreases more slowly. Because of their relatively small size, the ovaries are less consistently identified sonographically in postmenopausal women than in menstruating women. About 82% to 87% are seen with transvaginal scanning, and 48% to 87% are visualized with transabdominal imaging.[37–41] Postmenopausal ovarian volume ranges widely in reported series, from 0.4 to 14.1 cm³ (mean, ± 2SD).[30, 34, 37–41] This wide range results in part from gradual postmenopausal shrinkage, making it difficult to define the upper limit of normal. Based on my review of the medical literature, I consider 3 cm³ to be the upper limit of normal for ovarian volume 5 or more years after menopause.

Cyclical follicle development is not a normal feature of postmenopausal ovaries; therefore, ovarian cysts must always be regarded with concern in postmenopausal patients, even though most cysts turn out to be benign.[41, 51]

CUL-DE-SAC FLUID

A small volume of free intraperitoneal fluid may be observed sonographically in the pelvis of menstrual-age women at any stage of the menstrual cycle. Fluid is most commonly seen just after ovulation or within 5 days preceding menstruation. The source of this fluid is unknown. Normal pelvic fluid is anechoic and moves freely with respiration or changes in patient position.[19, 52]

UTERINE AND OVARIAN VESSELS

The increasing use of Doppler sonography for female pelvic diagnosis requires basic familiarity with the arterial supply and venous drainage of the uterus and ovaries.

Arteries

The uterine arteries[2, 53–56] are the principal sources of blood flow to the uterus, the fallopian tubes, and the ovaries. The ovarian arteries also supply a variable portion of blood flow to the ovaries and adnexa. The anatomy of the uterine and ovarian arteries is illustrated in Figure 27–16.[20, 53–56] Please review this figure before proceeding as the contents are not repeated in the text.

The uterine arteries may be identified with color duplex sonography along the lateral surface of the uterus at the broad ligament attachment. Since these arteries are quite tortuous, only small segments are visible. The Doppler signals from these vessels exhibit a low-resistance flow pattern

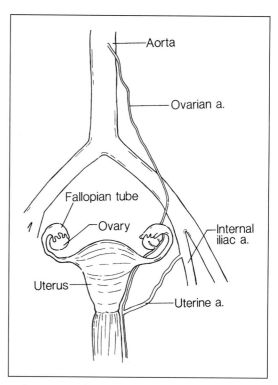

Figure 27–16—Uterine and Ovarian Vascular Anatomy. The uterine arteries arise from the internal iliac arteries and make contact with the uterus at the junction of the cervix and body. From this point, a branch from each uterine artery extends caudad along the cervix and vagina. A second branch extends cephalad along the lateral surface of the uterus to the fallopian tube. This cephalad-directed branch is embedded in the broad ligament adjacent to the uterus, and tributaries (not shown) extend into the myometrium.

Terminal branches of the uterine artery follow the fallopian tube to the ovary, where they freely anastomose with tributaries from the ovarian artery. The ovarian arteries arise from the aorta somewhere between the renal arteries and the inferior mesenteric artery (only one is shown here). They follow a variable course to the pelvic brim, where they join company with the ureters and the ovarian veins, and subsequently enter the ovaries via the infundibulopelvic ligaments (see Figure 27–13). The ovarian arteries often are small, and in such cases, the primary ovarian blood supply is via the uterine arteries.

similar to that shown previously for the renal arteries (Chapter 16).

Veins

The venous drainage of the female reproductive organs[2, 53, 56] generally parallels the arterial supply. The uterus is drained by a plexus of veins that consolidates along the lateral uterine surface and forms one, or several, large branches that empty into the internal iliac veins. The ovary is drained both by the uterine plexus and by a separate ovarian plexus that passes through the infundibulopelvic ligament to the pelvic side wall. From this point, the ovarian plexus consolidates to form either one or several veins that follow the ipsilateral ureter cephalad. The right ovarian vein(s) ultimately drains into the inferior vena cava at a variable point below the right renal vein. The left ovarian vein(s) drains into the left renal vein. The lengthy course of the ovarian veins and their relationship to the ureters are noteworthy. Thrombosis of these veins may cause abdominal pain distant from the pelvis, as well as ureteral obstruction.

Doppler Technique

Doppler interrogation of pelvic pathology may be conducted during either the transabdominal or transvaginal examination, but the latter is more common. Doppler flow assessment most commonly is used to assist with identification of an intrauterine or ectopic gestation, or to evaluate adnexal masses.[18–24] Details concerning these applications are covered in other chapters. The Doppler examination generally is focused directly on the structure of interest (e.g., the suspected ectopic gestation or adnexal mass), and not on large supply vessels such as the uterine artery. The color Doppler image is used to detect blood flow within the area of interest, and spectral Doppler is used subsequently to obtain quantitative flow information (e.g., pulsatility index) in areas where flow is visible. The instrument should be adjusted to detect relatively low-velocity flow, for the typical mean flow velocities are only 2 to 5 cm/sec in uterine and ovarian vessels.[22]

TECHNICAL OBJECTIVES

The objectives of pelvic sonography are the careful examination of the uterus and ovaries and evaluation of the entire pelvic cavity and the iliac fossa. When pathology is detected, the gross morphologic features of the lesion should be evaluated (e.g., solid, fluid-containing, thin-walled, smooth, irregular, and so on), and the origin of the pathology should be determined whenever possible.

TRANSABDOMINAL VERSUS TRANSVAGINAL SONOGRAPHY

The female pelvis is scanned routinely with both transabdominal and transvaginal° ultrasound techniques.[57–67] Transabdominal scanning through the distended bladder (Figs. 27–5 and 27–6) provides "the big picture" of the pelvic viscera, and frequently this approach best depicts the relationships between the pelvic organs and pathologic processes. Transabdominal imaging also is best for depicting a grossly enlarged uterus or a large pelvic mass. Furthermore, transabdominal scanning is the only means for examining the vagina, the upper reaches of the true pelvis, and the iliac fossae.

The disadvantages of transabdominal sonography are inferior image quality, as compared with transvaginal sonography, and the requirement for urinary bladder distention, which is uncomfortable and sometimes difficult to achieve. Patients prefer transvaginal sonography over transabdominal imaging at a rate of 82% to 93%, principally because of bladder-filling problems. Even patients with acute pelvic symptoms prefer transvaginal imaging by a wide margin.[28, 58, 59, 67]

The principal advantage of transvaginal sonography is the exquisite detail with which the uterus and ovaries can be visualized, as illustrated in Figure 27–17. The field of view of transvaginal instruments is small, however, and the resultant "postage stamp" perspective may create orientation problems and may obscure the origin of pelvic pathology. Field of view limitations, furthermore, may preclude visualization of normal ovaries that lie high in the pelvis, and they may cause pathologic findings to be overlooked if they are out of the range of the transducer.[34, 38–40, 51]

Transvaginal sonography provides more diagnostic information than transabdominal imaging in 24% to 70% of pelvic examinations, equivalent information in 15% to 36% of examinations, and less information in only 4% to 12% of examinations.† It might be assumed, based on these statistics, that transabdominal pelvic sonography is unnecessary; however, it is standard practice, as of this writing, to examine the pelvis with the bladder distended, have the patient void, and

---

°The terms "transvaginal" and "endovaginal" are used interchangeably in the medical literature, but the term "transvaginal" is preferred since it appears to be more precise linguistically than "endovaginal."[60]
†Refs. 28, 34, 38–40, 51, 58, 59, 61–64, 66, and 67.

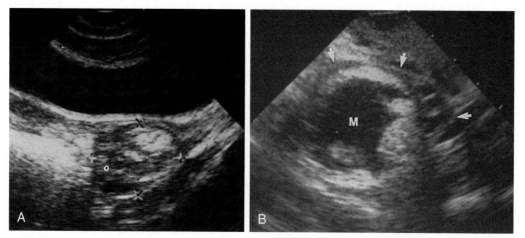

Figure 27-17—Superior Resolution with Transvaginal Sonography. (A) This left adnexal mass (cursors) was identified with transabdominal imaging, but its origin could not be determined. **(B)** With transvaginal sonography, a thin rim of ovarian tissue (arrows) was seen surrounding the mass (M), confirming ovarian origin. Furthermore, the borders and internal architecture of the mass were more clearly depicted with transvaginal imaging than with transabdominal sonography. The appearance of the mass, the age of the patient, and the clinical history were consistent with cystic teratoma, and this diagnosis was confirmed at surgery.

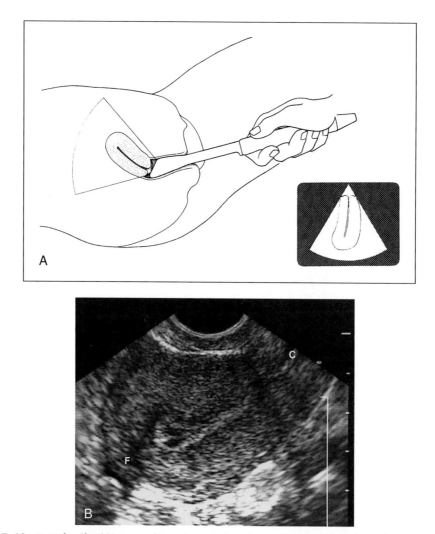

Figure 27-18—Longitudinal Transvaginal View of the Uterus. (A) Illustration of transducer position. Note that the thumb is up, corresponding to the plane of the image. **(B)** Representative transvaginal image of the uterus showing the cervix (C) and fundus (F). This uterus is more anteroflexed than that shown in **A**; hence the apex of the sector is at the body of the uterus rather than the cervix.

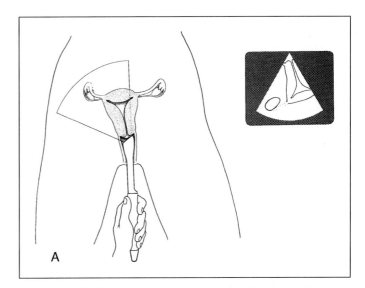

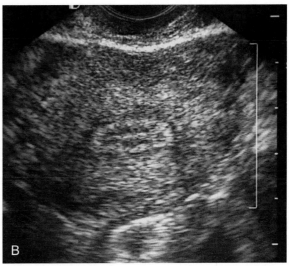

Figure 27-19—Coronal Transvaginal View of the Pelvis. (A) Illustration of transducer position. Note that the position of the operator's thumb correlates with the image plane. **(B)** Representative coronal transvaginal image of the uterus. In this case, the uterus is more anteroflexed than that shown in **A** and is sliced, therefore, almost at right angles to its long axis.

then examine the pelvis transvaginally to further delineate normal or abnormal features. This practice recognizes that transvaginal imaging occasionally provides less information than transabdominal scanning and occasionally overlooks pelvic pathology.[28, 62, 64] This is not to say that transvaginal imaging should never be used as the primary mode of pelvic sonography, but in such instances, *the pelvis, iliac fossa, and kidneys should always be examined transabdominally in conjunction with transvaginal pelvic examination.* Even with the bladder empty, this adjunctive examination will detect large-scale pathology that may be located out of the range of the transvaginal device. Furthermore, the kidneys should be examined as part of virtually all pelvic ultrasound examinations, whether transabdominal or transvaginal.

TRANSVAGINAL IMAGE PLANES

Transvaginal image planes are quite unlike other image planes used for abdominal and pelvic scanning, and the peculiarities of these planes takes a little "getting used to." First, the longitudinal images are oriented from caudad to cephalad, which is quite unique (Fig. 27–18). Second, "transverse" images are not really transverse but are coronal, more or less, as shown in Figure 27–19. Since the uterus usually is sharply anteroflexed, the coronal image often slices through the uterus at approximately right angles to the uterine long axis (Fig. 27–19*B*). As an aid to orientation, keep the thumb of the hand holding the transducer in line with the image plane, and be sure that the left side of the image display

Table 27-2. Protocol for Pelvic Sonography

Transabdominal Component	Transvaginal Component
Longitudinal uterine and vaginal examination • Measure uterine length (external os to fundus). • Survey for pathology. • Obtain hard copy of normal and pathologic features.	Uterine examination • Use longitudinal and coronal image planes. • Scrutinize myometrial and endometrial structure for normal features and evidence of pathology. • Measure endometrial thickness, if of clinical importance. • Evaluate the gross morphology of uterine lesions, if present. • Obtain hard copy of normal and pathologic features.
Transverse uterine examination • Measure AP and transverse dimensions as needed.° • Survey for pathology. • Obtain hard copy of normal and pathologic features.†	Adnexal examination • Scrutinize each ovary in coronal and transverse planes for normal features and evidence of pathology. • Measure long- and short-axis dimensions of the ovaries. • Identify the fallopian tubes, if possible. • Scrutinize adnexal pathology for gross features and site of origin. • Obtain hard copy of normal and pathologic features.
Adnexal examination • Visualize each ovary in long-axis and short-axis planes. • Measure long- and short-axis dimensions of ovaries.‡ • Survey ovaries and adnexal areas for pathology. • Obtain hard copy of normal ovaries (long axis) and pathologic features.	Doppler examination • Visualize blood flow with color Doppler sonography. • Assess pulsatility and other flow characteristics with Doppler spectrum analysis. • Obtain hard copy of color Doppler and Doppler spectral features.
Pelvic and iliac fossa survey • Get the "global perspective" by sweeping back and forth through the pelvis, using longitudinal and transverse images. • Obtain hard copy of pathologic features.	
Kidney survey • Visualize both kidneys in long-axis planes. • Survey kidneys for pathology. • Obtain hard copy of normal and pathologic features.	

°AP and transverse dimensions are not obtained routinely.
†A single transverse view high in the uterine body suffices in normal cases.
‡Delete measurements if transvaginal examination is anticipated.

represents the right side of the patient (and vice versa). This orientation will seem logical as you move the transducer about and is the standard method for orienting ultrasound images.

EXAMINATION PROTOCOL

The scope of this text does not permit detailed description of ultrasound scanning technique. The protocol for pelvic sonography that I recommend is presented in Table 27-2 and is offered as a technical guideline.

REFERENCES

1. Grant JCB, Basmajian JV: Grant's Method of Anatomy. Baltimore, Williams and Wilkins, 1965, pp 310–337.
2. Grant JCB, Basmajian JV: Grant's Method of Anatomy. Baltimore, Williams and Wilkins, 1965, pp 338–356.
3. Auh YH, Rubenstein WA, Schneider M, Reckler JM, Whalen JP, Kazam E: Extraperitoneal paravesical spaces: CT delineation with US correlation. Radiology 159:319–328, 1986.
4. Sample FW, Lippe BM, Gyepes MT: Gray-scale ultrasonography of the normal female pelvis. Radiology 125:477–483, 1977.
5. Stanhope R, Adams J, Jacobs HS, et al: Ovarian ultrasound assessment in normal children, idiopathic precocious puberty, and during low-dose pulsatile gonadotropin-releasing hormone treatment of hypogonadotropic hypogonadism. Arch Dis Child 60:116–119, 1985.
6. Orsini LF, Salardi S, Pilu G, Bovicelli L, Cacciari E: Pelvic organs in premenarcheal girls: Real-time ultrasonography. Radiology 153:113–116, 1984.
7. Salardi S, Orsini LF, Cacciari E, et al: Pelvic ultrasonography in premenarcheal girls: Relation to puberty and sex hormone concentrations. Arch Dis Child 60:120–125, 1985.
8. Kangerloo H, Sarti DA, Sample WF: Ultrasound of the pediatric pelvis. Semin Ultrasound 1:51–60, 1980.
9. Bundscherer F, Deeg K-H: Die sonographische Beurteilung der Uterusentwicklung im Kindesalter. Monatsschr Kinderheilkd 136:246–250, 1988.
10. Ivarsson S-A, Nilsson KO, Persson P-H: Ultrasonography of the pelvic organs in prepubertal and postpubertal girls. Arch Dis Childhood 58:352–354, 1983.
11. Siegel MJ: Pediatric gynecologic sonography. Radiology 179:593–600, 1991.
12. Nussbaum AR, Sanders RC, Jones MD: Neonatal uterine morphology as seen on real-time US. Radiology 160:641–643, 1996.
13. Zemlyn S: The length of the uterine cervix and its significance. J Clin Ultrasound 9:267–269, 1981.
14. Viscomi GN, Gonzalez R, Taylor KJW: Ultrasound detection of uterine abnormalities after diethylstilbestrol (DES) exposure. Radiology 136:733–735, 1980.
15. DuBose TJ, Hill LW, Hennigan HW, Nichols DH, Mezaraups GG, Porter L, Marley L, Butschek CM, Karnaze GC, Walser E, Reyes K, Cunyus JA: Sonography of arcuate uterine blood vessels. J Ultrasound Med 4:229–233, 1985.
16. Fleischer AC, Pittaway DE, Beard LA, et al: Sonographic depiction of endometrial changes occurring with ovulation induction. J Ultrasound Med 3:341–346, 1984.

17. Thickman D, Arger P, Tureck R, et al: Echographic assessment of the endometrium in patients undergoing in vitro fertilization. J Ultrasound Med 5:197–201, 1986.

18. Brandt TD, Levy EV, Grant TH, et al: Endometrial echo and its significance in female infertility. Radiology 157:225–229, 1985.

19. Pupols AZ, Wilson SR: Ultrasonographic interpretation of physiological changes in the female pelvis. J Can Assoc Radiol 35:34–39, 1984.

20. Fleischer AC, Kalemeris GC, Machin JE, et al: Sonographic depiction of normal and abnormal endometrium with histopathologic correlation. J Ultrasound Med 5:445–452, 1986.

21. Fleischer AC, Kalemeris GC, Entman SS: Sonographic depiction of the endometrium during normal cycles. Ultrasound Med Biol 12:271–277, 1986.

22. Forrest TS, Elyaderani MK, Muilenburg MI, Bewtra C, Kable WT, Sullivan P: Cyclic endometrial changes: US assessment with histologic correlation. Radiology 167:233–237, 1988.

23. Mitchell DG, Schonholz L, Hilpert PL, Pennell RG, Blum L, Rifkin MD: Zones of the uterus: Discrepancy between US and MR images. Radiology 174:827–831, 1990.

24. Lin MC, Gosink BB, Wolf SI, Feldesman MR, Stuenkel CA, Braly PS, Pretorius DH: Endometrial thickness after menopause: Effect of hormone replacement. Radiology 180:427–432, 1991.

25. Warwick R, Williams PL: Gray's Anatomy. London, Longman, 1973, pp 1354–1356.

26. Tessler FN, Perrella RR, Fleischer AC, Grant EA: Endovaginal sonographic diagnosis of dilated Fallopian tubes. AJR Am J Roentgenol 153:523–525, 1989.

27. Patten RM, Vincent LM, Wolner-Hanssen P, Thorpe E: Pelvic inflammatory disease: Endovaginal sonography with laparoscopic correlation. J Ultrasound Med 9:681–689, 1990.

28. Bulas DL, Ahlstrom PA, Sivit CJ, Nussbaum Blask AR, O'Donnell RM: Pelvic inflammatory disease in the adolescent: Comparison of transabdominal and transvaginal sonographic evaluation. Radiology 183:435–439, 1992.

29. Lawson TL, Albarelli JN: Diagnosis of gynecologic pelvic masses by gray scale ultrasonography: Analysis of specificity and accuracy. AJR Am J Roentgenol 128:1003–1006, 1977.

30. Campbell S, Goessens L, Goswamy R, Whitehead M: Real-time ultrasonography for determination of ovarian morphology and volume. Lancet 1:425–426, 1982.

31. Ritchie WGM: Sonographic evaluation of normal and induced ovulation. Radiology 161:1–10, 1986.

32. Yeh H-C, Futterweit W, Thornton JC: Polycystic ovarian disease: US features in 104 patients. Radiology 163:111–116, 1987.

33. Pache TD, Waldimiroff JW, Hopp WCJ, Fauser BCJM: How to discriminate between normal and polycystic ovaries: Transvaginal US study. Radiology 183:421–423, 1992.

34. Goswamy R, Campbell S, Whitehead M: Screening of ovarian cancer. Clin Obstet Gynecol 10:621–643, 1983.

35. Nicolini U, Ferrazzi E, Bellotti M, Travaglini P, Elli R, Scapperrotta RC: The contribution of sonographic evaluation of ovarian size in patients with polycystic ovarian disease. J Ultrasound Med 4:347–351, 1985.

36. Munn CS, Kiser LC, Wetzner SM, Baer JE: Ovary volume in young and premenopausal adults: US determination. Radiology 159:731–732, 1986.

37. Hall DA, McCarthy KA, Kopans DB: Sonographic visualization of the normal postmenopausal ovary. J Ultrasound Med 5:9–11, 1986.

38. Granberg S, Wikland M: A comparison between ultrasound and gynecological examination for detection of enlarged ovaries in a group of women at risk for ovarian carcinoma. J Ultrasound Med 7:59–63, 1988.

39. Cohen HL, Tice HM, Mandel FS: Ovarian volumes measured by US: Bigger than we think. Radiology 177:189–192, 1990.

40. Rodriguez MH, Platt LD, Medearis AL, Lacarra M, Lobo RA: The use of transvaginal sonography for the evaluation of postmenopausal ovarian size and morphology. Am J Obstet Gynecol 159:810–814, 1988.

41. Higgins RV, van Nagell JR, Donaldson ES, Gallion HH, Pavlik EJ, et al: Transvaginal sonography as a screening method for ovarian cancer. Gynecol Oncol 34:402–406, 1989.

42. Hall D: Sonographic appearance of the normal ovary, of polycystic ovarian disease, and of functional cysts. Semin Ultrasound 4:149–165, 1983.

43. Simkins CS: Development of the human ovary from birth to sexual maturity. Am J Anat 51:465–493.

44. Hackelör BJ, Fleming R, Robinson HP, et al: Correlation of ultrasonic and endocrinologic assessment of human follicular development. Am J Obstet Gynecol 135:122–128, 1979.

45. Kerin JF, Edminds DK, Warnes GM, et al: Morphological and functional evaluation of Graafian follicle growth to ovulation in women using ultrasonic, laparoscopic and biochemical measurements. Br J Obstet Gynecol 88:81–90, 1981.

46. Lenz S: Ultrasonic study of follicular maturation, ovulation and development of corpus luteum during normal menstrual cycles. Acta Obstet Gynecol Scand 64:15–19, 1985.

47. Mendelson EB, Friedman H, Nieman HL, et al: The role of imaging in infertility management. AJR Am J Roentgenol 144:414–420, 1985.

48. Zandt-Stastny D, Thorsen MK, Middleton WD, Aiman J, Zion A, McAsey M, Harms L: Inability of sonography to detect imminent ovulation. AJR Am J Roentgenol 152:91–95, 1989.

49. Hilgers TW, Dvorak AD, Tamisiea DF, Ellis RL, Yaksich PJ: Sonographic definition of the empty follicle syndrome. J Ultrasound Med 8:411–416, 1989.

50. Fleischer AC, Herbert CM, Hill GA, Kepple KM, Worrell JA: Transvaginal sonography of the endometrium during induced cycles. J Ultrasound Med 10:93–95, 1991.

51. Hall DA, McCarthy KA: The significance of the postmenopausal simple adnexal cyst. J Ultrasound Med 5:503–505, 1986.

52. Davis JA, Gosink BB: Fluid in the female pelvis: Cyclic patterns. J Ultrasound Med 5:75–79, 1986.

53. Hollingshead WH: Textbook of Anatomy. 3rd ed. Hagerstown, MD, Harper & Row, 1974, pp 521–523.

54. Taylor KJW, Burns PN, Woodcock JP, et al: Blood flow in deep abdominal and pelvic vessels: Ultrasonic pulsed Doppler analysis. Radiology 154:487–493, 1985.

55. Zwiebel WJ, Fruechte DF: Basics of abdominal and pelvic duplex: Instrumentation, anatomy, and vascular Doppler signals. Semin Ultrasound CT MRI 13:3–21, 1992.

56. Fleischer AC, Keppel DM: Transvaginal color duplex sonography: Clinical potentials and limitations. Semin Ultrasound CT MRI 13:69–81, 1992.

57. Schwimer SR, Lebovic J: Transvaginal pelvic ultrasonography. J Ultrasound Med 3:381–383, 1984.

58. Vilaro MM, Rifkin MD, Pennell RG, Baltarowich OH, Needleman L, Kurtz AB, Goldberg BB: Endovaginal ultrasound. A technique for evaluation of nonfollicular pelvic masses. J Ultrasound Med 6:697–701, 1987.

59. Nyberg DA, Mack LA, Jeffrey RB, Laing FC: Endovaginal sonographic evaluation of ectopic pregnancy: A prospective study. AJR Am J Roentgenol 149:1181–1186, 1987.

60. Mendelson EB, Bohm-Velez M, Nieman HL, Russo J: Transvaginal sonography in gynecologic imaging. Semin Ultrasound CT MRI 9:102–121, 1988.

61. Dashefsky SM, Lyons EA, Levi CS, Lindsay DJ: Suspected ectopic pregnancy: Endovaginal and transvesical US. Radiology 169:181–184, 1988.

62. Fleischer AC, Gordon AN, Entman SS: Transabdominal and transvaginal sonography of pelvic masses. Ultrasound Med Biol 15:529–533, 1989.

63. Tessler FN, Schiller VL, Perrella RR, Sutherland ML, Grant EG: Transabdominal versus endovaginal pelvic sonography: Prospective study. Radiology 170:553–556, 1989.

64. Andolf E, Jörgensen C: A prospective comparison of transabdominal and transvaginal ultrasound with surgical findings in gynecologic disease. J Ultrasound Med 9:71–75, 1990.

65. Laing FC: Technical aspects of vaginal ultrasound. Semin Ultrasound CT MRI 11:4–11, 1990.

66. Thorsen MK, Lawson TL, Aiman EJ, Miller DP, McAsey ME: Diagnosis of ectopic pregnancy: Endovaginal vs. transabdominal sonography. AJR Am J Roentgenol 155:307–310, 1990.

67. Pennell RG, Needleman L, Pajak T, Baltarowich O, Vilaro M, Goldberg BB, Kurtz AB: Prospective comparison of vaginal and abdominal sonography in early pregnancy. J Ultrasound Med 10:63–67, 1991.

68. Schaaps JP, Soyeur D: Pulsed Doppler on a vaginal probe—necessity, convenience, or luxury? J Ultrasound Med 8:315–320, 1989.

Chapter 28

Pelvic Congenital Anomalies and Pubertal Disorders

William J. Zwiebel

EMBRYOLOGY

The fallopian tubes, the uterus, and the superior portion of the vagina originate from paired tubular structures called the müllerian ducts.[1, 2] These ducts persist superiorly as the fallopian tubes, but the more inferior portions fuse to form the uterus and upper vagina. In the course of the fusion process, the original duct lumens are obliterated and a new lumen is formed. This new lumen ultimately becomes the uterine, cervical, and vaginal cavities.

The ovaries originate from the inner lining of the embryonic coelomic cavity and develop near the upper end of the müllerian ducts. Ovarian development is independent of müllerian development, however, and the ovaries may be present in patients with müllerian anomalies, as discussed in the next section.

MÜLLERIAN ANOMALIES

The most common anomalies of the female reproductive organs result from failed development or fusion of the müllerian ducts.[1–11] Four principal types of müllerian anomalies occur, as illustrated in Figure 28–1.

1. One of the müllerian ducts may fail to form, producing a unicornuate uterus and absent fallopian tube.
2. Agenesis or atresia may occur in any of the müllerian segments, causing isolated absence of that segment. Agenesis may result in absence of the upper vagina, uterus, or a fallopian tube. Figure 28–2 is an illustration of uterine agenesis.
3. The müllerian ducts may fuse incompletely, causing a wide variety of septation anomalies potentially involving the uterus, cervix, and vagina.
4. The fused müllerian components may fail to recanalize, causing vaginal or cervical obstruction.

NON-MÜLLERIAN ANOMALIES

The principal non-müllerian anomalies of the female genital tract are ovarian agenesis and maldevelopment of the lower two thirds of the vagina (remember, the upper third is müllerian). Ovarian agenesis results from failure of germ cell development and may be unilateral or bilateral.[1, 2] Because ovarian development and müllerian development are not directly linked, a fallopian tube may form normally in spite of absence of an ovary, or vice versa. Malformation of the lower portion of the vagina results from anomalous cloacal development, which is considerably less common than müllerian abnormality.[1, 2, 10]

ASSOCIATED URINARY TRACT ANOMALIES

Anomalies of the müllerian system are frequently associated with urinary tract anomalies, including renal agenesis, collecting system duplication, and ectopic ureteral insertion.[1, 2] In light of this association, the kidneys should be examined carefully when anomalies are discovered in the female reproductive organs.

PRESENTATION AND DIAGNOSIS

Congenital anomalies of the female genital tract tend to present clinically in four settings: (1) at birth in infants with ambiguous genitalia; (2) in the neonatal period with genital tract obstruction (e.g., hydrocolpos); (3) in the teenage years because of delayed puberty or menstruation; and (4) in relation to pregnancy, because of infertility, habitual abortion, premature labor, or other pregnancy complications.[2–10]

Sonographic assessment of female reproductive organ anomalies[2, 5–9] should focus on four important points: first, whether or not the genital tract is complete; second, whether the *external* configuration of the uterus is normal or abnor-

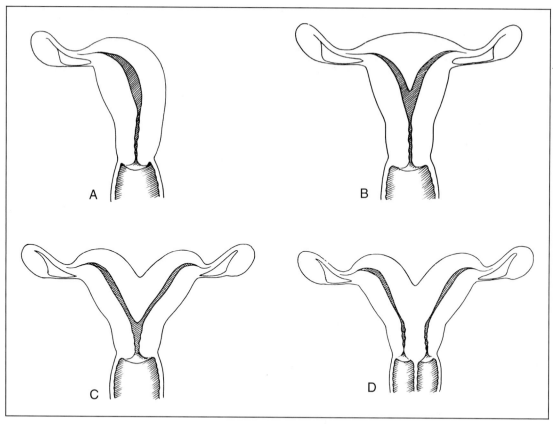

Figure 28-1—Illustration of Müllerian Abnormalities. (A) Unicornuate or single horn uterus. **(B)** Septate uterus. Note that the exterior surface is normal. **(C)** Bicornuate uterus (fundus is indented). **(D)** Didelphic uterus, with two endometrial and cervical canals.

mal; third, whether the *internal* configuration of the uterus (uterine cavity) is normal or abnormal; and fourth, whether or not there are coexistent renal anomalies. Therefore, the structure of the reproductive organs should be examined in detail, the external dimensions of the uterine body and cervix should be measured, and the ovarian volume should be calculated and compared with reference standards (Chapter 27). In cases of uterine septation or duplication, the degree of duplication should be defined as precisely as possible, and it should be determined whether duplication is purely internal or whether there is visible external duplication (Fig. 28–1). In cases of organ agenesis, efforts should be made to determine which structures are present and which are absent. Finally, if the reproductive organs are distended with fluid, anatomic landmarks should be sought to define the point of obstruction (e.g., vagina, cervix, or uterus).

The features that define major müllerian anomalies are summarized in Table 28–1 and illustrated in Figures 28–1 through 28–5.[2–11] Please review this material carefully as it is not repeated in the text. It is noteworthy that precise sonographic classification of genital tract anomalies often is not possible, and complete assessment often requires hysterosalpingography and magnetic resonance imaging (MRI). References 5, 6, 8, 9, and 11 are suggested for further reading on this subject.

PUBERTAL DISORDERS

In this section we will consider four conditions; ambiguous genitalia, true precocious puberty, premature thelarche/adrenarche, and precocious pseudopuberty. Before proceeding to the specifics, however, it will be helpful to review the general principles of imaging assessment of pubertal disorders.[1, 8, 9, 12–19]

Sonography plays a major role in the clinical evaluation of pubertal disorders by providing a noninvasive "window" through which the reproductive organs can be examined in detail. This window provides much more detail than pelvic examination; furthermore, pelvic examination is inappropriate in many pediatric patients. The general objectives of sonography are the following: (1) to establish that the ovaries, uterus, and

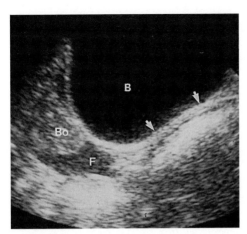

Figure 28-2—Absence of the uterus in a 16 year old, amenorrheic girl. This longitudinal sonogram showed a small amount of fluid (F) and bowel (Bo) posterior to the bladder (B). The vagina is visible (arrows), but the uterus is congenitally absent. Both ovaries (not shown) were identified sonographically and were normal in size and appearance.

vagina are present and have an age-appropriate appearance; (2) to determine whether puberty-related changes have occurred in the uterus and ovaries; and (3) to detect specific causes of pubertal disorders, such as anomalies, tumors, or functional cysts.

In the ideal world, pubertal disorders would be evaluated in a logical and orderly manner, with biochemical tests performed before imaging studies. As a time-saving expedient, however, imaging studies and biochemical tests often are conducted contemporaneously. The sonographer, therefore, should "cover all the bases" by looking for all diagnostic possibilities, including ovarian and adrenal tumors or cysts that might be hormonally active.

Other imaging studies used for diagnosis of pubertal disorders are radiographic bone age and cranial magnetic resonance imaging (MRI). Skeletal maturation characteristically is advanced in true precocious puberty and may be advanced in precocious pseudopuberty (defined later). Cranial MRI is used to search for central nervous system tumors and anomalies that may cause precocious puberty.

Ambiguous Genitalia

Patients with ambiguous genitalia typically are evaluated in the neonatal period so that gender may be correctly chosen. In some cases, however, patients may not be seen until pubertal changes occur along unexpected lines, e.g., breast development in a young man.[12, 16, 18] The principal role of ultrasound is to determine whether or not a

uterus and gonads are present within the pelvis. Sonography also is used to search for undescended gonads within the inguinal canals, and for adrenal tumors that may cause abnormal genital development through secretion of androgenic steroids. Two points should be noted with respect to these tasks. First, in utero exposure to high material levels of estrogen and progesterone may give the neonatal uterus a somewhat adult-like configuration that disappears during the first few months of life.* Second, a gonad does not equal an ovary or a testis (Fig. 28–6)! An individual with hermaphroditism may have an ovary on one side of the pelvis or in one scrotal sac and a testis on the other side. Alternatively, one or both

*If you are unfamiliar with the normal appearance of the uterus and ovaries at different ages, please see Chapter 27.

Table 28-1. Sonographic Features of Selected Müllerian Anomalies

Anomaly	Sonographic Features
Unicornuate uterus	Sausage-like uterine configuration
	Superior end of uterus points to right or left pelvic side wall
	Diameter of uterine body and cervix similar
	Uterine body and endometrial cavity *circular* in cross section
Uterus didelphys	Uterine body and cervix completely divided into right and left components
	Angle between the horns generally greater than 105°, but this is not specific
	Each horn is circular on transverse images
	Two cervical canals present
	Possible upper vaginal septum
Bicornuate uterus	Uterine body divided into right and left horns, which unite at or above the cervix
	Angle between the horns generally more than 105°, but this is not specific*
	Separate, circular horns seen on high-uterine transverse images
	Single or double cervical canal(s)
Septate uterus†	Uterine cavity divided to various degrees by a longitudinal septum
	Septate uterus suggested if angle between uterine cavities does not exceed 75°
	Normal external uterine configuration confirms septate diagnosis

*If the angle between the endometrial cavities does not exceed 75°, septate uterus is suggested. If the angle is 105° or greater, the uterus probably is bicornuate and may be didelphic, but these findings are not conclusive.[7] Other imaging modalities such as MRI are needed in many cases to accurately differentiate septate uterus from other anomalies.

†Septate appearance means that the external configuration is normal but the uterine cavity is partially divided into right and left compartments by a longitudinal muscular septum.

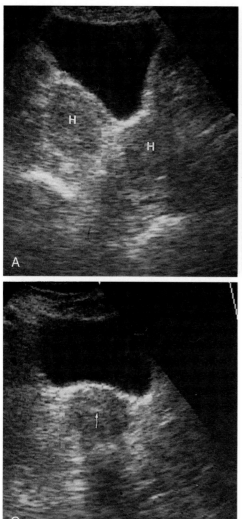

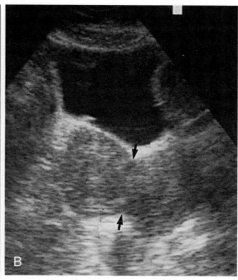

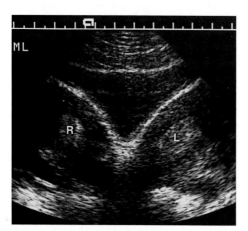

Figure 28-3—Bicornuate Uterus. (A) A transverse sonogram demonstrates two separate uterine horns (H). **(B)** A section slightly inferior to **A** demonstrates the point of fusion of the two horns (arrows). **(C)** A transverse scan farther inferior shows a single cervix with a central canal (arrow). Because there was obvious external division and the horns were separated widely, this was thought to be a bicornuate uterus, but the appearance at hysterosalpingography suggested a deeply septated uterus.

Figure 28-4—Bicornuate Uterus. A transabdominal sonogram in the transverse plane shows wide separation of the right (R) and left (L) horns of a bicornuate uterus. (Kindly provided by Paula Woodward, MD, University of Utah Medical Center, Salt Lake City.)

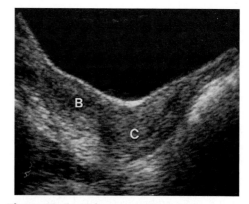

Figure 28-5—Unicornuate Uterus. On a longitudinal image, the uterine body (B) in this adult patient is smaller in its anteroposterior dimension than the cervix (C) and appears to taper at its superior end. The body was circular in cross-section (not shown) and deviated far to the left. The findings were correctly interpreted as unicornuate uterus. Two ovaries and two kidneys were present.

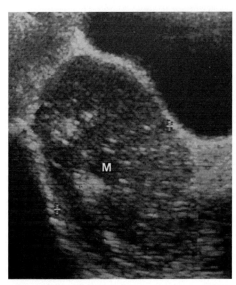

Figure 28-6—Dysgerminoma (Arising in a Pelvic Testis.) A longitudinal sonogram demonstrates a 12-cm, solid mass (M) with strong echogenic components probably due to calcification. This tumor occurred in a 21 year old woman with ambiguous genitalia and testicular feminization who had not previously received medical care for her condition. A vestigial uterus was found at surgery, as well as a nonmalignant dysgerminoma in a pelvic testis.

gonads may contain both ovarian and testicular tissue.[16, 18] The sonographic texture of the gonads should be assessed, therefore, for typical ovarian or testicular features.

True Precocious Puberty

True precocious puberty[12–17] in girls is defined as early development of the gonads and secondary sexual characteristics, accompanied by ovulation prior to the age of 8 years. This is a hypothalamic-pituitary disorder characterized by an elevated serum level of gonadotropin-releasing hormone. Skeletal age is advanced because of gonadotropic effects, and premature closure of sutures may lead to short stature without proper therapy. Most cases of true precocious puberty in female patients are idiopathic, but central nervous system tumors are a serious consideration (Table 28–2) and often are sought with MRI (Fig. 28–7).

Ultrasound findings in true precocious puberty consist of a "hormonally stimulated" appearance of the ovaries and uterus (Fig. 28–8). The ovaries are enlarged and may be adult size. Graafian follicles of adult proportion (1 or more cm) may be present in the ovaries. The uterus is larger than normal for the patient's age, and it has adult features that include a bulbous uterine body and a body-to-cervix ratio greater than 1 (i.e., the

Table 28-2. Causes of Precocious Puberty

	Girls (%)	Boys (%)
True Precocious Puberty		
Idiopathic	74	41
Central nervous system lesion	7	26
Precocious Pseudopuberty		
Ovarian neoplasm or cyst	11	—
Testicular neoplasm	—	10
Adrenal neoplasm	2	22
Other	6	1

Data from Speroff L, Glass RH, Kase NG: Clinical Gynecologic Endocrinology and Infertility, 5th ed. Baltimore, Williams and Wilkins, 1994, pp. 321–456.

body of the uterus is longer than the cervix). The uterus does not usually reach full adult proportions, however, in precocious puberty patients. The principal role of ultrasound[12–17, 19] is to detect these gonadotropin-mediated ovarian and uterine changes. The *presence* of such changes strongly suggests true precocious puberty. The *absence* of such changes mediates strongly against *true* precocious puberty and suggests instead the following mimickers of this condition.

Premature Thelarche and Adrenarche. The main conditions that mimic true precocious puberty are premature thelarche (breast development) and premature adrenarche (pubic hair development). In patients with these idiopathic conditions, the ovaries and uterus are normal in size and appearance for the patient's

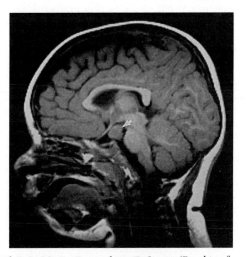

Figure 28-7—Precocious Puberty (Resulting from a Central Nervous System Tumor). This 9 month old infant developed heterosexual pubertal changes. MRI revealed a 2-cm mass (arrow) in the area of the hypothalamus (sagittal, T1-weighted image), confirmed at surgical resection. The histologic diagnosis was hamartoma. (Image kindly contributed by Douglas Brockmeyer, MD, Primary Children's Medical Center, Salt Lake City.)

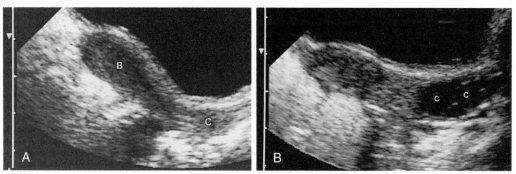

Figure 28-8—True (Idiopathic) Precocious Puberty. This 5 year old girl was evaluated for sudden growth acceleration and breast development. Serum gonadotropins were elevated and ultrasound demonstrated the following pubertal changes in the uterus and ovaries. **(A)** The uterine body (B) was bulbous and considerably longer than the cervix (C) (longitudinal image). **(B)** Several large cysts (C) were present in the left ovary, which had a calculated volume of 1.6 ml, far exceeding the normal range for 5 years (see Chapter 27). The right ovary (not shown) was similar in size and appearance. A clinical diagnosis of idiopathic, true precocious puberty was made, and the patient was treated with gonadotropin-suppressing drugs. Follow-up ultrasound scans showed gradual return of the uterus and ovaries to a prepubertal appearance. (Images kindly contributed by Mary Murray, MD, Baystate Medical Center, Springfield, MA.)

age. This finding, in conjunction with normal skeletal age and absence of elevated gonadotropin levels, effectively excludes true precocious puberty.[12, 13, 15, 16]

Precocious Pseudopuberty. This condition[12–14, 16, 17] is an additional category of precocious pubertal development that is *not* hypothalamic in origin and therefore is not "true" precocious puberty. Gonadotropin levels are low, ovulation does not occur, and various hormonal patterns may be found, none of which are seen in normal puberty or true precocious puberty. A wide range of disorders may cause precocious pseudopuberty, including ovarian and adrenal neoplasms, central nervous system disorders, and neurofibromatosis (Table 28–2). Ultrasound may or may not show pubertal changes in the ovaries and uterus in patients with precocious pseudopuberty, and if these changes are present, they generally are not as pronounced as in true precocious puberty. Because some pubertal ovarian and uterine changes may occur, sonographic findings alone cannot differentiate between precocious pseudopuberty and true precocious puberty. Functional ovarian cysts, ovarian neoplasms (benign, malignant, cystic, or solid), and adrenal tumors may secrete hormones that cause precocious pseudopuberty; therefore, it is important to search for such lesions in precocious puberty patients.[12–14, 16, 17]

DELAYED PUBERTY

Failure of onset of menses *or* the absence of other manifestations of puberty by age 16 years is abnormal and is termed "delayed puberty." Delays in puberty may be idiopathic or may result from genital tract obstruction, gonadal dys-

genesis, uterine agenesis, or hermaphroditism. Alternatively, delayed puberty may be idiopathic.[9, 12, 13, 16, 18, 19] The objectives for sonographic examination in cases of delayed puberty are threefold: (1) to exclude obstructive processes, including hematocolpos and hematometros; (2) to establish that the ovaries, uterus, and vagina are present; and (3) to determine whether the uterus and ovaries have a prepubertal or adult configuration.

In patients with idiopathic delayed menarche, both the ovaries and the uterus are present but are prepubertal in size and shape. With uterine agenesis, the uterus cannot be detected sonographically (Fig. 28–2), but the ovaries typically are seen. With genital tract obstruction, the vagina and uterus are prominently distended with fluid (see Figure 29–1).

Failure to detect the ovaries by the teenage years is an ominous finding suggesting gonadal dysgenesis or hermaphroditism.[18] The uterus is present in gonadal dysgenesis, but it is small in size and prepubertal in shape. The uterus is absent in hermaphroditism, and the vagina ends as a blind pouch. The most frequently cited form of hermaphroditism is the testicular feminization syndrome, in which a genetic male develops the primary and secondary sexual characteristics of a female. The testes, in such cases, frequently are located in the pelvis and may be mistaken for ovaries, unless it is noted that the sonographic texture is inappropriate. Neoplastic degeneration of a pelvic testis (see Figure 28–6) is a recognized complication of testicular feminization.

SECONDARY AMENORRHEA

Patients with secondary amenorrhea[12, 16] exhibit normal pubertal development, including menarche, but menstruation ceases at some time following menarche. The most common causes of secondary amenorrhea in teenagers are pregnancy and functional cysts. Less common causes are benign or malignant ovarian neoplasms or central nervous system lesions. Sonography has obvious value in the diagnosis of pregnancy, ovarian cysts, and ovarian neoplasms, and the detection of these conditions should be the focus of ultrasound examination.

REFERENCES

1. Kraus FT: Female genitalia. *In* Kissane JM (ed): Anderson's Pathology. 8th ed. St. Louis, CV Mosby, 1985, pp 1451–1455.
2. Baramki TA: Treatment of congenital anomalies in girls and women. J Reprod Med 29:376–384, 1984.
3. Gilsanz V, Cleveland RH: Duplication of the Müllerian ducts and genitourinary malformations, part 1. Radiology 144:793–796, 1982.
4. Gilsanz V, Cleveland RH, Reid BS: Duplication of the Müllerian ducts and genitourinary malformations, part 2. Radiology 144:797–801, 1982.
5. Malini S, Valdes C, Malinak R: Sonographic diagnosis and classification of anomalies of the female genital tract. J Ultrasound Med 3:397–404, 1984.
6. Valdes C, Malini S, Malinak LR: Ultrasound evaluation of female genital tract anomalies: A review of 64 cases. J Obstet Gynecol 149:285–292, 1984.
7. Reuter KL, Daly DC, Cohen SM: Septate versus bicornuate uteri: Errors in imaging diagnosis. Radiology 172:749–752, 1989.
8. Blask ARN, Sanders RC, Gearhart JP: Obstructed uterovaginal anomalies: Demonstration with sonography. Part I. Neonates and infants. Radiology 179:79–83, 1991.
9. Blask ARN, Sanders RC, Rock JA: Obstructed uterovaginal anomalies: Demonstration with sonography. Part II. Teenagers. Radiology 179:84–88, 1991.
10. Hricak H, Chang YCF, Thurnher S: Vagina: Evaluation with MR imaging. Part I. Normal anatomy and congenital anomalies. Radiology 169:169–174, 1988.
11. Carrington BM, Hricak H, Nuruddin RN, Secaf E, Laros RK, Hill EC: Müllerian duct anomalies: MR imaging evaluation. Radiology 176:715–720, 1990.
12. Hedlund GL, Royal SA, Parker KL: Disorders of puberty: A practical imaging approach. Semin Ultrasound CT MRI 15:49–77, 1994.
13. Speroff L, Glass RH, Kase NG: Clinical Gynecologic Endocrinology and Infertility. 5th ed. Baltimore, Williams and Wilkins, 1994, pp 321–456.
14. Stanhope R, Adams J, Jacobs HS, et al: Ovarian ultrasound assessment in normal children, idiopathic precocious puberty, and during low-dose pulsatile gonadotropin-releasing hormone treatment of hypogonadotropic hypogonadism. Arch Dis Child 60:116–119, 1985.
15. Shawker TH, Comite F, Rieth KG, Dwyer AJ, Cutler GB, Loriaux DL: Ultrasound evaluation of female isosexual precocious puberty. J Ultrasound Med 3:309–316, 1984.
16. Siegel MJ: Pediatric gynecologic sonography. Radiology 179:593–600, 1991.
17. Fakhry J, Khoury A, Kotval PS, Noto RA: Sonography of autonomous follicular ovarian cysts in precocious pseudopuberty. J Ultrasound Med 7:597–603, 1988.
18. Eberenz W, Rosenberg HK, Moshang T, Chatten J, Keating MA: True hermaphroditism: Sonographic demonstration of ovotestes. Radiology 179:429–431, 1991.
19. Dietrich RB, Kangarloo H: Pelvic abnormalities in children: Assessment with MR imaging. Radiology 163:367–372, 1987.

Chapter 29

Vaginal and Uterine Pathology

William J. Zwiebel

VAGINAL AND UTERINE FLUID COLLECTIONS

The terms "hydrocolpos," "hydrotrachelos," and "hydrometra" refer to the accumulation of watery fluid in the vagina, cervix, and uterus, respectively.[1, 2] Analogous terms using the prefix "hemato-" (e.g., hematocolpos) refer to the accumulation of blood in the corresponding cavities.[1] Similarly, the prefix "muco-" refers to mucus and the prefix "pyo-" refers to pus.[1] Large intracavitary fluid collections are always pathologic, and such collections usually are associated with partial or complete obstruction of the genital tract. The etiology of pathologic intracavitary fluid is age related. In girls from infancy to puberty, the usual cause is congenital obstruction of the genital tract. During the childbearing years, intracavitary fluid generally is related to menstruation, pregnancy, or infection. After the menopause, fluid collections typically are related to neoplasms.[2–12]

Sonographic Findings

The sonographic features of intracavitary fluid are nonspecific and do not differentiate one type of fluid from another.[2–13] Most collections are anechoic, but mixed or dependent echogenicity may be seen when the fluid contains particulate matter such as intracavitary blood or pus. The presence of intracavitary fluid is a cause for thorough ultrasound investigation that may indicate the cause of fluid accumulation (Figs. 29–1 through 29–3). The sonographer should begin by determining where the fluid is located (vagina, uterus, or fallopian tube), and then should search for related pathology, such as: (1) an obstructive congenital anomaly (Chapter 28); (2) an obstructing mass; (3) endometrial thickening and other signs of endometrial neoplasia (considered later); (4) pelvic inflammatory disease (Chapter 31); and (5) intrauterine or ectopic pregnancy (Chapter 36).[2–4, 6, 7, 14, 15]

Caveats

Ultrasound diagnosis of intracavitary fluid generally is straightforward, but the following caveats are noteworthy.[4, 6, 7, 9, 13]

1. One can differentiate between uterine and vaginal collections by noting the thickness of the wall surrounding the collection. Only a thin wall surrounds a vaginal collection, whereas a uterine collection is surrounded by a thick, muscular wall (the myometrium). The vagina, furthermore, is much more distensible than the uterus, allowing the fluid-filled vagina to achieve massive proportions compared with the adjacent uterus (Fig. 29–1).

2. Blood, mucus, and pus may occasionally be highly echogenic, in which case the intracavitary fluid may blend in with the normal endometrium and be difficult to detect.[4, 6, 9, 13]

3. An intrauterine fluid collection may, in fact, be a gestational sac or a pseudogestational sac of ectopic pregnancy (Chapter 36).

4. Urine may leak from the distended urinary bladder and collect in the vagina, mimicking a pathologic fluid collection. Alternatively, fluid may be introduced into the vagina iatrogeni-

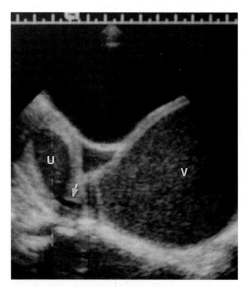

Figure 29-1—Hematocolpometra (12 year old girl with primary amenorrhea and abdominal pain). A longitudinal scan demonstrates massive distention (7.7 cm AP) of the vagina (V) due to accumulated menses. The uterus (U) and cervical canal (arrow) are less distended because their rigid muscular walls resist expansion. The cause of hematocolpometra in this case was imperforate hymen. The medium-level echogenicity is typical of accumulated menses.

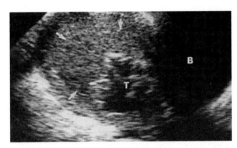

Figure 29-2—Retained Products of Conception Resulting in Pyometrium (longitudinal image 1 week postsuction curettage for elective abortion). The uterine cavity (arrows) is distended with moderately echogenic material. A mass of retained tissue (T) from the pregnancy is present in the lower portion of the uterine cavity. B = bladder.

cally (usually during attempted filling of the bladder).

RETAINED PRODUCTS OF CONCEPTION

Gestational tissue may remain within the uterine cavity following spontaneous or induced abortion or normal delivery. Such material must be removed by suction or sharp curettage. The principal clinical differential for retained products of conception is endometritis, which is considered later.

The products of conception that may be retained include fetal parts, placental fragments, or pieces of the chorioamniotic membranes. The following features suggest the presence of retained gestational material: (1) visible fetal structures within the uterine cavity; (2) heterogeneous intracavitary material (Fig. 29–2); (3) any intrauterine material that has mass effect; and (4) "endometrial" thickness greater than 5 mm (actually endometrium plus retained tissue). Sonography cannot always confirm that gestational products have been "left behind" because clotted blood or other intracavitary fluid may resemble gestational tissue.[16–18] The mere presence of endometrial fluid is *not* helpful in identifying retained conception products. Conversely, however, the presence of a thin endometrium and little or no fluid *is* helpful for *excluding* retained material.

ENDOMETRITIS

The term "endometritis" refers to infection of the endometrium, or more generally, of the uterus. Endometritis may result from sexually transmitted infection, but it also occurs following recent delivery, spontaneous or induced abortion, or after uterine instrumentation in nonpregnant patients.

The only ultrasound finding specifically suggesting endometritis is the presence of strong reflections within the uterine wall at the margin of the endometrial cavity.[16–18] These reflections are produced by microscopic, bacterium-generated gas bubbles that are too small to be resolved per se but make the endometrium unusually bright. Gas also may accumulate as "macroscopic" bubbles within the endometrium (Fig. 29–3) or the uterine cavity. Intracavitary gas is less diagnostic than the "bright endometrium," as gas may enter the uterine cavity through instrumentation or bowel fistulization (Fig 29–4),

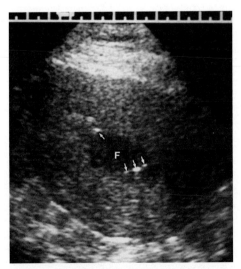

Figure 29-3—Endometritis (10 days after cesarean section). Fluid (F) is present in the endometrial cavity. Macroscopic gas bubbles (arrows) are present in the uterine wall adjacent to the uterine cavity. These bubbles were not free within the uterine cavity.

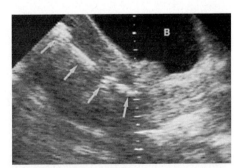

Figure 29-4—Intracavitary Gas. This longitudinal sonogram of the uterus demonstrates bright reflections (arrows) within the uterine cavity due to accumulated gas. The uterine cavity is not distended. In this patient with rectal carcinoma, the gas gained entry to the uterus via a fistula within the colon. B = bladder.

as well as endometritis. Intracavitary gas, therefore, is nonspecific but can be consistent with endometritis in the proper clinical setting. Certain additional nonspecific findings[16-18] also suggest endometritis. These findings result from inflammation, and include endocavitary fluid (Figs. 29-2, 29-3), poor definition of the endometrium and its margins,* uterine enlargement, and indistinct extrinsic uterine borders. Infection-related adnexal abnormalities also may be seen, as described in Chapter 31.

ENDOMETRIAL THICKENING

Conditions that may cause endometrial thickening include (1) pregnancy, (2) physiologic hypertrophy, (3) hyperplasia, (4) adenomatous polyp, and (5) endometrial carcinoma.[19] Pregnancy and physiologic hypertrophy represent normal growth of the endometrium in response to hormonal stimulation. Hyperplasia is a benign overgrowth caused by excessive or prolonged estrogen stimulation. Adenomatous polyps are benign neoplasms usually heralded by abnormal uterine bleeding. Endometrial carcinoma is a malignant neoplasm that most commonly affects menopausal or postmenopausal women. This tumor typically produces abnormal uterine bleeding, leading to early detection and a good prognosis.[19]

As stated in Chapter 27, the normal thickness

*These also may be normal findings in the immediate postmenstrual period.

of the endometrium (myometrium to myometrium) is 6.2 to 13 mm in menstruating women and 4 to 8 mm in postmenopausal women (including individuals receiving replacement estrogen).* Abnormal endometrial thickness suggests any of the aforementioned pathologic conditions, but sonographic findings generally cannot distinguish among these etiologies.[4, 9, 11, 13, 20-23] Furthermore, the accumulation of ectogenic mucus, pus, or blood within the endometrial cavity may occasionally mimic endometrial thickening, as noted previously.[3-5, 9, 13]

These diagnostic limitations notwithstanding, it is very important to recognize sonographic findings that suggest endometrial carcinoma.[4, 13, 21, 22] This diagnosis should come to mind when the endometrium is *thickened and heterogeneous*, when intracavitary fluid accompanies endometrial thickening, when the patient is postmenopausal, and particularly when there is evidence of *myometrial invasion*. The earliest evidence of such invasion is obliteration of the sonolucent line that normally marks the endometrial/myometrial junction. More advanced invasion is represented by irregularity of the endometrial/myometrial boundary or frank extension of endometrial tissue into the myometrium. In advanced cases, a large intracavitary mass (Fig. 29-5) may be present, or tumor may extend beyond the confines of the uterus.[9, 13, 20, 21, 23-26]

*Note that these are myometrium-to-myometrium measurements that represent the combined thickness of both "layers" of the endometrium.

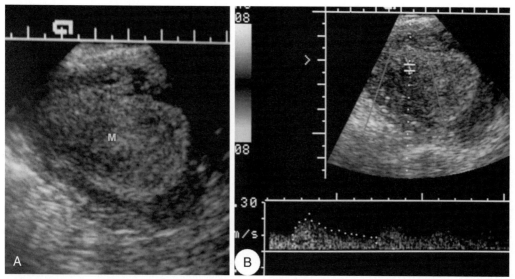

Figure 29-5—Endometrial Carcinoma. (A) A large, slightly heterogeneous mass (M) is seen within the uterine cavity in this 80 year old woman. Note that the mass is well defined on the right side of the image but is poorly defined on the left side, suggesting that it is invasive on the left. **(B)** Low-resistance arterial Doppler signals are present in the mass, consistent with (but not specific for) a malignant tumor.

CERVICAL CARCINOMA

Cervical carcinoma[19, 27] originates in the endothelial lining of the cervix and may remain silent until it has spread locally or even distantly. Sonography is only rarely used for assessment of cervical carcinoma, since the tumor usually is detected clinically and staged with physical examination, computed tomography (CT), or magnetic resonance imaging (MRI). Sonographic findings[27] consist principally of cervical enlargement or a soft tissue mass arising from the cervix. The mass may distort the contours of the cervix, the uterine body, or the vagina and may extend into the parametria or perirectal area, obscuring the origin of the tumor. Pelvic and para-aortic adenopathy occur commonly and may be detected sonographically.

NABOTHIAN CYSTS

Nabothian cysts are mucous retention cysts of the cervical mucosa[19] that are visualized as small (6 to 20 mm), rounded, anechoic areas within the cervical endometrium (Fig. 29–6). Several cysts are visible in most cases,[28] but these often are unsuspected clinically as they are located well within the cervical canal and are invisible during speculum examination. Nabothian cysts are common but harmless, and they should not be mistaken for significant pathology.

LEIOMYOMA

Leiomyomas[29–41] are benign neoplasms of myometrial origin that occur in 20% to 40% of women older than 35 to 40 years.[19] These tumors are composed principally of smooth muscle cells and are uniform histologically, except for occasional areas of hyaline degeneration and calcification. The great majority of leiomyomas are located in the uterine body or fundus. Cervical

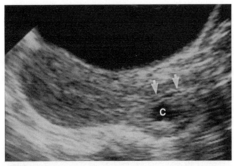

Figure 29-6—Nabothian Cyst. An anechoic cyst (C) with distal acoustic enhancement is seen adjacent to the endocervical canal (arrows). This is the typical location and appearance for a nabothian cyst.

leiomyomas occur infrequently but are particularly important during pregnancy because they may obstruct the birth canal. Leiomyomas may enlarge rapidly during pregnancy or in response to hormonal therapy.[19, 27, 33–35]

Most leiomyomas are asymptomatic, but tumors that deform the endometrial cavity may cause hypermenorrhea or infertility. Large leiomyomas also may cause pelvic pain or symptoms related to visceral compression. Abrupt, severe pain may result from hemorrhage into a leiomyoma (particularly apt to occur during pregnancy) and from torsion of an exophytic leiomyoma.[19, 27, 33–35]

Sonographic Findings

Leiomyomas are classified as subserosal, intramural, or submucosal, according to their location within the uterine wall.

1. Subserosal leiomyomas (Fig. 29–7A) arise from the outer surface of the myometrium and grow away from the uterus, into the peritoneal cavity. Occasionally, these exophytic tumors are pedunculated and may seem to be separate from the uterus. In such cases, they usually are mistaken for an ovarian tumor or other pelvic organ.
2. Intramural leiomyomas (Fig. 29–7B) are the standard-variety tumors that are predominantly located in the substance of the myometrium. The identity of intramural leiomyomas is seldom in doubt.
3. Submucosal leiomyomas arise from the inner portion of the myometrium (near the endometrial lining) and enlarge into the endometrial cavity. These tumors may distend the uterine cavity (Fig. 29–7C) and may be mistaken for endometrial masses or even for endometrial fluid collections.

Most leiomyomas are hypoechoic relative to the myometrium (Fig. 29–7B), but they also may be iso- or hyperechoic. Sizeable areas of hemorrhage or hyaline degeneration in large leiomyomas, may produce discrete, hypoechoic zones (Fig. 29–8). Rarely, leiomyomas with extensive degeneration may resemble cysts, causing diagnostic confusion.[38] Focal dystrophic calcification is common in leiomyomas and produces typical strong reflections and acoustic shadows[27, 33, 34] (Fig. 29–9).

Most leiomyomas are discrete, rounded masses with smooth, well-defined borders (Fig. 29–7B), but these features vary, and some leiomyomas "blend in" with the myometrium, making them difficult to identify. In such cases, the only evidence of leiomyomas is in indirect findings, such

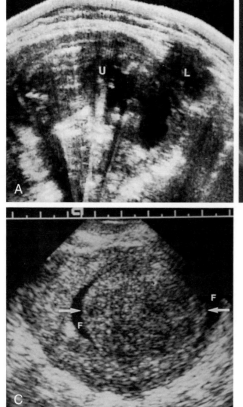

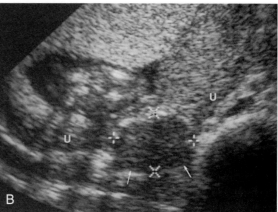

Figure 29-7—Uterine Leiomyoma Locations. (A) A pedunculated, subserosal leiomyoma (L) is visible adjacent to the pregnant uterus (U) on this transverse static scan. The leiomyoma moved freely with manual pressure, indicating that it was attached to the uterus only by a pedicle. **(B)** An intramural leiomyoma (cursors) projects extrinsically (arrows) from the uterine wall (U) in a 12-week pregnant uterus. **(C)** An endocavitary leiomyoma (arrows) is illustrated in this coronal transvaginal image. The tumor originated in a submucous location and grew into the uterine cavity. A small amount of fluid (F) separates a portion of the tumor from the uterine wall.

as distortion of the extrinsic uterine contours or the endometrial cavity, focal alterations of the myometrial "texture," and uterine enlargement.[27, 33–38]

Diagnostic Accuracy

Owing to the aforementioned subtle presentation of some leiomyomas and the small size of others, ultrasound detects only 62% to 78% of these tumors and is especially insensitive for tumors smaller than 3 cm.[30, 33, 40] In addition to this sensitivity problem, sonography often cannot define clearly the location of leiomyomas relative to the endometrial lining and cannot differentiate leiomyomas from adenomyosis (see below).[30–32, 41] These deficiencies are of more than academic interest. The effectiveness of the endoscopic myomectomy hinges on the number, size, and location of leiomyomas, as well as the differentiation of leiomyomas and adenomyosis.[30–32] Accurate

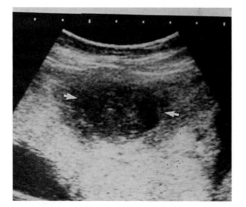

Figure 29-8—Hemorrhagic Leiomyoma. A large area of sonolucency (arrows), attributed to hemorrhage, is evident in the center of this leiomyoma, which is located in the wall of a gravid uterus. Acute pain at the site of the leiomyoma prompted ultrasound examination.

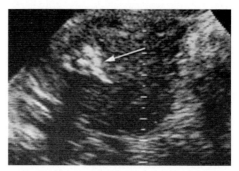

Figure 29-9—Calcified Leiomyoma. Dystrophic Calcification (arrow) is seen in an otherwise unremarkable uterine leiomyoma.

pre-operative assessment, therefore, is important.

The diagnostic sensitivity of MRI for leiomyomas approaches 100%, and studies have shown that MRI is far more accurate than sonography for determining the number and location of leiomyomas[36, 39–41] and for differentiating between adenomyosis and leiomyomatosis.[29, 30] Because of these advantages, MRI may be the procedure of choice in selected situations when precise information about leiomyomas is needed.

ADENOMYOSIS

Adenomyosis[29–32] is also called internal endometriosis, for it is characterized by ectopic growth of endometrial tissue (non-neoplastic) within the myometrium. The incidence of this condition is not precisely known, but it is recognized as a common and important cause of menometrorrhagia. Both endovaginal ultrasound and MRI are used to diagnose this condition, and it appears that the accuracy of these modalities is similar. The reported sensitivity and specificity of ultrasound for adenomyosis is as high as 89%,[30, 32] but one series reported only a 53% sensitivity.[31] A high level of ultrasound sensitivity necessitates in-person sonologist examination, or video tape recording of the examination for subsequent sonologist review. Hard copy film does not adequately display the subtle findings in this condition.[32]

The sonographic diagnosis of adenomyosis is based on the presence of poorly defined areas of heterogeneity within the myometrium.[30, 32] The heterogeneous areas generally exhibit decreased echogenicity relative to normal myometrium and are never increased in echogenicity. In some cases, 1- to 3-mm lucent areas may be present in the affected areas; these are thought to be small cysts.[30] Uterine enlargement is another possible finding, but this is nonspecific. Differentiation between adenomyosis and leiomyoma is based on the following: Areas of adenomyosis do not have focal mass effect and are poorly margined. They do not distort the uterine contours, although the uterus may be enlarged overall.

MYOMETRIAL CALCIFICATIONS

Myometrial calcifications are seen occasionally in the uterine body on high-quality sonograms (particularly on transvaginal images). It is important to recognize these calcifications, for they are of no clinical consequence and should not be mistaken for significant pathology. Two varieties

of calcifications occur: phleboliths located in the arcuate uterine veins, and dystrophic subendometrial calcifications that appear to result from prior instrumentation (e.g., dilatation and curettage).[42, 43] Arcuate vein phleboliths (see Figure 27–7) are *peripheral* within the myometrium, are relatively *large,* and may cast acoustic shadows. Instrumentation-related subendometrial calcifications are *central* in location (subendometrial) and *tiny*. The latter calcifications may produce reverberation artifacts or acoustic shadows, but in some cases they produce only focal bright dots.

INTRAUTERINE CONTRACEPTIVE DEVICES

Sonography is a safe, painless, and reliable method for determining the location of intrauterine contraceptive devices (IUD).[44–49] These devices are no longer used widely in women of childbearing age because they facilitate sexually transmitted infection of the uterus and adnexa. As a consequence, they may secondarily cause infertility and ectopic pregnancy. IUDs are currently used, however, in women who have completed their family and are sexually monogamous. Clinical concern about the location of IUDs occurs in the following circumstances:

1. The strings attached to the device cannot be identified manually within the vagina. In such cases, the IUD may have been expelled, the strings may have detached or withdrawn into the uterine cavity, or the device may have penetrated into or through the myometrium (pulling the strings along).
2. An IUD cannot be removed with gentle traction on the strings. In such cases the IUD may be deeply embedded within the endometrium or may have penetrated into the myometrium.
3. A patient becomes pregnant in spite of IUD use. In such cases the device may have been expelled unnoticed, may have penetrated into or through the myometrium, or may remain within the uterine cavity with the gestation.

Sonographic Localization

Ultrasound localization[44–47] is aided by knowledge of the type and shape of the IUD that is sought. Both transabdominal and transvaginal ultrasound should be used as needed. In most cases it is not sufficient merely to know that some part of the IUD lies within the uterine cavity, but it must be determined that *all* the device is within the uterine cavity. Only in this way can endometrial embedding or myometrial penetration be excluded. The sonographer can best assure that the *entire* IUD lies within the uterine cavity if the shape is known.

Hysterosalpingography or MRI may be used if ultrasound does not reveal the location of the IUD relative to the uterine cavity.[47] If an IUD cannot be identified at all with ultrasound, then it may have penetrated the uterus. A radiograph should be obtained to determine whether or not the device is within the abdominal cavity.[47]

REFERENCES

1. Taylor JE (ed): Dorland's Illustrated Medical Dictionary. 27th ed. Philadelphia, WB Saunders, 1985, pp 741, 742, 783, 785, 1058, 1395.
2. Pretorius DH, Dennis MA, Manco-Johnson ML, Gottesfield KR: Ultrasound diagnosis of hematotrachelos: A case report. Am J Obstet Gynecol 151:1080–1082, 1985.
3. Breckenridge JW, Kurtz AB, Ritchie WGM, et al: Postmenopausal uterine fluid collections: Indicator of carcinoma. AJR Am J Roentgenol 139:529–534, 1982.
4. McCarthy KA, Hall DA, Kopans DB, et al: Postmenopausal endometrial fluid collections: Always an indicator of malignancy? J Ultrasound Med 5:647–649, 1986.
5. Rubin D, Graham MF, Cronhilm C, et al: Ectogenic hematometra mimicking endometrial carcinoma. J Ultrasound Med 4:47–48, 1985.
6. Laing FC, Filly RA, Marks W, et al: Ultrasonic demonstration of endometrial fluid collections unassociated with pregnancy. Radiology 137:471–474, 1980.
7. Schaffer RM, Taylor C, Haller JO, et al: Nonobstructive hydrocolpos: Sonographic appearance and differential diagnosis. Radiology 149:273–278, 1983.
8. Yaghoobian J, Yankelevitz DF, Pinck RL, et al: Pyometrium in a three-year-old girl: Sonographic findings. AJR Am J Roentgenol 138:517–518, 1981.
9. Johnson MA, Graham MF, Cooperberg PL: Abnormal endometrial echoes: Sonographic spectrum of endometrial pathology. J Ultrasound Med 1:161–166, 1982.
10. Pupols AZ, Wilson SR: Ultrasonographic interpretation of physiological changes in the female pelvis. J Can Assoc Radiol 35:34–39, 1984.
11. Fleischer AC, Pittaway DW, Beard LA, et al: Sonographic depiction of endometrial changes occurring with ovulation induction. J Ultrasound Med 3:341–436, 1984.
12. Thickman D, Arger P, Tureck R, et al: Echographic assessment of the endometrium in patients undergoing in vitro fertilization. J Ultrasound Med 5:197–201, 1986.
13. Fleischer AC, Kalemeris GC, Machin JE, et al: Sonographic depiction of normal and abnormal endometrium with histopathologic correlation. J Ultrasound Med 5:445–452, 1986.
14. Nussbaum Blask AR, Sanders RC, Gearhart JP: Obstructed uterovaginal anomalies: Demonstration with sonography. Part I. Neonates and infants. Radiology 179:79–83, 1991.
15. Nussbaum Blask AR, Sanders RC, Gearhart JP: Obstructed uterovaginal anomalies: Demonstration

16. Patten RM, Vincent LM, Wolner-Hanssen P, Thorpe E: Pelvic inflammatory disease: Endovaginal sonography with laparoscopic correlation. J Ultrasound Med 9:681–689, 1990.
17. Hertzberg BS, Bowie JD: Ultrasound of the postpartum uterus. J Ultrasound Med 10:451–456, 1991.
18. Kurtz AB, Shlansky-Goldberg RD, Choi HY, Needleman L, Wapner RJ, Goldberg BB: Detection of retained products of conception following spontaneous abortion in the first trimester. J Ultrasound Med 10:387–395, 1991.
19. Kraus FT: Female genitalia. *In* Kissane JM (ed): Anderson's Pathology. St Louis, CV Mosby, 1985, pp 1451–1455.
20. Requard CK, Widkc JD, Mettler FA, et al: Ultrasonography in the staging of endometrial carcinoma. Radiology 140:781–785, 1981.
21. Fleischer AC, Dudley BS, Entman SS, Baxter JW, Kalemeris GC, James AE: Myometrial invasion by endometrial carcinoma: Sonographic assessment. Radiology 162:307–310, 1987.
22. Fleischer AC, Mendelson EB, Bohm-Velez M, Entman SS: Transvaginal and transabdominal sonography of the endometrium. Semin Ultrasound CT MRI 9:81–101, 1988.
23. Lien HH, Blomlie V, Tropé C, Kaern J, Abeler VM: Cancer of the endometrium: Value of MR imaging in determining depth of invasion into the myometrium. AJR Am J Roentgenol 157:1221–1223, 1991.
24. Hricak H, Rubinstein LV, Gherman GM, Karstaedt N: MR imaging evaluation of endometrial carcinoma: Results of an NCI cooperative study. Radiology 179:829–832, 1991.
25. Granai CO, Allee P, Doherty F, Madoc-Jones H, Curry SL: Ultrasound used for assessing the in situ position of intrauterine tandems. Gynecol Oncol 18:334–338, 1984.
26. Brascho DJ, Kim RY, Wilson EE: Use of ultrasonography in planning intracavitary radiotherapy of endometrial carcinoma. Radiology 129:163–167, 1978.
27. Walsh JW, Brewer WH, Schneider V: Ultrasound diagnosis in diseases of the uterine corpus and cervix. Semin Ultrasound 1:30–40, 1980.
28. Fogel SR, Slasky BS: Sonography of nabothian cysts. AJR Am J Roentgenol 138:927–930, 1982.
29. Togashi K, Ozasa H, Konishi I, et al: Enlarged uterus: Differentiation between adenomyosis and leiomyoma with MR imaging. Radiology 171:531–534, 1989.
30. Fedele L, Bianchi S, Dorta M, et al: Transvaginal ultrasonography in the differential diagnosis of adenomyoma versus leiomyoma. Am J Obstet Gynecol 167:603–606, 1992.
31. Ascher SM, Arnold LL, Patt DH, et al: Adenomyosis: Prospective comparison of MR imaging and transvaginal sonography. Radiology 190:803–806, 1994.
32. Reinhold C, McCarthy S, Bret PM, et al: Diffuse adenomyosis: Comparison of endovaginal US and MR imaging with histopathologic correlation. Radiology 199:151–158, 1996.
33. Gross BH, Silver TM, Jaffe MH: Sonographic features of uterine leiomyomas: Analysis of 41 proven cases. J Ultrasound Med 2:401–406, 1983.
34. Smith JP, Weiser EB, Karnei RF, et al: Ultrasonography of rapidly growing uterine

leiomyomata associated with anovulatory cycles. Radiology 134:713–716, 1980.

35. Mack LA, Gottesfeld K, Johnson ML: Ultrasonic evaluation of a cervical mass in pregnancy. J Clin Ultrasound 9:49–50, 1981.

36. Lehrman BJ, Nisenbaum HL, Glasser SC, Najar D, Rosen M: Uterine myolipoma: Magnetic resonance imaging, computed tomographic, and ultrasound appearance. J Ultrasound Med 9:665–668, 1990.

37. Soyer PH, Harry G, Cazier A, Masselot J, Vanel D: Uterine fibromyolipoma: Uncommon imaging features. Eur J Radiol 13:67–68, 1991.

38. Green WJ, Fendley SM, Wintzell EC, Green AE, Lorino CO, Rodning CB: Cystic degeneration of a large uterine leiomyoma: Radiologic and surgical analyses. Invest Radiol 8:626–629, 1989.

39. Weinreb JC, Barkoff ND, Megibow A, Demopoulos R: The value of MR imaging in distinguishing leiomyomas from other solid pelvic masses when sonography is indeterminate. AJR Am J Roentgenol 154:295–299, 1990.

40. Hricak H, Tscholakoff D, Heinrichs L, Fisher MD, Dooms GC, Reinhold C, Jaffe RB: Uterine leiomyomas: Correlation of MR, histopathologic findings, and symptoms. Radiology 158:385–391, 1986.

41. Dudiak CM, Turner DA, Patel SK, Archie JT, Silver B, Norusis M: Uterine leiomyomas in the infertile patient: Preoperative localization with MR imaging versus US and hysterosalpingography. Radiology 167:627–630, 1988.

42. Occhipinto K, Kutcher R, Rosenblatt J: Sonographic appearance and significance of arcuate artery calcification. J Ultrasound Med 10:97–100, 1991.

43. Burks DD, Stainken BF, Burkhard TK, Balsara ZN: Uterine inner myometrial ectogenic foci: Relationship to prior dilatation and curettage and endocervical biopsy. J Ultrasound Med 10:487–492, 1991.

44. Callen PW, Filly RA, Munyer TP: Intrauterine contraceptive devices: Evaluation by sonography. AJR Am J Roentgenol 135:797–800, 1980.

45. Najarian KE, Kurtz AB: New observations in the sonographic evaluation of intrauterine contraceptive devices. J Ultrasound Med 5:205–210, 1986.

46. Abramovici H, Sorokin Y, Bornstein J, Auslander R: A partial uterine perforation (type 2) by a copper-T IUD: Sonographic diagnosis and management. J Ultrasound Med 4:381–383, 1985.

47. Rosenblatt R, Zakin D, Stern WZ, Kutcher R: Uterine perforation and embedding by intrauterine device: Evaluation by US and hysterography. Radiology 157:765–770, 1985.

48. Shalev J, Greif M, Ben-Rafael Z, Itzchak Y, Serr DM: Continuous sonographic monitoring of IUD extraction during pregnancy: Preliminary report. AJR Am J Roentgenol 139:521–523, 1982.

49. Ylöstalo PR, Nilsson CG, Hieta-Heikurainen MH: Ultrasonically controlled removal of an intrauterine contraceptive device. J Clin Ultrasound 12:505–506, 1984.

Chapter 30

Ovarian Enlargement and Solid Extrauterine Pathology

William J. Zwiebel

The term "solid extrauterine pathology," as used in the title of this chapter, may seem a little odd, but this term represents the diagnostician's real-life view of pelvic pathology. When a pelvic lesion is detected, the sonographer first attempts to determine whether the lesion is uterine or extrauterine in origin. If extrauterine, the next step is to determine whether or not the pathology is related to the ovaries. In some cases it can be determined that an extrauterine mass clearly does or does not arise from an ovary. In others, the ovary simply cannot be detected, and it is unclear whether the ovary is the site of origin or is simply displaced by the mass. Therefore, the term "extrauterine" is used herein to avoid the misleading assumption that anything outside the uterus is ovarian.

DIFFERENTIAL CONSIDERATIONS

The differential diagnosis for solid extrauterine masses is presented in Table 30–1.[1-4] Some of the entities in this listing also appear in the differential list for cystic extrauterine pathology presented in the next chapter. These dual listings, in some cases, are histologically based, for some neoplasms may be solid or cystic. In other instances, dual listing is related to sonographic variability, as is the case with endometriomas or abscesses, which may appear either solid or cystic, depending on the properties of their contents.

The length of the differential list for solid extrauterine lesions (Table 30–1) is somewhat daunting, especially considering that sonographic features are nonspecific. But this list can be culled substantially. Certain of these lesions are primary diagnostic considerations, simply because they are more common than others. These are hematomas related to ectopic pregnancy (Chapter 36), primary ovarian neoplasms (Fig. 30–1), ovarian inflammation (from pelvic inflammatory disease), ovarian torsion, lymphoma, metastasis, and bowel-related masses (inflammatory or neoplastic). The differential listing can be culled further by considering three key elements

of pelvic diagnosis: whether or not the mass arises from an ovary, the age of the patient, and the clinical history. Patient age is particularly helpful; for example, ovarian carcinoma would be a serious consideration in a 55-year-old woman with an ovarian mass, but an ovarian teratoma would be much more likely in a 17-year-old patient.

OVARIAN ENLARGEMENT

Ovarian enlargement may be unilateral or bilateral and is a common cause of solid extrauterine masses. Unilateral enlargement occurs with functional cysts, neoplasms, inflammation, torsion, and polycystic ovary disease that happens to be asymmetric. Bilateral enlargement occurs with endocrinopathies including polycystic ovary

Table 30-1. Sonographic Differential Diagnosis of Solid-Appearing,° Extrauterine Pathology

Ovarian lesions
　Massive ovarian inflammation (PID)
　Torsed ovary
　Primary ovarian neoplasm
　Secondary ovarian neoplasm (including lymphoma)
　Polycystic ovary disease
　Hemorrhagic cyst
Pelvic abscess°
　Sexually transmitted
　Other sources, especially diverticulitis
Endometrioma°
Lymphadenopathy
Bowel lesions
　Neoplasm
　Crohn disease
　Diverticulitis
Hematoma
　Related to ectopic pregnancy
　Related to trauma (violent or surgical)
Pedunculated uterine leiomyoma†
Drop metastasis‡
Musculoskeletal tumor (pelvic floor or side wall)
Bladder tumor

°Although some lesions are solid appearing by sonographic standards of echogenicity, they may contain thick fluid that is echogenic.
　†Although a pedunculated leiomyoma is uterine in origin, it appears extrauterine.
　‡Intraperitoneal tumor spread to the pelvis.
　PID, pelvic inflammatory disease.

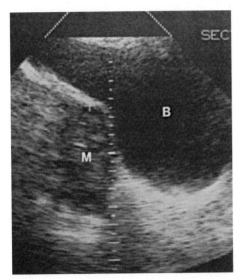

Figure 30-1—Epithelial Carcinoma of the Ovary. A 6-cm-long, slightly heterogeneous, solid mass (M) is seen on this longitudinal sonogram in a 69 year old woman with abdominal swelling. The margins of the mass are poorly defined, and no cystic elements are present. B = bladder. Ascites (not shown) was the cause of abdominal swelling. Diffuse peritoneal studding was found at surgery, but the tumor implants were too small for sonographic visualization.

disease, exogenous hormone administration, and neoplasms. The differential considerations for unilateral and bilateral ovarian enlargement are presented in Table 30–2. Please review this table as the contents are not repeated in the text. The noteworthy diagnostic features of selected conditions listed in Table 30–2 are presented below.

OVARIAN TORSION

Ovarian torsion is an uncommon but important cause of unilateral (and solid-appearing) ovarian enlargement. In this condition, the ovary twists about its ligamentous attachments, with the result that the arterial supply or venous drainage, or both, are impeded.[5–8] The initial effect of torsion is ovarian congestion (edema, hyperemia), but persistent venous and arterial occlusion causes ischemia and leads ultimately to hemorrhagic necrosis. Torsion may cut off blood flow to the ovary alone, or to both the ovary and the distal portion of the fallopian tube, depending on the location of adnexal twisting. Adnexal torsion occurs principally in adolescent patients, and in such cases there generally is no identifiable cause. The opposite is true for adult women in whom ovarian torsion usually is precipitated by an ovarian tumor or cyst. The expedient diagnosis of ovarian torsion is critical, because the ovary

may be saved if surgery is performed promptly to untwist the pedicle and restore blood flow.

Adnexal torsion is heralded by acute pain and tenderness. The signs and symptoms are apt to mimic appendicitis, and torsion may not even be a clinical consideration when the patient presents for sonographic examination.

The most consistent finding in ovarian torsion[5–8] is unilateral ovarian enlargement, and this may be the only finding. In about half of patients, the torsed ovary retains its ovoid configuration, which is helpful for confirming that the visualized structure is the ovary rather than another adnexal mass.[7] In the remaining cases, the torsed ovary has a rounded configuration, and it is more difficult to confirm that the mass is the ovary. The visualization of small peripheral cysts, representing graafian follicles, also helps confirm that the mass is the ovary. Such cysts are seen in about three fourths of ovarian torsion cases.[7]

The torsed ovary usually retains its typical echogenicity and sharp margination.[6] Echogenicity is variable, however, and ranges from hypoechoic (Fig. 30–2) to moderately echogenic. The "texture" of the ovary generally is homogeneous or slightly heterogeneous, and a small-to-moderate volume of pelvic fluid is present in about one third of torsion cases.[5, 7]

Although our experience is limited, Doppler sonography appears to be of great value in the diagnosis of ovarian torsion. Diminished or absent arterial flow signals are present in the torsed ovary compared with the unaffected ovary. A point of caution is noteworthy, however: torsion may incompletely obstruct arterial flow; hence, arterial signals may be detected even though clinically significant torsion is present. As of this writing, no published information on this subject could be found.

NEOPLASTIC OVARIAN ENLARGEMENT

Most ovarian neoplasms present as cystic ovarian masses, but solid ovarian neoplasms also oc-

Table 30-2. Causes of Ovarian Enlargement

Unilateral

Functional cyst
Primary or secondary neoplasm
Torsion
Asymmetric polycystic ovary disease
Infection (usually sexually transmitted)

Bilateral

Primary or secondary neoplasm
Endocrinopathy (especially polycystic ovary disease)
Exogenous hormone administration
Infection (usually sexually transmitted)
Ovarian hyperstimulation

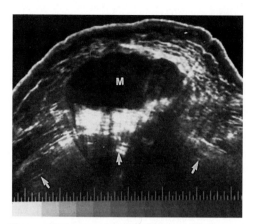

Figure 30-2—Ovarian Torsion (grossly obese, 35 year old pregnant woman). A transverse static scan shows a 17-cm mass (M) representing a torsed, infarcted ovary lying in an anterior abdominal wall hernia! A large portion of the mass is anechoic as a result of hemorrhagic necrosis, but overall the mass retains an ovoid configuration. (Arrows = border between abdominal wall musculature and peritoneal space.)

cur, and these may cause unilateral or bilateral enlargement. The common primary ovarian tumors, carcinoma and teratoma, usually are cystic, but they also may be predominantly or completely solid. These tumors are considered in detail in the following chapter. Lymphoma and metastases also are solid, as are many germ cell and stromal ovarian tumors.[1, 2] These tumors will not be considered in detail since they are relatively uncommon. The following points are noteworthy, however. First, with neoplastic enlargement the ovoid shape of one or both ovaries generally is lost, and the affected ovary may be irregular in configuration. The adage here is, "Beware the round or irregular ovary." Second, lymphoma may occur as a primary ovarian neoplasm, in which case it presents with massive unilateral ovarian enlargement (Fig. 30–3). Third, ovarian metastases may be unilateral but commonly are bilateral, as discussed next. Finally, germ cell and stromal neoplasms (Fig. 30–4; also see Figure 27–6) are major considerations when a large (e.g., 10 to 15 cm), predominately solid ovarian mass is identified in a young patient, yet the mass does not have features of a teratoma (see following chapter). These tumors often are malignant and often are heralded by endocrine activity.[1–4, 9–12]

BILATERAL OVARIAN ENLARGEMENT

Bilateral ovarian enlargement[1, 2, 13–24] is an unusual sonographic finding that may be caused by endogenous hormonal abnormalities, hormone therapy, or ovarian neoplasia. Endocrine causes of bilateral ovarian enlargement include polycystic ovarian disease, Cushing disease, pituitary adenoma, and exogenous hormone administration (usually clomiphene citrate or menotropins, as used in fertility-enhancement efforts).[13, 14] Ovaries that enlarge in response to hormonal stimuli retain their normal ovoid shape, and they may either may have a uniform solid appearance or may contain multiple cysts.[2, 13, 15]

POLYCYSTIC OVARY DISEASE

Polycystic ovary disease (POD)[1, 15, 17–24] is a complex endocrine disorder of unknown etiology

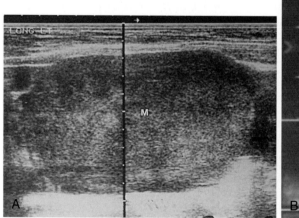

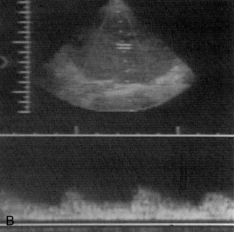

Figure 30-3—Primary Ovarian Lymphoma (18 year old woman, 13 weeks pregnant). **(A)** A longitudinal, composite view demonstrates a 13-cm-long, homogeneous left adnexal mass (M). The hypoechoic, homogeneous texture of this mass is typical of lymphoma. **(B)** The presence of arterial flow signals clearly indicates that the mass is solid (i.e., not a cyst with echogenic contents). The low-resistance flow pattern is typical of a neoplasm.

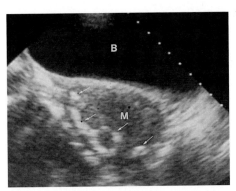

Figure 30-4—Ovarian Fibroma (19 year old woman with an asymptomatic left adnexal mass). An oblique view of the left adnexa demonstrates a solid ovoid mass (M) measuring 9 cm in length. Large, serpentine areas of calcification are evident (arrows). The uterus and right ovary were normal (not shown). B = bladder.

associated with ovarian enlargement and the development of multiple small ovarian cysts that classically are peripheral (subserosal) in location. These cysts are thought to be graafian follicles that persist in arrested states of development because of low levels of follicle-stimulating hormone. Although this is a "cystic" condition, the predominant finding is ovarian enlargement rather than cysts per se, and for this reason POD is included in this chapter.

The clinical signs and symptoms of POD include obesity, hirsutism, menstrual irregularity, oligomenorrhea, and infertility. The term "polycystic ovary disease" may be applied when any of these symptoms and signs occur with two additional findings: (1) polycystic ovaries, and (2) hormonal abnormalities that specifically include elevated levels of androgenic steroids and luteinizing hormone.[24] It is important to note that the presence of polycystic ovaries alone does not constitute the polycystic ovary syndrome. Approximately 75% of patients with polycystic ovaries on ultrasound examination have clinical abnormalities, and some of these patients may have the requisite diagnostic features of POD. The remaining 25% of individuals with polycystic ovaries have regular menstrual cycles, and some may have no features of the POD syndrome.[15, 17–19, 24] Note also that the presence of *normal* ovaries does not exclude POD either, for about one third of patients with clinical and endocrine manifestations of POD have sonographically normal ovaries.[19, 21–23]

These are the classic sonographic features of polycystic ovaries (Fig. 30–5): (1) bilateral enlargement, usually symmetric (mean, 13 to 14 cm); (2) multiple- 2 to 6-mm cysts; (3) the absence of cysts greater than 1.5 cm in diameter; (4) smooth ovarian contours (in spite of peripheral cysts); and (5) hyperechoic ovarian stroma.[15, 18–23]

In 20% of POD cases, the ovaries are significantly asymmetric in size (one ovary may be 50% larger than the other).[4] In some cases, the

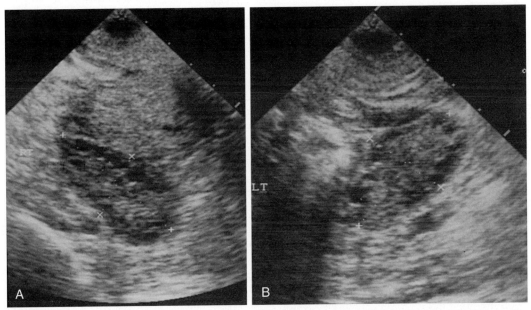

Figure 30-5—Polycystic Ovary Disease. Typical features of polycystic ovary disease are seen in this 32 year old infertility patient. Both the right (**A**) and left (**B**) ovaries (cursors) contain multiple small peripheral cysts that measure up to 7 mm. Note that the contours of the ovaries are smooth in spite of the peripheral cysts. The ovaries are large but do not exceed the upper limit of normal for volume. (Right: 47 × 22 mm, volume 11.4 cm³. Left: 40 × 24 mm, volume 11.5 cm³.)

smaller ovary may fall within the normal range for ovarian size, and the condition may appear to be unilateral.

The cysts that characterize POD are small and do not project from the ovarian surface, as normal graafian follicles do, because the serosal covering of the ovary is thick.[15, 18, 19] The cysts typically are peripheral, but they may be dispersed throughout the ovarian parenchyma. In some patients with POD, cysts may not be seen with ultrasound, apparently because they are too small to be resolved. The stroma of more than 90% of polycystic ovaries is hyperechoic, due to the acoustic effect of multiple unresolved cysts.[15, 18, 19, 23]

BILATERAL OVARIAN NEOPLASIA

Ovarian neoplasms may cause bilateral ovarian enlargement by two mechanisms.[1, 2, 15, 16] First, a tumor in one ovary may secrete hormones that cause enlargement of the other ovary. Second, the tumor may occur bilaterally. Various primary and secondary ovarian neoplasms tend to occur bilaterally, but principal among these are ovarian teratoma (8% to 15% bilateral) and dysgerminoma (15% to 17% bilateral).[1] Since teratoma is a common ovarian tumor (20% of ovarian neoplasms in adults and 50% in children), it is the most likely diagnosis when tumors are present bilaterally.[1] Ovarian metastases usually originate from the thyroid, breast, or colon and are bilateral in 60% to 80% of cases, but they represent only 6% of all ovarian neoplasms.[1] The incidence of bilaterality for ovarian leukemia and lymphoma is not defined, but it may be assumed to be quite high. Burkitt lymphoma, in particular, exhibits a predilection for ovarian involvement.

POSTMENOPAUSAL OVARIAN ENLARGEMENT

As noted in Chapter 27, the ovaries normally "shrink" substantially following menopause; nonetheless, they can be detected regularly with transabdominal and transvaginal sonography. They do not usually exceed 3 cm³ in volume 5 years or longer after the menopausal period, *even in patients receiving estrogen supplementation*.[14, 25–31] Any departures from the usual norms for ovarian size, shape, and texture are cause for concern in a post-menopausal woman. In this respect, note that cystic ovarian activity does not occur normally after the menopause,[27, 28, 30–34] and in most cases, therefore, a postmenopausal cyst must be investigated as a possible ovarian carci-noma. Fortunately, the majority of postmenopausal cysts are benign.[32]

REFERENCES

1. Kraus FT: Female genitalia. *In* Kissane JM (ed): Anderson's Pathology. 8th ed. St Louis, CV Mosby, 1985, pp 1451–1456.
2. Barber HRK: Ovarian cancer. Ca Cancer J Clin 36:148–184, 1986.
3. Williams AG, Mettler FA, Wicks JD: Cystic and solid ovarian neoplasms. Semin Ultrasound 4:166–183, 1983.
4. Cassoff J, Hanna T: Grey-scale ultrasonography for assessment of gynecologic pelvic masses. Can Med Assoc J 120:38–46, 1979.
5. Farrell TP, Boal DK, Teele RL, Ballantine TV: Acute torsion of normal uterine adnexa in children: Sonographic demonstration. AJR Am J Roentgenol 139:1223–1225, 1982.
6. Han BK, Babcock DS: Ultrasonography of torsion of normal uterine adnexa. J Ultrasound Med 2:321–323, 1983.
7. Graif M, Shalev J, Strauss S, Engelberg S, Mashiach S, Itzchak Y: Torsion of the ovary: Sonographic features. AJR Am J Roentgenol 143:1331–1334, 1984.
8. Worthington-Kirsch RL, Raptopoulos V, Cohen IT: Sequential bilateral torsion of normal ovaries in a child. J Ultrasound Med 5:663–664, 1986.
9. Stephenson WM, Laing FC: Sonography of ovarian fibromas. AJR Am J Roentgenol 144:1239–1240, 1985.
10. Athey PA, Siegel MF: Sonographic features of Brenner tumor of the ovary. J Ultrasound Med 6:367–372, 1987.
11. Athey PA, Malone RS: Sonography of ovarian fibromas/thecomas. J Ultrasound Med 6:431–436, 1987.
12. Brammer HM, Buck JL, Hayes WS, Sheth S, Tavassoli FA: Malignant germ cell tumors of the ovary: Radiologic-pathologic correlation. RadioGraphics 10:715–724, 1990.
13. Mendelson EB, Friedman H, Neiman HL, Calenoff L, Vogelzang RL, Cohen MR: The role of imaging in infertility management. AJR Am J Roentgenol 144:415–420, 1985.
14. Goldstein SR: The postmenopause. Appl Radiol 77:37–47, 1991.
15. Swanson M, Sauerbrei EE, Cooperberg PL: Medical implications of ultrasonically detected polycystic ovaries. J Clin Ultrasound 9:219–222, 1981.
16. Athey PA, Butters HE: Sonographic and CT appearance of Krukenberg tumors. J Clin Ultrasound 12:205–210, 1984.
17. McKenna TJ: Pathogenesis and treatment of polycystic ovary syndrome. N Engl J Med 318:558–562, 1988.
18. Parisi L, Tramonti M, Derchi LE, Casciano S, Zurli A, Rocchi P: Polycystic ovarian disease: Ultrasonic evaluation and correlations with clinical and hormonal data. J Clin Ultrasound 12:21–26, 1984.
19. Hann LE, Hall DA, McArdle CR, Seibel M: Polycystic ovarian disease: Sonographic spectrum. Radiology 150:531–534, 1984.
20. el Tabbakh GH, Lofty I, Azab I, Rahman HA, Southren AL, Aleem FA: Correlation of the ultrasonic appearance of the ovaries in polycystic ovarian disease and the clinical, hormonal, and

laparoscopic findings. Am J Obstet Gynecol 154:892–895, 1986.

21. Nicolini U, Ferrazzi E, Bellotti M, Travaglini P, Elli R, Scaperrotta RC: The contribution of sonographic evaluation of ovarian size in patients with polycystic ovarian disease. J Ultrasound Med 4:347–351, 1985.

22. Yeh H-C, Futterweit W, Thornton JC: Polycystic ovarian disease: US features in 104 patients. Radiology 163:111–116, 1987.

23. Pache TD, Wladimiroff JW, Hop WCJ, Fauser BCJM: How to discriminate between normal and polycystic ovaries: Transvaginal US study. Radiology 183:421–423, 1992.

24. Franks S: Polycystic ovary syndrome. N Engl J Med 333:853–861, 1995.

25. Campbell S, Goessens L, Goswamy R, Whitehead M: Real-time ultrasonography for determination of ovarian morphology and volume. Lancet 2:425–426, 1982.

26. Goswamy R, Campbell S, Whitehead M: Screening of ovarian cancer. Clin Obstet Gynecol 10:621–643, 1983.

27. Hall D: Sonographic appearance of the normal ovary, of polycystic ovarian disease, and of functional cysts. Semin Ultrasound 4:149–165, 1983.

28. Granberg S, Wikland M: A comparison between ultrasound and gynecological examination for detection of enlarged ovaries in a group of women at risk for ovarian carcinoma. J Ultrasound Med 7:59–63, 1988.

29. Cohen HL, Tice HM, Mandel FS: Ovarian volumes measured by US: Bigger than we think. Radiology 177:189–192, 1990.

30. Rodriguez MH, Platt LD, Medearis AL, Lacarra M, Lobo RA: The use of transvaginal sonography for the evaluation of postmenopausal ovarian size and morphology. Am J Obstet Gynecol 159:810–814, 1988.

31. Higgins RV, van Nagell JR, Donaldson ES, Gallion HH, Pavlik EJ, et al: Transvaginal sonography as a screening method for ovarian cancer. Gynecol Oncol 34:402–406, 1989.

32. Hall DA, McCarthy KA: The significance of the postmenopausal simple adnexal cyst. J Ultrasound Med 5:503–505, 1986.

33. Wolf SI, Gosink BB, Feldesman MR, Lin MC, Stuenkel CA, Braly PS, Pretorious DH: Prevalence of simple adnexal cysts in postmenopausal women. Genitourin Radiol 180:65–71, 1991.

34. Fleischer AC, McKee MS, Gordon AN, Page DL, Kepple DM, Worrell JA, Jones HW, Burnett LS, James AE: Transvaginal sonography of postmenopausal ovaries with pathologic correlation. J Ultrasound Med 9:637–644, 1990.

Chapter 31

Cystic Extrauterine Pathology

William J. Zwiebel

Myriad extrauterine pelvic lesions may exhibit a cystlike appearance on sonographic examination.[1-6] As noted in Table 31–1, these lesions include functional ovarian cysts, non-gynecologic cysts, abscesses, endometrial cysts, and ovarian neoplasms. With rare exceptions, the sonographic features of these lesions are nonspecific; nonetheless, the differential diagnosis usually can be focused somewhat on the basis of certain sonographic findings, as outlined in Table 31–2. The differential considerations for cystic lesions can often be narrowed further if the sonographic features are considered in conjunction with the patient's age, the history of illness, the physical findings, and laboratory data.[3] Indeed, I feel that the latter information should be available before any ultrasound diagnosis of pelvic pathology is rendered.

Table 31–1. Cystic Extrauterine Pelvic Pathology

Ovarian Origin

Functional cysts
Cystadenoma
Cystadenocarcinoma
Cystic teratoma
Other primary ovarian neoplasms (usually solid)
Cystic ovarian metastases (usually solid)
Lymphoma (may appear cystic if very hypoechoic)

Uterine or Fallopian Origin

Exophytic leiomyoma that is necrotic or hemorrhagic
Hydrosalpinx

Inflammatory Origin

Tubo-ovarian abscess
Pyosalpinx
Abscesses from other organs or sources

Endometriosis

Endometrioma (chocolate cyst)

Pregnancy-Related

Corpus luteum cyst (functional cyst)
Ectopic pregnancy (gestational sac, hematoma, or
 cul-de-sac blood)

Miscellaneous

Fluid-filled bowel
Cul-de-sac fluid
Parovarian cysts
Inclusion cysts and lymphocele (postsurgical)
Developmental cysts
Bladder diverticulum
Urachal cyst

In this chapter, we review the ultrasound findings that help characterize the more common lesions listed in Tables 31–1 and 31–2. These are functional cysts, parovarian cysts, neoplastic cysts, abscesses, and endometriomas. Before proceeding, the reader is encouraged to review Tables 31–1 and 31–2 to obtain an overview of cystic pelvic pathology. Some of the material included in these tables is not repeated in the text.

FUNCTIONAL OVARIAN CYSTS

Functional ovarian cysts[1-7] are *not* neoplasms; rather, they are normal physiologic cysts that have accumulated excessive amounts of fluid or have failed to involute during the course of the menstrual cycle. These cysts are extremely common and usually occur during the early childbearing years. Three different types of functional cysts may be encountered: follicular cysts, corpus luteum cysts, and theca lutein cysts. No specific sonographic findings differentiate among these three histologic types.

Follicle Cysts

Follicle cysts are nonovulatory graafian follicles that have failed to rupture and have enlarged to a size exceeding 3 cm, which is the upper limit for normal graafian follicles. The typical size of follicular cysts at the time of clinical discovery is 6 to 8 cm. These cysts usually present clinically with pelvic pain or with menstrual disorders, which result from excessive estrogen production by the cyst. Follicular cysts may be complicated by rupture, hemorrhage into the cyst, or ovarian torsion, but such complications are uncommon, and most follicular cysts regress when hormonal therapy is administered (typically in the form of oral contraceptives).

Corpus Luteum Cyst

The corpus luteum, which is the postovulatory remnant of the graafian follicle, may evolve normally into a small cyst 2 to 3 cm in diameter. If pregnancy does not occur, this cyst involutes within 14 days of ovulation. A corpus luteum cyst of 2 to 3 cm is a commonly seen, normal feature

Table 31-2. Differential Features of Cystic
Extrauterine Pathology

1. Thin-walled, anechoic cyst with minimal or no septation
   Most likely: Functional cyst, cystadenoma, parovarian cyst
   Also possible: Cystadenocarcinoma, abscess, endometrial cyst, bladder diverticulum
2. Thick-walled cyst, irregular inner border, anechoic or with internal echoes
   Most likely: Abscess, hemorrhagic functional cyst, cystic neoplasm
   Also possible: Hematoma, endometrial cyst
3. Highly loculated cyst
   Most likely: Cystadenoma, cystadenocarcinoma, other ovarian or nonovarian neoplasm
   Also possible: Chronic abscess, hemorrhagic functional cyst, endometrial cyst, necrotic leiomyoma
4. Thin-walled cyst with diffuse or dependent, low-level echogenicity
   Most likely: Endometrial cyst
   Also possible: Abscess, hemorrhagic functional cyst, hematoma, cystic teratoma, other cystic neoplasm
5. Cyst containing strongly echogenic elements with acoustic shadowing, or strongly echogenic layered contents
   Most likely: Cystic teratoma
   Also possible: Calcified ovarian or nonovarian neoplasms, gas-containing abscess, dilated or pathologic bowel
6. Principally solid mass with cystic components
   Most likely: Primary ovarian neoplasm
   Also possible: Leiomyoma, nonovarian neoplasm, chronic abscesses, hematoma

of the first trimester of pregnancy. During the first trimester, the corpus luteum provides progestational steroids that maintain the proliferative state of the endometrial lining.

A corpus luteum cyst is considered pathologic in a non-pregnant woman if it fails to regress during the menstrual cycle. Such cysts are less common than follicular cysts but tend to be larger (5 to 11 cm in diameter). Symptoms include pelvic pain, as well as menstrual disturbances related to persistent progesterone production by the cyst. Serious complications are more common with corpus luteum cysts than with follicular cysts and include intracyst hemorrhage, rupture, and torsion. Rupture is a particularly frequent complication and may cause acute symptoms mimicking ectopic pregnancy.

Theca Lutein Cyst

Theca lutein cysts are large follicles in which the theca cells have become luteinized through excessive stimulation by human chorionic gonadotropin (hCG). These cysts occur only in the presence of abnormal quantities of hCG, which may be secreted by a gestational trophoblastic neoplasm or introduced iatrogenically in the course of infertility therapy. Theca lutein cysts

are the largest of functional cysts and are especially prone to rupture because of their size. They are distinctive among functional cysts because they are frequently bilateral and multiple. Massive ovarian enlargement due to multiple theca lutein cysts occurs in the "ovarian hyperstimulation syndrome," which is a complication of infertility therapy. This subject is discussed in Chapter 32.

The Role of Sonography in Functional Cyst Management

When an adnexal cyst that is thought to be a functional cyst is detected on physical examination, the role of sonography is to confirm that the gross appearance of the lesion matches the clinical diagnosis. If this is the case, then the lesion may be followed conservatively and surgery is avoided. In one study of palpable adnexal masses *not* examined with ultrasound, 65% were found to be normal ovaries or functional cysts at surgery.[4] In contrast, only 8% of lesions were determined to be functional cysts at surgery in a group of patients examined sonographically.[4]

An uncomplicated functional cyst typically is unilocular, smoothly marginated, thin walled, and anechoic (Fig. 31–1). Deviation from this appearance suggests complications such as cyst hemor-

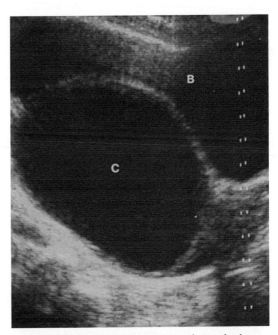

Figure 31-1—Functional Cyst. A longitudinal transabdominal image shows a 9-cm functional cyst (C). The margins of the cyst are smooth, and the contents are anechoic. Enhanced through-transmission is evident. The cyst resolved completely with oral contraceptive therapy in this 27 year old woman with pelvic pain. B = bladder.

rhage or that the lesion is not, in fact, a functional cyst. A functional cyst should decrease in size and should be less than 7 cm in diameter after one cycle of oral contraceptive therapy.[5, 7–9]

Cyst Hemorrhage

Intracyst hemorrhage drastically changes the sonographic appearance of functional cysts.[5, 7–9] Hemorrhage (Fig. 31–2) may cause cyst wall thickening, irregular borders, septation, or a loculated appearance. In addition, thrombus may form a dependent, echogenic layer, or may even "ball up," mimicking a focal mass within the cyst. In rare cases, the hemorrhagic cyst may appear entirely echoic. In the presence of these dramatic alterations of cyst architecture, hemorrhagic functional cysts may readily be mistaken for neoplastic cysts or even for solid masses. Echoes occasionally are present in nonhemorrhagic functional cysts (Fig. 31–3), and the cause of such echoes is unknown.

PAROVARIAN CYSTS

Pelvic cysts that originate from structures near to, but distinct from, the ovary are generally lumped together as "parovarian" cysts.[10, 11] In this context, the term "parovarian" means situated beside the ovary.[12] This term is a bit confusing, however, since "parovarian cyst" also refers to a specific type of cyst arising in a vestigial mesonephric (wolffian duct) structure.[12] We will use the term "parovarian cyst" in the broad sense, meaning any pelvic cyst originating from a structure near the ovary. In this context, about 70%

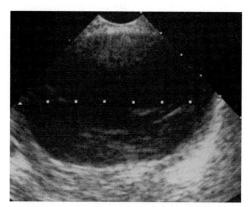

Figure 31-3—Nonhemorrhagic, Echoic Functional Cyst. This transverse sonogram, in a 22 year old woman with acute pelvic pain, demonstrates a 7-cm cyst with low-level, dependent internal echoes. These echoes were attributed to hemorrhage, but at pathologic examination the cyst contained clear fluid without visible debris. The echoes may have arisen from proteinaceous material within the fluid. Diagnosis: corpus luteum cysts with adnexal torsion.

of parovarian cysts arise from the mesothelium, and about 30% are müllerian in origin.[11] Parovarian cysts also may arise from the tubal fimbria (enlarged hydatids of Morgagni) or as peritoneal inclusion cysts that form in postsurgical pelvic adhesions.[13, 14]

Most parovarian cysts are unilocular, thin walled, sharply marginated, and anechoic. Since they are not associated with the ovary, they are not hormonally active and tend, therefore, to become quite large before discovery (average size, 6 cm).[10] The sonographic features of these cysts are indistinguishable from those of functional or neoplastic ovarian cysts, but two features assist with correct identification of these lesions. First, it sometimes is possible to demonstrate that the parovarian cyst is separate from the ovary and is not, therefore, ovarian in origin. Second, a full bladder tends to displace parovarian cysts superiorly out of the pelvis (Fig. 31–4). This is an uncommon location for ovarian cysts.

Peritoneal inclusion cysts (Fig. 31–5) are loculated accumulations of fluid that form among pelvic adhesions.[13] These collections do not resemble other parovarian cysts. They are irregularly shaped and tend to assume a configuration imposed by surrounding structures. They frequently are multilocular and are usually located deep within the true pelvis.

CYSTADENOMA AND CYSTADENOCARCINOMA

We now shift our attention from non-neoplastic cysts to true neoplasms. Table 31–3 presents

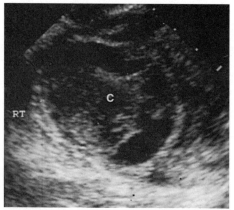

Figure 31-2—Hemorrhagic Functional Cyst. Transvaginal sonographic image of a 6-cm functional cyst (C) related to ovulation induction in a 30 year old woman. Heterogeneous echogenic components are seen in the center of the cyst, and the cyst wall is somewhat thickened. The appearance is consistent with retracted thrombus. The cyst resolved completely on follow-up examination. RT = right side of patient.

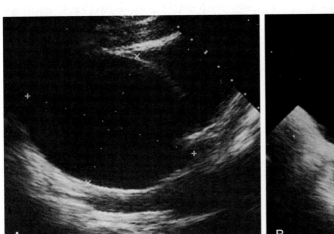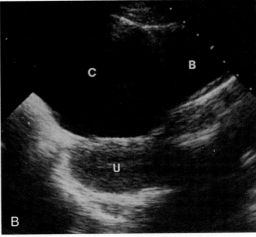

Figure 31-4—Parovarian Cyst. (A) A longitudinal transabdominal sonogram in a 22 year old woman with an asymptomatic pelvic mass reveals a 9-cm, anechoic, thin-walled cyst (cursors) that was shown to be separate from the ovaries. **(B)** Note that the cyst (C) lies anterosuperior to the uterus (U) and bladder (B) (longitudinal image). Such a position is typical, although not specific, for a parovarian cyst. Pathologic diagnosis: broad ligament parovarian cyst.

an abbreviated classification of primary ovarian neoplasms.[1, 2, 5] Please review this table, as the overview provided is important for understanding the material that follows. We will principally consider cystadenoma and cystadenocarcinoma, the common epithelial neoplasms of the ovary, and cystic teratoma. These three tumors usually contain large cystic components or are entirely cystic. The other neoplasms listed in Table 31–3 are uncommon and, for the most part, are solid lesions.

The surface of the ovary is covered by a thin layer of coelomic epithelium that gives rise to 65% of all ovarian neoplasms and 95% of all malignant ovarian tumors.[1, 2, 5] Cystadenoma and cystadenocarcinoma are predominant among the epithelial tumors. The former are benign and

the latter are malignant. These neoplasms either contain viscid, mucinous fluid or more watery fluid. Those with mucinous contents are named with the prefix "mucinous," as in mucinous cystadenoma, whereas those with watery contents are named with the prefix "serous." Malignancy is less common in mucinous than in serous varieties.

Ultrasound Findings

Mucinous and serous tumors of the ovary range widely in size and sonographic features,[5,

Table 31-3. Classification of Ovarian Neoplasms

Epithelial Neoplasms

Serous and mucinous cystadenoma (benign, cystic)
Serous and mucinous cystadenocarcinoma (malignant, cystic)
Other types of adenocarcinoma (malignant, cystic or solid)
Endometrioid carcinoma (malignant, cystic)

Germ Cell Neoplasms (origin: immature ova)

Teratoma (usually benign and cystic)
Dysgerminoma (malignant, solid)
Endometrial sinus tumor (malignant, solid with cystic degeneration)

Sex Cord Tumors (stromal origin)

Granulosa theca cell tumors (usually benign and cystic)
Sertoli–Leydig cell tumor (usually benign and solid)

Mesenchymal Neoplasms

Fibroma (benign, solid)
Lymphoma (malignant, solid)
Mixed mesenchymal sarcoma (malignant, cystic, or solid)

Compiled from Granberg S, Wikland M: A comparison between ultrasound and gynecologic examination for detection of enlarged ovaries in a group of women at risk for ovarian carcinoma. J Ultrasound Med 7:59–64, 1988; and Swayne LC, Love MB, Karasick SR: Pelvic inflammatory disease: Sonographic-pathologic correlation. Radiology 151:751–755, 1984.

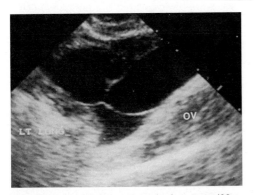

Figure 31-5—Peritoneal Inclusion Cyst (36 year old woman with primary infertility). A transvaginal sonogram shows a loculated, irregular fluid collection adjacent to the left ovary (OV). Note that the collection appears to assume the shape of surrounding structures. Laparoscopic examination revealed fibrous peritoneal adhesions with entrapped fluid.

[6, 15–20] as illustrated in Figures 31–6 through 31–8. Most contain large cyst spaces, but some, particularly the malignant varieties, may be largely or completely solid (see Figure 30–1). Mucinous tumors tend to be larger than serous tumors, and very large lesions (over 15 cm) are likely to be the mucinous variety. Mucinous tumors also tend to be more loculated than serous tumors. In spite of these differences, sonographic features do not distinguish between the mucinous and serous varieties.

Features of Benignity or Malignancy

The inability of sonography to separate mucinous from serous tumors is unimportant. What is important is to identify characteristics that suggest benignity or malignancy,[15, 18–22] which are outlined in Table 31–4. The reader should review Table 31–4 carefully, as the sonographic features included therein are of great importance. Approximately 95% of unilocular, completely anechoic *neoplastic* cysts are benign, if no solid components are evident.[15, 18] The benignity rate falls to 85% for neoplastic cysts with up to 5% solid components, and malignancy becomes increasingly likely as the degree of loculation or the percentage of solid elements increases.

The use of transvaginal sonography appears to enhance the accuracy of ultrasound classification of benign and malignant lesions, for the architectural features of these masses often are most clearly seen with transvaginal imaging.[20] Doppler sonography has been used to assess the malignant potential of ovarian cysts, but with mixed results.[21, 22] A high-resistance flow pattern (pulsatility index greater than 2 or resistive index° greater than 0.5) in vessels at the margin of an adnexal mass suggests benignity. A low-resistance pattern (pulsatility index 1 or less, or resistive index less than 0.5) suggests malignancy. Low-flow resistance is not specific for malignancy, however, since inflammatory lesions or ectopic pregnancy also may have low-resistance blood flow.

Computed tomography (CT) and magnetic resonance imaging (MRI) may be used to characterize ovarian pathology further, and these imaging techniques appear to be particularly valuable when ultrasound findings are indeterminate.[18, 23, 24]

Peritoneal Metastasis

Cystic epithelial ovarian neoplasms may metastasize to local pelvic lymph nodes or to distant sites, such as the liver, via the blood stream. Epithelial tumors are particularly prone, however, to seed the peritoneal space diffusely with metastatic cells,[1, 2, 25] and these tumors are particularly deadly because this mode of spread frequently is coupled with late diagnosis. It is interesting that peritoneal metastases may be seen following rupture of benign cystadenomas as well as with spread of malignant ovarian tumors.

Ascites is the primary sonographic manifestation of peritoneal tumor metastasis from serous or mucinous carcinomas, and in many cases this

---

°These methods of assessing flow resistance are defined in Chapter 18.

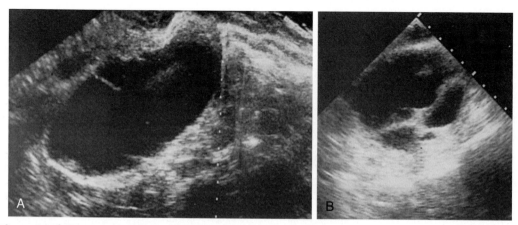

Figure 31-6—Examples of Benign Epithelial Ovarian Neoplasms. (A) A transverse sonogram through the iliac fossa in a 25 year old asymptomatic woman demonstrates a portion of a 20-cm, unilocular cystic mass. Note that the wall is smooth and relatively thin. Several incomplete septa project into the cyst. Echoes seen in the cyst are artifactual. Diagnosis: mucinous cystadenoma. **(B)** Oblique sonogram of an 8-cm-diameter, multilocular cystic ovarian mass in a 31 year old pregnant woman (15 weeks). Both the septations and the wall of the mass are fairly thick, suggesting malignancy, but a mucinous cystadenoma was diagnosed at laparotomy.

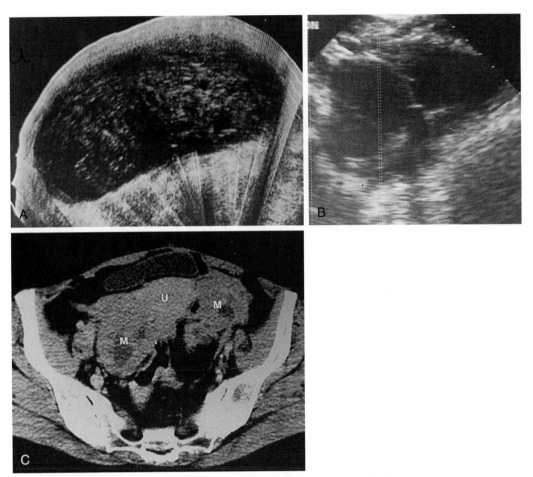

Figure 31-7—Examples of Malignant Epithelial Ovarian Neoplasms. (A) This transverse static sonogram at the umbilical level in a 56 year old woman with increasing abdominal girth demonstrates a well-circumscribed, heterogeneous mass with the appearance of multiple cysts embedded in a solid stroma. Diagnosis: mucinous cystadenocarcinoma. **(B)** Oblique sonogram and **(C)** contrast-enhanced computed tomogram in a 49 year old woman with a palpable abdominal mass. The sonogram shows a portion of a multiloculated tumor with thick, shaggy walls and poorly defined exterior margins. The CT scan shows a portion of this extensive mass (M), which filled much of the true and false pelvis and was adherent to the bowel and uterus (U). Diagnosis: serous cystadenocarcinoma.

is the only finding since the peritoneal tumor deposits are too small to be seen directly. When peritoneal tumor deposits are seen, they are manifested as small nodules located on the inner surface of the abdominal wall, among bowel loops, or on the surface of the liver. Tumor deposits also may produce omental thickening (the omental "tumor cake"). Direct visualization of peritoneal tumor deposits is achieved more commonly with CT than with ultrasound.

In some cases, mucinous tumors produce multilocular cystic metastases that may be localized or diffuse. When these cystic masses are extensive, they fill the peritoneal space with a form of mucinous ascites known as pseudomyxoma peritonei.[19, 25–28] Visualization of mucin balls within the ascites is diagnostic of this condition, as illustrated in Figure 31–8.

Surveillance for Ovarian Carcinoma

Ovarian carcinoma is almost universally fatal and has a median survival period, following diagnosis, of only 1.6 years.[2] The dismal prognosis for patients with this tumor is principally the result of late diagnosis. Between one half and two thirds of ovarian cancers have metastasized by the time of discovery. Because of these statistics, considerable interest has been expressed in the use of ultrasound as a surveillance mechanism for ovarian carcinoma in postmenopausal patients (in whom the great majority of tumors occur).[29–32] There seems little doubt that sonography would be an effective medium for identifying occult ovarian carcinomas, particularly if transvaginal imaging were employed routinely. Unfor-

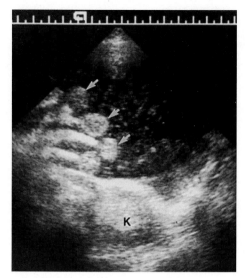

Figure 31-8—Pseudomyxoma Peritonei. A transverse sonogram demonstrates several bowel loops (arrows) floating in ascites that contains rounded mucin balls. The latter are a characteristic feature of pseudomyxoma peritonei. K = left kidney.

tunately, however, it is likely that most of the ovarian lesions picked up by this approach would be benign, rather than malignant, leading to unnecessary surgery. Jacobs and associates[33] estimate that the consequences of these false-positive diagnoses would be significant. If 100,000 women were screened, 40 ovarian carcinomas would be detected, but 5,389 nonmalignant ad-

nexal lesions also would be found. Surgical assessment of these nonmalignant lesions would be expensive, but perhaps more importantly, surgery would cause 120 complications, among which 21 would be major. The glamor of ovarian carcinoma screening is dimmed when viewed from this perspective, and it is not clear that sonography will be accepted as a screening tool for this tumor.

Staging and Follow-up of Ovarian Malignancies

Except in selected situations,[34] staging and post-therapeutic follow-up of epithelial ovarian malignancies is best performed with CT or MRI. As compared with ultrasound, both these modalities clearly are more accurate for staging and more sensitive for detecting recurrence or metastasis.[18, 19, 28, 35]

OVARIAN TERATOMAS

Teratomas of ovarian origin[1, 2, 5] are common tumors accounting for 20% of ovarian neoplasms in adults and 50% in children and adolescents. Fortunately, less than 2% of these tumors are malignant. Ovarian teratomas are worthy of the reader's attention, both because they are common and because they may exhibit specific sonographic findings.

Table 31-4. Sonographic Features of Ovarian Masses Suggesting Benignity or Malignancy

Proportion of solid components	Cysts with less than 5% solid components are probably benign. The likelihood of malignancy increases with the proportion of solid elements.
Loculation	Little or no cyst loculation suggests benignity. Extensive loculation suggests malignancy. Septa with a thickness of 1 mm or less suggest benignity. Thicker septa suggest malignancy.
Size	Cyst diameter 5 cm or less suggests benignity. Cyst diameter of 10 cm or greater suggests malignancy, except for thin-walled unilocular cysts.
Internal surfaces	Smooth cyst surfaces suggest benignity. Irregularity suggests malignancy. Papillary projections into a cyst are particularly suggestive of malignancy but can be seen in cystic teratoma (usually benign).
Debris	Dependent debris may be seen in both benign and malignant cysts. Large amount of debris favors malignancy, but debris may be present in cystic teratoma or hemorrhagic functional cysts.
Regression	Substantial regression of cyst size in response to hormonal therapy is an excellent sign of benignity.
Doppler°	Benign—RI > 0.5, PI >2. Malignant—RI < 0.5, PI ≤1.

°RI, resistivity index; PI, pulsatility index.

Pathology

Ovarian teratomas may contain ectodermal, mesodermal, and endodermal components in any combination.[1, 2] The great majority of ovarian teratomas are cystic, at least in part, because the epithelial elements secrete sebaceous material, water-based proteinaceous fluids, or mixtures of these secretions. Other tumor contents include hair, cellular debris, hemorrhagic debris, teeth, bone, or focal heterogeneous calcification. Because epithelial components predominate in most cystic teratomas, these tumors often are called dermoids or dermoid cysts.

Cystic teratomas are usually encountered in adolescence, but they may occur at any age. Most cystic teratomas measure 5 to 10 cm at the time of discovery, but even larger lesions may occur. Overall, about one third of ovarian teratomas are predominantly cystic, one third are predominantly solid, and one third contain an equal mixture of cystic and solid components. Completely solid lesions are rare.[36–47]

Sonographic Findings

The sonographic diagnosis of cystic teratomas (Fig. 31–9) is based on the detection of a mass with one or more of the following features:[36–46]

1. A cyst containing a smooth, rounded, tissue mass that projects into the lumen from the inner cyst surface. This tissue mass, which is called the "dermoid plug," is considered to be characteristic for cystic teratomas, but it is not often seen with ultrasound.
2. A cyst containing fine, bright dots and fine lines generated by hair within the cyst contents. These features are seen only with transvaginal sonography and appear to be characteristic, since hair is not found in other tumors.[45]
3. A mass with focal, highly echogenic components that produce acoustic shadows. These components are teeth, bone, or amorphous calcification, and they typically are located in the "dermoid plug."
4. A cyst containing layers or balls of highly echogenic material (fat or hair). In some cases the more echogenic components are supernatant, and in other cases the more echogenic contents are dependent.
5. A mass with homogeneous, diffuse, high-level echogenicity generated by fat and/or hair.

Diagnostic Accuracy

Hair is said to be visible, as just described, in about 85% of cystic teratomas examined transva-ginally; therefore, this feature should permit the accurate identification of about 85% of cystic teratomas.[45] The other "characteristic" ultrasound features just listed can be identified in only 38% to 44% of cystic teratomas,[38, 46, 47] and the remaining teratomas exhibit nonspecific features of fluid-filled or solid masses. Computed tomography is reported to identify characteristic features of cystic teratoma in 98% of cases and is, therefore, the examination of choice for confirming this diagnosis.[39, 44, 47]

Ironically, the strongly echogenic appearance of some cystic teratomas limits the diagnostic potential of ultrasound. In some instances, the tumor may be overlooked sonographically because only the highly echogenic components are visualized, and these are mistaken for gas-filled bowel. This deceptive feature (Fig. 31–10) is called the "tip of the iceberg sign,"[37] since only the highly echogenic "leading edge" of the neoplasm is seen and not the bulk of the tumor.

PELVIC INFLAMMATORY DISEASE

The term "pelvic inflammatory disease" (PID) refers to pyogenic infection of the female reproductive organs. PID is included in this chapter since a common manifestation of this condition is a cystic pelvic mass resulting from abscess formation. Appendicitis, diverticulitis, and Crohn disease are other common causes of pelvic abscess,[1, 48, 49] but PID is particularly important sonographically since it is a common condition frequently evaluated with ultrasound.[48–56]

Pathology

Bacterial infections of the female reproductive tract are commonly lumped together under the diagnosis PID, which ignores the fact that the extent and seriousness of such infections vary greatly.[1, 48, 49, 51, 52] Most cases of PID are caused by *Neisseria gonorrhoeae* or *Chlamydia trachomatis*. The bacteria ascend from the vagina into the uterus and thence into the fallopian tubes. The invading organism may cause cervicitis, endometritis, or salpingitis. The infection, and accompanying inflammatory reaction, may be confined to the endometrium, or it may spread full thickness through the muscular layers of the uterus and tubes to the serosal surfaces. Pus may distend the uterine cavity (pyometrium) or the fallopian tubes (pyosalpinx).

The bacterial infection may spread from the ampullary end of the fallopian tubes to the ovaries and adjacent peritoneal surfaces. In some cases, one or both ovaries may become grossly

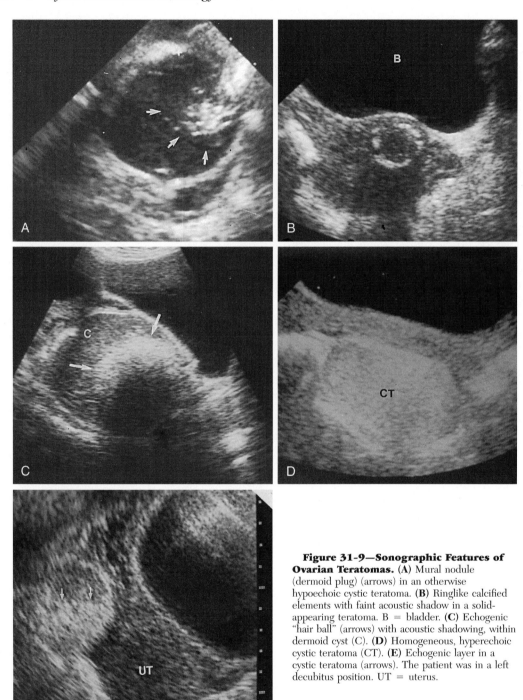

Figure 31-9—Sonographic Features of Ovarian Teratomas. (A) Mural nodule (dermoid plug) (arrows) in an otherwise hypoechoic cystic teratoma. **(B)** Ringlike calcified elements with faint acoustic shadow in a solid-appearing teratoma. B = bladder. **(C)** Echogenic "hair ball" (arrows) with acoustic shadowing, within dermoid cyst (C). **(D)** Homogeneous, hyperechoic cystic teratoma (CT). **(E)** Echogenic layer in a cystic teratoma (arrows). The patient was in a left decubitus position. UT = uterus.

infected and inflamed, and pus may become loculated in the vicinity of the ovary and the tubal fimbria, forming a tubo-ovarian abscess.[48, 49, 52] Abscesses from tubal spillage also may develop elsewhere within the pelvis and are particularly apt to occur within the cul-de-sac of Douglas, which is the most dependent portion of the peritoneal space.

Objectives of Sonography

The first objective of sonography is to define the severity and extent of pelvic inflammatory disease. In this regard, *it is most important to detect massive ovarian inflammation, pyosalpinx, and abscess formation.* Physical examination does not differentiate well between these serious con-

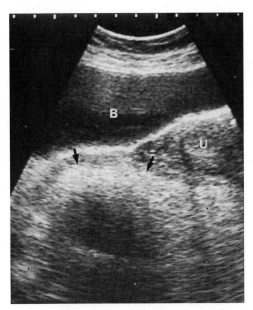

Figure 31-10—Tip of the Iceberg Sign. A transverse sonogram demonstrates a vague echogenic area (arrows) with some acoustic shadowing. A 12-cm cystic teratoma was found at surgery, but this mass is difficult to appreciate sonographically and might easily be mistaken for air-containing bowel. U = uterus; B = bladder.

sequences of PID and less serious types of infection. The second objective is to differentiate between PID and other causes of acute pelvic pain, especially ovarian torsion, complicated functional cyst, and ectopic pregnancy. Transvaginal sonography is clearly superior to transabdominal imaging for meeting both of these objectives.[52, 53]

Uterine Findings

Ultrasound is only about 25% sensitive for uterine abnormalities related to PID.[52] Enlargement of the uterus, due to generalized inflammation, is the most easily recognized finding.* Additional uterine abnormalities may include: (1) indistinct endometrial boundaries, resulting from endometritis; (2) fluid in the endometrial cavity, resulting from accumulated pus; and (3) ill-defined external uterine contours, resulting from inflammatory serosal adhesions.

Tubal Findings

With close scrutiny, transvaginal sonography is said to reveal abnormalities in about 90% of infected fallopian tubes.[52] The most important tubal finding may be easy recognition of a fallopian tube, in contrast to the normal situation in

which the fallopian tubes cannot be seen because of their small size.[52] The undistended but inflamed tube is seen as a thick-walled, linear structure extending from the uterine cornua to the ovary. If the tube is distended with pus, it may be sausage shaped or may have a distinctive hornlike appearance (Fig. 31–11). Dilated fallopian tubes generally can be distinguished from dilated bowel loops by lack of peristaltic activity and by anatomic association with the uterus. Purulent tubal distention (pyosalpinx), resulting from acute infection, is indistinguishable sonographically from chronic, nonpurulent distention (hydrosalpinx) related to chronic scarring and entrapment of secretions.[51]

Ovarian Findings

Transvaginal sonography is about 90% sensitive for PID-related abnormalities of the ovary and its environs. These abnormalities are divided, according to severity, into two classes, the tubo-ovarian complex and the tubo-ovarian abscess.[52]

The "tubo-ovarian complex"[52] refers to the inflammatory changes that occur with PID in the fimbriated portion of the tube, the ovary, and the adjacent serosal structures (Fig. 31–12A). This inflammatory complex is manifested by ovarian enlargement, loss of definition of the ovarian borders, parovarian tissue thickening, and parovarian fluid accumulation. Tubal abnormalities, as described, also are present in most cases.[52, 53]

The term "tubo-ovarian abscess" refers to a more severe form of parovarian inflammation in which the predominant finding is an adnexal mass (frank abscess), and the anatomic boundaries of the ovary and tube are obscure. A walled-off, purulent collection is present, with the variable sonographic manifestations of an abscess, as described later. In some cases it may not be possible to identify the ovary as a discrete structure.[49, 52, 53]

Pelvic Abscesses

In general, sonographic findings do not indicate the etiology of a pelvic abscess, and sonographic features do not differentiate with certainty between abscess and other forms of pelvic pathology such as hematoma or complicated ovarian cyst.[48–50, 52, 53] Nonetheless, abscess detection is very important in the clinical management of patients with PID. Most pelvic abscesses (Fig. 31–12) are ovoid or spherical and have a mean diameter of 4 to 5 cm. The inner margin of an abscess usually is irregular, and dependent debris commonly is present. Loculation also is common, particularly with chronic abscesses (Fig. 31–

---

*Transabdominal images may be superior to transvaginal scans for detection of uterine enlargement.

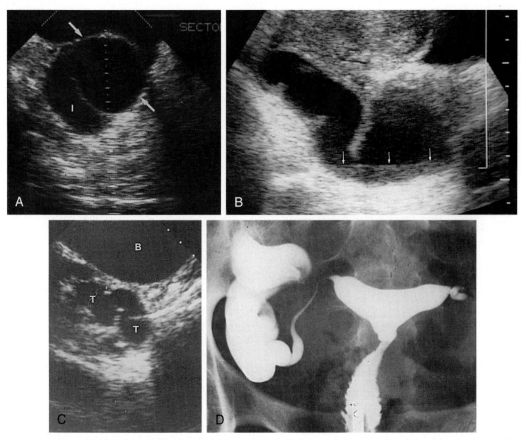

Figure 31-11—Examples of Dilated Fallopian Tubes. (A) "Cornucopia" appearance. The dilated isthmic (I) portion leads to a bulbous infundibular portion (arrows). **(B)** A debris level (arrows) is visible in this dilated tube. **(C)** Vermiform appearance of a dilated right fallopian tube (T). B = bladder. **(D)** Hysterosalpingogram corresponding to **C.**

12C). Rarely, a pelvic abscess may appear solid[49, 50] because it contains thick, echogenic pus or is actually a nonsuppurative phlegmonous area (i.e., tubo-ovarian complex). The ultrasound features of an abscess clearly are affected by its age. An acute abscess may appear as a focal, thin-walled, anechoic collection (Fig. 31–12A) that is indistinguishable from an ovarian cyst.[48, 49, 52, 53] In contrast, a large, chronic abscess may fill the pelvis with loculated, thick-walled material that mimics the appearance of a malignant cystic neoplasm (Fig. 31–12F).

Free Pelvic Fluid

Pelvic abscesses should be differentiated from free fluid within the cul-de-sac of Douglas, which is seen in about 70% of patients with PID.[52] This fluid is hemorrhagic or purulent at laparotomy; hence, faint echoes or septa may be seen within PID-related cul-de-sac collections. Generally, this fluid can be displaced, which is not the case with abscess fluid.

ENDOMETRIOSIS

Endometriosis[1, 57–64] is a common disorder in which foci of normal endometrium are ectopically located on the pelvic peritoneal surfaces.* In response to hormonal changes that occur during the menstrual cycle, these foci cause localized inflammation and, in some cases, the accumulation of hemorrhagic debris. Two clinical/pathologic forms of endometriosis occur.[1, 57] In the diffuse form, multiple small implants are scattered throughout the pelvis. In the focal form, only one or a few implants are present, which develop into cystic masses called endometrial cysts, endometriomas, or chocolate cysts. These cysts are, in essence, hematomas encapsulated by a thin, fibrous wall. The term "chocolate cysts" is used because they contain dark brown, hemorrhagic debris.[1] The diffuse form of endometriosis is much more common than the focal form and is more likely to be symptomatic. Symptoms may

---

*Endometrial tissue also may be ectopic to the myometrium in the condition called adenomyomatosis, which is discussed in Chapter 29.

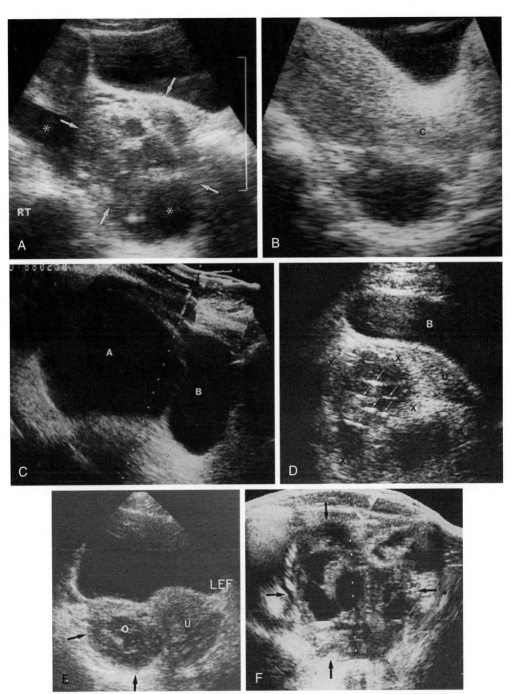

Figure 31-12—Examples of Tubo-ovarian Abscesses. (A) Tubo-ovarian complex (31 year old woman with pelvic pain, fever, nausea, vomiting; surgically confirmed). A heterogeneous mass (arrows) represents the inflamed right ovary and adjacent tubal structures. The lucent areas (asterisks) are portions of a pyosalpinx. **(B)** Typical pelvic abscess with a poorly defined "shaggy" wall, which is located posterior to the cervix (C) in the cul-de-sac of Douglas. **(C)** Longitudinal sonogram showing a 12-cm, unilocular, anechoic abscess (A), which mimics a functional cyst, in a 42 year old woman, with 10 days of pelvic infection symptoms. B = bladder. **(D)** A transverse scan shows a gas-containing abscess (arrows = air bubbles) in a patient with chronic pelvic inflammatory disease. U = uterus; B = bladder. **(E)** A transverse sonogram demonstrates an echogenic right adnexal tubo-ovarian complex (arrows) mimicking a solid mass. The ovary (O) is central within the abscess. (Approximately 2 weeks of pelvic infection symptoms.) U = uterus. **(F)** A transverse sonogram demonstrates a massive, complex pelvic abscess (arrows) in a 23 year old woman with recurrent pelvic inflammatory disease symptoms of over 1 month's duration. Fifteen hundred ml of pus was drained at surgery, and both tubes and ovaries were involved.

include dysmenorrhea, infertility, and dyspareunia.

Diagnosis

Sonographic abnormalities are detected in only about 10% of surgically proved cases of endometriosis,[58] because the implants of the common "diffuse" form are too small for sonographic detection. Therefore, ultrasound is not a primary diagnostic tool in patients clinically suspected of endometriosis. Ultrasound is more commonly used to determine whether a mass detected on physical examination has typical features of an endometrial cyst or appears to be another form of pathology. The best imaging technique for detecting and characterizing the lesions of endometriosis is MRI. Unfortunately, the sensitivity of MRI (71% to 90%) is not sufficiently high to supplant laparoscopy for clinical staging, which is required to determine whether or not therapy is needed.[62-64]

Ultrasound Findings

Endometrial cysts[57, 59-61] range widely in size, but most are 4 to 8 cm in diameter. A spherical shape is the rule, but a few may be lobulated. Eighty to ninety-eight percent of these cysts appear fluid-filled on sonographic examination; 80% are thin-walled, but 20% have thicker walls. About 40% are septated and some may be multilocular. In 60% of cases, the cyst fluid exhibits low-level echogenicity (Fig. 31–13), focally, diffusely, or as dependent debris. Approximately 20% of endometrial cysts are entirely echogenic, and these lesions may be mistaken for solid masses. Conversely, 15% of endometrial cysts are anechoic, unilocular, and thin walled and are identical, therefore, to functional or neoplastic ovarian cysts. In rare cases, extensive cystic endometriosis may distort pelvic anatomy so severely that normal structures, such as the ovaries and uterus, are difficult to identify.[57, 59-61]

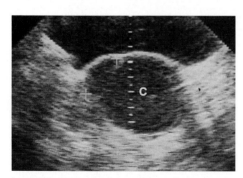

Figure 31-13—Endometrial Cyst. A transverse sonogram in this 27 year old patient with pelvic pain demonstrates a well-defined, 3-cm endometrial cyst (C) with uniform low-level echoes. Cursors = ovary.

REFERENCES

1. Krause FT: Female genitalia. *In* Kissane JM (ed): Anderson's Pathology. St. Louis, CV Mosby, 1985, pp 1451–1455.
2. Barber HRK: Ovarian cancer. Cancer J Clin 36:148–184, 1986.
3. Hernandez E, Miyazawa K: The pelvic mass: Patients' ages and pathologic findings. J Reprod Med 33:361–364, 1988.
4. Eriksson L, Kjellgren O, von Shoultz B: Functional ovarian cancer: Histopathological findings during surgery. Gynecol Obstet Invest 19:155–158, 1985.
5. Williams AG, Mettler FA, Wicks JD: Cystic and solid ovarian neoplasms. Semin Ultrasound 4:166–183, 1983.
6. Cassoff J, Hanna T: Grey-scale ultrasonography for assessment of gynecologic pelvic masses. Can Med Assoc J 120:38–46, 1979.
7. Hall DA: Sonographic appearance of the normal ovary, of polycystic ovary disease, and of functional ovarian cysts. Semin Ultrasound 4:149–165, 1983.
8. Bass IS, Haller JO, Friedman AP, Twersky J, Balsam D, Gottesman R: The sonographic appearance of the hemorrhagic ovarian cyst in adolescents. J Ultrasound Med 3:509–513, 1984.
9. Baltarowich OH, Kurtz AB, Pasto ME, Rifkin MD, Needleman L, Goldberg BB: The spectrum of sonographic findings in hemorrhagic ovarian cysts. AJR Am J Roentgenol 148:901–905, 1987.
10. Alpern MB, Sandler MA, Madrazo BL: Sonographic features of parovarian cysts and their complications. Am J Roentgenol 143:157–160, 1984.
11. Athey PA, Cooper NB: Sonographic features of parovarian cysts. Am J Roentgenol 144:83–86, 1985.
12. Dorland's Illustrated Medical Dictionary. Philadelphia, WB Saunders, 1985, pp 572, 1233.
13. Hoffer FA, Kozakewich H, Colodny A, Goldstein DP: Peritoneal inclusion cysts: Ovarian fluid in peritoneal adhesions. Radiology 169:189–191, 1988.
14. Schiebler ML, Dotters D, Baudoin L, Keefe B: Sonographic diagnosis of hydatids of Morgagni of the fallopian tube. J Ultrasound Med 11:115–116, 1992.
15. Miene HB, Jarrant P, Guha T: Distinction of benign from malignant ovarian cysts by ultrasound. Br J Obstet Gynecol 85:893–899, 1978.
16. Demand M, Fried A, van Nagell JR, et al: Ultrasonography in the diagnosis of tumors of the ovary. Surg Gynecol Obstet 148:346–348, 1979.
17. Moyle JW, Rochester D, Sider L, et al: Echography of ovarian tumors: Predictability of tumor type. AJR Am J Roentgenol 141:985–991, 1983.
18. Buy J-N, Ghossain MA, Sciot C, et al: Epithelial tumors of the ovary: CT findings and correlation with US. Radiology 178:811–818, 1991.
19. Finkler NJ, Benacerraf B, Lavin PT, Wojciechowski C, Knapp RC: Comparison of serum CA 125, clinical impression, and ultrasound in the preoperative evaluation of ovarian masses. Obstet Gynecol 72:659–664, 1988.
20. Granberg S, Norstöm A, Wikland M: Comparison of endovaginal ultrasound and cytological evaluation of cystic ovarian tumors. J Ultrasound Med 10:9–14, 1991.
21. Kurjak A, Zalud I, Alfirevic Z, Jurkovic D: The

assessment of abnormal pelvic blood flow by transvaginal color and pulsed Doppler. Ultrasound Med Biol 16:437–442, 1990.

22. Fleischer A, Rodgers WH, Rao BK, Kepple DM, Worrell JA, Williams L, Jones HW: Assessment of ovarian tumor vascularity with transvaginal color Doppler sonography. J Ultrasound Med 10:563–568, 1991.

23. Dooms GC, Hricak H, Tscholakoff D: Adnexal structures: MR imaging. Radiology 158:639–646, 1986.

24. Stevens SK, Hricak H, Stern JL: Ovarian lesions: Detection and characterization with Gadolinium-enhanced MR imaging at 1.5 T. Radiology 181:481–488, 1991.

25. Seshul MB, Coulam CM: Pseudomyxoma peritonei: Computed tomography and sonography. AJR Am J Roentgenol 136:803–806, 1981.

26. Paling MR, Shawker TH: Abdominal ultrasound in advanced ovarian carcinoma. J Clin Ultrasound 9:435–441, 1981.

27. Wicks JD, Mettler FA, Hilgers RD, Ampuero F: Correlation of ultrasound and pathologic findings in patients with epithelial carcinoma of the ovary. J Clin Ultrasound 12:397–402, 1984.

28. Murolo C, Costantini S, Foglia G, Guido T, Odicino F, Pace M, Parodi S, Pino G, Ragni N, Repetto L, Sala P, Tomao S, Valenzano M, Conte PF: Ultrasound examination in ovarian cancer patients: A comparison with second look laparotomy. J Ultrasound Med 8:441–443, 1989.

29. Hall DA, McCarthy KA, Kopans DB: Sonographic visualization of the normal postmenopausal ovary. J Ultrasound Med 5:9–11, 1986.

30. Rodriguez MH, Platt LD, Medearis AL, Lacarra M, Lobo RA: The use of transvaginal sonography for evaluation of postmenopausal ovarian size and morphology. Am J Obstet Gynecol 159:810–814, 1988.

31. Granberg S, Wikland M: A comparison between ultrasound and gynecologic examination for detection of enlarged ovaries in a group of women at risk for ovarian carcinoma. J Ultrasound Med 7:59–64, 1988.

32. Hogans RV, van Nagell JR, Donaldson ES, Gallion HH, Pavlik EJ, Endicott B, Woods CH: Transvaginal sonography as a screening method for ovarian cancer. Gynecol Oncol 34:402–406, 1989.

33. Jacobs I, Bridges J, Reynolds C, Stabile I, Kemsley P, et al: Multimodal approach toward screening for ovarian cancer. Lancet 2:268–271, 1988.

34. Meanwell CA, Rolfe EB, Blackledge G, Docker MF, Lawton FG, Mould JJ: Recurrent female pelvic cancer: Assessment with transrectal ultrasonography. Radiology 162:278–281, 1987.

35. Bies JR, Ellis JH, Kopecky KK, Sutton GP, Klatte EC, Stehman FB, Ehrlich CE: Assessment of primary gynecologic malignancies: Comparison of 0.15-T resistive MRI with CT. AJR Am J Roentgenol 143:1249–1257, 1984.

36. Hutton L, Rankin R: The fat-fluid level: Another feature of dermoid tumors of the ovary. J Clin Ultrasound 7:215–216, 1979.

37. Guttman PH: In search of the elusive benign cystic ovarian teratoma: Application of the ultrasound "tip of the iceberg" sign. J Clin Ultrasound 5:403, 1977.

38. Sandler MA, Silver TM, Karo JJ: Gray-scale ultrasonic features of ovarian teratomas. Radiology 131:705–707, 1979.

39. Friedmen AC, Pyatt RS, Hartman DS, Downey EF,

Olson WB: CT of benign cystic teratomas. AJR Am J Roentgenol 138:659–665, 1982.

40. Nicolet V, Ethier S, Lamarre L: Sonographic appearances of the wall of ovarian dermoid cysts. J Can Assoc Radiol 35:375–377, 1984.

41. Yaghoobian J, Pinck RL, Woodrow P: The fat-fluid level in an ovarian dermoid. Med Ultrasound 8:157–159, 1984.

42. Quinn SF, Erickson S, Black WC: Cystic ovarian teratomas: The sonographic appearance of the dermoid plug. Radiology 155:477–478, 1985.

43. Sisler CL, Siegel MJ: Ovarian teratomas: A comparison of the sonographic appearance in prepubertal and postpubertal girls. AJR Am J Roentgenol 154:139–141, 1990.

44. Dodd GD, Budzik RF: Lipomatous tumors of the pelvis in women: Spectrum of imaging findings. AJR Am J Roentgenol 155:317–322, 1990.

45. Bronshtein M, Yoffe N, Brandes JM, Blumenfeld M: Hair as a sonographic marker of ovarian teratomas: Improved identification using transvaginal sonography and simulation model. J Clin Ultrasound 19:351–355, 1991.

46. Laing FC, Van Dalsem VF, Marks WM, et al: Dermoid cysts of the ovary: Their ultrasonographic appearance. Obstet Gynecol 57:99–104, 1981.

47. Buy J-N, Ghossain MA, Moss AA, Bazot M, Doucet M, Hugol D, Truc JB, Poitout P, Ecoiffier J: Cystic teratoma of the ovary: CT detection. Radiology 171:697–701, 1989.

48. Spiegel RM, Ben-Ora A: Ultrasound in inflammatory disease of the pelvis. Semin Ultrasound 1:41–50, 1980.

49. Swayne LC, Love MB, Karasick SR: Pelvic inflammatory disease: Sonographic-pathologic correlation. Radiology 151:751–755, 1984.

50. Lavery JP, Howell RS, Shaw L: Ultrasonic demonstration of a phlegmon following Cesarean section. J Clin Ultrasound 13:134–136, 1985.

51. Tessler FN, Perrella RR, Fleischer AC, Grant EG: Endovaginal sonographic diagnosis of dilated fallopian tubes. AJR Am J Roentgenol 153:523–525, 1989.

52. Patten RM, Vincent LM, Wolner-Hanssen P, Thorpe J: Pelvic inflammatory disease: Endovaginal sonography with laparoscopic correlation. J Ultrasound Med 9:681–689, 1990.

53. Bulas DI, Ahlstrom PA, Sivit CJ, Blask ARN, O'Donnell RM: Pelvic inflammatory disease in the adolescent: Comparison of transabdominal and transvaginal sonographic evaluation. Radiology 183:435–439, 1992.

54. Worthen NJ, Gunning JE: Percutaneous drainage of pelvic abscesses: Management of the tubo-ovarian abscess. J Ultrasound Med 5:551–556, 1986.

55. Nosher JL, Needell GS, Amorosa JK, Krasna IH: Transrectal pelvic abscess drainage with sonographic guidance. AJR Am J Roentgenol 146:1047–1048, 1986.

56. van Sonnenberg E, D'Agostino HB, Casola G, Goodacre BW, Sanchez RB, Taylor B: US-guided transvaginal drainage of pelvic abscesses and fluid collections. Radiology 181:53–56, 1991.

57. Birnholz JC: Endometriosis and inflammatory disease. Semin Ultrasound 4:184–192, 1983.

58. Friedman H, Vogelzang RL, Mendelson EB, Neiman HL, Cohen M: Endometriosis detection by US with laparoscopic correlation. Radiology 157:217–220, 1985.

59. Sandler MA, Karo JJ: The spectrum of ultrasonic

findings in endometriosis. Radiology 127:229–231, 1978.

60. Coleman BG, Arger PH, Mulhern CB: Endometriosis: Clinical and ultrasonic correlation. AJR Am J Roentgenol 132:747–749, 1979.
61. Athey PA, Diment DD: The spectrum of sonographic findings in endometriomas. J Ultrasound Med 8:487–491, 1989.
62. Zawin M, McCarthy S, Scoutt L, Comite F:

Endometriosis: Appearance and detection at MR imaging. Radiology 171:693–696, 1989.
63. Arrivé L, Hricak H, Martin MC: Pelvic endometriosis: MR imaging. Radiology 171:687–692, 1989.
64. Togashi K, Nishimura K, Kimura I, Tsuda Y, Yamashita K, Shibata T, Nakano Y, Konishi J, Konishi I, Mori T: Endometrial cysts: Diagnosis with MR imaging. Radiology 180:73–78, 1991.

William J. Zwiebel

The treatment of infertility has achieved a position of great importance in Western medical practice,[1-5] and for this reason sonographers and sonologists alike should have a basic understanding of the role that ultrasound plays in the diagnosis and treatment of this disorder. It is useful to think of infertility in light of six potential causes: (1) cervical disorders, (2) uterine/endometrial disorders, (3) tubal disorders, (4) ovarian disorders, (5) peritoneal disorders, and (6) male disorders.[1] Ultrasound has a limited role with respect to some of these disorders and a major role with respect to others; nonetheless, we will consider all six, at least briefly.

CERVICAL DISORDERS

The properties of the cervical mucus influence the migration of sperm from the vagina to the reproductive tract. Fertility may be affected if the cervical mucus contains sperm antibodies (which "attack" sperm), or other agents that are detrimental to sperm viability or motility. Sperm antibodies alone are thought to account for 10% of infertility cases.[1] The only role played by ultrasound with respect to the cervical disorders is to assist with timing for postcoital cervical mucus testing. Such testing must be performed as close to ovulation as possible, and ultrasound may be used to monitor follicle development in order to predict when ovulation is imminent.[1]

Ultrasound also is used for a procedure called gamete intrafallopian transfer (GIFT),[1, 2, 5] which is used to circumvent cervical mucus problems as well as cervical stenosis, oligospermia, or endometriosis. GIFT refers to the catheter transfer of ova and spermatozoa to the fimbriated end of the fallopian tube. In the GIFT procedure, ultrasound is used to monitor follicle development (discussed later), to guide the harvesting of ova from the ovaries, and to guide the insertion of the fallopian tube catheter. Fertilization occurs naturally with the GIFT technique, and the embryo migrates down the fallopian tube and into the uterine cavity in the same way as in unaided fertilization. Obviously, tubal occlusion or significant tubal scarring is a contraindication for the GIFT procedure.

UTERINE/ENDOMETRIAL DISORDERS

Uterine/endometrial disorders are a relatively uncommon cause of infertility. The first to be considered is anomalous uterine development. A unicornuate, septate, or bicornuate configuration (Chapter 28) can affect implantation and cause recurrent pregnancy loss. In strict terms, this is not an infertility problem, since pregnancy and implantation do occur, but recurrent pregnancy loss clearly affects fecundity, or the ability to produce viable offspring. Ultrasound is a valuable method for screening for uterine abnormalities that may cause recurrent abortion, as discussed in Chapter 28.

Two additional uterine disorders that may cause infertility are leiomyomas and adenomyosis, either of which reduce the "receptivity" of the endometrium for the conceptus. By an unknown mechanism, these disorders reduce the likelihood of implantation, resulting in expulsion of the conceptus from the uterine cavity. Ultrasound has an obvious role in the detection of leiomyomas in the infertile patient and also may detect adenomyosis, as presented in Chapter 29.

Endometrial receptivity also is reduced by endocavitary scarring related to previous uterine instrumentation or infection. Strands of scar, called synechiae, may form within the endometrial cavity. If extensive, these scars crisscross and segment the cavity into multiple compartments. The end result is interference with implantation of the conceptus. Ultrasound occasionally has a role in the detection of uterine synechiae, which can impart a bizarre, multilocular appearance to the endometrial cavity, as shown in Figure 32-1. In most cases, however, the status of the uterine cavity is investigated with hysterosalpingography.

The final uterine/endometrial disorder that may affect fertility is the physiologic receptivity of the endometrium for the conceptus. Although aberrations of endometrial physiology are uncommon causes of infertility, they are cured readily. Ultrasound has been studied as a method for assessing the physiologic status of the endometrium in relation to follicle development, ovulation, and implantation potential. Both the thickness of the endometrium and its echogeni-

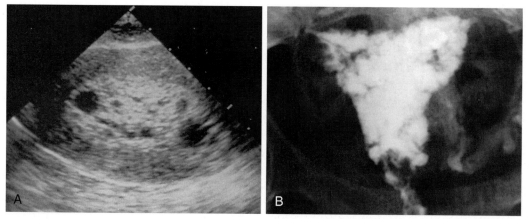

Figure 32-1—Endocavitary Synechiae. (**A**) A transvaginal sonogram shows a "cystic"-appearing endometrium caused by entrapped fluid. (**B**) A hysterosalpingogram shows that the endometrial cavity is segmented by innumerable adhesions.

city have been examined, but it has not yet been shown that ultrasound findings are of benefit in circumventing physiologic disorders of the endometrium.

TUBAL DISORDERS

Tubal disorders are of great importance, as they are the most common cause of infertility in women (accounting for 40% of cases).[1] In almost all instances, tubal dysfunction results from the destructive sequelae of salpingitis, which include tubal obstruction, mucosal scarring, glandular damage, and other adverse effects. This damage interferes with migration of the conceptus to the uterine cavity and contributes to the occurrence of ectopic implantation of the pregnancy (Chapter 36). The mainstay of tubal imaging is hysterosalpingography. Ultrasound has been proposed as an alternative in which transvaginal color Doppler ultrasound is used to detect flow within the tubes as saline is instilled into the uterine cavity. Visualization of flow and the absence of tubal dilatation implies tubal patency.[1] This technique is not used widely, and as of this writing, the primary role of ultrasound with respect to tubal injury is the detection of hydrosalpinx, as illustrated in Chapter 31.

Although ultrasound does not have a great role in the diagnosis of tubal disease, it has a major role in in vitro fertilization, which is the principal method for circumventing the effects of tubal obstruction. Ultrasound functions as follows in the in vitro fertilization process.

First, ultrasound is used to monitor ovarian follicle development,[1, 3–12] as illustrated in Figure 32–2. A drug called clomiphene citrate (discussed later) typically is administered prior to ovum harvesting to encourage the development of several follicles, which permits the fertilization

of several ova, in turn enhancing the prospects for implantation. To "mature" the follicles, and increase the potential for fertilization, an injection of human chorionic gonadotropin (hCG) is administered about 36 hours prior to ova harvesting. The trick is to determine when the follicles are ready for hCG and subsequent harvesting. This determination is based on follicle size and number, as ascertained by serial ultrasound studies, as well as on serum estradiol levels. When ultrasound shows four to six follicles of about 20 mm in diameter and the estradiol level is appropriate, hCG is administered.

The second role of ultrasound is to guide transvaginal harvesting (aspiration) of the mature follicle contents, which include the ova (Fig. 32–3). Ova thus obtained are mixed with sperm, incubated, and then reintroduced transcervically into the endometrial cavity, in the hope that implantation will take place.

A third role of ultrasound in the in vitro fertilization process has been suggested. This is to assess the readiness of the endometrium for implantation. Both the endometrial thickness and echogenicity have been evaluated to determine whether the endometrium is in an optimal state for embryo implantation, but the value of such assessment remains questionable.[5, 13–15]

The final role of ultrasound in in vitro fertilization is the confirmation of intrauterine pregnancy and the determination of the number of gestations. As noted, several fertilized ova are introduced into the uterine cavity, because the likelihood of implantation of any single ovum is relatively low. The result of this practice is a slight risk of multiple gestations.

OVARIAN DISORDERS

After tubal disorders, ovarian disorders are the second most important cause of female infertility,

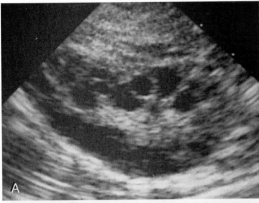

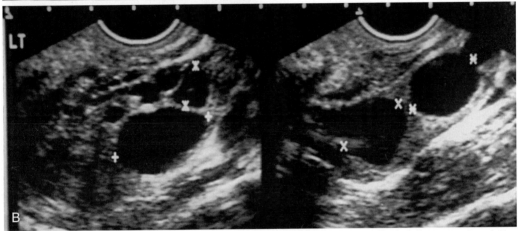

Figure 32-2—Follicle Monitoring.
(A) A long axis view of the left ovary on day 5 of menotropin therapy shows multiple follicles of about 5-mm diameter. (B) On day 12, two views of the left ovary show three large (mature) follicles ranging from 16 to 19 mm. Several smaller follicles also are visible.

accounting for about 20% of cases. Infertile patients with ovarian disorders fall into two general categories: those with relatively mild disruption and those with severe disruption of the hypothalamic/ovarian function.[1–5, 7]

Fertility Drugs

Mild ovulatory disorders may be treated with a drug called clomiphene citrate (Marion Merrell Dow, Kansas City, MO, USA; Serono Labora-

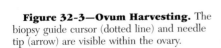

Figure 32-3—Ovum Harvesting. The biopsy guide cursor (dotted line) and needle tip (arrow) are visible within the ovary.

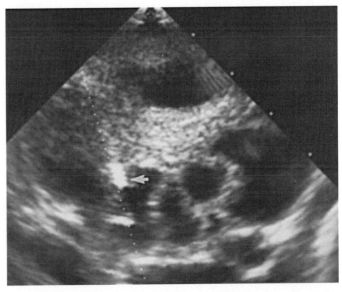

tories, Norwell, MA, USA). This drug is an estrogen antagonist that acts indirectly to promote pituitary secretion of follicle-stimulating hormone (FSH) and luteinizing hormone (LH). In some women, the elevation of serum FSH and LH levels may result in follicle development and ovulation without further therapy. In others, it may be necessary to induce ovulation through administration of human chorionic gonadotropin after clomiphene has induced follicle development.

More severe ovulatory disorders are not amenable to clomiphene citrate therapy (e.g., some patients with polycystic ovarian disease). In these conditions, follicle development usually is induced directly through the administration of FSH and LH. These gonadotropins are extracted from the urine of postmenopausal women and are sold under the generic name "menotropins" (trade name, Pergonal; Serono Laboratories, Norwell, MA, USA). Menotropins must be administered by intramuscular injection. A second drug is used less commonly in patients with serious ovulatory disturbances. This drug is a gonadotropin-releasing hormone (GnRH) analogue (trade name, Lupron; TAP Pharmaceuticals, Deerfield, IL, USA), which directly affects the hypothalamus, causing the release of FSH and LH.

Both of the drugs used for severe ovulatory disorders induce follicle development but do not cause ovulation. In normal women, ovulation occurs in response to a massive preovulatory release of LH by the hypothalamus (Chapter 27). This "LH surge" is often absent in women with ovulatory disorders, and in such cases, human chorionic gonadotropin (hCG) is used as a substitute. hCG is a normal hormone of pregnancy, but it also exhibits a dramatic LH effect, which causes ovulation in mature graafian follicles. hCG, which is derived from the urine of pregnant women, must be administered by injection.

Ultrasound Follicle Monitoring

Sonography generally is not used during clomiphene therapy, unless hCG induction of ovulation is needed. In such cases, ultrasound is used to monitor follicle growth as described later for menotropin therapy.

During menotropin or GnRH therapy, ultrasound is used to keep track of the number and size of graafian follicles (Fig. 32–2) in order to optimize ovulation-induction with hCG.[1–5, 7–12] A graafian follicle is deemed to be mature and capable of ovulation if its maximum diameter exceeds 15 mm. In measuring follicles, consider-

ation must be given to the effects of compression of one follicle by another. If follicular shape is markedly distorted by compression, an average diameter should be used. Besides follicle size, two additional ultrasound findings have been said to predict follicle maturity. These are the visualization of the cumulus oophorus, which is the cluster of cells surrounding the preovulatory ovum, and/or visualization of low-level echoes within the fluid contents of the follicle.[5, 7–12] Unfortunately, neither the cumulus oophorus nor preovulatory echogenicity is seen with sufficient frequency to be of value in predicting follicular maturity.[5, 8, 10–12]

Follicular development also is assessed during menotropin or Lupron therapy, with serial measurement of the serum estradiol concentration. Serum estradiol level is affected by both the number and size of follicles, however, and multiple small, immature follicles may produce as much estradiol as several large, mature follicles. For this reason, the serum estradiol concentration is not sufficient for timing ovulation. Menotropin therapy, furthermore, typically induces the growth of numerous follicles, creating the risk of multiple gestations. In monitoring the number as well as the size of follicles, ultrasound assesses the risk for multiple gestations. In some instances, the ovulating dose of hCG is withheld if ultrasound shows more than three large follicles.

Ovarian Hyperstimulation

Ovarian hyperstimulation refers to gonadotropin-induced, massive ovarian enlargement that results from the development of multiple theca lutein cysts, as well as edema of the ovarian stroma.[3–5, 16–18] This condition is seen most commonly with menotropin-mediated ovulation induction. Less commonly, clomiphene citrate and Lupron also may hyperstimulate the ovary. Ovarian hyperstimulation occurs rarely in the first trimester of normal pregnancy, or in association with hydatidiform mole.

Two mechanisms contribute to ovarian hyperstimulation: excessive serum levels of gonadotropins, or excessive sensitivity of the ovaries to these hormones. Because two causative mechanisms exist, it is difficult to eliminate the risk of this condition during infertility therapy, but some risk reduction is effected by monitoring serum estradiol concentration. If the estradiol level exceeds 1000 pg/mL, the ovulation dose of hCG is withheld.[17] Ovarian hyperstimulation occurs only *after* ovulation, and hyperstimulation can be prevented, therefore, by preventing ovulation.

Hyperstimulation of the ovaries may be accompanied by an aberration of fluid balance called the ovarian hyperstimulation syndrome, which is characterized by third-space fluid accumulation (including ovarian stromal edema), ascites, pleural effusion, and generalized soft tissue edema. The hyperstimulation syndrome is the product of an unexplained global increase in capillary permeability. The syndrome generally is more severe if pregnancy follows ovulation, but the severity of the condition varies greatly and is not predictable on a patient-by-patient basis. In severe cases, third-space fluid accumulation may be refractory to diuretics and supportive efforts and may result in hemoconcentration, hypotension, oliguria, and electrolyte imbalance. Deaths have occurred from this syndrome.

As seen with ultrasound, the hyperstimulated ovary is massively enlarged by the presence of myriad cysts separated by thick septa of edematous stroma[3–5, 18] (Fig. 32–4). In general, the size of the cyst is proportionate to the severity of the condition. In severe cases, individual cysts may be as large as 7 cm.[18] Sonographic follow-up reveals gradual regression of the cysts and the return to a normal ovarian appearance.

Ultrasound generally is not needed for diagnosis of ovarian hyperstimulation, as associated peripheral edema and weight gain are obvious clinically. Ultrasound findings are most useful for categorizing the severity of the disease and for following its progression or regression.[3–5, 16, 18]

Mild cases are characterized by minimal weight gain and a maximal ovarian dimension of up to 5 cm.* Moderate cases are classified as weight gain up to 10 pounds and ovarian size not exceeding 10 cm. Some ascites may be evident in moderate cases. With severe hyperstimulation, weight gain exceeds 10 pounds, the ovaries exceed 10 cm in size, ascites is readily apparent, and pleural fluid may be present.[16]

Protocol for Follicle Monitoring

The protocol I recommend for initial patient assessment, as well as monitoring during follicle induction, is presented in Table 32–1.[3]

PERITONEAL DISORDERS

The main peritoneal disorder that contributes to infertility is scarring, either in the form of postinflammatory adhesions or endometriosis. Such scarring may reduce fertility directly by impeding the movement of sperm or the conceptus. In the case of endometriosis, fertility also may be reduced indirectly through poorly understood hormonal effects.[1] Ultrasound does not play much of a role in the diagnosis or manage-

---

*The maximal dimension of the largest ovary, not the sum of ovarian dimensions.

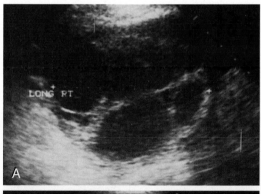
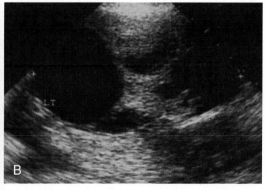
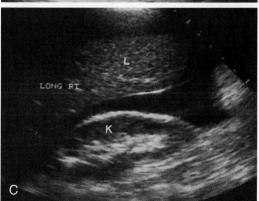

Figure 32-4—Ovarian Hyperstimulation (32 year old ovulation induction [menotropin] patient, 3 days post β-hCG administration). Massive cystic enlargement is evident in both the right (**A**) and left (**B**) ovaries (cursors), as seen on transverse transvaginal images. (Right ovary, 8 cm; left ovary, 11 cm.) (**C**) A moderate volume of ascites is evident on this longitudinal scan through the right kidney (K) and liver (L).

Table 32-1. Protocol for Infertility Assessment and Monitoring in Women[4, 5]

Baseline Assessment
Transabdominal and transvaginal evaluation of the uterus, fallopian tubes, ovaries, and kidneys for normality or pathology, as well as unexpected intrauterine pregnancy

Follicle Monitoring
Day 1: Obtain baseline ultrasound study as described in the text and look for "leftover" ovarian cysts from the preceding cycle of therapy.
Day 5: Check follicular size, which typically is small at this stage. Menotropin therapy may be adjusted accordingly.
Days 8, 10, 12, etc.: Recheck follicle size and number. As follicles approach desired size (15–20 mm), begin every-day assessment so that follicles do not become too large (transform to follicular cysts).
Confirm number of large follicles prior to inducing ovulation with hCG.

Harvesting
Utilize ultrasound for follicle harvesting (in vitro fertilization or GIFT).

Postfertilization
Confirm the number and "viability" of intrauterine gestations.
Search for extrauterine pregnancies.
Assist with selective pregnancy reduction of multiple gestations if needed.

ment of peritoneal factor infertility. Although adhesion-related peritoneal inclusion cysts may be seen occasionally with ultrasound (Fig. 32–4), most adhesions are not detectable with imaging methods. Also not detected with ultrasound is the diffuse form of endometriosis, which is more commonly associated with infertility than the cystic form that is detectable with ultrasound (Chapter 31).

MALE DISORDERS

Lest we give an impression of sexism, we will conclude this section of the text by pointing out that male factors cause infertility in about 50% of couples.[1] The immediate causes of male infertility include a low number of sperm, absence of sperm, sperm motility disorders, and other sperm abnormalities.[2] Ultrasound has several potential roles in male infertility.

First, it serves the functions described previously for in vitro fertilization or GIFT therapy.

Second, ultrasound serves to maximize the chances of natural fertilization, through the prediction of imminent ovulation. The previously described features of follicle maturity are used in this case to predict the optimum time for insemination.

Third, ultrasound can be used to detect varicoceles that can reduce sperm production. See Chapter 48 for details.

Finally, transrectal ultrasound may be used to detect potentially correctable causes of obstruction in sperm-carrying conduits such as the ejaculatory ducts and seminal vesicles.

REFERENCES

1. Collins JI, Woodward PJ: Radiological evaluation of infertility. Semin Ultrasound CT MRI 16:304–316, 1995.
2. Seibel MM: A new era in reproductive technology: In vitro fertilization, gamete intrafallopian transfer, and donated gametes and embryos. N Engl J Med 318:828–834, 1988.
3. Haning RV, Zwiebel WJ: Ultrasound assistance in clinical management of infertility. Semin Ultrasound 4:226–234, 1983.
4. Hann LE, Crivello M, McArdle C, Seibel M, Fein V, Taylor M: In vitro fertilization: Sonographic perspective. Radiology 163:665–668, 1987.
5. Fleischer AC, Herbert CM, Hill GA, Kepple DM: Transvaginal sonography: Applications in infertility. Semin Ultrasound CT MR 11:71–81, 1990.
6. Schwimer SR, Lebovic J: Transvaginal pelvic ultrasonography: Accuracy in follicle and cyst size determination. J Ultrasound Med 4:61–63, 1985.
7. Mendelson EB, Friedman H, Nieman HL, et al: The role of imaging in infertility management. AJR Am J Roentgenol 144:414–418, 1985.
8. Hackelor BJ, Fleming R, Robinson HP, et al: Correlation of ultrasonic and endocrinologic assessment of human follicular development. Am J Obstet Gynecol 135:122–128, 1979.
9. Kerin JF, Edminds DK, Warnes GM, et al: Morphological and functional evaluation of Graafian follicle growth to ovulation in women using ultrasonic, laparoscopic and biochemical measurements. Br J Obstet Gynaecol 88:81–90, 1981.
10. Lenz S: Ultrasonic study of follicular maturation, ovulation and development of corpus luteum during normal menstrual cycles. Acta Obstet Gynecol Scand 64:15–19, 1985.
11. Hilgers TW, Dvorak AD, Tamisiea DF, Ellis RL, Yaksich PJ: Sonographic definition of the empty follicle syndrome. J Ultrasound Med 8:411–416, 1989.
12. Zandt-Stastny D, Thorsen MK, Middleton WD, Aiman J, Zion A, McAsey M, Harms L: Inability of sonography to detect imminent ovulation. AJR Am J Roentgenol 152:91–95, 1989.
13. Thickman D, Arger P, Tureck R, Blasco L, Mintz M, Coleman B: Sonographic assessment of the endometrium in patients undergoing in vitro fertilization. J Ultrasound Med 5:197–201, 1986.
14. Brandt TD, Levy EB, Grant TH, Marut E, Leland J: Endometrial echo and its significance in female infertility. Radiology 157:225–229, 1985.
15. Fleischer AC, Herbert CM, Hill GA, Kepple DM, Worrell JA: Transvaginal sonography of the endometrium during induced cycles. J Ultrasound Med 10:93–95, 1991.
16. Cowan BD: Ovarian hyperstimulation syndrome. Female Patient 16:37–44, 1991.
17. Haning RV, Austin CW, Kuzma KL, Shapiro SS, Zwiebel WJ: Ultrasound evaluation of estrogen monitoring for induction of ovulation with menotropins. Fertil Steril 37:627–632, 1982.
18. Rankin RN, Hutton LC: Ultrasound in the ovarian hyperstimulation syndrome. J Clin Ultrasound 9:473–476, 1981.

Section 8
Obstetric Ultrasound

Early on in its development, diagnostic ultrasound was recognized to have considerable potential for assessment of the pregnant uterus. After all, the pregnant uterus previously was impervious diagnostically to all modes except x-ray, which provided little information. In 1966 I (WJZ) was first involved with ultrasound (as a medical student), and I can assure you that early investigators did not imagine the importance that ultrasound would ultimately have in obstetric practice. Nor did they envision the image quality that would be obtained with ultrasound instruments like those currently available.

Ultrasound is invaluable for the modern practice of obstetrics, but for all of its rewards, obstetric imaging remains one of the most challenging applications of ultrasound. Excellent sonographic technique and solid knowledge of ultrasound diagnosis are needed for successful obstetric ultrasound practice. To this end, this portion of the text emphasizes technique, the requisites of a thorough examination, and basic diagnostic principles. It is not our goal to teach "referral center" obstetric sonography. Rather, we teach herein a brand of sonography that, we hope, will allow the practitioner to perform reliable ultrasound examinations in a community obstetric setting.

Chapter 33
Obstetric Primer and Ultrasound Examination Guidelines

Roya Sohaey

OBSTETRIC PRIMER

The effective use of ultrasound in obstetrics requires a basic foundation of clinical obstetric principles. To this end, we begin by reviewing selected obstetric concepts and terms.[1]

Pregnancy Dating

It is important to realize that clinicians using the term "gestational age" actually are referring to menstrual age, and in this text we will follow suit. The "menstrual age" is measured from the *first day* of the menstrual period that preceded fertilization. The true gestational age, based on the date of fertilization, is 2 weeks less than the menstrual age, because fertilization occurs about 2 weeks after the first day of menstruation. It would be preferable to date pregnancies from fertilization, but there is no marker for fertilization in most cases (except during in vitro fertilization or a similar procedure). Menstrual age, therefore, is used routinely in obstetric practice, even though this dating method has two recognized deficiencies. First, the length of the menstrual cycle varies from one woman to another, and this affects the accuracy of the menstrual age. The usual menstrual cycle of 28 days is assumed, but some women may have longer cycles, in which case the time from the first day of menses to fertilization is longer than expected (and the gestation is younger than its stated menstrual age). Second, some women may have irregular or infrequent cycles that preclude accurate estimation of the time of fertilization.

Due Date

The "due date" is more correctly called the estimated date of delivery (EDD). The old term was the estimated date of confinement (EDC). Fortunately, we no longer confine women for delivery, so the EDC has become the EDD. The EDD can be calculated quickly with the 7 and 3 rule: add 7 days to the first day of the last menstrual period and then subtract 3 months; presto, you have the EDD.

Growth

Fetal growth refers to the *age-related* change in the size or weight of the fetus. Growth cannot be assessed accurately if the age of the fetus (the gestational age) is unknown or imprecise (Chapter 34). By definition, a newborn infant is considered "growth retarded" if its birth weight falls below the tenth percentile for term infants. ("Term" is defined in the next paragraph.) A newborn infant is "macrosomic" if its weight exceeds the 90th percentile at term. The concepts of growth retardation and macrosomia originally were defined in neonates, but the same concepts now are used during the prenatal period as well, because ultrasound permits the assessment of fetal growth in utero.

Duration of Pregnancy

Normal pregnancy in humans encompasses 9 calendar months, or 40 weeks' menstrual age. This 40-week period is divided into three equal segments, or "trimesters." The first trimester extends through week 13, the second trimester from the 14th through 26th weeks, and the third trimester from the 27th week to term. A pregnancy is said to be at "term" in the 38th through 41st weeks of gestation, and it is considered post-term thereafter. Generally it is not desirable for a pregnancy to extend into the 42nd week, due to a substantial increase in delivery and postpartum complications.

Term and lung maturity are not entirely interchangeable concepts. The lungs of virtually all fetuses are sufficiently mature at term to sustain life in the postnatal period, but the lungs may be mature *before* term in some cases. The ratio of lecithin to sphingomyelin (L/S ratio) in amniotic fluid is used to evaluate fetal lung maturity. If the L/S ratio is 2.0 or greater, then it is highly likely that the lung maturity is sufficient to support life even if the fetus has not reached term. Respiratory distress is likely with a ratio of less than 1.0. The phosphatidylglycerol content of the amniotic fluid also is used to evaluate lung maturity. Respiratory distress is unlikely if the amniotic fluid concentration of this phospholipid is 3% or greater.

Clinical Landmarks

The status of a pregnancy is evaluated clinically with certain developmental landmarks. Fetal cardiac activity generally can be detected with a Doppler stethoscope by 9 to 12 weeks' menstrual age and with a standard stethoscope by 18 to 20 weeks. The patient experiences "quickening" or the perception of fetal motion by 16 to 20 weeks (earlier in multiparous patients and later in primiparous patients). The height of the uterine fundus (as measured from the symphysis pubis) is a mainstay for clinical assessment of the status of the pregnancy. The fundal height in centimeters is equivalent to the menstrual age in weeks (e.g., at 16 weeks, fundal height should be 16 cm above the symphysis pubis). The fundus reaches the level of the umbilicus at about 20 weeks. The term "large for dates" refers to a fundal height greater than expected for the menstrual age, and "small for dates" refers to the opposite. Fundal height is a valuable means of pregnancy assessment but is affected by many biologic variables and may be misleading in some cases.

Number of Pregnancies

A primigravida is a woman who is pregnant for the first time. A primipara (slang, "primip") is a woman who has carried a pregnancy for the first time to the age of viability, and a multipara (slang, "multip") has carried more than one pregnancy to that stage. A women who has had four pregnancies, a spontaneous abortion at 12 weeks, and three live births at term would be described as gravida 4, para 3.

Lie and Presentation

Fetal lie describes the orientation of the fetus relative to the mother. The only options permitted are longitudinal, transverse, or oblique. Fetal presentation refers to the part of the fetus that is closest to the birth canal. For ultrasound purposes, it generally is sufficient to determine whether presentation is cephalic (head down), which is normal, or breech (head up). The term "cephalic" should be used rather than "vertex," as the latter term describes a specific presentation that is not usually confirmed with ultrasound. Detailed information about presentation can be obtained with ultrasound, such as the type of breech presentation, and this information

sometimes is important for planning the method of delivery.

Common Obstetric Problems

Ultrasound is used to address a wide range of obstetric problems, but certain of these occur commonly and are particularly noteworthy. The obstetric questions commonly addressed with ultrasound are reviewed briefly in Table 33–1. Please review this material as it is not repeated in the text.

OBSTETRIC ULTRASOUND SCREENING

The role of ultrasound as a tool for screening a low-risk obstetric population is controversial.[2–4] The controversy stems from the relatively poor anomaly detection rate noted in several large screening studies. In a series of European trials, fetal anomaly detection was 51% whereas the largest United States study to date showed a dismal 17% detection rate.[2,3] The latter was the much publicized RADIUS study (Routine Antenatal Diagnostic Imaging with Ultrasound), which evaluated the effect of prenatal ultrasound screening on perinatal outcome.[2] The low anomaly detection rate in the RADIUS study should not be interpreted as the best that can be done with ultrasound screening. There were significant differences in anomaly detection rates between referral centers and primary care centers in the RADIUS study despite the fact that all the centers used identical imaging protocols.[2–4] Obviously, fetal anatomic evaluation is not easy, and the RADIUS study confirms that the training and experience of sonographers and sonologists is germane to how well the obstetric examination is performed. In the near future, certification of obstetric imaging practices may be mandated. Currently, the American Institute of Ultrasound in Medicine (AIUM) and the American College of Radiology (ACR) offer voluntary certification for ultrasound departments performing obstetric sonography.

OBSTETRIC ULTRASOUND GUIDELINES

A variety of medical practitioners perform obstetric ultrasound. To standardize the examination, specific guidelines have been established by leaders in the field of obstetric imaging. These guidelines are updated at intervals of 3 to 5 years and are published by the AIUM and the ACR (both sets of standards are substantially the

Table 33-1. Common Obstetric Problems Addressed with Ultrasound

1. Number of Gestations	Ultrasound is accurate for determining the number of gestations when the uterus is large for dates or following fertility enhancement procedures (e.g., in vitro fertilization).
2. Pregnancy Location	Ultrasound can determine accurately whether or not a pregnancy is located normally within the uterine cavity, or whether it is ectopic.
3. Uncertain Dates	The most common reason for ultrasound examination is to establish the gestational age. Accurate determination of gestational age is essential for assessment of fetal growth and well-being.
4. Uterus Small for Dates	This is a common indication for ultrasound. Differential considerations include incorrect dates, growth retardation, anomalous fetal development, chromosome abnormalities, and oligohydramnios (reduced amniotic fluid volume). The latter may be caused by spontaneous rupture of membranes, placental insufficiency, or fetal urinary tract problems.
5. Uterus Large for Dates	This is another common indication for ultrasound. Possible diagnoses include incorrect dates, multiple gestations, hydatidiform mole, large uterine leiomyoma or other pelvic mass, polyhydramnios from a wide range of causes (including congenital anomalies, hemolytic disorders, and intrauterine infection), and maternal diabetes mellitus (large fetus, large placenta, and polyhydramnios).
6. Risk of Fetal Anomaly	A focused ultrasound examination is an accurate means for detecting and excluding many fetal anomalies and is indicated when the risk of anomaly is high because of family history, exposure to toxic chemicals, or exposure to infectious diseases, or when clinical findings raise a question of fetal abnormalities (e.g., uterus too large or small for dates).
7. Vaginal Bleeding	In the first trimester, vaginal bleeding may be incidental or may indicate pregnancy failure. Ultrasound can assess pregnancy viability, detect intrauterine hemorrhage, and diagnose an embryonic pregnancy or missed abortion. Later in pregnancy, ultrasound is used to search for placenta previa or placental abruption, either of which may cause vaginal bleeding.
8. Pain During Pregnancy	Obstetric causes of pain that can be detected sonographically include placental abruption, hemorrhagic uterine leiomyoma, and ovarian tumors or cysts. Nonobstetric causes of pain that can be detected with ultrasound include appendicitis and acute cholecystitis.
9. Possible Fetal Demise	If fetal cardiac activity cannot be detected at the appropriate stage of pregnancy, or if fetal motion ceases later in pregnancy, ultrasound can be used to determine whether the fetus is alive.
10. Presentation and Lie	The orientation of the fetus within the uterine cavity can usually be determined clinically, but ultrasound is helpful to confirm fetal position when clinical examination is compromised, before cesarean section, or when detailed positional information is needed that cannot be determined clinically.

same).[5, 6] The AIUM/ACR guidelines describe the measurements and sonographic images that should be obtained routinely. It is essential that ultrasound practitioners follow these guidelines, but note that only the minimum required views are addressed in the AIUM guidelines. I feel that additional views and measurements should also be obtained on a regular basis. The AIUM guidelines and suggested additional views are presented below in outline, and illustrated in Figures 33–1 through 33–16.[5] Please review this material thoroughly, as it is fundamental to the practice of obstetric ultrasound. Note also that first-trimester ultrasound guidelines are listed in this chapter for the sake of completeness, but this material is illustrated and discussed in detail in Chapter 36.

Equipment and Documentation

Real Time Sonography. This is needed to confirm cardiac activity, fetal movement, and overall level of fetal activity.

Appropriate Transducers. Use 3 to 5 MHz for transabdominal scanning; 5 to 7.5 MHz usually is adequate for transvaginal scanning.

Documentation. A permanent record of images is required. The images and other material are labeled with date, patient identification, and image orientation (if needed). A formal written report is generated.

First-Trimester Examination

(Illustrated in Chapter 36)

Transabdominal Versus Transvaginal. If one method fails to provide diagnostic information, the other method should be performed.

Gestational Sac (GS). Document the location of the GS and the presence or absence of an embryo. If no embryo, document the presence of a yolk sac. Measure the mean diameter of the GS. Differentiate between the GS and other intrauterine fluid collections by documenting structures within the sac.

Embryo. Determine whether cardiac activity is present. Document embryo crown-rump length (CRL). Embryonic demise is diagnosed if the CRL is greater than 5 mm without cardiac activity.

Multiple Gestations. Document the fetal number. Wait until multiple embryos can be seen to confirm the number of gestations, because incomplete membrane fusion or subchorionic hemorrhage can mimic a gestational sac.

Uterus, Adnexa, and Cervix. Document the presence, location, and size of leiomyomas, adnexal masses, or other pathologic findings. Docu-

ment the presence or absence of fluid in the cul-de-sac of Douglas.

Gestational Age. The CRL is a more accurate indicator of gestational age than the mean GS diameter. Late in the first trimester, use the biparietal diameter and other fetal measurements presented later to establish the gestational age.

Clinical Correlation. Correlate the gestational age and other findings, e.g., the presence or absence of yolk sac or embryo is correlated with the menstrual age (if known), the clinical history, and serum hormone levels.

Second- and Third-Trimester Examination

Document Fetal Life. Note the presence of fetal cardiac activity and overall fetal activity. Report abnormal heart rate or rhythm, or both.

Presentation, Lie, and Number. Note the presentation and lie of the fetus (except early in the second trimester when the fetus is very mobile).

Multiple Pregnancies. Document the number of gestational sacs, the number of placentas, and the presence of dividing membrane(s) separating fetuses. Determine sex (genitalia) of each fetus. Compare fetal size, and the volume of amniotic fluid about each fetus.

Amniotic Fluid Volume. Determine whether amniotic fluid volume is increased, decreased, or normal with respect to the gestational age (Chapter 35).

Placenta. Determine the location and appearance of the placenta. Use abdominal, transperineal, or vaginal views to show the relationship of the placenta to the internal cervical os.

Gestational Age. Use cranial and limb measurements for determining the gestational age (GA). The initial (earliest) ultrasound examination is used to establish the GA; subsequent examinations are for evaluating fetal growth. Once the gestational age is established, it is never changed on subsequent examinations.

Biparietal Diameter (BPD). Measure the BPD on an axial image that includes the thalamus (Fig. 33–1). Measure *only* the skull.

Head Circumference (HC). Use the same image as the BPD but *include* the soft tissues in the HC measurement (Fig. 33–2). HC may be more accurate than BPD if the head is dolichocephalic (long and thin) or brachycephalic (short and broad), as discussed in Chapter 34.

Femur Length (FL). Measure as shown in Figure 33–3. There is considerable variation in femur length late in pregnancy.

Abdominal Circumference (AC). Measure

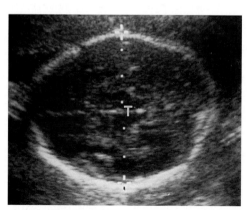

Figure 33-1—Biparietal Diameter (BPD). Axial image of the fetal head at the level of the thalamus (T). The measurement is taken from the outer edge of the near skull margin to the inner edge of the far skull margin (calipers). The soft tissues are *excluded* in measuring the BPD. The hypoechoic thalamus is clearly seen.

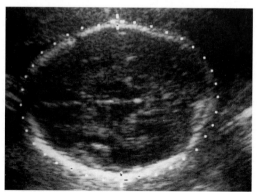

Figure 33-2—Head Circumference (HC). The HC is measured on the same image as the BPD. The soft tissues are *included* in this perimeter measurement (dotted line). If the fetal head is dolichocephalic (long and thin) or brachycephalic (round and broad), the HC measurement may be a more accurate estimation of gestational age than the BPD.

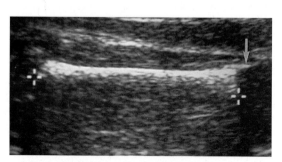

Figure 33-3—Femur Length (FL). Determine the longest measurement (calipers) of the femur that is closest to the transducer. Only the femoral shaft is measured. An echogenic line from a femoral epiphysis (arrow) may be seen and should *not* be included in the FL measurement. Linear and curvilinear transducers are preferable for measuring the FL, and the long axis of the femur should be roughly perpendicular to the ultrasound beam.

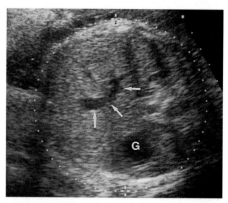

Figure 33-4—Abdominal Circumference (AC). This transverse image illustrates the desired level for the AC view. The abdomen is round (not oblique) and includes the fluid-filled gastric fundus (G). The junction of the left and right portal veins is visible (arrows) and forms a C or J shape. If the portal vein is linear or extends to the skin, then the plane is incorrect.

Figure 33-5—Cervix. Midline sagittal view of the lower uterine segment shows the cervix (calipers) and cervical canal (arrows). The internal os should be clear of placenta (as shown here) during the third trimester. The cervix is usually seen well using a partially filled maternal bladder (B) as an acoustic window. Care should be taken to not overdistend the maternal bladder, which may compress the lower uterine segment and artifactually elongate the cervix. Translabial or transvaginal imaging may be needed to visualize the cervix adequately. Placenta previa and specialized imaging techniques for the cervix are discussed further in Chapter 44.

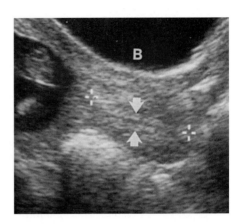

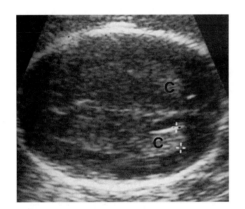

Figure 33-6—Cerebral Ventricles. An axial scan of the fetal head superior to the usual BPD/HC view shows the choroid plexus (C) filling the lateral ventricles. The transverse dimension of the lateral ventricle at the level of the atria (calipers) is measured, when necessary, to assess ventricular size. In normal fetuses, this measurement remains constant, at under 10 mm, throughout pregnancy.

Figure 33-7—Posterior Fossa (PF) and Nuchal Thickness (NT). The PF/NT view is best obtained by angling the transducer 10 to 15 degrees posteriorly from the standard BPD/HC view (Figs. 33–1, 33–2). The cerebellar hemispheres (C), cisterna magna (+ calipers), and nuchal skin (x calipers) are best evaluated with this view. The thalamus (T) is visible, as well as the cisterna magna (CM), which is the fluid collection directly posterior to the cerebellar midline. The CM should measure between 3 and 10 mm during the second and third trimesters. A compressed CM suggests the presence of a spinal defect, and a large CM should raise suspicion for a Dandy Walker anomaly. In our institution, the nuchal skin thickness is measured routinely prior to 20 weeks (not required by the AIUM or the ACR). The measurement is made from the outer margin of the skull to the outer margin of the skin (x cursors) and does not normally exceed 6 mm between 16 and 20 weeks' menstrual age. The nuchal thickness may be exaggerated if the imaging angle is excessively coronal. Nuchal thickening has been associated with an increased risk for aneuploidy, particularly trisomy 21.

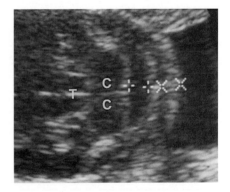

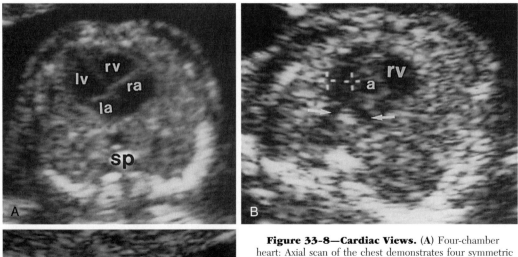

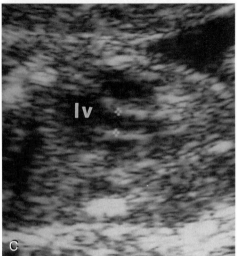

Figure 33-8—Cardiac Views. (A) Four-chamber heart: Axial scan of the chest demonstrates four symmetric cardiac chambers, with normal position of the heart in the chest (rv = right ventricle, lv = left ventricle, ra = right atrium, la = left atrium, sp = spine). Although ventricular outflow tract views are not required by the AIUM/ACR guidelines, I believe that they can be obtained easily (with practice) and increase sensitivity for detecting cardiac anomalies. **(B)** Right ventricular outflow tract (RVOT). From the four-chamber view, the transducer is angled toward the fetal head and turned toward the right ventricle to obtain the RVOT view. The main pulmonary artery (PA) (calipers) forms a semicircle anterior to the aorta (a) and branches into the right and left PA trunks (arrows) posterior to the aorta. **(C)** Left ventricular outflow tract (LVOT). From the four-chamber view, the transducer is turned a quarter turn toward the fetal right side. The left atrium disappears from view and the LVOT becomes apparent (calipers). lv = left ventricle. A detailed discussion of normal cardiac views and cardiac anomalies follows in Chapter 40.

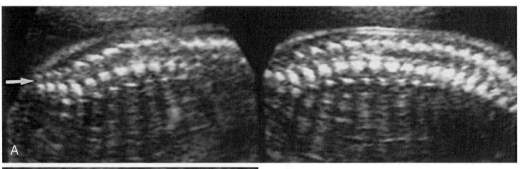

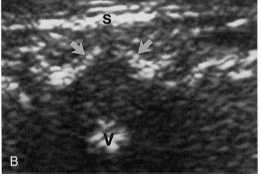

Figure 33-9—Spine. (A) A coronal view through the posterior elements of the spine reveals the normal spine curvature and the distal point of the sacrum (arrow). This view by itself, however, may miss spinal defects. **(B)** A transverse view shows convergence of the posterior elements (arrows) of the vertebra, and skin (S) covering the spine (V = vertebral body in cross section). The normal posterior elements may be parallel or convergent, but *never divergent*. The cervical, thoracic, lumbar, and sacral spine should be evaluated in both coronal and transverse planes, with representative images obtained at each level.

Figure 33-10—Kidneys. Normal fetal kidneys may be difficult to discern from other fetal tissue in the abdomen. This transverse image shows normal kidneys (K), which are mildly hypoechoic compared with surrounding tissue. A specular echo is generated from the interface between Gerota's fascia (arrows) and the peritoneal space. (s = spine.)

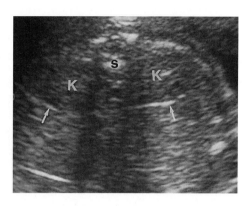

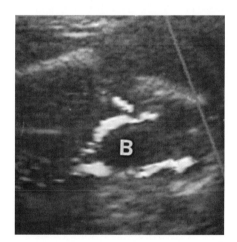

Figure 33-11—Urinary Bladder. A transverse, color Doppler image through the fetal pelvis shows a urine-filled bladder (B) with umbilical arteries (white) flanking the lateral aspect of the bladder. A fluid-filled urinary bladder should be seen after 13 weeks, and its absence should alert the sonographer of possible renal anomalies.

Figure 33-12—Cord Insertion. A transverse image of the abdomen shows a normal umbilical cord (C) insertion site. Care should be taken to show the skin/cord junction (arrows), since gastroschisis defects can be subtle.

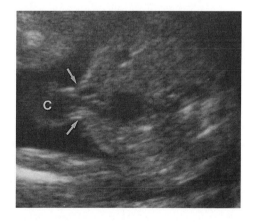

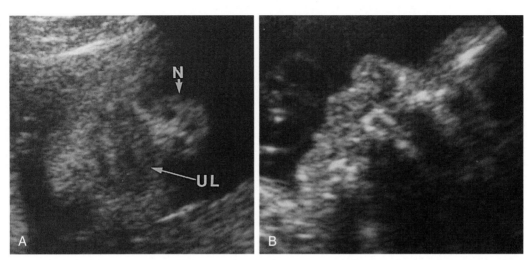

Figure 33-13—Face. (A) A coronal oblique view through the nose (N) and lips shows the intact upper lip margin (UL), helping to exclude cleft lip anomalies. (B) Normal sagittal image of the face. Anomalies, such as micrognathia (small jaw), can be diagnosed if this view is obtained routinely.

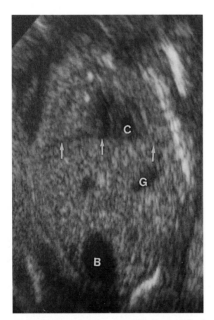

Figure 33-14—Diaphragm. The normal fetal diaphragm is a thin, hypoechoic line (arrows) located between the chest and abdomen, seen best on coronal or sagittal images. A coronal image of the diaphragm is an informative view, because it shows the relationships among the cardiac apex, stomach, and bladder. This image demonstrates a normal left-sided cardiac apex (C), a left-sided gastric fundus (G) located *below* the diaphragm, and a fluid-filled bladder (B).

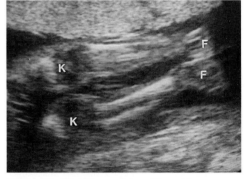

Figure 33-15—Extremities. Normal lower extremities are illustrated, as confirmed by normal shin/foot orientation. (K = knees, F = feet.)

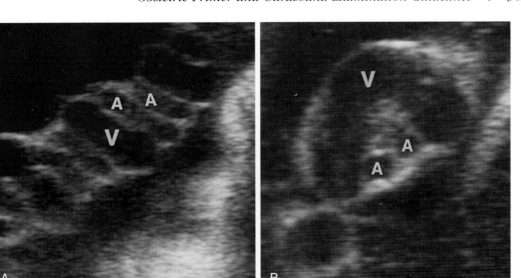

Figure 33-16—Umbilical Cord. (**A**) Longitudinal and (**B**) transverse images of a normal umbilical cord confirm the presence of two arteries (A) and one vein (V). If there is confusion about the number of vessels in the umbilical cord, a Doppler examination at the level of the fetal bladder should help delineate the number of arteries present.

on a true transverse view (not oblique) at the level of the gastric fundus and the junction of the right and left portal veins (Fig. 33–4). The AC is the best measurement for assessing fetal weight.

Interval Growth. Compare fetal measurements on successive examinations to evaluate the appropriateness of interval growth.

Uterus, Cervix, and Adnexa. Record the presence, location, and size of myomas, adnexal masses, and other pathology. Transvaginal or transperineal scanning may be needed to help visualize the cervix (Fig. 33–5).

Fetal Anatomy. Confirm normality (minimum requirements) of the cerebral ventricles (Fig. 33–6); posterior fossa (Fig. 33–7); four-chamber heart (Fig. 33–8*A*); spine (Fig. 33–9); stomach (Fig. 33–4); kidneys (Fig. 33–10); urinary bladder (Fig. 33–11); and cord insertion site (Fig. 33–12).

Nonvisualized Anatomy. The written report should note what structures were not well seen.

Abnormal Anatomy. A targeted evaluation of the areas of concern may be required.

Additional Views Recommended by Author

Nuchal Thickness. A nuchal skin measurement should be obtained on the posterior fossa view (Fig. 33–7) for fetuses between 16 and 20 weeks' gestational age.

Face. Document facial structure with sagittal and oblique coronal views through the nose and lips (Fig. 33–13).

Cardiac Ventricle. Use oblique images at the level of the ventricles (Fig. 33–8*B,C*) to show the position and size of the ventricular outflow tracts.

Diaphragm. Document the presence of the diaphragm, when possible, with a coronal image through the chest and abdomen (Fig. 33–14).

Extremities. Document the presence of two arms and two legs (Fig. 33–15) and show that the proportions of extremity parts are grossly normal.

Three-Vessel Cord. Demonstrate the number of cord vessels on a free-floating loop of cord or at the level of the urinary bladder (Fig. 33–16).

REFERENCES

1. Scott JR, Disaia PJ, Hammond CB, Spellacy WN (eds): Danforth's Obstetrics and Gynecology, 7th ed. Philadelphia, JB Lippincott, 1994, pp 67–128, 163–174, 269–316, 501–520.
2. Ewigman BG, Crane JP, Frigoletto FD, et al: Effect of prenatal ultrasound screening on perinatal outcome. N Engl J Med 329:821–827, 1993.
3. Finberg HJ: Obstetrics. *In* Merritt CRB (ed): Yearbook of Ultrasound 1994. St Louis, Mosby–Year Book, 1994, pp 1–7.
4. Crane JP, LeFevre ML, Winborn RC, et al: A randomized trial of prenatal ultrasonographic screening: Impact on the detection, management, and outcome of anomalous fetuses. Am J Obstet Gynecol 171:3921–3929, 1994.
5. American Institute of Ultrasound in Medicine: 1994 Guidelines for Performance of the Antepartum Obstetrical Ultrasound Examination. AIUM Executive Office, 14750 Sweitzer Lane, Suite 100, Laurel, MD 20707–5906.
6. American College of Radiology: ACR Standard for Antepartum Obstetrical Ultrasound, 1995. American College of Radiology, 1891 Preston White Drive, Reston, VA 22091.

Chapter 34

Fetal Growth

Roya Sohaey

Ultrasound plays a major role in confirming or determining the gestational age, which is a central factor in obstetric management. The sonographer, therefore, must be intimately familiar with the techniques and limitations of ultrasound in dating a pregnancy. The first goal of this chapter is to introduce fetal biometric tables used to establish the gestational age. The limitations of these tables will be presented, as well as guidelines for their use in dating pregnancies. The tables will help the sonographer understand the connection between fetal size and fetal age in normal pregnancy.

The second goal of this chapter is to provide guidelines for the identification of abnormal growth patterns, such as intrauterine growth retardation (IUGR) and macrosomia. I will emphasize the concept that growth is an age-related change in size or weight of the fetus. Growth, therefore, can be assessed accurately only when the gestational age is known. Remember that gestational age is measured as "menstrual age"; that is, in relation to the first day of the last menstrual period preceding pregnancy (see preceding chapter). The terms "menstrual age" and "gestational age" are used interchangeably in this text.

FETAL BIOMETRY

"Bio" refers to life, and "metry" to measurement, so biometry means "life measurement" in a literal sense. Current application of this term, however, implies the use of statistical methods in measuring living things. This statistical sense is appropriate for gestational biometry, since we measure the gestational sac or the fetus and then use statistics to determine the gestational age and to evaluate fetal growth.

The best time to establish the gestational age with ultrasound is during the first trimester, at the earliest time that the living embryo or fetus is seen.[1, 2] Statistically, the size/gestational age relationship is most precise during the first trimester, when the entire fetus (or embryo) can be measured via the crown-rump length. For technical details about first-trimester dating, see Chapter 36. In today's health care environment, with emphasis on limiting cost, most women with

uncomplicated pregnancies have only one ultrasound examination, usually in the second trimester. It is fortunate, therefore, that fetal biometry used in the second trimester is also an excellent way to determine the gestational age.

After the first trimester, the fetus is too large to measure in its entirety with ultrasound, so selected fetal structures, such as the head and abdomen, are measured instead. A variety of structures can be measured, since anatomic visualization with ultrasound is excellent, but the routine measurements are the biparietal diameter (BPD) of the fetal head, the head circumference (HC), the abdominal circumference (AC), and the femur length (FL). These measurements correspond well with the menstrual age in normal fetuses.[2–6] In a normal pregnancy, there is no advantage in obtaining additional biometric values,[2] but other measurements, such as kidney size, chest size, and cardiac chamber size, can be obtained when needed for special problems. Tables with measurements of these structures are provided in subsequent chapters. Using the BPD, HC, AC, and FL, the sonographer can assess all aspects of fetal size. Because these measurements are the basis for both gestational age and growth evaluation, care must be taken to obtain correct images and measurements. *Examples of the images used for fetal biometry are shown in Chapter 33.* These examples should be reviewed by readers who are unfamiliar with fetal measurement technique.

Biparietal Diameter and Head Circumference

Biometric data for the BPD and HC are presented in Figure 34–1. The BPD and HC are equally accurate measurements for assessing the menstrual age when the head shape is normal. In cases of dolichocephaly (long and narrow head) or brachycephaly (short and broad head), the BPD is an inaccurate measurement and the HC should be used instead. If the sonographer is unsure as to whether the head shape is normal, the cephalic index can be computed, as illustrated in Figure 34–2. The cephalic index is age independent and ranges from 73.9 to 82.8 (mean, 78.3).[7] If the cephalic index is abnormal, the

Menstrual Age (wks)	Biparietal Diameter (cm)*	Head Circumference (cm)†	Abdominal Circumference (cm)‡	Femur Length (cm)§
12.0	1.7	6.8	4.6	0.7
12.5	1.9	7.5	5.3	0.9
13.0	2.1	8.2	6.0	1.1
13.5	2.3	8.9	6.7	1.2
14.0	2.5	9.7	7.3	1.4
14.5	2.7	10.4	8.0	1.6
15.0	2.9	11.0	8.6	1.7
15.5	3.1	11.7	9.3	1.9
16.0	3.2	12.4	9.9	2.0
16.5	3.4	13.1	10.6	2.2
17.0	3.6	13.8	11.2	2.4
17.5	3.8	14.4	11.9	2.5
18.0	3.9	15.1	12.5	2.7
18.5	4.1	15.8	13.1	2.8
19.0	4.3	16.4	13.7	3.0
19.5	4.5	17.0	14.4	3.1
20.0	4.6	17.7	15.0	3.3
20.5	4.8	18.3	15.6	3.4
21.0	5.0	18.9	16.2	3.5
21.5	5.1	19.5	16.8	3.7
22.0	5.3	20.1	17.4	3.8
22.5	5.5	20.7	17.9	4.0
23.0	5.6	21.3	18.5	4.1
23.5	5.8	21.9	19.1	4.2
24.0	5.9	22.4	19.7	4.4
24.5	6.1	23.0	20.2	4.5
25.0	6.2	23.5	20.8	4.6
25.5	6.4	24.1	21.3	4.7
26.0	6.5	24.6	21.9	4.9
26.5	6.7	25.1	22.4	5.0
27.0	6.8	25.6	23.0	5.1
27.5	6.9	26.1	23.5	5.2
28.0	7.1	26.6	24.0	5.4
28.5	7.2	27.1	24.6	5.5
29.0	7.3	27.5	25.1	5.6
29.5	7.5	28.0	25.6	5.7
30.0	7.6	28.4	26.1	5.8
30.5	7.7	28.8	26.6	5.9
31.0	7.8	29.3	27.1	6.0
31.5	7.9	29.7	27.6	6.1
32.0	8.1	30.1	28.1	6.2
32.5	8.2	30.4	28.6	6.3
33.0	8.3	30.8	29.1	6.4
33.5	8.4	31.2	29.5	6.5
34.0	8.5	31.5	30.0	6.6
34.5	8.6	31.8	30.5	6.7
35.0	8.7	32.2	30.9	6.8
35.5	8.8	32.5	31.4	6.9
36.0	8.9	32.8	31.8	7.0
36.5	8.9	33.0	32.3	7.1
37.0	9.0	33.3	32.7	7.2
37.5	9.1	33.5	33.2	7.3
38.0	9.2	33.8	33.6	7.4
38.5	9.2	34.0	34.0	7.4
39.0	9.3	34.2	34.4	7.5
39.5	9.4	34.4	34.8	7.6
40.0	9.4	34.6	35.3	7.7

* BPD = $-3.08 + 0.41$ (MA) $- 0.000061$ MA^3; $r^2 = 97.6\%$; 1 SD = 3 mm.
† HC = $-11.48 + 1.56$ (MA) $- 0.0002548$ MA^3; $r^2 = 98.1\%$; 1 SD = 1 cm.
‡ AC = $-13.3 + 1.61$ (MA) $- 0.00998$ MA^2; $r^2 = 97.2\%$; 1 SD = 1.34 cm.
§ FL = $-3.91 + 0.427$ (MA) $- 0.0034$ MA^2; $r^2 = 97.5\%$; 1 SD = 3 mm.

Figure 34-1—Predicted Fetal Measurements at Specific Menstrual Age. (Reprinted with permission from Hadlock FP, Deter LR, Harrist RB, et al: Estimating fetal age: Computer-assisted analysis of multiple fetal growth parameters. Radiology 152:497–501, 1984.)

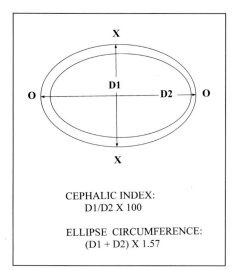

CEPHALIC INDEX:
D1/D2 X 100

ELLIPSE CIRCUMFERENCE:
(D1 + D2) X 1.57

Figure 34-2—Calculation of the Cephalic Index and Ellipse Circumference (for Head and Abdominal Circumference Measurements). The outer-to-outer calvarial biparietal diameter (the X-X distance, or D1) and the occipital frontal diameter (the O-O distance, or D2) are used to calculate the cephalic index. The normal range for the cephalic index is 78.3 +/− 4.3.

head circumference, not the BPD, should be used in determining the fetal head size.[7, 8] The HC is best estimated by drawing an ellipse around the fetal calvarium. If the ultrasound instrument does not have ellipsoid measurement capabilities, the following formula for an ellipse can be used:

$$Circumference = (D1 + D2) \times 1.57$$

where D1 and D2 are the perpendicular measurements of the long and short axes of the calvarium (Fig. 34–2).

If the fetal head is low in the maternal pelvis and the BPD or HC measurements cannot be obtained, other cranial measurements have been shown to be accurate indicators of gestational age. The binocular distance (BOD) can be obtained when the head is in a direct occiput posterior position (face up), and the transverse cerebellar diameter can be obtained when the head is in the occiput anterior (face down) position.[9, 10] Tables for these anatomic measurements are provided in Chapter 37.

Abdominal Circumference

Biometric data for the abdominal circumference (AC) are presented in Figure 34–1. The abdominal circumference is technically the most difficult fetal measurement to obtain. It is also the most important measurement for assessing

fetal weight and well-being, particularly in the late second and third trimesters.[11, 12] I recommend obtaining two to three AC measurements per examination, especially for inexperienced sonographers. The AC measurement shows the most variability in some series.[2, 13] This variability is thought to be secondary to technical difficulties, as well as to distortion of the fetal abdomen by crowding, oligohydramnios, and a narrow anteroposterior diameter of the maternal abdomen. The distorted abdomen is difficult to measure accurately. The AC is optimally measured with an electronic ellipse. If the ultrasound instrument does not have this capability, the formula presented previously, for calculating the head circumference, may be used (Fig. 34–2).

Femur Length

Biometric data for fetal femur length are presented in Figure 34–1. The femur length is used to evaluate fetal length, as the overall length of the fetus is proportionate to the length of the long bones. After 32 weeks, the femoral epiphyses are visualized with ultrasound, but these *must not* be included in the femur length measurement (see Figure 33–3, Chapter 33).

DATING THE PREGNANCY

In a woman with unsure menstrual dates or irregular cycles, ultrasound may be the only way to determine the gestational age (menstrual age). As stated previously, the best time to date the pregnancy is the first time a living embryo or fetus is seen, since variability in fetal size is least at that point and increases as pregnancy advances (Fig. 34–3).[1-6] In the late third trimester, normal fetuses can vary in size by the equivalent of 3 to 3.5 weeks' menstrual age.[2, 14] Obviously, this is the worst time to try to determine the gestational age from a single ultrasound examination, since the actual gestational age may be up to 3.5 weeks greater or less than the ultrasound estimate! If, for example, the fetus is 3.5 weeks "small" relative to the last menstrual period–based gestational age, there is no way to determine whether the fetus is growth retarded or whether the discrepancy is due to normal variation. Variability in fetal size is related to population and hereditary factors that affect the size of all human beings.

To reduce the effects of biometric variability in obtaining a "best guess" gestational age from a single ultrasound study, the gestational age estimates for each of the routine measurements (BPD, HC, AC, FL) should be averaged (Fig. 34–3).[2] Each of the four measurements carries inherent variability. Simple averaging of the four

Fetal Parameters	Subgroup Variability (±2 SD) in Weeks				
	12–18 Weeks (N = 43)	18–24 Weeks (N = 69)	24–30 Weeks (N = 76)	30–36 Weeks (N = 95)	36–42 Weeks (N = 78)
BPD	±1.19	±1.73	±2.18	±3.08	±3.20
HC	±1.19	±1.48	±2.06	±2.98	±2.70
AC	±1.66	±2.06	±2.18	±2.96	±3.04
FL	±1.38	±1.80	±2.08	±2.96	±3.12
BPD, AC	±1.26	±1.68	±1.92	±2.60	±2.88
BPD, HC	±1.08	±1.49	±1.99	±2.86	±2.64
BPD, FL	±1.12	±1.46	±1.84	±2.60	±2.62
HC, AC	±1.20	±1.52	±1.98	±2.68	±2.52
HC, FL	±1.08	±1.34	±1.86	±2.52	±2.28
AC, FL	±1.32	±1.64	±1.88	±2.66	±2.60
BPD, AC, FL	±1.20	±1.52	±1.82	±2.50	±2.52
BPD, HC, FL	±1.04	±1.35	±1.81	±2.52	±2.34
HC, AC, FL	±1.14	±1.46	±1.86	±2.52	±2.34
HC, AC, BPD	±1.21	±1.58	±1.94	±2.60	±2.52
BPD, HC, AC, FL	±1.08	±1.40	±1.80	±2.44	±2.30

Figure 34-3—Subgroup Variability in Predicting Menstrual Age. Example, the gestational age variance, based on the BPD, is ± 1.19 weeks, if the fetus is examined during the 12th to 18th weeks of pregnancy. The variance is ± 3.2 weeks if the fetus is examined between 36 and 42 weeks. (BPD = biparietal diameter; HC = head circumference; AC = abdominal circumference; FL = femur length.) (Reprinted with permission from Hadlock FP, Deter LR, Harrist RB, et al: Estimating fetal age: Computer-assisted analysis of multiple fetal growth parameters. Radiology 152:497–501, 1984.)

age estimates has been found to improve accuracy, and a simple average is as accurate as complex regression equations for estimating the menstrual age.[2, 15] I recommend, therefore, that the gestational age reported to the referring practitioner should be the average of the gestational ages represented by the BPD, HC, AC, and FL.

Case Example

The following example illustrates the use of biometric concepts. A woman with irregular menstrual periods presents for her first obstetric ultrasound examination. The menstrual age, based on her last menstrual period (LMP), is 20 weeks. The following biometric data are obtained:

- BPD: 23.5 weeks
- HC: 25.0 weeks
- AC: 26.2 weeks
- FL: 25.2 weeks
- Average: 25.0 weeks

The fetal head is slightly dolichocephalic, but in this case the cephalic index falls within normal limits. The BPD is included, therefore, in the average gestational age, which is 25.0 ± 1.5 weeks. The gestational age of 20 weeks, based on the menstrual history, is deemed inaccurate. Any subsequent ultrasound examinations of this patient would be used to evaluate the growth of the fetus. *The pregnancy would never be redated on future examinations.*

FETAL GROWTH

The objective standard for the diagnosis of fetal growth disturbance is the fetal weight percentile, the calculation of which requires three steps.[16] First, the gestational age must be determined with accuracy. Second, a fetal weight estimate is established. Third, a weight percentile is calculated, by comparing the gestational age and the fetal weight. Many formulas exist for the estimation of fetal weight. The formula of Dr. Hadlock and colleagues,[11] using all fetal biometric data (BPD, HC, AC, FL), is sensitive to 7.5% of actual fetal weight (1 SD). The Hadlock formula is as follows:

$$\text{Log 10 Birth Weight} = 1.5662 - 0.0108 \, (\text{HC}) + 0.0468 \, (\text{AC}) + 0.171 \, (\text{FL}) + 0.00034 \, (\text{HC})^2 - 0.003685 \, (\text{AC} \times \text{FL})$$

With a computer, routine use of this equation is easy. Alternatively, the fetal weight estimate may be derived from a table. Hadlock found that the best results for estimating fetal weight are obtained using all four biometric parameters. The next best results used three parameters, followed by the use of only the AC and FL measurements. When the fetal head cannot be measured, or when a computer program is not available, the AC and FL regression model can be used to estimate fetal weight, as illustrated in Figure 34–4.

Once the fetal weight is calculated and compared with the menstrual age, a fetal weight percentile can easily be established (Fig. 34–5).[7]

FL (cm)	AC (cm) 20.0	20.5	21.0	21.5	22.0	22.5	23.0	23.5	24.0	24.5	25.0	25.5	26.0	26.5	27.0	27.5	28.0	28.5	29.0	29.5	30.0
4.0	663	691	720	751	783	816	851	887	925	964	1006	1048	1093	1139	1188	1239	1291	1346	1403	1463	1525
4.1	680	709	738	769	802	836	871	907	946	986	1027	1070	1115	1162	1211	1262	1315	1371	1429	1489	1551
4.2	697	726	757	788	821	855	891	928	967	1007	1049	1093	1138	1186	1235	1287	1340	1396	1454	1515	1578
4.3	715	745	776	808	841	875	912	949	988	1029	1071	1116	1162	1209	1259	1311	1365	1422	1480	1541	1605
4.4	734	764	795	827	861	896	933	971	1010	1051	1094	1139	1185	1234	1284	1336	1391	1448	1507	1568	1632
4.5	753	783	815	847	882	917	954	993	1033	1074	1118	1163	1210	1259	1309	1362	1417	1474	1534	1596	1660
4.6	772	803	835	868	903	939	976	1015	1056	1098	1142	1187	1235	1284	1335	1388	1444	1501	1561	1623	1688
4.7	792	823	856	889	924	961	999	1038	1079	1122	1166	1212	1260	1310	1361	1415	1471	1529	1589	1652	1717
4.8	812	844	877	911	947	984	1022	1062	1103	1146	1191	1237	1286	1336	1388	1442	1498	1557	1618	1681	1746
4.9	833	865	899	933	969	1007	1046	1086	1128	1171	1216	1263	1312	1363	1415	1470	1527	1585	1647	1710	1776
5.0	855	887	921	956	993	1031	1070	1111	1153	1197	1243	1290	1339	1390	1443	1498	1555	1615	1676	1740	1806
5.1	877	910	944	980	1016	1055	1095	1136	1179	1223	1269	1317	1367	1418	1471	1527	1584	1644	1706	1770	1837
5.2	899	933	967	1004	1041	1080	1120	1162	1205	1250	1296	1344	1395	1447	1500	1556	1614	1674	1737	1801	1868
5.3	922	956	992	1028	1066	1105	1146	1188	1232	1277	1324	1373	1423	1476	1530	1586	1645	1705	1768	1833	1900
5.4	946	981	1016	1053	1091	1131	1172	1215	1259	1305	1352	1401	1452	1505	1560	1617	1675	1736	1799	1865	1933
5.5	971	1005	1041	1079	1118	1158	1199	1242	1287	1333	1381	1431	1482	1535	1591	1648	1707	1768	1832	1897	1966
5.6	995	1031	1067	1105	1144	1185	1227	1271	1316	1362	1411	1461	1513	1566	1622	1679	1739	1801	1864	1931	1999
5.7	1021	1057	1094	1132	1172	1213	1255	1299	1345	1392	1441	1491	1544	1598	1654	1712	1772	1834	1898	1964	2033
5.8	1047	1084	1121	1160	1200	1242	1285	1329	1375	1422	1472	1523	1575	1630	1686	1744	1805	1867	1932	1999	2068
5.9	1074	1111	1149	1188	1229	1271	1314	1359	1406	1454	1503	1555	1608	1663	1719	1778	1839	1902	1966	2034	2103
6.0	1102	1139	1178	1217	1258	1301	1345	1390	1437	1485	1535	1587	1641	1696	1753	1812	1873	1936	2002	2069	2139
6.1	1130	1168	1207	1247	1289	1331	1376	1421	1469	1518	1568	1620	1674	1730	1788	1847	1908	1972	2038	2105	2175
6.2	1160	1198	1237	1278	1319	1363	1408	1454	1501	1551	1602	1654	1709	1765	1823	1882	1944	2008	2074	2142	2212
6.3	1189	1228	1268	1309	1351	1395	1440	1487	1535	1585	1636	1689	1744	1800	1858	1919	1981	2045	2111	2180	2250
6.4	1220	1259	1299	1341	1384	1428	1473	1520	1569	1619	1671	1724	1779	1836	1895	1956	2018	2082	2149	2218	2289
6.5	1251	1291	1332	1373	1417	1461	1507	1555	1604	1655	1707	1760	1816	1873	1932	1993	2056	2121	2188	2256	2328
6.6	1284	1324	1365	1407	1451	1496	1542	1590	1640	1691	1743	1797	1853	1911	1970	2031	2094	2160	2227	2296	2367
6.7	1317	1357	1399	1441	1486	1531	1578	1626	1676	1728	1780	1835	1891	1949	2009	2070	2134	2199	2267	2336	2408
6.8	1351	1391	1433	1477	1521	1567	1615	1663	1713	1765	1819	1873	1930	1988	2048	2110	2174	2240	2307	2377	2449
6.9	1385	1427	1469	1513	1558	1604	1652	1701	1752	1804	1857	1913	1970	2028	2089	2151	2215	2281	2348	2418	2490
7.0	1421	1463	1506	1550	1595	1642	1690	1740	1791	1843	1897	1953	2010	2069	2130	2192	2256	2322	2391	2461	2533
7.1	1458	1500	1543	1588	1633	1681	1729	1779	1830	1883	1938	1994	2051	2110	2171	2234	2299	2365	2433	2504	2576
7.2	1495	1538	1581	1626	1673	1720	1769	1819	1871	1924	1979	2035	2093	2153	2214	2277	2342	2408	2477	2547	2620
7.3	1534	1577	1621	1666	1713	1761	1810	1861	1913	1966	2021	2078	2136	2196	2258	2321	2386	2453	2521	2592	2665
7.4	1573	1616	1661	1707	1754	1802	1852	1903	1955	2009	2065	2122	2180	2240	2302	2365	2431	2498	2566	2637	2710
7.5	1614	1657	1702	1749	1796	1845	1895	1946	1999	2053	2109	2166	2225	2285	2347	2411	2476	2543	2612	2683	2756
7.6	1655	1699	1745	1791	1839	1888	1939	1990	2043	2098	2154	2211	2270	2331	2393	2457	2523	2590	2659	2730	2803
7.7	1698	1742	1788	1835	1883	1933	1983	2035	2089	2144	2200	2258	2317	2378	2440	2504	2570	2638	2707	2778	2851
7.8	1741	1786	1833	1880	1928	1978	2029	2082	2135	2191	2247	2305	2365	2426	2488	2553	2618	2686	2755	2827	2899
7.9	1786	1832	1878	1926	1975	2025	2076	2129	2183	2238	2295	2353	2413	2474	2537	2602	2668	2735	2805	2876	2949
8.0	1832	1878	1925	1973	2022	2073	2124	2177	2232	2287	2344	2403	2463	2524	2587	2652	2718	2785	2855	2926	2999
8.1	1879	1926	1973	2021	2071	2121	2173	2227	2281	2337	2394	2453	2513	2575	2638	2702	2769	2837	2906	2977	3050
8.2	1928	1974	2022	2070	2120	2171	2224	2277	2332	2388	2446	2504	2565	2626	2690	2754	2821	2889	2958	3029	3102
8.3	1978	2024	2072	2121	2171	2223	2275	2329	2384	2440	2498	2557	2617	2679	2743	2807	2874	2942	3011	3082	3155

A

Figure 34-4—(A and B) Estimation of Fetal Weight (in Grams) Based on Abdominal Circumference (AC) and Femur Length (FL). (Reprinted with permission from Hadlock FP, Harrist RB, Carpenter RJ, et al: Sonographic estimation of fetal weight: The value of femur length in addition to head and abdomen measurements. Radiology 150:535–540, 1984.)

AC (cm)

FL (cm)	30.5	31.0	31.5	32.0	32.5	33.0	33.5	34.0	34.5	35.0	35.5	36.0	36.5	37.0	37.5	38.0	38.5	39.0	39.5	40.0
4.0	1590	1658	1729	1802	1879	1959	2042	2129	2220	2314	2413	2515	2622	2734	2850	2972	3098	3230	3367	3511
4.1	1617	1685	1756	1830	1907	1987	2071	2158	2249	2344	2442	2545	2652	2764	2880	3002	3128	3260	3397	3540
4.2	1644	1712	1783	1858	1935	2016	2100	2187	2279	2373	2472	2575	2683	2794	2911	3032	3159	3290	3427	3570
4.3	1671	1740	1812	1886	1964	2045	2129	2217	2308	2404	2503	2606	2713	2825	2942	3063	3189	3321	3458	3600
4.4	1699	1768	1840	1915	1993	2075	2159	2247	2339	2434	2533	2637	2744	2856	2973	3094	3220	3352	3488	3630
4.5	1727	1797	1869	1944	2023	2105	2189	2278	2370	2465	2565	2668	2776	2888	3004	3125	3251	3383	3519	3661
4.6	1756	1826	1898	1974	2053	2135	2220	2309	2401	2497	2596	2700	2807	2919	3036	3157	3283	3414	3550	3692
4.7	1785	1855	1928	2004	2084	2166	2251	2340	2432	2528	2628	2732	2840	2952	3068	3189	3315	3446	3582	3723
4.8	1814	1885	1959	2035	2115	2197	2283	2372	2464	2560	2660	2764	2872	2984	3100	3221	3347	3478	3613	3754
4.9	1845	1916	1990	2066	2146	2229	2315	2404	2497	2593	2693	2797	2905	3017	3133	3254	3380	3510	3645	3786
5.0	1875	1947	2021	2098	2178	2261	2347	2437	2530	2626	2726	2830	2938	3050	3166	3287	3412	3542	3677	3818
5.1	1906	1978	2053	2130	2210	2294	2380	2470	2563	2659	2760	2864	2972	3084	3200	3320	3445	3575	3710	3850
5.2	1938	2010	2085	2163	2243	2327	2413	2503	2597	2693	2794	2898	3006	3117	3234	3354	3479	3608	3743	3882
5.3	1970	2043	2118	2196	2277	2360	2447	2537	2631	2728	2828	2932	3040	3152	3268	3388	3513	3642	3776	3915
5.4	2003	2076	2151	2229	2311	2395	2482	2572	2665	2762	2863	2967	3075	3186	3302	3422	3547	3676	3809	3948
5.5	2036	2109	2185	2264	2345	2429	2516	2607	2700	2797	2898	3002	3110	3221	3337	3457	3581	3710	3843	3981
5.6	2070	2143	2220	2298	2380	2464	2552	2642	2736	2833	2933	3038	3145	3257	3372	3492	3616	3744	3877	4015
5.7	2104	2178	2254	2333	2415	2500	2587	2678	2772	2869	2970	3074	3181	3293	3408	3527	3651	3779	3911	4048
5.8	2139	2213	2290	2369	2451	2536	2624	2714	2808	2905	3006	3110	3218	3329	3444	3563	3686	3814	3946	4082
5.9	2175	2249	2326	2405	2488	2573	2660	2751	2845	2942	3043	3147	3254	3366	3480	3599	3722	3849	3981	4117
6.0	2211	2286	2363	2442	2525	2610	2698	2789	2883	2980	3080	3184	3292	3403	3517	3636	3758	3885	4016	4151
6.1	2248	2323	2400	2480	2562	2647	2736	2827	2921	3018	3118	3222	3329	3440	3554	3673	3795	3921	4052	4186
6.2	2285	2360	2438	2518	2600	2686	2774	2865	2959	3056	3157	3260	3367	3478	3592	3710	3832	3957	4087	4222
6.3	2323	2398	2476	2556	2639	2725	2813	2904	2998	3095	3195	3299	3406	3516	3630	3747	3869	3994	4124	4257
6.4	2362	2437	2515	2595	2678	2764	2852	2943	3037	3134	3235	3338	3445	3555	3668	3785	3906	4031	4160	4293
6.5	2401	2477	2555	2635	2718	2804	2892	2983	3077	3174	3274	3378	3484	3594	3707	3824	3944	4069	4197	4329
6.6	2441	2517	2595	2675	2759	2844	2933	3024	3118	3215	3315	3418	3524	3633	3746	3863	3983	4106	4234	4366
6.7	2481	2557	2636	2716	2800	2885	2974	3065	3159	3256	3355	3458	3564	3673	3786	3902	4021	4144	4271	4402
6.8	2523	2599	2677	2758	2841	2927	3016	3107	3200	3297	3397	3499	3605	3714	3826	3941	4060	4183	4309	4439
6.9	2564	2641	2719	2800	2884	2969	3058	3149	3242	3339	3438	3541	3646	3754	3866	3981	4100	4222	4347	4477
7.0	2607	2683	2762	2843	2927	3012	3101	3192	3285	3381	3481	3583	3688	3796	3907	4022	4140	4261	4386	4514
7.1	2650	2727	2806	2887	2970	3056	3144	3235	3328	3424	3523	3625	3730	3838	3948	4062	4180	4300	4425	4552
7.2	2694	2771	2850	2931	3014	3100	3188	3279	3372	3468	3567	3668	3772	3880	3990	4104	4220	4340	4464	4591
7.3	2739	2816	2895	2976	3059	3145	3233	3323	3416	3512	3610	3712	3816	3922	4032	4145	4261	4381	4503	4629
7.4	2785	2861	2940	3021	3105	3190	3278	3369	3461	3557	3655	3756	3859	3966	4075	4187	4303	4421	4543	4668
7.5	2831	2908	2987	3068	3151	3236	3324	3414	3507	3602	3700	3800	3903	4009	4118	4230	4344	4462	4583	4708
7.6	2878	2955	3034	3115	3198	3283	3371	3461	3553	3648	3745	3845	3948	4053	4161	4272	4387	4504	4624	4747
7.7	2926	3003	3081	3162	3245	3331	3418	3508	3600	3694	3791	3891	3993	4098	4205	4316	4429	4545	4665	4787
7.8	2974	3051	3130	3211	3294	3379	3466	3555	3647	3741	3838	3937	4039	4143	4250	4360	4472	4588	4706	4827
7.9	3024	3100	3179	3260	3343	3427	3514	3604	3695	3789	3885	3984	4085	4188	4295	4404	4515	4630	4748	4868
8.0	3074	3151	3229	3310	3392	3477	3564	3653	3744	3837	3933	4031	4131	4234	4340	4448	4559	4673	4790	4909
8.1	3125	3202	3280	3360	3443	3527	3614	3702	3793	3886	3981	4079	4179	4281	4386	4493	4604	4716	4832	4950
8.2	3177	3253	3332	3412	3494	3578	3664	3752	3843	3935	4030	4127	4226	4328	4432	4539	4648	4760	4875	4992
8.3	3230	3306	3384	3464	3546	3630	3716	3803	3893	3985	4080	4176	4275	4376	4479	4585	4693	4804	4918	5034

B

Figure 34-4 *Continued*

351

Menstrual Week	Percentiles (g)				
	3rd	10th	50th	90th	97th
10	26	29	35	41	44
11	34	37	45	53	56
12	43	48	58	68	73
13	55	61	73	85	91
14	70	77	93	109	116
15	88	97	117	137	146
16	110	121	146	171	183
17	136	150	181	212	226
18	167	185	223	261	279
19	205	227	273	319	341
20	248	275	331	387	414
21	299	331	399	467	499
22	359	398	478	559	598
23	426	471	568	665	710
24	503	556	670	784	838
25	589	652	785	918	981
26	685	758	913	1,068	1,141
27	791	876	1,055	1,234	1,319
28	908	1,004	1,210	1,416	1,513
29	1,034	1,145	1,379	1,613	1,724
30	1,169	1,294	1,559	1,824	1,649
31	1,313	1,453	1,751	2,049	2,189
32	1,465	1,621	1,953	2,285	2,441
33	1,622	1,794	2,162	2,530	2,703
34	1,783	1,973	2,377	2,781	2,971
35	1,946	2,154	2,595	3,036	3,244
36	2,110	2,335	2,813	3,291	3,516
37	2,271	2,513	3,028	3,543	3,785
38	2,427	2,686	3,236	3,786	4,045
39	2,576	2,851	3,435	4,019	4,294
40	2,714	3,004	3,619	4,234	4,524

Figure 34-5—Estimated Fetal Weight Percentiles Based on in Utero Ultrasound Measurements.
(Reprinted with permission from Hadlock FP, Harrist RB, Martinez-Poyer J: In utero analysis of fetal growth: A sonographic weight standard. Radiology 181:129–133, 1991.)

Normal growth implies that the calculated fetal weight falls between the 10th and 90th percentiles. A fetus is considered small or large for gestational age if the calculated weight is less than the 10th percentile or more than the 90th percentile, respectively. Abnormally small or large fetuses are at an increased risk for a poor outcome; therefore, their identification in utero is very important.[16–19]

Note that fetal weight is the only fetal biometric parameter that uses the 10th and 90th percentiles as the normal range. This practice is based on the original clinical definition of growth retardation and macrosomia: under the 10th percentile or above the 90th percentile (respectively), for a term neonate. The normal range for the BPD, HC, AC, and FL is the 5th to 95th percentiles.

GROWTH PATTERNS

An accurate representation of fetal growth can be obtained only if the biometric parameters are plotted against gestational age in a graphic format. In clinical practice, five primary growth patterns are seen repeatedly in graphic plots of fetal growth. Most normal and abnormal pregnancies fall into one of these patterns, and for that reason these patterns should be recognized and understood by all ultrasound practitioners.

1. **Normal for age and staying normal**. This is the normal pattern (Fig. 34–6) that all expectant mothers and obstetricians hope for. (Keep up the good work, baby!)
2. **Small but stable**. The initial ultrasound examination plots the fetal size at the lower limit of normal or perhaps a little below normal. Subsequent examinations show a growth pattern that follows the normal curves but remains in the low range (Fig. 34–7). This small but stable pattern suggests that the original estimate of the gestational age was incorrect. Alternatively, the fetus may be small for constitutional reasons but is normal.
3. **Small and getting smaller**. This is the most ominous of all patterns (Fig. 34–8). If the fetus is small early in pregnancy and shows progressive worsening of growth rate, a significant abnormality probably exists. Although placental insufficiency or maternal nutritional factors may be issues, the likely cause is an inherent abnormality of the fetus. A chromo-

some abnormality is of particular concern, but an early infectious insult to the pregnancy can also result in this pattern of growth.
4. **Normal, then dropping off**. This ominous pattern (Fig. 34–9), in which fetal size is normal early in pregnancy but the fetal growth rate drops off later in pregnancy, is typical of placental insufficiency. Such fetuses must be monitored closely for signs of hypoxia.
5. **Normal and getting big**. This pattern (Fig. 34–10) is typical of the macrosomic fetus. Close monitoring of fetal weight during the third trimester is important to ensure that the fetus does not get too big, as discussed at the end of this chapter.

INTRAUTERINE GROWTH RETARDATION

A fetus that is estimated to be less than the 10th percentile in weight is considered small for gestational age (SGA). A fetus with intrauterine growth retardation (IUGR) is a fetus whose size or growth is suboptimal.[18, 20] Although the SGA fetus may *not* have IUGR, it is difficult to determine whether the fetus is small but has reached is potential size or whether it is small because it is growth retarded. Therefore, most ultrasound

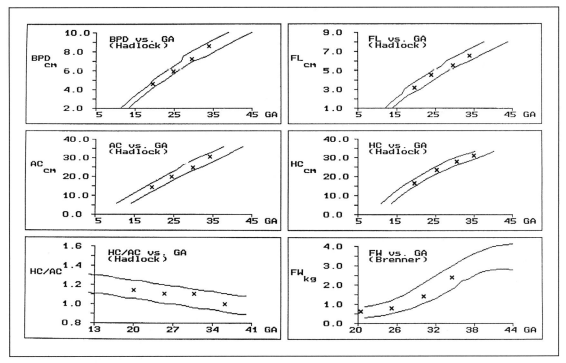

Figure 34-6—Graphic Plot of Normal Growth. On the initial examination, the fetus measures as expected for menstrual age. Subsequent examinations show normal interval growth for all measured parameters.

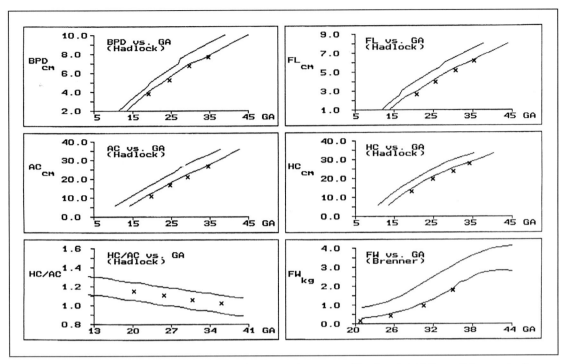

Figure 34-7—Graphic Plot of Small but Stable Growth Pattern. The fetus is initially small for menstrual age but subsequent examinations show normal interval growth. The original estimate of gestational age may have been incorrect, or the constitutionally small fetus is probably normal.

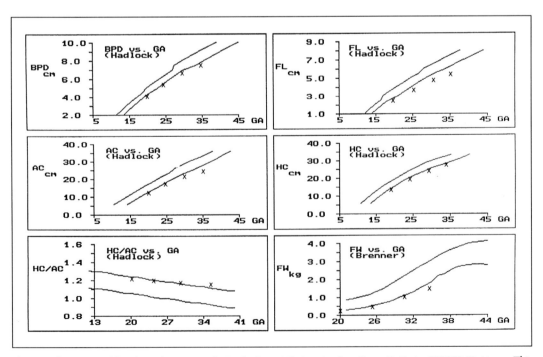

Figure 34-8—Graphic Plot of Symmetric Early-Onset Intrauterine Growth Rate (IUGR) Pattern. This initially small fetus does not exhibit normal interval growth and continues to "become smaller," dropping off the plot. This pattern is more typical for an early insult in pregnancy, such as infection or a chromosomally abnormal fetus, and is a more ominous pattern than that seen in Figure 34–7.

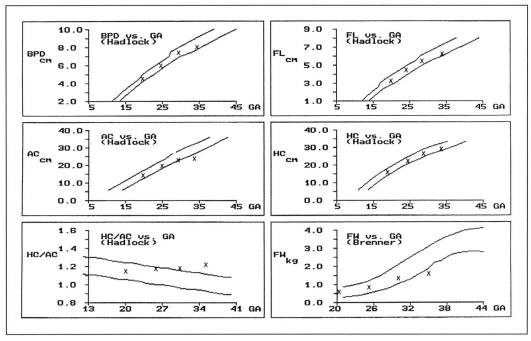

Figure 34-9—Graphic Plot of the Asymmetric Late-Onset IUGR Pattern. The fetus is initially normal in size but subsequently develops IUGR. Abdominal circumference growth is the most severely affected while the fetal head measurements remain normal. This head-sparing pattern is typical for placental insufficiency.

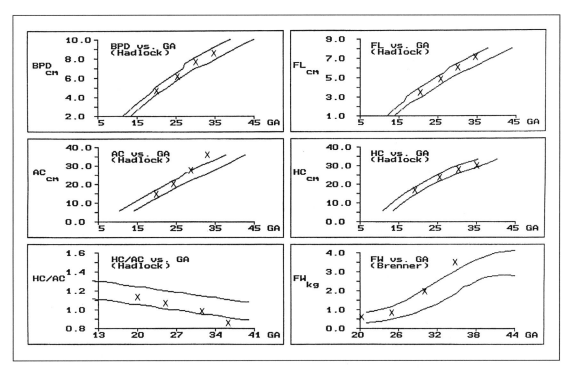

Figure 34-10—Graphic Plot of Macrosomia. Initially, the fetal size is normal. As pregnancy advances, the abdominal circumference growth is greater than expected and the estimated fetal weight exceeds the 90th percentile. This pattern is typical for macrosomia from maternal diabetes.

Table 34-1. Intrauterine Growth Retardation: Causes and Patterns

Causes	Classic Patterns
Primary placental insufficiency	Late onset; asymmetric
Maternal causes:	Late onset; asymmetric
Hypertension	
Collagen vascular disease	
Renal disease	
Uterine anomalies	
Uterine fibroids	
Chronic abruptions	
Poor nutrition	
Smoking, alcohol	
Pregnancy causes:	Early onset; symmetric
Infection	
Fetal causes:	Early onset; symmetric
Chromosomal anomalies (trisomy 18, trisomy 13, triploidy)	

practitioners and literature references use the terms SGA and IUGR synonymously.[16, 18, 21, 22] The most inclusive definition of IUGR is preferable, so that all fetuses at risk can be identified regardless of the cause of IUGR.[18] In our practice, we diagnose an increased risk for IUGR when a fetus is below the 10th percentile for gestational age, and we follow these pregnancies carefully. By definition, IUGR is seen in 10% of term pregnancies; however, the incidence is only 3% to 5% in a well-nourished, healthy population, and the incidence approaches 25% in women with hypertension or a previous IUGR fetus.[23–26]

IUGR Causes and Patterns

IUGR can result from many maternal or fetal causes, as outlined in Table 34–1, but placental insufficiency is the most common etiology.[18, 26] Primary placental insufficiency is a diagnosis of exclusion. Secondary placental insufficiency can result from maternal conditions such as hypertension, smoking, uterine anomalies, leiomyomas, and collagen vascular disease, to name but a few. Fetal or pregnancy-related causes of placental insufficiency include infection and chromosomal abnormalities. Trisomy 18, trisomy 13, and triploidy karyotypes, in particular, are associated with severe IUGR.[18, 26, 27]

Not all fetal body parts are symmetrically affected by growth retardation, and two IUGR patterns have been noted: the "head sparing" asymmetric pattern (Fig. 34–9), and the symmetric IUGR pattern, in which the fetus is uniformly small (Fig. 34–8).[18, 26–28] With asymmetric IUGR, the fetal abdomen is the smallest measurement, while the extremities and head measurements

remain normal for a longer period of time (until IUGR is quite severe). This pattern, dubbed "spare the head to spite the body," is explained by the following theory: The cross-section of the abdomen used for the AC measurement principally contains the liver (see Figure 33–4, Chapter 33). As the glycogen stores of the liver are depleted in the undernourished fetus, the liver decreases in size, and the AC, therefore, is the first measurement affected.[29] Symmetric IUGR, on the other hand, tends to involve the head, extremities, and abdomen. Even in symmetric IUGR, however, the abdomen is usually the most severely affected measurement.

In practice, the subdivision of IUGR into the symmetric and asymmetric varieties is not always possible or even helpful.[18, 20] Doubilet and Benson[18] plotted the HC/AC ratio in a large population of fetuses with growth retardation. Instead of the expected bimodal distribution, the HC/AC ratio showed a unimodal distribution, suggesting that the symmetric/asymmetric categories are, in fact, artifactual. We and others[18] find that the *time of onset* and the *severity* of the growth abnormality are more helpful for determining the cause and outcome of IUGR than the asymmetric/symmetric pattern. Severe, early IUGR is associated with a poorer prognosis than later-onset IUGR. Symmetric IUGR associated with chromosomal abnormalities carries a dismal prognosis and tends to occur early; therefore, we recommend genetic amniocentesis for all early IUGR cases (evident by 24 weeks). Late-onset IUGR (late third-trimester) is more likely associated with placental insufficiency, and with careful monitoring it has a better prognosis. The IUGR growth pattern also is helpful in determining the prognosis. The "small and getting smaller" fetus carries a poorer prognosis than the "initially normal but getting small" fetus.

Monitoring the IUGR Fetus

Weekly or semiweekly ultrasound examinations typically are needed for cases of *third-trimester* IUGR.[18] Monitoring of fetal growth (not more than once a week), amniotic fluid,

Table 34-2. Macrosomia Causes

Multiparity
Maternal age greater than 35 years
Maternal height greater than 169 cm
Prepregnancy weight greater than 70 kg
Post-term fetus (greater than 7 days)

Data from Spellacy WN, Miller S, Winegar A, et al: Macrosomia: Maternal characteristics and infant complications. Obstet Gynecol 66:158–161, 1985.

biophysical profile score, and umbilical artery Doppler waveforms is recommended. The trend in these measurements helps identify the fetus that may benefit from early delivery. The details of these monitoring efforts are discussed in Chapter 35.

MACROSOMIA

A fetus is considered macrosomic, or large for gestational age, if the estimated fetal weight is greater than the 90th percentile.[29-31] A birth weight greater than 4000 grams is also considered evidence for macrosomia.[32] The causes for macrosomia are summarized in Table 34–2.[33] An association between maternal diabetes and fetal macrosomia has been well established, yet only 2% of macrosomic babies are born to diabetic mothers.[32] Basically, most large babies are born to large mothers.[33]

Macrosomia, like IUGR, can also be categorized as symmetric or asymmetric. Macrosomia from diabetes tends to be asymmetric, with greater than expected fetal abdominal circumference measurements.[29] It is very important for the sonographer to identify the large-for-gestational age fetus so that early delivery may be planned, before the fetus reaches severely large proportions (greater than 4500 gm).

REFERENCES

1. Hadlock FP, Shah YP, Kanon DJ, et al: Fetal crown rump length: Evaluation of relation to menstrual age (5–18 weeks) with high resolution real US. Radiology 182:501–505, 1992.

2. Hadlock FP, Deter RL, Harrist RB, et al: Estimating fetal age: Computer-assisted analysis of multiple fetal growth parameters. Radiology 152:497–501, 1984.

3. Hadlock FP, Deter RL, Harrist RB, et al: Fetal biparietal diameter: A critical re-evaluation of the relation to menstrual age using real time ultrasound. J Ultrasound Med 1:97–104, 1982.

4. Hadlock FP, Deter RL, Harrist RB, et al: Fetal head circumference: Relation to menstrual age. AJR Am J Roentgenol 138:649–653, 1982.

5. Hadlock FP, Deter RL, Harrist RB, et al: Fetal abdominal circumference as a predictor of menstrual age. AJR Am J Roentgenol 139:367–370, 1982.

6. Hadlock FP, Deter RL, Harrist RB, et al: Fetal femur length as a predictor of menstrual age: Sonographically measured. AJR Am J Roentgenol 138:875–878, 1982.

7. Hadlock FP, Deter RL, Carpenter RJ, et al: The effect of head shape on the accuracy of BPD in estimating fetal gestational age. AJR Am J Roentgenol 137:83–85, 1981.

8. Gray DL, Songster GS, Parvin CA, et al: Cephalic index: A gestational age-independent biometric parameter. Obstet Gynecol 74:600–603, 1989.

9. Jeanty P, Cantraine F, Cousaert E, et al: The binocular distance: A new way to estimate fetal age. J Ultrasound Med 3:241–243, 1984.

10. Hill LM, Guzick D, Fries J, et al: The transverse cerebellar diameter in estimating gestational age in the large for gestational age fetus. Obstet Gynecol 75(6):981–985, 1990.

11. Hadlock FP, Harrist RB, Carpenter RJ, et al: Sonographic estimation of fetal weight: The value of femur length in addition to head and abdomen measurements. Radiology 150:535–540, 1984.

12. Campbell S, Wilkin D: Ultrasonic measurement of fetal abdominal circumference in the estimation of fetal weight. Br J Obstet Gynecol 82:689–697, 1975.

13. Hill LM, Guzick D, Hixson J, et al: Composite assessment of gestational age: A comparison of institutionally derived and published regression equations. Am J Obstet Gynecol 166:551–555, 1992.

14. Benson CB, Doubilet PM: Sonographic prediction of gestational age: Accuracy of second and third trimester fetal measurements. AJR Am J Roentgenol 157:1275–1277, 1991.

15. Hadlock FP, Harrist RB, Shah YP, et al: Estimating fetal age using multiple parameters: A prospective evaluation in a racially mixed population. Am J Obstet Gynecol 156:955–957, 1987.

16. Benson CB, Doubilet PM: Fetal measurements: Normal and abnormal fetal growth. *In* Rumack C, Charboneau W, Wilson S (eds): Diagnostic Ultrasound. St. Louis, Mosby–Year Book, 1992, pp 723–728.

17. Hadlock FP, Harrist RB, Martinez-Poyer J: In utero analysis of fetal growth: A sonographic weight standard. Radiology 181:129–133, 1991.

18. Doubilet PM, Benson CB: Sonographic evaluation of intrauterine growth retardation. AJR Am J Roentgenol 164:709–717, 1995.

19. Harvey D, Prince J, Bunton J, et al: Abilities of children who were small for gestational age babies. Pediatrics 69:296–300, 1982.

20. Chang TC, Robson SC, Boys RJ, et al: Prediction of the small for gestational age infant: Which ultrasonic measurement is best? Obstet Gynecol 80:1030–1038, 1992.

21. Doubilet PM, Benson CB: Fetal growth disturbances. Semin Roentgenol 15:309–316, 1990.

22. Romero R, Jeanty P: The detection of fetal growth disorders. Semin Ultrasound CT MR 5:130–143, 1984.

23. Lugo G, Cassady G: Intrauterine growth retardation: Clinicopathologic findings in 233 consecutive infants. Am J Obstet Gynecol 109:615–622, 1971.

24. Galbraith RS, Karchmar EJ, Piercy WN, et al: The clinical prediction of intrauterine growth retardation. Am J Obstet Gynecol 133:281–286, 1979.

25. Simon NC, Surosky BA, Shearer DM, et al: Effect of the pretest probability of intrauterine growth retardation on the predictiveness of sonographic estimated fetal weight in detecting IUGR: A clinical application of Bayes' theorem. J Clin Ultrasound 18:145–153, 1990.

26. Brar HS, Rutherford SE. Classification of intrauterine growth retardation. Semin Perinat 12:2–10, 1988.

27. Nyberg DA, Crane JP: Chromosome abnormalities. *In* Nyberg DA, Mahony BS, Pretorius DH (eds): Diagnostic Ultrasound of Fetal Anomalies: Text and Atlas. St Louis, CV Mosby, 1990, pp 676–724.

28. Crane JP, Kopta MM: Comparative newborn anthropometric data in symmetric versus

asymmetric intrauterine growth retardation. Am J Obstet Gynecol 138:518–522, 1980.

29. Hadlock FP: Ultrasound evaluation of fetal growth. *In* Callen PW (ed): Ultrasonography in Obstetrics and Gynecology. 3rd ed. Philadelphia, WB Saunders, 1994, pp 129–143.

30. Benson CB, Doubilet PM, Saltzman DH: Intrauterine growth retardation: Predictive value of US criteria for antenatal diagnosis. Radiology 160:415–417, 1986.

31. Hadlock FP, Deter RL, Harrist RB: Ultrasound detection of abnormal fetal growth patterns. *In* Platt LD (ed): Clinical Obstetrics and Gynecology. Philadelphia, JB Lippincott, 1984.

32. Boyd ME, Usher RH, McLean FH: Fetal macrosomia: Prediction risks, proposed management. Obstet Gynecol 61:715–722, 1983.

33. Spellacy WN, Miller S, Winegar A, et al: Macrosomia: Maternal characteristics and infant complications. Obstet Gynecol 66:158–161, 1985.

Chapter 35

Amniotic Fluid and Fetal Well-Being

Roya Sohaey

The objective for assessing fetal well-being is to identify the fetus at risk for in utero death or injury. Fetuses may be at risk because of maternal disease (such as diabetes or hypertension), fetal disease (e.g., anemia), or pregnancy-related disease (e.g., premature membrane rupture). With the use of real-time ultrasound, direct visualization of the fetus and its environment is possible, and an indirect "physical examination" can be conducted that provides important clues about how well the fetus is faring in its environment. These clues include the status of fetal growth, the environment itself (namely, the amniotic fluid status), the presence of fetal anomalies or other disorders, and certain aspects of fetal activity and physiology. Specific diagnostic tests (e.g., the Nonstress test, the Biophysical Profile, and umbilical artery Doppler) may be used to evaluate the physiologic status of the fetus and identify the fetus at risk for a poor outcome.

The goal of this chapter is to familiarize the ultrasound practitioner with assessment of amniotic fluid volume, with the clinical implications of oligo- and polyhydramnios, and with methods for assessing fetal well-being. It may seem odd to combine amniotic fluid and fetal well-being in a single chapter, but the fluid volume and well-being are closely linked, as you will quickly appreciate.

AMNIOTIC FLUID

Human embryos and fetuses are surrounded by amniotic fluid, the volume and composition of which change throughout pregnancy. The amniotic fluid volume increases steadily during the first half of pregnancy.[1]* In the second half of pregnancy, the fluid volume reaches a stable plateau and then declines sharply after 39 weeks. On average, the amniotic fluid volume is 777 ml between 22 and 39 weeks. Since the fluid volume is relatively stable and the fetal volume (size) increases steadily, the fetus occupies proportion-

ately more of the uterine cavity as the pregnancy progresses, and the volume of fluid *appears* to decrease. In fact, however, the 500-gm, 22-week fetus has an amniotic fluid volume (500 ml) that is similar to the 3500-gm, 39-week fetus (750 gm)![1] Considerable variability in amniotic fluid volume occurs from one pregnancy to another at any gestational age, and large variations occur even within the same pregnancy on serial measurements.[1, 2] The greatest variation occurs in the third trimester.[1] The cause for this variability is unknown, but the implications are clear: amniotic fluid flux is complex, and it is difficult to define normal parameters for ultrasound fluid assessment.

Fluid Composition and Production

The composition of amniotic fluid varies with the gestational age and with the mode of fluid production.[3] In the first trimester, amniotic fluid is isotonic with fetal and maternal blood, because the fluid represents a transudate from trophoblastic and fetal tissue.[4-6] The fluid easily crosses the embryonic or fetal skin before the skin cornifies (around 23 to 25 weeks).[7] Amniotic fluid generation gradually shifts from transudation to renal production at the end of the first and the beginning of the second trimesters.[3-7] At 10 to 11 weeks, the fetal kidneys begin excreting urine, and thereafter the kidneys play an increasing role in fluid generation.[8] The fetal kidneys are the main contributors to amniotic fluid production throughout the second and third trimesters,* and during this period, the fluid is hypo-osmolar, compared with fetal and maternal plasma.[4-6, 9] Hypo-osmolality is a key factor in fluid volume regulation, as will be seen later. The complexity of amniotic fluid volume regulation is illustrated by the fact that the fluid volume remains relatively stable even though fetal urinary output is

---

*Rate of increase is 25 ml per week during weeks 11 to 15, and 50 ml per week during weeks 15 to 28.

*If the idea of the fetus floating in a bath of urine sounds pretty gross, be comforted by the fact that metabolic waste products are removed by the placenta, and the composition of amniotic fluid is far different from urine produced in postnatal life.

estimated to increase from 5 ml per hour (120 ml per day) at 20 weeks to 51 ml per hour (1224 ml per day) at 40 weeks.[10]

The fetal lungs also contribute significantly to amniotic fluid production, beginning after 7 weeks, when communication is established between the posterior pharynx and the trachea. Whereas some amniotic fluid moves into the lungs, the net movement is *out* of the lungs and averages 10% of the fetal body weight *per day* in animal studies.[3, 8] The amount of amniotic fluid contributed by the lungs, therefore, is significant.

Fluid Removal

Fetal swallowing is the major means for amniotic fluid removal in the second and third trimesters, and it is estimated that fetal swallowing removes 200 to 500 ml of fluid per day near term.[11, 12] Swallowed amniotic fluid distends the fetal stomach, making the fluid-filled stomach visible on ultrasound as early as 9 weeks.[13] Nonvisualization of the fetal stomach later in gestation suggests swallowing problems or esophageal anomalies and is associated with significant morbidity.[14]

Urinary and pulmonary amniotic fluid production greatly exceed the rate of fluid removal by fetal swallowing; therefore, other important pathways for fluid removal must exist. By far the most important of these is intramembranous absorption at the fetal surface of the placenta, where fluid traverses the membranes directly and enters fetal blood perfusing the placenta.[15] This transfer occurs for two reasons; first, because a large osmotic gradient drives fluid from the amniotic space into fetal vessels (recall that amniotic fluid is hypo-osmolar), and second, because the placenta provides a fetal/maternal interface from which the fluid can ultimately be transferred to the maternal circulation. Intramembranous absorption volumes of 200 ml per day have been measured in sheep, accounting for the aforementioned difference between urinary and respiratory fluid production and removal by fetal swallowing.[15–17]

A much less important pathway for amniotic fluid removal is the transmembranous route, in which fluid crosses the amniotic membranes and enters the maternal circulation directly through vessels lining the uterine wall.[3, 17] The osmotic gradient, once again, favors fluid movement away from the amniotic cavity. This is a minor pathway compared with the intramembranous route described previously.

Table 35–1 summarizes the routes of amniotic fluid production and removal. An understanding of these pathways is important since it permits

Table 35-1. Second Trimester Amniotic Fluid Production and Removal

Production	Removal

Fetal kidneys:
  5 ml/hr at 20 wk
  50 ml/hr at 40 wk
Fetal lungs:
  10% of body weight/day
	Fetal swallowing:
	  10–20 ml/hr near term
	Intramembranous absorption:
	  Via placental surface
	Transmembranous absorption:
	  Via membranes

the ultrasound practitioner, in some cases, to suggest causes for an abnormal amniotic fluid volume.

ULTRASOUND ASSESSMENT OF AMNIOTIC FLUID

The direct measurement of amniotic fluid volume requires amniocentesis with dye instillation, followed by repeat amniocentesis and the calculation of dye dilution.[1, 18] Obviously, this method is impractical for everyday patient care. Ultrasound is a convenient alternative for fluid assessment, and the volume of fluid should be evaluated during every second or third trimester ultrasound study.[19, 20] A number of ultrasound techniques have been described for evaluating the fluid volume, but we will discuss only the three methods that are used most commonly.

Subjective Assessment

Subjective assessment of amniotic fluid relies on the ability of the sonographer to sense the overall amount of amniotic fluid present. Obviously, only experienced sonographers should use this technique. Early in the second trimester, the volume occupied by the fetus is about equal to the volume of amniotic fluid, and the fetus "swims" freely in a bath of fluid. Throughout the second and third trimesters, the relative volume of the fetus increases in comparison with the volume of fluid, and there is progressively more fetus than fluid. As the second trimester progresses, the fetus no longer "floats" freely. Late in pregnancy, the volume of fluid appears small in comparison with the fetus, and some fetal parts are almost always in contact with the anterior uterine wall.

Using the subjective ultrasound method of fluid assessment, oligohydramnios, or decreased amniotic fluid, is diagnosed when (1) there is obvious, marked lack of amniotic fluid; (2) when pockets of amniotic fluid are inordinately small; (3) when the volume of fluid is small relative to the fetal volume and the gestational age; and (4) when there is a sense of crowding of the fetus. Even in the third trimester, the sonographer should be able to identify oligohydramnios correctly if there is a sense of fetal crowding, or if sizable pockets of fluid cannot be found anywhere in the uterine cavity.[21] Polyhydramnios, or excessive fluid, is diagnosed subjectively when the overall fluid volume is disproportionately large with respect to the fetal volume and gestational age, and when the pockets of fluid are inordinately large.

The experienced sonographers at our institution use the subjective method for amniotic fluid assessment for routine ultrasound examination. Objective measurements (described next) are utilized when the fluid volume appears decreased or increased and in complicated obstetric cases, such as a uterus measuring small or large for dates, a fetus with intrauterine growth retardation, or a maternal condition such as hypertension.

Maximum Vertical Pocket

The maximum vertical pocket measurement is an objective means for assessing amniotic fluid volume. This method is based on a single measurement of the anteroposterior dimension (or "depth") of the largest pocket of amniotic fluid. The fluid pocket must be *void of fetal parts or umbilical cord*; color Doppler imaging is sometimes helpful in identifying, and thus avoiding, the umbilical cord. A pocket measuring between 2 and 8 cm is considered normal during the second and third trimesters. Oligo- or polyhydramnios is diagnosed when the largest pocket measures less or greater than the normal values, respectively.[22, 23] A pitfall of this method is lack of compensation for the gradual increase in amniotic fluid volume that occurs with advancing gestational age. Furthermore, the definition of oligohydramnios with this method is controversial and ranges from a pocket depth of less than 3 cm to less than 1 cm.[24]

In our institution, we use less than 2 cm as the cut-off, because this number corresponds to the "inadequate" fluid level defined in the biophysical profile scoring system (discussed later). Polyhydramnios may be characterized as mild, moderate, or severe: mild, vertical pocket 8 to 12 cm; moderate, between 12 and 16 cm; severe, greater than 16 cm.[25]

Amniotic Fluid Index

The amniotic fluid index (AFI) is another objective method for assessing amniotic fluid volume. The AFI is calculated from the sum of maximum fluid pockets in four quadrants of the uterus.[26, 27] The uterus is divided into four equal parts, as illustrated in Figure 35–1. In each quadrant, the largest pocket of amniotic fluid *void of fetal parts and umbilical cord* is measured, as just described for the maximum vertical pocket method. The sum of these measurements yields the amniotic fluid index (AFI), which varies with gestational age as shown in Figure 35–2. As a rule of thumb, the AFI is between 10 and 24 cm after 30 weeks' gestational age.

Oligohydramnios and polyhydramnios are suggested when the AFI is less than the 5th percentile or greater than the 95th percentile, respectively, for gestational age.[27] Some investigators suggest a diagnosis of oligohydramnios when the AFI is less than 5 cm, regardless of the gestational age.[28, 29]

The AFI is the most reproducible and valid of the three commonly used methods for assessing the volume of amniotic fluid,[19, 27, 30] and I recommend using the AFI when objective assessment of fluid volume is needed. It should be noted, however, that the AFI is more accurate for identifying normal fluid volume and polyhydramnios than for identifying oligohydramnios.[31, 32]

OLIGOHYDRAMNIOS

Oligohydramnios, defined as a deficiency in amniotic fluid, occurs in 0.5% to 5.5% of all

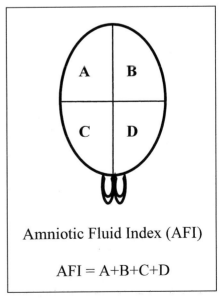

Figure 35-1—Amniotic Fluid Index (AFI) Calculation. Scheme of the uterus divided into four quadrants. The largest vertical pocket of fluid in each quadrant is measured in centimeters (A, B, C, D). This measurement should not include any fetal parts or umbilical cord, *only fluid*. The AFI is the sum of the four measurements.

	2.5th	5th	50th	95th	97.5th	n
16	73	79	121	185	201	32
17	77	83	127	194	211	26
18	80	87	133	202	220	17
19	83	90	137	207	225	14
20	86	93	141	212	230	25
21	88	95	143	214	233	14
22	89	97	145	216	235	14
23	90	98	146	218	237	14
24	90	98	147	219	238	23
25	89	97	147	221	240	12
26	89	97	147	223	242	11
27	85	95	146	226	245	17
28	86	94	146	228	249	25
29	84	92	145	231	254	12
30	82	90	145	234	258	17
31	79	88	144	238	263	26
32	77	86	144	242	269	25
33	64	83	143	245	274	30
34	72	81	142	248	278	31
35	70	79	140	249	279	27
36	68	77	138	249	279	39
37	66	75	135	244	275	36
38	65	73	132	239	269	27
39	64	72	127	226	255	12
40	63	71	123	214	240	64
41	63	70	116	194	216	162
42	63	69	110	175	192	30

Figure 35-2—Comparison of Amniotic Fluid Index (AFI) Values with Gestational Age (Weeks). The AFI can be compared with the gestational age (left vertical column) in order to diagnose oligohydramnios or polyhydramnios accurately. A value less than the 5th or greater than the 95th percentile is considered abnormal. (With permission from Moore TR, Gayle JE: The amniotic fluid index in normal human pregnancy. Am J Obstet Gynecol 162:1168–1173, 1990.)

pregnancies.[24] It can be devastating, as indicated by a perinatal mortality rate (for severe cases) that is 40 to 50 times greater than that of normal pregnancies.[22, 24] Many potential causes for oligohydramnios exist,[25] as summarized in Table 35–2, and the sonographer should search diligently for any cause that can be identified with ultrasound.

Premature Rupture of Membranes

Premature rupture of membranes (PROM) occurs in 10% of pregnancies and represents one of the most common causes of oligohydramnios.[33] PROM is associated with an increased risk of maternal and fetal sepsis, premature delivery, and perinatal mortality. The severity of oligohydramnios has a direct bearing on the severity of PROM complications[24, 34, 35]; therefore, ultrasound fluid assessment is central in following pregnancies complicated by PROM. At our institution, women with viable fetuses (greater than 24 weeks) and PROM are examined with ultrasound at least weekly, and often twice a week, to monitor the amniotic fluid volume. PROM per

Table 35-2. Common Causes of Oligohydramnios

Pregnancy-related
 Premature rupture of membranes
 Postdate pregnancy

Fetal Causes
 Congenital anomalies: Genitourinary
 Chromosomal abnormalities
 Fetal demise
 Intrauterine growth retardation (IUGR)

Maternal Causes
 Placental insufficiency: Primary or secondary
 Placental abruption

Pharmaceutical Causes
 Prostaglandin synthetase inhibitors
 Angiotensin-converting enzyme inhibitors

Idiopathic

se is not an ultrasound diagnosis; therefore, from an ultrasound perspective, PROM is a diagnosis of exclusion, and other causes for oligohydramnios should always be considered. The diagnosis of PROM requires the evaluation of vaginal pool material for alkaline pH and ferning.[33] Definitive diagnosis may require ultrasound-guided intra-amniotic injection of 5ml of indigo carmine dye followed by observation for leakage of blue-colored vaginal secretions.

Fetal Anomalies

The majority of anomalies associated with oligohydramnios involve the genitourinary tract, and these are discussed in detail in Chapter 42. Anomalies resulting in deficient fetal urine production include bilateral renal agenesis or dysplasia, obstruction of urinary outflow, and nephropathy resulting from vesicoureteral reflux.[24, 25] Since amniotic fluid production early in pregnancy does not involve the kidneys,[4-6] fetuses with renal anomalies can have a normal fluid volume early in pregnancy and oligohydramnios in the second and third trimesters (Fig. 35–3).

Severe oligohydramnios may limit the visualization of fetal anatomy, making it difficult to diagnose urinary tract or other anomalies. In such cases, warm, sterile, normal saline or an isotonic electrolyte solution may be instilled into

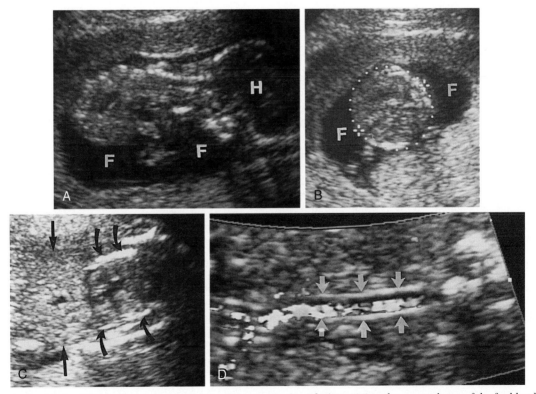

Figure 35-3—Oligohydramnios from Renal Agenesis. (A and B) At 13.5 weeks, a sagittal view of the fetal head (H) and chest and also a transverse view of the fetal abdomen (ellipse) show amniotic fluid (F) surrounding the fetus. At this stage, a substantial amount of amniotic fluid production is still from transudation via fetal skin, and the fetal kidneys play a lesser role in fluid production. **(C)** At 21 weeks, a coronal view through the fetal chest (curved arrows) and trunk (straight arrows) shows complete absence of amniotic fluid. No fetal bladder or kidneys were seen. **(D)** Color Doppler investigation of the aorta (arrows) shows absence of renal arteries. The diagnosis of renal agenesis was confirmed at autopsy.

the amniotic cavity to facilitate sonographic visualization.[36] In addition, transvaginal ultrasound may enhance visualization of fetal anatomy.[37] With these techniques, it may be possible to answer the all-important question: "Are fetal kidneys present?" If ultrasound is unsuccessful, in our institution we use magnetic resonance imaging to look for the fetal kidneys, but this approach usually is not needed.

Intrauterine Growth Retardation

Oligohydramnios is often associated with intrauterine growth retardation (IUGR),[24, 25] which is considered in Chapter 34. In essence, any condition that causes IUGR also causes oligohydramnios. Conversely, oligohydramnios is a clinical hallmark for IUGR, and its presence helps identify the growth-retarded fetus. Oligohydramnios probably occurs in the IUGR fetus because of hypoxia. The fetus tries to "fight" hypoxia through redistribution of blood flow to the brain, resulting in decreased profusion of the kidneys and lungs.[24, 38] Studies have documented reduced urine production in growth-retarded fetuses.[9, 39, 40]

Postdate Pregnancy

In the last few weeks of pregnancy, the amniotic fluid volume declines normally, at an estimated rate of 33% per week.[24, 41] Changes in amniotic fluid volume can occur quickly, however, in the postdate pregnancy, and these pregnancies are at an increased risk for developing rapid and severe oligohydramnios that is closely linked with serious complications, including fetal acidosis, fetal distress, and low Apgar scores.[42] Postdate pregnancies with normal amounts of amniotic fluid are at much less risk for such complications. Frequent ultrasound examinations are warranted in postdate pregnancies to assess both the amniotic fluid volume and fetal well-being.

POLYHYDRAMNIOS

Polyhydramnios, or an excess of amniotic fluid, is a common problem that complicates 1% to 4% of all pregnancies.[43] Polyhydramnios, like oligohydramnios, is associated with significant maternal and fetal morbidity; therefore, prenatal identification of this condition is important. Objective ultrasound measurements of amniotic fluid volume should be made whenever subjective assessment suggests polyhydramnios. In addition, the cause of polyhydramnios should be diligently sought.

The causes of polyhydramnios can be categorized as idiopathic, maternal, and fetal, as summarized in Table 35–3. Factors that suggest the cause of polyhydramnios include the gestational age at which the fluid volume becomes excessive, the severity of polyhydramnios, the size of the fetus, the maternal medical history, and the presence of fetal anomalies. The age of onset and the severity of polyhydramnios are predictive of both the cause of the condition and the prognosis. Early onset is associated with increased likelihood of serious problems, such as infection or severe congenital anomaly. Severe polyhydramnios also predicts significant problems and is associated with a postnatal fetal survival rate of only 46% (principally because of a high incidence of congenital anomalies). In comparison, a survival rate of 81% can be expected with mild polyhydramnios, which is less commonly associated with congenital anomalies and life-threatening conditions.[25, 44]

Idiopathic Polyhydramnios

Most cases of polyhydramnios are idiopathic, and generally these cases are mild in severity. Conversely, two thirds of mild polyhydramnios cases are idiopathic.[44] An association has been shown recently between idiopathic polyhydramnios and large-for-gestational-age fetuses, even in the absence of maternal diabetes.[43, 45] This association suggests that idiopathic polyhydramnios may simply represent the somewhat overhydrated state of the larger-than-expected fetus. As the severity of polyhydramnios increases, it becomes more likely that the condition is due to a maternal or fetal abnormality—i.e., is not idiopathic.[44]

Table 35-3. Causes of Polyhydramnios

Idiopathic
   60%–70% of all cases
   Associated with large fetuses
   Usually mild or moderate

Maternal Condition
   Diabetes mellitus: Primary or gestational
                        15–23% of all cases
   Rh incompatibility: Less than 1% of all cases

Pregnancy Causes
   Infection: Cytomegalovirus, toxoplasmosis, others
   Twin-twin Transfusion: Larger twin with
                            polyhydramnios
                          Smaller twin with
                            oligohydramnios

Fetal Anomalies:
   See Table 35–4

Maternal and Pregnancy Causes

Gestational diabetes and insulin-dependent diabetes account for 15% to 25% of polyhydramnios cases and represent the most common maternal cause of excessive amniotic fluid.[44, 46] Polyhydramnios may be severe in these cases. The incidence of polyhydramnios is reduced in diabetic mothers by rigid glucose control during pregnancy.[25, 44] Erythroblastosis fetalis is another well-recognized maternal cause of polyhydramnios. This condition results from Rh blood incompatibility between the mother and fetus, causing fetal red blood cell destruction, anemia, fetal hydrops, and associated polyhydramnios. Rh incompatibility accounted for 12% of polyhydramnios cases in 1970, but less than 1% of cases in 1987 owing to the widespread use of Rh immune globulin.[44, 46] Overall, the prevalence of polyhydramnios from maternal causes should continue to decrease in the future as pregnancies are monitored more carefully and women seek prenatal care earlier.

Pregnancy-related causes of polyhydramnios include congenital infections and the twin-twin transfusion syndrome. Cytomegalovirus, toxoplasmosis, listeriosis, and congenital hepatitis are a few of the viral diseases that may infect a pregnancy and cause polyhydramnios.[25] Sonographic clues that suggest infection include growth retardation and fetal cranial or liver calcifications. The twin-twin transfusion syndrome is an uncommon entity caused by communication between the placental circulations of twins. This condition results in massive polyhydramnios in one twin's gestation and severe oligohydramnios, as discussed in Chapter 44.

Fetal Anomalies

Severe polyhydramnios is associated with an increased risk of fetal chromosome anomalies,[44] but chromosome anomalies are only evident sonographically when they cause secondary structural abnormalities in the fetus. In general, fetal anomalies causing polyhydramnios tend to involve the central nervous system, the gastrointestinal tract, the cardiovascular system, the musculoskeletal system, and the genitourinary tract.[25, 47] Basically, any anomaly that tips amniotic fluid balance toward increased production *or* decreased resorption of fluid can cause polyhydramnios. The anomalies that produce polyhydramnios and associated causes of excess fluid are outlined in Table 35–4. Please review this table for important details not included in the text. Ultrasound can correctly identify 90% to 95% of fetal anomalies causing severe polyhydramnios (Fig. 35–4).[47]

DETECTING FETAL DISTRESS

As mentioned previously, ultrasound-based fetal assessment allows for in utero "physical examination" that may be used to identify the distressed fetus that is at risk for a poor outcome. Many situations put the fetus at risk, but three major categories of disease particularly threaten the fetus: (1) fetal asphyxiation; (2) fetal anoma-

Table 35–4. Fetal Anomalies Associated with Polyhydramnios

Fetal Anomaly	Cause for Polyhydramnios
Central Nervous System Disorder	Fetal swallowing depressed Polyhydramnios seen after 25 wk
Gastrointestinal Disorders Bowel atresia: Esophageal, duodenal, jejunal, ileal Bowel obstruction: Volvulus, meconium ileus, abdominal wall defects, diaphragmatic hernia	Amount of amniotic fluid swallowed greater than amount of amniotic fluid absorbed
Facial and Neck Disorders Neck masses: Teratoma, goiter Facial clefts	Obstruction to swallowing Ineffective swallowing
Fetal Masses	Masses produce fluid or may cause bowel obstruction
Cardiovascular Anomalies	Heart failure causes decreased renal perfusion and hydrops
Hydrops: Any cause	Polyhydramnios often the earliest finding, high-output state
Unilateral Renal Anomaly Ureteropelvic junction obstruction, multicystic dysplastic kidney	Glomerular hypertrophy Hormonally induced polyuria
Skeletal Anomalies Dwarfism, osteogenesis imperfecta, arthrogryposis	Etiology unknown: Normal fetal movement seems to be necessary for normal amniotic fluid volume

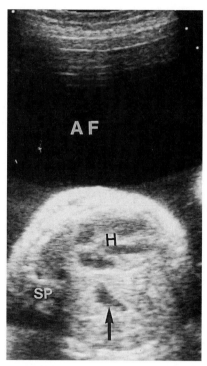

Figure 35-4—Polyhydramnios. A large amount of amniotic fluid (AF) is present, and the fetus is displaced from the anterior uterine wall. Transverse view of the fetal chest (SP = spine) shows that the heart (H) is displaced to the right because the fetal stomach (arrow) is in the chest in this fetus with a large, left-sided diaphragmatic hernia. The mass effect upon the esophagus leads to a decreased amount of swallowed fluid and subsequent polyhydramnios.

lies; and (3) diseases acquired in utero.[48] When prenatal testing is not utilized, fetal asphyxia is the most frequent immediate cause of fetal morbidity and mortality,[48, 49] but the fetal death rate from asphyxia is decreased substantially when the biophysical profile examination (described later) is used to detect physiologic depression that is a sign of asphyxia.[48–50]

Fetal Asphyxia

Asphyxia, which occurs when the fetus does not receive enough oxygen, may be transient or chronic. Either multiple transient episodes of asphyxia or continuous chronic asphyxia may lead to changes in fetal activity and amniotic fluid status. Asphyxia affects many organ systems, and as an adaptive measure, the fetus can shunt blood from "nonvital" organs (such as kidneys) to supply more "vital" organs such as the brain.[48–51] The redistribution of blood flow may lead to diminished amniotic fluid production by the kidneys and severe oligohydramnios.[22, 48] Even though the fetus does its best to protect the brain, this organ is sensitive to even mild

degrees of hypoxemia or acidosis. The results of cerebral hypoxemia include apnea (cessation of breathing movement in utero), decreased fetal movement and tone, and reduced variability of the fetal heart rate.[48–56] A strong correlation has been demonstrated between the biophysical profile score and umbilical cord blood pH (proving acidosis and asphyxia).[57]

The Biophysical Profile

Many parameters of fetal activity can be monitored to detect the adverse effects of asphyxia, but at our institution we have chosen the time-tested, well-documented parameters that Manning defined as the fetal biophysical profile (BPP).[48] A summary of this technique is presented in Table 35–5. In total, five variables are assessed that reflect the physiologic state of the fetus: the amniotic fluid volume, fetal movement, fetal tone, fetal breathing, and heart rate variability. Each of the five variables is scored as 2 points if the fetus meets the diagnostic criteria for that parameter. A score of 0 is given if the fetus "fails" the test. The final BPP score is the sum of the individual variables, and it may range from 0 to 10.

Before presenting the technical details of the

Table 35-5. The Biophysical Profile Test

Fetal Parameter (30 min. observation)	Score: 2 or 0
Amniotic Fluid	At least one pocket of fluid measuring 2 cm in perpendicular planes = 2 points No pockets measuring 2 cm in perpendicular planes = 0 points
Fetal Movement	At least three discrete gross body (limb and/or trunk) movements = 2 points Less than three movements = 0 points
Fetal Tone	At least one episode of limb extension (from flexion) with return to flexion = 2 points No extension/flexion or sluggish movement with failure to fully flex = 0 points
Fetal Breathing	At least one episode of breathing lasting 30 seconds = 2 points No breathing or breathing lasting less than 30 seconds = 0 points
Nonstress Test	At least two episodes of heart rate acceleration greater than 15 bpm for at least 15 sec duration = 2 points Less than above = 0 points

biophysical profile, you should understand three things. First, the goal of the test is to identify the at-risk fetus for which intervention is possible. Therefore, BPP testing at our institution (and at Manning's) is rarely performed prior to 25 weeks, since postnatal survival is unlikely prior to that gestational age. Second, the BPP examination must be conducted precisely and knowledgeably, since many important obstetric decisions are based on the BPP score. Everyone involved with the care of the patient, including the sonographer, must know how to perform the test correctly and what the scoring means. Third, fetuses, like all humans, have times of rest and times of activity. Therefore, a "quick" BPP examination is usually not possible, and both patience and attention are prerequisites for this test. The fetus is allowed 30 minutes to try to meet the physiologic criteria.

Variable One, Amniotic Fluid Volume. An inadequate fluid volume is the most significant (ominous) finding in the BPP test.[22, 54] For the pregnancy to receive a normal score of 2, at least one pocket of amniotic fluid (free of umbilical cord and fetal parts) should be seen that measures 2 cm or greater in vertical and transverse planes that are perpendicular. If the amount of fluid does not meet this strict criterion, the score is 0.

Variable Two, Fetal Breathing. Breathing movements are a normal feature of second- and third-trimester fetal life, but they are not present continuously. These movements are seen easily with ultrasound on coronal or sagittal planes that include the fetal diaphragm (Chapter 33). To receive a score of 2, at least one episode of breathing movement lasting at least 30 seconds should be seen during a 30-minute observation period. A score of 0 is given if this criterion is not met. Absence of fetal breathing movements is a relatively early sign of hypoxemia, whereas decreased fetal movement and tone are more indicative of chronic hypoxemia.[23, 50]

Variables Three and Four, Fetal Movement and Tone. Gross fetal body movements are common after the first trimester. To receive a BPP score of 2, the fetus must demonstrate at least three discrete gross body movements during a 30-minute period. A single movement that involves both the trunk and a limb is considered one gross body movement, not two. Furthermore, the movements should be separated by a time interval, albeit usually small. A long episode of continuous activity is regarded as only one movement.

Gross fetal body movement is not the same as fetal tone. A fetus with normal tone assumes a flexed position overall and frequently flexes and

extends its extremities. For a score of 2 in the tone category, the fetus must demonstrate at least one episode, during 30 minutes of observation, of active extension of a limb or the trunk, followed by *prompt* return to flexion (i.e., flexion to extension and back to flexion). When the amniotic fluid volume is low and fetal motion is restricted by limited space, opening and closing of a hand is considered normal tone. The fetus receives a score of 0 if extension is sluggish, if the return to flexion is partial, or if flexion-extension movements are absent.

Variable Five, The Nonstress Test. This examination usually is not performed by a sonographer or with the aid of ultrasound imaging. Although the nonstress test (NST) is an important BPP variable, this component often is excluded if the sonographic variables previously discussed are normal.[48] In this circumstance, the NST adds little information about fetal well-being.[23]

The NST uses nonimaging Doppler ultrasound to record fetal heart rate and a tocodynamometer to document fetal movements. Fetal heart rate reactivity is considered normal, and is given a score of 2, if at least two accelerations (exceeding 15 beats per minute and lasting 15 or more seconds) occur in association with fetal movement during a 30-minute observation period. The score for the NST is 0 if, after 30 minutes of monitoring, the fetus does not demonstrate the requisite two episodes of heart rate acceleration.

Clinical Significance of the BPP Score

Once again, let us stress that the amniotic fluid score is the most important indicator of fetal well-being. If the amniotic fluid volume is scored as 2, an overall BPP score of 8/10 holds the same prognostic significance as a score of 10/10, and in that circumstance the 8/10 score is considered normal.[48] If all the sonographic criteria are met, the NST often is excluded, as discussed previously. The resultant BPP score is 8/10 (still normal). If, on the other hand, the ultrasound score is 6/8 (e.g., absent fetal breathing movements), an NST would be performed immediately at our institution. If the NST is normal, then the score 8/10 would be considered normal. The risk for fetal asphyxia is extremely low (perinatal mortality, 1 per 1000 within 1 week of examination), with a normal BPP score defined as 10/10, 8/10 with normal fluid, or 8/8 without an NST.[48]

The presence of oligohydramnios, regardless of the BPP score, is associated with increased perinatal mortality. For example, a score of 8/10 or 6/10 with oligohydramnios implies a perinatal mortality rate of 89/1000 without intervention and is an indication for delivery.[48] On the other hand, a score of 6/10, with normal fluid, is equivocal. In this circumstance, most obstetricians choose to deliver the fetus if lung maturity is likely. Alternatively, the fetus may be followed closely with a repeat BPP within 24 hours, if lung maturity is not assured.

A BPP score of 4/10 or less is associated with a higher risk for fetal asphyxia. Perinatal mortality is reported as 91 per 1000 for a score of 4/10, 125 per 1000 for 2/10, and 600 per 1000 for 0/10. Fetuses with scores of 4 or less usually are delivered immediately, without much concern for lung maturity test results.

The greatest strength of the BPP is a very low false-negative rate (0.68/1000).[55, 56] That is to say: if the test is normal, there is little chance that the fetus is hypoxemic. Since 98% of BPP tests in a high-risk population are normal,[48] the clinician can feel justified in practicing conservative management for the pregnancy until lung maturity or a favorable cervix is achieved.

Fetal Doppler Examination

Considering the importance of identifying the hypoxic fetus, the sonographer should use all the tools available for identifying fetal asphyxia. In addition to the BPP, Doppler ultrasound assessment of the fetoplacental circulation can help identify the hypoxic fetus noninvasively. Umbilical artery Doppler examination has been shown to be a sensitive indicator of fetal acidosis (related to hypoxemia) in fetuses without structural anomalies.[58] Absolute blood flow volume through the umbilical cord is difficult to determine with Doppler techniques, because umbilical cord tortuosity precludes the accurate assignment of a Doppler angle. On the other hand, Doppler waveform analysis, such as the systolic/diastolic (S/D) ratio, does not require Doppler angle correction. Umbilical artery waveform analysis is easy to perform, and represents a practical way to assess the fetoplacental circulation. It is used in most clinical centers.[59–61] The S/D ratio compares the peak systolic frequency with the end diastolic frequency, as shown in Figure 35–5. With advancing gestational age, flow resistance in the placental circulation decreases, and as a result the S/D ratio decreases as the fetus matures. This normal decrease in the S/D ratio occurs because decreased resistance is accompanied by increased diastolic flow. After 30 weeks, the S/D ratio normally is less than 3.[61] Falsely elevated S/D ratios may be obtained if the fetus is breathing rapidly or experiencing fetal brady-

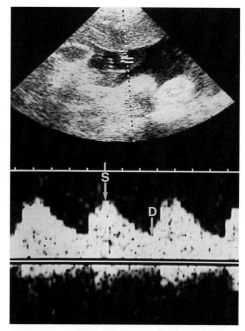

Figure 35-5—Normal Umbilical Cord Doppler Waveform. Pulsed Doppler interrogation of a free loop of umbilical cord shows this normal arterial waveform. The peak systolic/end diastolic ratio can be calculated by dividing the frequency value at peak systole (S) by the frequency value at end diastole (D). After 30 weeks, the S/D ratio is usually less than 3.0, as seen in this case.

cardia (heart rate less than 110) at the time of sampling[62]; therefore, sampling should be performed during fetal "quiet time" when possible. A free loop of cord should be sampled with a sample volume of 5 to 10 mm, excluding venous flow. If the umbilical artery is sampled too close to the fetal abdomen, the resistance may be falsely elevated. Alternatively, sampling too close to the placenta may yield a falsely low resistive pattern.[61]

An abnormal umbilical Doppler examination in a high-risk pregnancy should alert the sonographer to an increased risk for fetal compromise (Fig. 35–6). Absent end diastolic flow or reversed diastolic flow in the umbilical artery is an ominous finding that correlates with increased fetal morbidity and mortality.[56, 63, 64] In one series, absent end diastolic flow was associated with a 16% mortality rate,[63] and in another series, reversed diastolic flow was associated with a 50% fetal mortality rate.[64] We find the cord Doppler assessment a valuable complement to the BPP when the amniotic fluid volume is borderline, or when the BPP score is 6 (equivocal examination). In these cases, the Doppler examination provides another clue about whether the fetus is doing poorly in its environment.

As mentioned, the compromised fetus has the

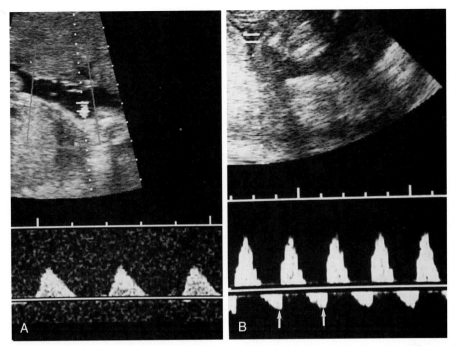

Figure 35-6—Abnormal Umbilical Cord Doppler Waveforms. (A) The umbilical artery waveform in this fetus with severe intrauterine growth retardation shows a very high resistive pattern with absent diastolic flow (compare with Figure 35–5). (B) The umbilical artery waveform in this fetus with twin-twin transfusion syndrome shows reversal of diastolic flow (arrows), an ominous sign often associated with fetal demise. The twins were too young to deliver, and this fetus died 48 hours after the ultrasound examination. The other twin survived.

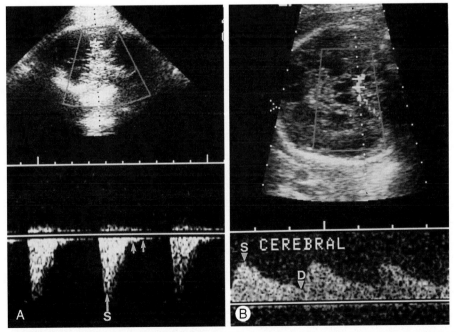

Figure 35-8—Middle Cerebral Artery (MCA) Doppler Waveform. In the third trimester, the normal MCA waveform shows a high resistive flow pattern (A), with little diastolic flow seen. Typically, the S/D ratio in the MCA is greater than 4.0. Compare this waveform with Figure 35–5. (S = peak systolic frequency, arrows = small amount of diastolic flow.) (B) The compromised fetus, in "brain-sparing" mode, demonstrates a lower than expected resistive flow pattern in the brain (note the increased diastolic flow). This fetus with intrauterine growth retardation had a high resistive pattern in the cord (same fetus as in Figure 35–6A). The reversal in ratios (between cord and brain Doppler) is associated with an increased risk for perinatal death. This fetus was delivered within hours after the ultrasound examination and survived. (S = systolic peak; D = end diastole.)

ability to spare its brain when "the going gets tough." Doppler examination of the brain circulation allows the sonographer to document this phenomenon. By obtaining an axial image at the skull base, the circle of Willis can usually be seen well with color Doppler (see Figure 35–7, following page 268). The middle cerebral artery, as it exits from the circle of Willis, can be sampled and waveform analysis performed. In the well-oxygenated fetus, the middle cerebral artery S/D ratio is greater than 4.0, and little diastolic flow is present.[65] Thus, the normal fetal brain exhibits relatively high flow resistance. The compromised fetus, in the "brain-sparing" mode, demonstrates lower than expected middle cerebral artery flow resistance and a lower S/D ratio (Fig. 35–8). The normal umbilical cord S/D ratio is usually *less than* the middle cerebral artery S/D ratio, but this relationship is reversed in the severely compromised fetus. The reversal of these ratios seems to be a good predictor for outcome in stressed fetuses. In a study of 120 small-for-gestational-age fetuses, perinatal fetal deaths occurred only in fetuses in which the relationship between flow resistance in the umbilical artery and the middle cerebral artery was reversed.[65, 66]

REFERENCES

1. Brace RA, Wolf EJ: Characterization of normal gestational changes in amniotic fluid volume. Am J Obstet Gynecol 161:382–388, 1989.
2. Queehnan JT, Thompson W, Whitfield CR, et al: Amniotic fluid volumes in normal pregnancies. Am J Obstet Gynecol 114:34–38, 1972.
3. Gilbert WM, Brace RA: Amniotic fluid volume and normal flows to and from the amniotic cavity. Semin Perinat 17:150–157, 1993.
4. Lind T, Cheyne GA: Biochemical and cytological changes in liquor amnii with advancing gestation. J Obstet Gynaecol Br Commonw 76:673–683, 1969.
5. Gillibrand PN: Changes in the electrolytes, urea and osmolality of the amniotic fluid with advancing pregnancy. J Obstet Gynaecol Br Commonw 76:898–905, 1969.
6. Benzie RJ, Doran TA, Harkin JL, et al: Composition of the amniotic fluid and maternal serum in pregnancy. Am J Obstet Gynecol 119:798–810, 1974.
7. Parmley TH, Seeds AE: Fetal skin permeability to isotopic water (THO) in early pregnancy. Am J Obstet Gynecol 108:128–131, 1970.
8. Moore KL: The urogenital system. *In* The Developing Human: Clinically Oriented Embryology. 4th ed. Philadelphia, WB Saunders, 1988, pp 246–285.
9. Wladimiroff JW, Campbell S: Fetal urine production rates in normal and complicated pregnancy. Lancet 1:151–154, 1974.
10. Rabinowitz R, Peters MT, Vyas S, et al: Measurement of fetal urine production in normal pregnancy by real time ultrasonography. Am J Obstet Gynecol 161:1264–1266, 1989.
11. Abramovich DR, Garden A, Jancial L, et al: Fetal swallowing and voiding in relation to hydramnios. Obstet Gynecol 54:15–20, 1979.
12. Pritchard JA: Deglutition by normal and anencephalic fetuses. Obstet Gynecol 25:289–297, 1965.
13. Goldstein I, Reede EA, Yarkoni S, et al: Growth of the fetal stomach in normal pregnancy. Obstet Gynecol 70:641–644, 1987.
14. Millener PB, Anderson NG, Chisholm RJ: Prognostic significance of nonvisualization of the fetal stomach by sonography. AJR Am J Roentgenol 160:827–830, 1993.
15. Gilbert WM, Brace RA: The missing link in amniotic fluid volume regulation: Intramembranous absorption. Obstet Gynecol 74:748–754, 1989.
16. Gilbert WM, Brace RA: Novel determination of filtration coefficient of ovine placenta and intramembranous pathway. Am J Physiol 259:R1281–1288, 1990.
17. Gilbert WM, Moore TR, Brace RA: Amniotic fluid volume dynamics. Fetal Med Rev 3:89–104, 1991.
18. Williams K: Amniotic fluid assessment. Obstet Gynecol Surv 48:795–800, 1993.
19. American Institute of Ultrasound in Medicine: 1994 Guidelines for Performance of the Antepartum Obstetrical Ultrasound Examination. AIUM Executive Office, 14750 Sweitzer Lane, Suite 100, Laurel, MD 20707–5906.
20. American College of Radiology: ACR Standards for Antepartum Obstetrical Ultrasound, 1995. American College of Radiology, 1891 Preston White Drive, Reston, VA 22091.
21. Phillipson EH, Sokol RJ, Williams T: Oligohydramnios: Clinical associations and predictive value for intrauterine growth retardation. Am J Obstet Gynecol 146:271–278, 1983.
22. Chamberlain PF, Manning FA, Morrison I, et al: Ultrasound evaluation of amniotic fluid volume. I: The relationship of marginal and decreased amniotic fluid volumes to perinatal outcome. Am J Obstet Gynecol 150:245–249, 1984.
23. Manning FA, Platt LD, Sipos L: Antepartum fetal evaluation: Development of a fetal biophysical profile. Am J Obstet Gynecol 136:787–795, 1980.
24. Piepert JF, Donnenfeld AE: Oligohydramnios: A review. Obstet Gynecol Surv 46:325–339, 1991.
25. Hill LM: Abnormalities of amniotic fluid. *In* Nyberg DA, Mahony BS, Pretorius DH (eds): Diagnostic Ultrasound of Fetal Anomalies: Text and Atlas. St Louis, CV Mosby, 1990, pp 38–66.
26. Phelan JP, Smith CV, Broussard P, et al: Amniotic fluid volume assessment with the four quadrant technique at 36–42 weeks' gestation. J Reprod Med 32:540–542, 1987.
27. Moore TR, Gayle JE: The amniotic fluid index in normal human pregnancy. Am J Obstet Gynecol 162:1168–1173, 1990.
28. Nimrod C, Varela-Gittings F, Machin D, et al: The effect of very prolonged membrane rupture on fetal development. Am J Obstet Gynecol 148:540–543, 1984.
29. Phelan JP, Ahn O, Smith CV, et al: Amniotic fluid index measurements during pregnancy. J Reprod Med 32:601–604, 1987.
30. Moore TR: Superiority of the four quadrant sum over the single deepest pocket technique in ultrasonographic identification of abnormal amniotic fluid volumes. Am J Obstet Gynecol 163:762–767, 1990.
31. Croom CS, Banias BB, Ramos-Santos E, et al: Do

semiquantitative amniotic fluid indexes reflect actual volume? Am J Obstet Gynecol 167:995–999, 1992.

32. Magann EF, Nolan TE, Hess LW, et al: Measurement of amniotic fluid volume: Accuracy of ultrasonography techniques. Am J Obstet Gynecol 167:1533–1537, 1992.

33. Mead PB: Management of the patient with premature rupture of the membranes. Clin Perinatol 7:243, 1980.

34. Gonik B, Bottoms SF, Cotton DB: Amniotic fluid volume as a risk factor in preterm premature rupture of the membranes. Obstet Gynecol 65:456–459, 1985.

35. Vintzileos AM, Campbell WA, Nochimson DJ, et al: Degree of oligohydramnios and pregnancy outcome in patients with premature rupture of the membranes. Obstet Gynecol 66:162–167, 1985.

36. Gembruch U, Hansmann M: Artificial instillation of amniotic fluid as a new technique for the diagnostic evaluation of cases of oligohydramnios. Prenat Diagn 8:33–45, 1988.

37. Benacerraf BR: Examination of the second trimester fetus with severe oligohydramnios using transvaginal scanning. Obstet Gynecol 75:491–493, 1990.

38. Manning FA, Hill LM, Platt LD: Qualitative amniotic fluid volume determination by ultrasound: Antepartum detection of intrauterine growth retardation. Am J Obstet Gynecol 139:254–258, 1981.

39. Kurjak A, Kirkinen P, Latin V, et al: Ultrasonic assessment of fetal kidney function in normal and complicated pregnancies. Am J Obstet Gynecol 144:266–270, 1982.

40. Deutinger J, Bartl W, Pfersman C, et al: Fetal kidney volume and urine production in cases of fetal growth retardation. J Perinat Med 15:307–315, 1987.

41. Elliot PM, Inman WHW: Volume of amniotic fluid in normal and abnormal pregnancy. Lancet 2:835–840, 1961.

42. Clement D, Schifirin BS, Kates RB: Acute oligohydramnios in post-date pregnancy. Am J Obstet Gynecol 157:884–886, 1987.

43. Sohaey R, Nyberg DA, Sickler GK: Idiopathic polyhydramnios: Association with fetal macrosomia. Radiology 190:393–396, 1994.

44. Hill LM, Breckle R, Thomas M, et al: Polyhydramnios: Ultrasonically detected prevalence and neonatal outcome. Obstet Gynecol 69:21–25, 1987.

45. Lazebnik N, Hill LM, Guzick D, et al: Severity of polyhydramnios does not affect the prevalence of large for gestational age newborn infants. J Ultrasound Med 15:385–388, 1996.

46. Queehnan JT, Gadow EC: Polyhydramnios: Chronic versus acute. Am J Obstet Gynecol 108:349–355, 1970.

47. Barkin SZ, Pretorius DH, Beckett MK, et al: Severe polyhydramnios: Incidence of anomalies. AJR Am J Roentgenol 148:155–159, 1987.

48. Manning FA: Dynamic ultrasound-based fetal assessment: The fetal biophysical profile score. Clin Obstet Gynecol 38:26–44, 1995.

49. Morrison I: Perinatal mortality: Basic considerations. Semin Perinat 9:144–150, 1985.

50. Manning FA, Morrison I, Lange IR, et al: Fetal assessment based on fetal biophysical profile scoring: Experience in 12,620 referred high-risk pregnancies. I: Perinatal mortality by frequency and etiology. Am J Obstet Gynecol 151:343–350, 1985.

51. Cohn HE, Sacks ET, Heyman MA, et al: Cardiovascular responses to hypoxemia and acidemia in fetal lambs. Am J Obstet Gynecol 120:817–824, 1974.

52. Manning FA, Platt LD: Maternal hypoxemia and fetal breathing movements. Obstet Gynecol 53:758–760, 1979.

53. Brown R, Patrick JE: The nonstress test: How long is enough? Am J Obstet Gynecol 141:646–651, 1981.

54. Manning FA, Baskett TF, Morrison I, et al: Fetal biophysical profile scoring: A prospective study in 1184 high-risk patients. Am J Obstet Gynecol 140:289–294, 1981.

55. Baskett TF, Allen AC, Gray JH, et al: Fetal biophysical profile scoring and prenatal death. Obstet Gynecol 70:357–360, 1987.

56. Manning FA, Morrison I, Harman CR, et al: Fetal assessment based on fetal biophysical profile scoring: Experience in 19,221 referred high-risk pregnancies. II: An analysis of false negative fetal death. Am J Obstet Gynecol 157:880–884, 1987.

57. Vintzileos AM, Gaffney SE, Salinger LM, et al: The relationships among the fetal biophysical profile, umbilical cord pH, and Apgar scores. Am J Obstet Gynecol 157:627–631, 1987.

58. Yoon BH, Syn HC, Kim SW: The efficacy of Doppler umbilical artery velocimetry in identifying fetal acidosis: A comparison with fetal biophysical profile. J Ultrasound Med 11:1–6, 1992.

59. Trudinger BJ, Cook CM, Jones R, et al: A comparison of fetal heart rate monitoring and umbilical artery waveforms in the recognition of fetal compromise. Br J Obstet Gynaecol 93:171–175, 1986.

60. Trudinger BJ: The umbilical circulation. Semin Perinat 11:311–321, 1987.

61. Nyberg DA, Finberg HJ: The placenta, placental membranes, and umbilical cord. In Nyberg DA, Mahony BS, Pretorius DH (eds): Diagnostic Ultrasound of Fetal Anomalies: Text and Atlas. St Louis, CV Mosby, 1990, pp 623–675.

62. Worrell JA, Fleisher AC, Drolshagon LF, et al: Duplex Doppler sonography of the umbilical arteries: Predictive value in IUGR and correlation with birth weight. Ultrasound Med Biol 17:207–210, 1991.

63. Johnston FD, Haddad NG, Hoskins P, et al: Umbilical artery Doppler flow velocity waveform: The outcome of pregnancies with absent end diastolic flow. Eur J Obstet Gynaecol 28:171–178, 1988.

64. Brar HS, Platt LD: Reverse end-diastolic flow velocity on umbilical artery velocimetry in high risk pregnancies: An ominous finding with adverse pregnancy outcome. Am J Obstet Gynecol 159:559–561, 1988.

65. Fleisher AC, Goldstein RB, Bruner JP, et al: Doppler sonography in obstetrics and gynecology. In Callen PW (ed): Ultrasonography in Obstetrics and Gynecology. 3rd ed. Philadelphia, WB Saunders, 1994, pp 503–523.

66. Arduini D, Rizzo G: Normal values of pulsatility index from fetal vessels: A cross-sectional study on 1556 healthy fetuses. J Perinat Med 18:165–172, 1990.

Chapter 36

The First Trimester

Roya Sohaey

EMBRYOLOGY

The first trimester of pregnancy is defined as the 13 weeks following the first day of the last menstrual period (LMP). Since the advent of transvaginal ultrasound, embryonic and fetal structures are seen routinely early in pregnancy, and familiarity with embryology is essential in order for sonologists to recognize normal and aberrant development. The first trimester of pregnancy is conveniently divided into the ovarian, conceptus, embryonic, and fetal periods, as outlined in Table 36–1.[1]

The ovarian period encompasses days 1 to 14 of the menstrual cycle, during which an ovarian follicle matures and ovulation occurs (usually on day 14). The ovarian cycle is gonadotropin dependent, with follicle-stimulating hormone (FSH) promoting the growth of a follicle, and with a luteinizing hormone (LH) surge resulting in ovulation. After ovulation, the corpus luteum forms at the previous ovulatory site and secretes progesterone, which prepares the endometrium for conceptus implantation. (See Chapter 27 for additional menstrual cycle details.)

Fertilization occurs during the third to fifth week and ushers in the conceptus period. Fertilization usually takes place when the ovum is in the ampulla of the fallopian tube, and is considered complete when the oocyte and sperm chromosomes intermingle. The fertilized ovum is transformed into the morula, a ball of 16 or more cells. Three days following fertilization, the morula enters the uterus and begins to implant into the endometrium. A blastocyst cavity forms and converts the morula into an inner embryoblast layer and an outer trophoblast layer. The embryoblast layer differentiates into a flat embryonic disc, and the trophoblast layer forms a primary yolk sac. When the blastocyst is wholly embedded within the endometrium (about week 4), implantation is complete.

The fourth menstrual week is a time of rapid trophoblastic proliferation and differentiation, resulting in the development of a primitive uteroplacental circulation. During week 4, the primary yolk sac also becomes smaller and gradually disappears as the secondary yolk sac develops. The embryoblast layer differentiates into a bilaminar embryo that lies between the secondary yolk sac and the developing amnion. Ultrasound now begins to visualize some of the anatomy of early pregnancy.[2]

The menstrual period is usually missed during week 5, and a woman may then start to suspect that she is pregnant. At this time, the embryo is converted to a structure with three layers (endoderm, mesoderm, and ectoderm). During week 5, neural tube, somite, and coelom formation begins, and blood vessels first appear on the yolk sac. At the site of the placenta formation, continued development of trophoblastic villi greatly increases the surface area between the chorion and endometrium.

The embryonic period begins with week 6 and continues through week 10. This is the most fascinating and critical part of human development, and disturbances during this time give rise to major malformation. In the embryonic period, the flat, trilaminar embryonic disc becomes a C-shaped embryo. A portion of the yolk sac is incorporated into the embryo, and the rest of the yolk sac becomes extra-amniotic. The amnion expands and forms an external investment for the umbilical cord and the embryo. As the major

Table 36-1. Embryology of Early Pregnancy

	Weeks	Features
Ovarian Period	1–2	Ovarian follicle matures ↓ Ovulation ↓ Corpus luteum
Conceptus Period	3–5	Fertilization ↓ Morula (16 cells) ↓ Blastocyst ↓ Trilaminar embryo (flat embryo)
Embryonic Period	6–10	C-shaped embryo ↓ Major organs develop ↓ Yolk sac detaches
Fetal Period	11–12	Fetal growth Amniotic cavity grows (chorioamniotic fusion by 17 wk)

organs organize and shift, the heart comes to lie ventrally, the brain lies cranially, and the limb buds become evident. By the end of the embryonic period (week 10), the major organ systems are established and the embryo appears human.

The 11th and 12th weeks represent the beginning of the fetal period, which is a time of rapid growth and differentiation. The crown-rump length doubles between week 11 and the end of the first trimester. The amniotic cavity continues to grow as the chorionic cavity shrinks. The amnion and chorion ultimately will fuse.[1]

GESTATIONAL SAC

An intrauterine gestational sac is the first landmark consistently seen with ultrasound in early pregnancy. With transvaginal scanning, the gestational sac can be visualized as early as 4.5 weeks, and the sac is seen consistently when it measures greater than 5 mm in diameter.[2, 3] Prior to the development of internal landmarks, the gestational sac can be confused with an endometrial fluid collection that does not represent an intrauterine pregnancy—i.e., a "pseudosac" of ectopic

pregnancy.[4, 5] Certain findings help confirm that a fluid collection truly is a gestational sac (Fig. 36–1): (1) round or oval configuration; (2) location within the fundus or midportion of the uterus; (3) echogenic borders (decidual reaction); (4) an eccentric position within the endometrial cavity; and (5) the double decidual sac appearance.[2] In addition, at very early stages of visualization (5 weeks), the sac is imbedded within the endometrium. The gestational sac is surrounded by echogenic tissue called the decidua. Three decidual components can be identified,[5] as discussed later.

YOLK SAC

The secondary yolk sac (hereafter simply called the "yolk sac") is the first structure to become visible *within* the gestational sac (Fig. 36–2). The yolk sac may be seen as soon as the gestational sac is visualized, but it should *always* be seen transvaginally when a gestational sac measures greater than 10 mm.[2, 3] A normal yolk sac is round and measures less than 6 mm in diameter.[6] The identification of a yolk sac is espe-

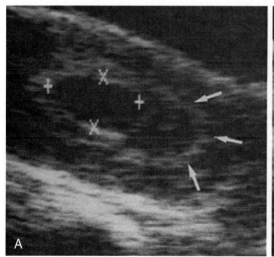

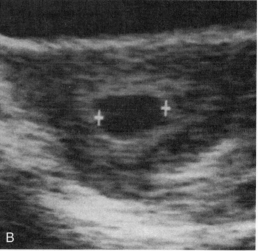

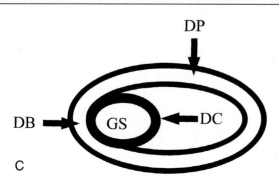

Figure 36-1—Normal Gestational Sac. Sagittal (**A**) and transverse (**B**) views through the gestational sac demonstrate the correct way to measure the gestational sac (calipers) in order to calculate the mean sac diameter. The decidual reaction is not included in the measurement. A double decidual sac sign is present in (**A**) (arrows indicate the decidua parietalis). (**C**) Schematic representation of the double decidual sac sign demonstrates the decidua basalis (DB), decidua capsularis (DC), and the decidua parietalis (DP). (With permission from Sohaey R, Woodward P, Zwiebel WJ: First-trimester ultrasound: The essentials. Semin Ultrasound CT MRI 17:2–14, 1996.)

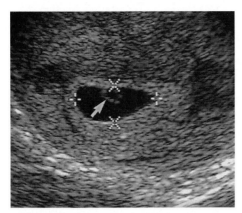

Figure 36-2—Yolk Sac. A normal yolk sac (arrow) is seen within an early gestational sac (calipers). The yolk sac should be round and measure less than 6 mm in diameter.

cially important, because it proves that the fluid collection within the uterus is a pregnancy rather than a pseudogestation or ectopic pregnancy or some other fluid collection.

EMBRYO

The second structure that becomes visible sonographically within the gestational sac is the embryo (Fig. 36–3), which should always be seen transvaginally when the gestational sac measures greater than 18 mm (7 weeks equivalent) and transabdominally when the gestational sac measures 25 mm (8 weeks).[7–10] Embryonic cardiac activity should always be seen when an embryo measures greater than 5 mm (crown-rump),[11] or the pregnancy is greater than 6 weeks and 4 days.[9] In some cases, the embryonic heart beat may be seen adjacent to the yolk sac even *before* the embryo is visible. Cardiac rates vary with menstrual age and increase from 100 to 110

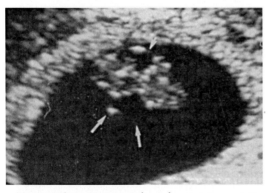

Figure 36-3—Embryo. The embryo is intra-amniotic (arrows point to the early amniotic cavity). (With permission from Sohaey R, Woodward P, Zwiebel WJ: First-trimester ultrasound: The essentials. Semin Ultrasound CT MRI 17:2–14, 1996.)

beats per minute (bpm) at 6 weeks to 150 to 170 bpm at 8 weeks.[12]

With improvements in ultrasound instrumentation, it now is possible to evaluate some embryonic and fetal structures during the first trimester. The embryonic cranium and brain are disproportionately large with respect to the trunk, and between 8 and 10 weeks the rhombencephalon, a fluid-filled cavity in the hindbrain, is easily identified (Fig. 36–4).[13] This chamber eventually becomes the fourth ventricle and central canal of the brain and spinal cord.[1] Normal physiologic bowel herniation is also seen routinely, as discussed in Chapter 41.

MEMBRANES AND PLACENTA

The amniotic cavity, the chorionic cavity, and the site of placentation are well seen with transvaginal ultrasound during the first trimester (Fig. 36–5). The (inner) amniotic cavity grows at a rate greater than the (outer) chorionic cavity, and as a result, the amnion eventually "grows" against the chorion, and the two membranes fuse.[14] Prior to fusion, the (outer) chorionic fluid is visibly more echogenic than the (inner) amniotic fluid, probably because of increased concentrations of protein and albumin within the chorionic cavity.[15] As the amnion grows, the yolk sac becomes detached from the embryo and lies between the chorion and the amnion.[1]

The decidua, which surrounds the gestational sac, begins as a diffusely thick, echogenic ring but changes to a focal area of thickening called the chorionic frondosum, which eventually becomes the placenta (Fig. 36–6).[1, 2, 16] Identification of the chorionic frondosum is important if chorionic villus sampling (CVS) is desired. The decidua has three components, as shown in Figure 36–1; the decidua basalis marks the site of placenta formation, the decidua capsularis surrounds the nonplacental side of the gestational sac, and the decidua parietalis represents the endometrial reaction surrounding the entire gestation.[5] The attachment of the umbilical cord to the developing placenta is easily identified, and the cord can be seen as early as 8 weeks' menstrual age (Fig. 36–7). The umbilical cord grows at a rate similar to the embryo with a 1:1 ratio reported between the cord length and the crown-rump length.[2]

FIRST-TRIMESTER PREGNANCY DATING

To assess the first-trimester pregnancy adequately, the gestational sac (GS) size or embryonic crown-rump (CRL) should be compared

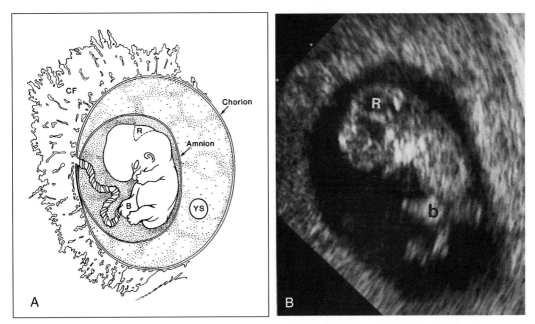

Figure 36-4—Normal Embryonic Anatomy. Schematic **(A)** and sonographic depiction **(B)** of embryonic anatomy. The rhombencephalon (R) becomes the fourth ventricle of the brain. Normal physiologic bowel herniation (B, b) can be seen and should resolve by 14 weeks. The yolk sac (YS) is extra-amniotic and the chorion frondosum (CF) becomes the placenta. (With permission from Sohaey R, Woodward P: The spectrum of first-trimester ultrasound findings. Curr Probl Diagn Radiol 25:53–76, 1996.)

with the menstrual age. The GS and CRL grow linearly and are excellent predictors of gestational age and fetal well-being.[2,9,17]

The GS should be measured in three orthogonal planes, and the mean sac diameter (MSD) should be calculated by averaging these measurements. Care should be taken to measure the chorionic tissue/fluid interface (see Figure 36–1)

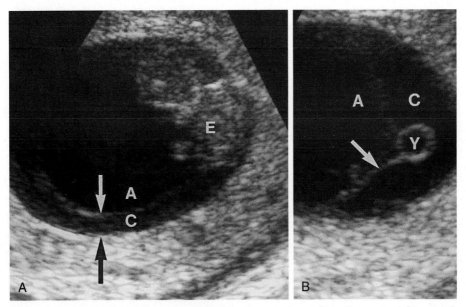

Figure 36-5—Amniotic and Chorionic Cavities. (A) Transvaginal scan shows the amnion (white arrow) and chorion (black arrow). The membranes have not fused yet. Note that the echogenicity in the chorionic cavity (C) is greater than that of the amniotic cavity (A). (E = embryo.) **(B)** The yolk sac (Y) is clearly detached and in the chorionic cavity. (A = amniotic cavity; C = chorionic cavity; *white arrow* = amnion.) (With permission from Sohaey R, Woodward P: The spectrum of first-trimester ultrasound findings. Curr Probl Diagn Radiol 25:53–76, 1996.)

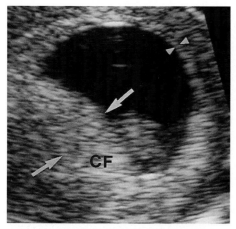

Figure 36-6—Early Placentation. The focally thickened area of decidual reaction (arrows) is the chorion frondosum (CF). The rest of the decidual reaction has become quite thin (arrowheads). Compare this figure from late in the first trimester with Figure 36-1 from early in the first trimester. At that time, the chorionic reaction was symmetric and the chorion frondosum had not yet formed.

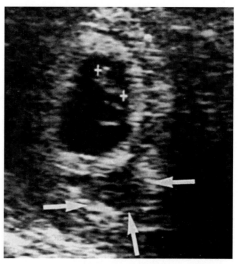

Figure 36-8—Early Crown-Rump Length. The greatest length of the embryonic pole (calipers) is measured in this early pregnancy. A small perigestational hemorrhage (arrows) is also seen. (With permission from Sohaey R, Woodward P, Zwiebel WJ: First-trimester ultrasound: The essentials. Semin Ultrasound CT MRI 17:2–14, 1996.)

and to exclude the decidual reaction or chorion. The MSD is especially useful for determining the menstrual age during the first 8 weeks, when the crown-rump length cannot be measured or is difficult to visualize. The equation *MSD + 30 = menstrual age (days)* can be applied when a chart of sac size is not easily accessible.[17]

The most accurate sonographic measurement correlating with menstrual dates is the CRL.[18] This measurement is the maximum visible length of the embryo or fetus. Care must be taken not to include the umbilical cord or yolk sac in the crown–rump measurement. Early in the first tri-

mester, the term "crown-rump" is a misnomer, as the embryo does not yet have a crown or rump, and this measurement actually represents the greatest length of the embryonic pole (Fig. 36–8). As the embryo flexes and becomes C-shaped, however, a true crown-rump length is measured (Fig. 36–9). Between 6 and 10 weeks there is little biologic variability in embryonic size, with the CRL = menstrual age in weeks ±4 to 5 days.[2] During the fetal period (between

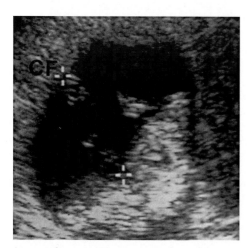

Figure 36-7—Umbilical Cord. The umbilical cord (calipers) attaches to the chorion frondosum (CF). (With permission from Sohaey R, Woodward P, Zwiebel WJ: First-trimester ultrasound: The essentials. Semin Ultrasound CT MRI 17:2–14, 1996.)

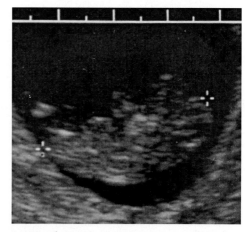

Figure 36-9—True Crown-Rump Length. Later in the first trimester, the embryo is more C shaped, and the CRL (calipers) is a true crown-rump length. Note that the measurement excludes the limb buds. (With permission from Sohaey R, Woodward P, Zwiebel WJ: First-trimester ultrasound: The essentials. Semin Ultrasound CT MRI 17:2–14, 1996.)

10 and 12 weeks), biologic size variation is more pronounced and may result from hereditary factors as well as flexion and extension of the fetus.

DISCRIMINATORY hCG LEVEL

Every ultrasound department should have tables available that correlate menstrual age with MSD and CRL measurements. In addition, the menstrual age may be correlated with the serum quantitative human chorionic gonadotropin (hCG) level (as summarized in Table 36–2).[19-21] In making such correlation, however, it is important to realize that different hCG preparations are in use that have different normal values. The two most common preparations are the first International Reference Preparation (First IRP) and the Second International Standard (2 IS). The First IRP values are approximately two times those of the 2 IS.

An important use of serum hCG levels in the first trimester concerns the discrimination between a normal intrauterine pregnancy and an abnormal pregnancy that may be ectopic. To this end, the so-called discriminatory hCG level has been defined.[2, 22] If the serum hCG concentration exceeds the discriminatory level [1800 units per liter (2 IS); or 2400 to 3600 units per liter (first IRP)], then an intrauterine gestational sac should be visible with *transabdominal* sonography. The corresponding values for transvaginal sonography are 800 to 1000 units per liter (2 IS) and 1000 to 2000 units per liter (First IRP).[2] If the hCG values exceed the discriminatory levels and an intrauterine gestational sac is not visible, then ectopic pregnancy or a recent spontaneous abortion is possible. Conversely, if the hCG level is low relative to the sac size and a fetal heart beat or embryo is not visible, then pregnancy failure is possible.

PREGNANCY FAILURE

Pregnancy failure is a common problem in the first trimester, with failure rates approaching 25%.[23-25] Almost 80% of early fertilized ova are lost before there is clinical recognition of a pregnancy.[26] In addition, women who are advanced in maternal age or have had previous miscarriages are at an increased risk of pregnancy failure from chromosome abnormalities in the conceptus.[27]

A threatened abortion is defined as bleeding and cramping in the first 20 weeks of a pregnancy. Ultrasound plays a key role in evaluating women with threatened abortion since hCG levels alone do not correlate well with a specific diagnosis.[23, 28] hCG levels that are falling may indicate a failed pregnancy, but hCG levels can also fall in ectopic pregnancy. Conversely, with an anembryonic gestation (blighted ovum) or with embryonic death, hCG levels may increase normally for a period of time.[29] Ultrasound, therefore, is needed to assess a pregnancy that is thought to be failing on clinical grounds.

Familiarity with normal first-trimester developmental landmarks (Table 36–3) is essential to diagnose a failing or nonviable pregnancy. High-resolution transvaginal ultrasound should be used, and sonographic findings should be compared with menstrual age and hCG levels. Common ultrasound findings in patients with threatened abortion are discussed next.

Developmental Landmarks Not Achieved

Failure to achieve expected developmental landmarks during early pregnancy suggests pregnancy failure, but when the observed anatomic landmarks indicate an earlier state of development than the LMP, it is important to remember that the LMP is not always accurate (for reasons discussed previously). The gestation may simply be "younger" than the LMP suggests. Before concluding that a gestation is failing or has failed because expected landmarks are absent, it may be advisable to re-examine the patient after a 1-week period. The gestational sac should increase in size in the interval, and developmental landmarks will be achieved if the pregnancy is normal; if not, then the failed or failing status of the pregnancy will be more clearly defined. The exception to the "wait and see" approach occurs in cases of possible ectopic pregnancy, in which more aggressive management may be warranted.

Poor Growth

First-trimester growth retardation is a sign of a failing pregnancy. Ultrasound demonstrates growth abnormalities better than serial hCG levels for reasons discussed previously.[30] Growth retardation is easily detected by comparing the MSD and the CRL, or by following these growth parameters serially. The MSD should be at least 4 mm larger than the CRL. A difference in size of less than 4 mm carries a high risk of subsequent demise.[31] In MSD/CRL discrepancy, a follow-up examination is recommended, and a guarded prognosis should be communicated to the referring practitioner.

Table 36-2. Combined Data Comparing Menstrual Age with Mean Gestational Sac Diameter, Crown-Rump Length, and hCG Levels*

Menstrual Age		Gestational Sac Size (mm)	Crown-Rump Length (cm)	hCG Level (First IRP)	
Days	Weeks			Mean (IU/l)	Range (IU/l)
30	4.3				
31	4.4				
32	4.6	3		1710	(1050–2800)
33	4.7	4		2320	(1440–3760)
34	4.9	5		3100	(1940–4980)
35	5.0	5.5		4090	(2580–6530)
36	5.1	6		5340	(3400–8450)
37	5.3	7		6880	(4420–10,810)
38	5.4	8		8770	(5680–13,660)
39	5.6	9		11,040	(7220–17,050)
40	5.7	10	0.2	13,730	(9050–21,040)
41	5.9	11	0.3	15,300	(10,140–23,340)
42	6.0	12	0.35	16,870	(11,230–25,640)
43	6.1	13	0.4	20,480	(13,750–30,880)
44	6.3	14	0.5	24,560	(16,650–36,750)
45	6.4	15	0.6	29,110	(19,910–43,220)
46	6.6	16	0.7	34,100	(25,530–50,210)
47	6.7	17	0.8	39,460	(27,470–57,640)
48	6.9	18	0.9	45,120	(31,700–65,380)
49	7.0	19	0.95	50,970	(36,130–73,280)
50	7.1	20	1.0	56,900	(40,700–81,150)
51	7.3	21	1.1	62,760	(45,300–88,790)
52	7.4	22	1.2	68,390	(49,810–95,990)
53	7.6	23	1.3	73,640	(54,120–102,540)
54	7.7	24	1.4	78,350	(58,100–108,230)
55	7.9	25	1.5	82,370	(61,640–112,870)
56	8.0	26	1.6	85,560	(64,600–116,310)
57	8.1	26.5	1.7		
58	8.3	27	1.8		
59	8.4	28	1.9		
60	8.6	29	2.0		
61	8.7	30	2.1		
62	8.9	31	2.2		
63	9.0	32	2.3		
64	9.1	33	2.4		
65	9.3	34	2.5		
66	9.4	35	2.6		
67	9.6	36	2.8		
68	9.7	37	2.9		
69	9.9	38	3.0		
70	10.0	39	3.1		
71	10.1	40	3.2		
72	10.3	41	3.4		
73	10.4	42	3.5		
74	10.6	43	3.7		
75	10.7	44	3.8		
76	10.9	45	4.0		
77	11.0	46	4.1		
78	11.1	47	4.2		
79	11.3	48	4.4		
80	11.4	49	4.6		
81	11.6	50	4.8		
82	11.7	51	5.0		
83	11.9	52	5.2		
84	12.0	53	5.4		

From Nyberg DA, Hill LM, Bohm-Velez M, et al: Normal early intrauterine pregnancy; Sonographic development and hCG correlation. *In* Patterson AS (ed): Transvaginal Ultrasound. St. Louis, Mosby–Year Book, Inc., 1992.

Table 36-3. Normal First-Trimester Landmarks

	Discriminatory Size
Yolk sac visible	GSD > 10 mm (TV)
Embryo visible	GSD > 18 mm (TV)
	GSD > 25 mm (TA)
Embryonic heart beat	CRL > 5 mm
GSD vs. CRL	CRL ≤ GS + 4 mm

GSD, mean gestational sac diameter; TV, transvaginal technique; TA, transabdominal technique; CRL, crown-rump length.

Anembryonic Pregnancy (Blighted Ovum)

Anembryonic pregnancy, or blighted ovum, is a form of failed pregnancy defined as a gestational sac in which the embryo failed to develop. The use of the term "blighted ovum" is discouraged. As E.A. Lyons, MD, of Winnipeg, Canada, has observed, "How do you know it was not a blighted sperm?"[32] With transvaginal ultrasound, embryonic remnants can sometimes be seen, but adequate development has not occurred, and expected sonographic landmarks (Table 36–3) are not met. A mean gestational sac diameter (GSD) greater than 18 mm (transvaginal technique) without a visualized embryo is unequivocal evidence of a failed, anembryonic pregnancy (Fig. 36–10).[27] An abnormally expanded amnion may be seen, with or without a visualized embryo. The latter situation is described as the "empty amnion" sign (Fig. 36–11).[33] Other findings associated with a poor outcome include an irregularly shaped gestational sac, heterogeneous tropho-

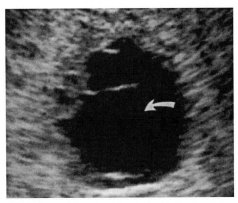

Figure 36-11—Empty Amnion Sign. Two cystic structures are seen in the gestational sac. The largest (curved arrow) most likely represents an expanded empty amnion, whereas the other is the yolk sac. If the amnion measures greater than 6 mm, an embryo should be present. (With permission from Sohaey R, Woodward P, Zwiebel WJ: First-trimester ultrasound: The essentials. Semin Ultrasound CT MRI 17:2–14, 1966.)

blastic reaction, and a gestational sac positioned low in the uterine cavity.[27]

Abnormal Yolk Sac

A failing or failed pregnancy is also suggested when the yolk sac is not visualized or is abnormal in size or shape. Large (greater than 6 mm), irregularly shaped, and calcified yolk sacs have all been found to correlate with early pregnancy failure (Fig. 36–12).[6, 27] Sometimes the distinction

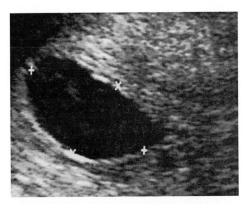

Figure 36-10—Anembryonic Pregnancy (Blighted Ovum). The gestational sac (calipers) shows a thin decidual reaction, has a mean sac diameter of 28 mm (transvaginal scanning), and does not contain any structures. These findings are diagnostic of a failed pregnancy (anembryonic). (With permission from Sohaey R, Woodward P, Zwiebel WJ: First-trimester ultrasound: The essentials. Semin Ultrasound CT MRI 17:2–14, 1996.)

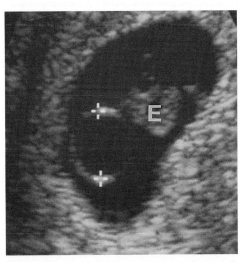

Figure 36-12—Enlarged Yolk Sac. A living embryo (E) was seen at the time of this examination; however, the yolk sac measured 8 mm and a follow-up examination was recommended. Seven days later, the embryo was dead. (With permission from Sohaey R, Woodward P: The spectrum of first-trimester ultrasound findings. Curr Probl Diagn Radiol 25:53–76, 1966.)

between an amniotic cavity or a yolk sac is difficult; however, any cystic structure in a gestational sac greater than 6 mm, *without* a living embryo, is strongly suggestive of abnormal development.[27]

Embryonic Demise and Bradycardia

The most convincing evidence that a pregnancy has failed is the visualization of embryonic demise. As stated previously, all embryos greater than 5 mm should demonstrate cardiac activity, indicating embryonic life. The confirmation of embryonic life does not ensure a viable pregnancy, but spontaneous abortion rates decrease steadily for living embryos as the gestational age increases. The demise rate for living embryos between 6 and 10 mm is only 0.5%.[34] At our institution, before an embryonic demise is diagnosed on the basis of absent cardiac activity, careful observation is performed by two experienced people, preferably sonographer and physician, for at least 3 minutes.

Embryonic bradycardia is a poor prognosticator of pregnancy viability and needs follow-up. An embryonic heart rate less than 90 beats per minute, in embryos of less than 8 weeks, is associated with an 80% rate of eventual embryonic demise, but pregnancy failure is not inevitable in such cases.[35]

Perigestational Hemorrhage

Perigestational hemorrhage, from the chorionic frondosum, commonly generates concern that a gestation is failing. Such hemorrhage is the most common source of vaginal bleeding during normal intrauterine pregnancy, and up to 20% of women with a threatened abortion have a subchorionic hematoma.[27] On ultrasound examinations, acute hemorrhage generally appears echogenic but becomes hypoechoic with subsequent liquefaction of the clot. Large perigestational hemorrhages have been associated with pregnancy loss even when a living embryo is seen at the time of ultrasound examination.[36] The prognosis is better for smaller perigestational hemorrhages, most of which resolve without sequelae (Fig. 36–13).[27]

ECTOPIC PREGNANCY

Ectopic pregnancy is a major health problem of increasing incidence, with 70,000 cases reported in the United States in the mid-1980s.[37] Women with a history of pelvic inflammatory disease, previous ectopic pregnancy, intrauterine contraceptive device use, and artificial insemina-

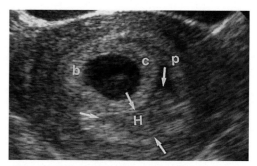

Figure 36-13—Perigestational Hemorrhage. A moderate-sized perigestational hemorrhage (arrows) is seen in this woman who presented to the emergency room with bleeding (threatened abortion). Since the hemorrhage (H) expands the endometrial cavity, decidual anatomy is seen well. (p = decidual parietalis; c = decidua capsularis; b = decidua basalis.) This pregnancy was successful. (With permission from Sohaey R, Woodward P: The spectrum of first-trimester ultrasound findings. Curr Probl Diagn Radiol 25:53–76, 1966.)

tion are at increased risk for an ectopic gestation. Early diagnosis and treatment result in a better chance for maintaining fertility.

The most reassuring sign that an ectopic pregnancy is *not* present is the sonographic demonstration of a normal intrauterine pregnancy. The presence of an intrauterine pregnancy decreases the risk of a concurrent ectopic pregnancy to 1 in 30,000 for a low-risk patient and 1 in 5000 for a high-risk patient.[38] In cases of suspected ectopic pregnancy, ultrasound findings should be correlated with serum hCG levels, as discussed previously. Unfortunately, as an expedient, ultrasound examination often is performed before the hCG results are available.

Transvaginal ultrasound, with a reported accuracy of greater than 90%,[39] should be used routinely in the evaluation of ectopic pregnancy. The diagnosis of ectopic pregnancy is not difficult when, for example, a living embryo is identified in an extrauterine gestational sac, adjacent to an ovary containing a corpus luteum (Fig. 36–14). Unfortunately, most cases are not so straightforward.

A variety of uterine findings can be seen with ectopic pregnancies.[40] Most frequently, the uterus is empty or a decidual reaction (thick endometrium) is present. The second most common finding, an endometrial fluid collection or pseudogestational sac, is seen in 10% to 20% of cases and should not be confused with an intrauterine gestational sac (Fig. 36–15).[41]

Adnexal findings in ectopic pregnancy also vary. In a recent study of 120 ectopic pregnancies visualized with ultrasound, only 17.5% showed a living ectopic embryo such as that seen in Figure 36–14. In 95% of cases, an adnexal mass was demonstrated, but this mass was reminiscent of a gestation sac in only 62% of cases.[42] In the remaining cases, a nonspecific, complex adnexal mass representing a hematoma was seen, and this in fact is the most common adnexal finding in ectopic pregnancy. An especially important adnexal finding in ectopic pregnancy is the adnexal ring (Fig. 36–16), which represents the decidual reaction surrounding an ectopic gestation. An exophytic ovarian corpus luteum can mimic the appearance of an adnexal ring; however, the corpus luteum usually contains more echoes than the adnexal ring and can be demonstrated to be intraovarian by transvaginal imaging. The majority of ectopic gestations are on the same side as the corpus luteum,[40] and we routinely try to identify the corpus luteum in our ectopic searches.

At the lowest hCG levels, the only sonographic finding in ectopic pregnancy may be blood—either distending the fallopian tube or free within the peritoneal space.[40, 43] Nonclotted, peritoneal space blood tends to be faintly echogenic at high gain levels (Fig. 36–17), and this sign suggests hemorrhage rather than serous fluid from a source other than ectopic pregnancy. The posterior cul-de-sac should be carefully investigated in every case when an ectopic pregnancy is suspected. Echogenic peritoneal fluid may be the only finding in 15% of ectopic pregnancies.[40]

Doppler ultrasound, particularly color Doppler, increases the sensitivity of ultrasound for detecting ectopic pregnancies.[44, 45] Color Doppler helps identify the echogenic and vascular "ring" of an ectopic pregnancy through the detection of

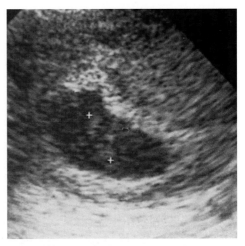

Figure 36-15—Pseudosac of Ectopic Pregnancy. This intrauterine fluid collection in a woman with an ectopic pregnancy initially fooled an inexperienced sonographer into believing it represented an embryo (calipers) within an intrauterine gestational sac. In actuality, the fluid is blood and the "embryo" is a blood clot. Note the absence of a double decidual reaction.

low-resistance blood flow. Without the use of color Doppler, 2% to 16% of ectopics may be overlooked.[44, 46] Once suspicious extrauterine flow is identified with color Doppler technique, waveform analysis and resistive index (RI)* calculations are made from the Doppler frequency spectrum. High-velocity (peak frequency, 2 to 4 kHz), low-resistance blood flow is typically seen in the trophoblastic or peritrophoblastic tissue of the ectopic gestation. This high-frequency, low-resistance flow pattern suggests ectopic gestation but is not specific for this diagnosis. The RI of blood flow around an ectopic gestation (range, 0.18 to 0.58) can overlap the RI of blood flow around a normal corpus luteum (range, 0.3 to 0.5).[44] Resistive index values less than 0.3 with high peak systolic frequency are more typical for ectopic pregnancies than for ovarian corpus luteum flow (Fig. 36–16); nonetheless, the gray scale image is the best means for differentiating between an ectopic gestation ring and an ovarian corpus luteum.[46]

The most common site for an ectopic pregnancy is within the fallopian tube. Nontubal sites, although less common, may result in greater morbidity and mortality, as the gestation may grow to a larger size before hemorrhage occurs.[47] Unusual sites include the uterine cornua (the pointed "corners" of the uterine cavity where the fallopian tubes attach), the intramural portion of the tubes (the portions surrounded by the

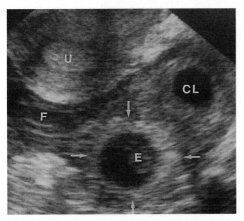

Figure 36-14—Living Ectopic Pregnancy. Transvaginal examination showing an empty uterus (U) with a prominent endometrium, echogenic fluid (F) in the cul-de-sac of the peritoneum, and a living embryo (E) within an ectopic gestational sac (arrows). Note the similarity in appearance between the echogenic ring of the ectopic pregnancy (arrows) and the ovarian corpus luteum cyst (CL) in this case.

---

*Resistive index: peak systolic velocity–end diastolic velocity/peak systolic velocity.

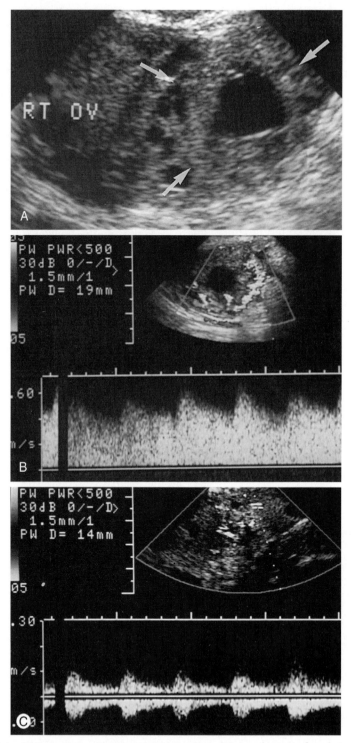

Figure 36-16—Ectopic Pregnancy: Doppler Interrogation. (**A**) An echogenic adnexal ring is seen adjacent to the right ovary (arrows). By gray scale imaging alone, it was difficult to determine whether this lesion represented an ovarian corpus luteum or an ectopic pregnancy. (**B**) The lesion "lit up" during color Doppler interrogation. Duplex Doppler was then used to study the Doppler waveform. High-velocity low-impedance blood flow is seen, which differed significantly from the lower-velocity higher-impedance blood flow seen in the ovary (**C**). In this case, Doppler helped correctly diagnose this early ectopic pregnancy.

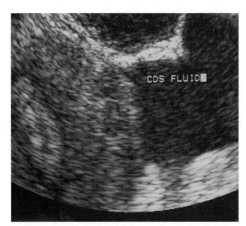

Figure 36-17—Ectopic Pregnancy: Echogenic Fluid. Transvaginal examination revealed diffusely echogenic fluid within the cul-de-sac (CDS). A small adnexal ring was subsequently found. (With permission from Sohaey R, Woodward P: The spectrum of first-trimester ultrasound findings. Curr Probl Diagn Radiol 25:53–76, 1966.)

myometrium), within the cervix, or on the surface of the ovary. Cornual pregnancies may be difficult to diagnose, since the gestational sac may be partially within the endometrium and its eccentric position may not be appreciated.[48] Cervical pregnancies are quite rare and may mimic a complex nabothian cyst or cystic malignancy. An attempt at curettage of a cervical ectopic pregnancy can lead to profound bleeding, and treatment with local methotrexate is preferable (Fig. 36–18).[49, 50]

Once diagnosed, ectopic pregnancy can be managed in several ways. Laparoscopic surgery is the mainstay for therapy; other options include medical treatment and expectant management.[46] With laparoscopic surgery, 86% of patients will subsequently have patent fallopian tubes. However, only 66% of these patients will become pregnant again, and 23% of subsequent pregnancies will be ectopic.[51] Less invasive medical treatment can be considered if certain criteria are met: (1) the patient is stable; (2) a living ectopic or growing pregnancy is confirmed (rising hCG levels or visualization of a living embryo); and (3) there is no evidence for tubal rupture on vaginal ultrasound examination (hematoma or echogenic pelvic fluid).[46, 52] Methotrexate is the drug most commonly used for nonsurgical treatment, and this drug can be administered locally (to the gestational sac) or systemically.[53, 54] Local therapy with methotrexate has been shown to result in higher subsequent pregnancy rates (82.5%) and lower recurrent ectopic rates (6%) than systemic methotrexate administration or laparoscopic surgery.[42] Obviously, the least invasive is the "wait and see" course. This therapy should be considered only for the asymptomatic or minimally symptomatic patient with a low hCG level (less than 1000), in whom the ectopic gestation is small (less than 3 cm overall size), there is no ultrasound evidence of a living embryo, and there are no signs of rupture. In a large series, 24% of ectopic gestations resolved spontaneously.[55] However, these patients require close monitoring and follow-up so that more invasive therapy can be instituted immediately, if needed.

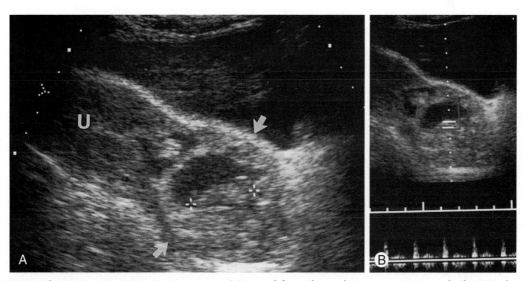

Figure 36-18—Cervical Ectopic Pregnancy. **(A)** Transabdominal view shows an empty uterine fundus (U), whereas the cervix is enlarged (arrows) from a gestational sac that contains an embryo (calipers). **(B)** Doppler examination demonstrates a living embryo. This patient was treated with local methotrexate and did well. (With permission from Sohaey R, Woodward P: The spectrum of first-trimester ultrasound findings. Curr Probl Diagn Radiol 25:53–76, 1966.)

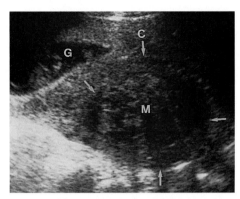

Figure 36-19—Cervical Myoma. A large cervical myoma (M, arrows) arising from the posterior lip of the cervix (C) precluded a vaginal delivery in this case. (G = gestational sac.) (With permission from Sohaey R, Woodward P: The spectrum of first-trimester ultrasound findings. Curr Probl Diagn Radiol 25:53–76, 1966.)

UTERINE ABNORMALITIES

Careful investigation of the uterus and adnexa is recommended as part of the routine first-trimester evaluation.[56] Myomas can grow during pregnancy,[57] and if they are located in the lower uterine segment they can obstruct the birth canal (Fig. 36–19). Uterine duplication anomalies are common and are associated with an increased risk of pregnancy loss. These anomalies generally are easiest to detect early in the first trimester (Fig. 36–20) and are more difficult to appreciate as pregnancy progresses. Of greatest concern is a septate uterus with placental implantation upon the septum. The septum cannot provide adequate perfusion for successful placentation, and this scenario is associated with a high pregnancy loss rate.[58]

Gestational Trophoblastic Disease

Gestational trophoblastic disease (GTD), or trophoblastic neoplasia, is an interesting disorder

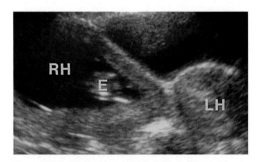

Figure 36-20—Uterus Didelphys. Transverse view shows two separate uterine horns. (RH = right horn, LH = left horn.) The pregnancy was in the right horn. (E = embryo.). (With permission from Sohaey R, Woodward P: The spectrum of first-trimester ultrasound findings. Curr Probl Diagn Radiol 25:53–76, 1996.)

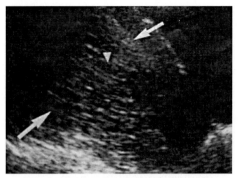

Figure 36-21—Gestational Trophoblastic Disease, Complete Mole. The uterine cavity (between arrows) contains a large mass containing innumerable cysts (arrowhead shows example of one of the cysts). (With permission from Sohaey R, Woodward P, Zwiebel WJ: First-trimester ultrasound: The essentials. Semin Ultrasound CT MRI 17:2–14, 1996.)

of pregnancy. The World Health Organization (WHO) has classified this group of disorders into five categories.[59] The most common is the "complete" hydatidiform mole, which represents trophoblastic neoplasia without an embryo. Complete moles are diploid in karyotype, but both sets of chromosomes are paternal in origin. With a "partial" mole, an abnormal embryo or fetus coexists with the mole. The karyotype is triploid, usually from two paternal sets of chromosomes and one maternal set.[60, 61] A mole is defined as "invasive" if it grows into the myometrium or beyond. Choriocarcinoma is a malignant mole that may metastasize to distant locations. An invasive mole or choriocarcinoma can occur after a normal pregnancy (1:160,000), abortion (1:15,400), or ectopic pregnancy (1:5300), but these neoplasms occur most commonly after a molar pregnancy (50% incidence).[62] A variant of GTD is a normal fetus with a coexistent mole. Such cases probably represent a complete mole in a twin pregnancy.

The classic findings in first-trimester molar pregnancy are uterine enlargement associated with a heterogeneous intrauterine mass (Fig. 36–21). Molar pregnancies have a variable sonographic appearance, however. Intrauterine findings range from an embryonic gestational sac to an endometrial mass, to a fetus (living or dead) accompanied by a mass or a thick "placenta."[63] Other findings associated with GTD include perigestational hemorrhage and ovarian theca lutein cysts. Theca lutein cysts occur in 50% of molar pregnancies and are thought to be secondary to abnormally high levels of circulating hCG. Sonographically, these cysts are large, bilateral, and multiseptate. Pathologically, they contain serosanguineous fluid.[64]

REFERENCES

1. Moore KL: The Developing Human: Clinically Oriented Embryology. Philadelphia, WB Saunders, 1977.
2. Nyberg DA, Hill LM, Bohm-Velez M, et al: Normal early intrauterine pregnancy: Sonographic development and hCG correlation. *In* Patterson AS (ed): Transvaginal Ultrasound. St. Louis, Mosby–Year Book, Inc., 1992, pp 64–85.
3. Fossum GT, Davagan V, Kletzky OA: Early detection of pregnancy with transvaginal US. Fertil Steril 49:788–791, 1988.
4. Marks WM, Filly RA, Callen PW, et al: The decidual cast of ectopic pregnancy: A confusing ultrasonographic appearance. Radiology 133:451–454, 1979.
5. Nyberg DA, Laing FC, Filly RA, et al: Ultrasonographic differentiation of the gestational sac of early intrauterine pregnancy from the pseudogestational sac of ectopic pregnancy. Radiology 146:755–759, 1983.
6. Lindsay DJ, Lovett IS, Lyons EA, et al: Yolk sac diameter and shape at endovaginal US: Predictors of pregnancy outcome in the first trimester. Radiology 183:115–118, 1992.
7. Cacciatore B, Titinen A, Stenman UH, et al: Normal early pregnancy: Serum hCG levels and vaginal ultrasonography findings. Br J Obstet Gynaecol 97:889–903, 1990.
8. Rempen A: Diagnosis of viability in early pregnancy with vaginal sonography. J Ultrasound Med 9:711–716, 1990.
9. Goldstein I, Zimmer EA, Tamir A, et al: Evaluation of normal gestational sac growth: Appearance of embryonic heartbeat and embryo body movements using the transvaginal technique. Obstet Gynecol 77(6):885–888, 1991.
10. Bernard KG, Cooperberg PL: Sonographic differentiation between blighted ovum and early viable pregnancy. AJR Am J Roentgenol 144:597–602, 1985.
11. Levi CS, Lyons EA, Zheng XH: Endovaginal US: Demonstration of cardiac activity in embryos of less than 5 mm in crown-rump length. Radiology 176:71–74, 1990.
12. Hertzberg BS, Mahony BS, Bowie JD: First trimester fetal cardiac activity: Sonographic documentation of a progressive early rise in heart rate. J Ultrasound Med 7:573–575, 1988.
13. Cyr DR, Mack LA, Nyberg DA, et al: Fetal rhombencephalon: Normal US findings. Radiology 166:691–692, 1988.
14. Burrows PE, Lyons EA, Phillips HJ, et al: Intrauterine membranes: Sonographic findings and clinical significance. J Clin Ultrasound 10:1, 1982.
15. Campbell J, Wathen N, Macintosh M, et al: Biochemical composition of amniotic fluid and extraembryonic coelomic fluid in the first trimester of pregnancy. Br J Obstet Gynaecol 99(7):563–565, 1992.
16. England MA: A Colour Atlas of Life Before Birth. Barcelona, Spain, Wolfe Medical Publications Ltd., 1983.
17. Nyberg DA, Mack LA, Laing FC, et al: Distinguishing normal from abnormal gestational sac growth in early pregnancy. J Ultrasound Med 6:23–27, 1987.
18. Ott WJ: Accurate gestational dating: Revisited. Am J Perinat 11(6):404–408, 1994.
19. Daya S, Woods S, Ward S, et al: Transvaginal ultrasound scanning in early pregnancy and correlation with human chorionic gonadotropin levels. J Clin Ultrasound 19:139–142, 1991.
20. Hadlock FP, Shah YP, Kanon DJ, et al: Fetal crown-rump length: Re-evaluation of relation to menstrual age (5–18 weeks) with high-resolution real time US. Radiology 182:501–505, 1992.
21. Robinson HP: "Gestation sac" volumes as determined by sonar in the first trimester of pregnancy. Br J Obstet Gynaecol 82:100–107, 1975.
22. Peisner DB, Timor-Tritsch IE: The discriminatory zone of beta hCG for vaginal probes. J Clin Ultrasound 18(4):280–285, 1990.
23. Hertz JB: Diagnostic procedures in threatened abortion. Obstet Gynecol 66:223, 1984.
24. Fantel AG, Shepard TH: Basic aspects of early (first-trimester) abortion. *In* Iffy L, Kaminetsky HA (eds): Principles and Practice of Obstetrics and Perinatology. Vol 1. New York, John Wiley & Sons, 1981, p 533.
25. Cavanagh D, Comas MR: Spontaneous abortion. *In* Danforth DN (ed): Obstetrics and Gynecology. Philadelphia, Harper & Row, 1982, p 378.
26. Roberts CJ, Lowe CR: Where have all the conceptions gone? Lancet 1:498–499, 1973.
27. Nyberg DA, Laing FC: Threatened abortion and abnormal first-trimester intrauterine pregnancy. *In* Patterson AS (ed): Transvaginal Ultrasound. St. Louis, Mosby–Year Book, Inc., 1992, pp 85–103.
28. Jouppila P, Huhtaniemi I, Tapanainen J: Early pregnancy failure: Study by ultrasonic and hormonal methods. Obstet Gynecol 55:42, 1980.
29. Nyberg DA, Filly RA, Duarte DL, et al: Abnormal pregnancy: Early diagnosis by ultrasound and serum chorionic gonadotropin levels. Radiology 158:393–396, 1986.
30. Jarjour L, Kletzky OA: Reliability of transvaginal ultrasound in detecting first-trimester pregnancy abnormalities. Fertil Steril 56(2):202–207, 1991.
31. Bromly B, Harlow BL, Laboda LA, et al: Small sac size in the first trimester: A predictor of poor fetal outcome. Radiology 178:375–377, 1991.
32. Lyons EA: Personal communication to William J. Zwiebel, 1990.
33. McKenna KM, Feldstein VA, Goldstein RB, et al: The "empty amnion": A sign of early pregnancy failure. J Ultrasound Med 14:117–121, 1995.
34. Goldstein SR: Embryonic death in early pregnancy: A new look at the first trimester. Obstet Gynecol 84(2):294–297, 1994.
35. Benson CB, Doubilet PM: Slow embryonic heart rate in early first trimester: Indicator of poor pregnancy outcome. Radiology 192(2):343–344, 1994.
36. Dickey RP, Olar TT, Curole DN, et al: Relationship of first-trimester subchorionic bleeding detected by color Doppler ultrasound to subchorionic fluid, clinical bleeding, and pregnancy outcome. Obstet Gynecol 80(3):415–420, 1992.
37. Centers for Disease Control: Current trends: Ectopic pregnancies—United States, 1979–1980. MMWR Morb Mortal Wkly Rep 33:201, 1984.
38. Van Dam PA, Vanderheyden JS, Uyttenbroeck F: Application of ultrasound in the diagnosis of heterotopic pregnancy: A review of the literature. J Clin Ultrasound 16:159–165, 1988.
39. Rempen A: Vaginal sonography in ectopic pregnancy. J Ultrasound Med 7:381–387, 1988.
40. Nyberg DA: Ectopic pregnancy. *In* Patterson AS

(ed): Transvaginal Ultrasound. St. Louis, Mosby–Year Book, Inc., 1992, pp 105–132.

41. Schaffer RM, Stein K, Shih YH, et al: The echoic pseudogestational sac of ectopic pregnancy simulating early intrauterine pregnancy. J Ultrasound Med 2:215–218, 1983.

42. Cacciatore B: Can the status of tubal pregnancy be predicted with transvaginal sonography? A prospective comparison of sonographic, surgical, and serum hCG findings. Radiology 177:481–484, 1990.

43. Cartwright PS, Morre RA, Dao AH, et al: Serum β-human chorionic gonadotropin levels relate poorly with the size of a tubal pregnancy. Fertil Steril 48:679–680, 1987.

44. Taylor KJW, Ramos IM, Feyock AL, et al: Ectopic pregnancy: Duplex Doppler evaluation. Radiology 173:93–97, 1989.

45. Pellerito JS, Taylor KJW, Quedens-Case C, et al: Ectopic pregnancy: Evaluation with endovaginal color flow imaging. Radiology 183:407–411, 1992.

46. Atri M, Leduc C, Gillet P, et al: Role of endovaginal sonography in the diagnosis and management of ectopic pregnancy. RadioGraphics 16:755–774, 1996.

47. Bayless R: Nontubal ectopic pregnancy. Clin Obstet Gynecol 30:191–199, 1987.

48. Beckman CRB, Sampson MB: Ultrasonographic diagnosis of interstitial ectopic pregnancy. J Clin Ultrasound 12:304, 1984.

49. Palti Z, Rowenn B, Goshen R, et al: Successful treatment of a viable cervical pregnancy with methotrexate. Am J Obstet Gynecol 161:1147–1148, 1989.

50. Marcovici I, Rosenzweig BA, Brill AI, et al: Cervical pregnancy: Case reports and a current literature review. Obstet Gynecol Surv 49:49–55, 1994.

51. Carson SA, Buster JE: Ectopic pregnancy. N Engl J Med 329:1174–1181, 1993.

52. Stovall TG, Ling FW: Single-dose methotrexate: An expanded clinical trial. Am J Obstet Gynecol 168:1759–1765, 1993.

53. Atri M, Bret PM, Tulandi T, et al: Ectopic pregnancy: Evolution after treatment with transvaginal methotrexate. Radiology 185:749–754, 1992.

54. Stovall TG, Ling FW, Gray LA: Single-dose methotrexate for treatment of ectopic pregnancy. Obstet Gynecol 77:754–757, 1991.

55. Atri M, Bret PM, Tulandi T: Spontaneous resolution of ectopic pregnancy: Initial appearance and evolution at transvaginal US. Radiology 186:83–86, 1993.

56. Guidelines for performance of the antepartum obstetrical ultrasound examination. J Ultrasound Med 10:577, 1991.

57. Lev-Toaff AS, Coleman BG, Arger PH, et al: Leiomyomas in pregnancy: Sonographic study. Radiology 164:375, 1987.

58. Fedele L, Dorta M, Brioschi D, et al: Pregnancies in septate uteri: Outcome in relation to site of uterine implantation as determined by sonography. AJR Am J Roentgenol 152:781–784, 1989.

59. World Health Organization Scientific Group: Gestational trophoblastic diseases. WHO Technical Report Series 692. Geneva, Switzerland, WHO, 1983.

60. Lawler SD, Fisher RA, Pickthall VJ, et al: Genetic studies on hydatidiform moles. I. The origin of partial moles. Cancer Genet Cytogenet 5:309–320, 1982.

61. Kajii T, Ohama K: Androgenetic origin of hydatidiform mole. Nature 268:633–634, 1977.

62. Hertig AT, Sheldon WH: Hydatidiform mole: A pathologicoclinical correlation of 200 cases. Am J Obstet Gynecol 53:1–36, 1947.

63. Woodward RM, Filly RA, Callen PW: First-trimester molar pregnancy: Nonspecific ultrasonographic appearance. Obstet Gynecol 55:315, 1980.

64. Krause FT: Female genitalia. *In* Anderson WAD, Kissane JR (eds): Pathology. 8th ed. St. Louis, CV Mosby, 1977, pp 1451–1456.

65. Sohaey R, Woodward P, Zwiebel WJ: First trimester ultrasound: The essentials. Semin Ultrasound CT MRI 17(1):2–14, 1996.

66. Sohaey R, Woodward PJ: The spectrum of first-trimester ultrasound findings. Curr Probl Diagn Radiol 25(2):53–76, 1996.

Chapter 37
The Neural Tube

Roya Sohaey

Among fetal head, neck, and spine anomalies, disorders affecting the central nervous system (CNS) potentially are among the most devastating, both physically for the fetus and emotionally for the family. Unfortunately, CNS anomalies also are relatively common. In this chapter, we discuss neural tube defects (NTD), since these are the most common class of CNS anomalies. Anomalies of the brain, face, and neck are discussed in Chapter 38. Readers who are unfamiliar with the standard ultrasound views of the fetal cranium and spine should review Chapter 33 before proceeding.

NEURAL TUBE DEFECTS

A sonographer will *not* have to perform large numbers of prenatal ultrasound scans before encountering a fetus with a neural tube defect (NTD). NTDs are common, occurring in 1:500 to 600 live births,[1] and are even more common prenatally. In 3% of all spontaneous abortions, a neural tube defect is found.[2] With the use of widespread alpha-fetoprotein screening and high resolution ultrasound, nearly all NTDs can be detected prior to viability.

The major types of NTDs are spina bifida, anencephaly, and encephalocele.[3, 4] Spina bifida and anencephaly occur with nearly equal frequency, most likely because of the embryology of neural tube closure.[1, 4] Normally, the central nervous system develops from a thickened area of ectoderm called the neural plate. A neural tube forms from the neural plate between 22 and 26 days after conception. The neural tube is open temporarily at both its cranial and caudal ends (Fig. 37–1). Normally, the cranial opening (the rostral neuropore) closes at 24 days after conception (5.5 weeks' menstrual age) and the caudal end (caudal neuropore) closes 26 days after conception (approximately 6 weeks' menstrual age).[5] Failure of rostral or caudal neuropore closure is thought to explain the pathogenesis of NTDs. This theory also explains why anencephaly and lumbosacral spina bifida are the most common central nervous system anomalies.[3, 5]

Neural tube defects tend to be sporadic, and multiple factors are cited as potential causes.[3]

The recurrence risk is estimated at 5%, but recurrence patterns fail to shed light on either a genetic or environmental cause.[1, 3] Certain maternal and environmental factors are associated, however, with an increased risk for NTDs, including maternal diabetes mellitus and the use of valproic acid (for seizures).[1, 3] Chromosome abnormalities associated with NTDs include trisomy 18, trisomy 13, and triploidy. Because of this association, chromosome analysis should be considered for fetuses with NTDs.[3] Recently, the use of high-dose folic acid has been shown to decrease the recurrence risk for NTDs. Some physicians now recommend routine use of folic acid during pregnancy, particularly in the first trimester and even before conception.[6]

Spina Bifida

Spina bifida refers to a split, or cleft, in the posterior elements of the spine. Spinal dysraphism is a related term meaning failure of closure of the spine. Open spina bifida is the most common type of NTD, and the lumbar or lumbosacral region is the most common site for this defect.[7, 8] A spina bifida is considered open if skin does not cover the divided (or dysraphic) portion of the spine. Two types of open defects are described: (1) a meningocele in which me-

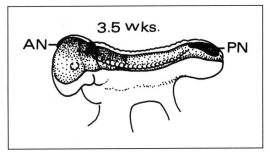

Figure 37-1—Neural Tube Embryology. Drawing of an embryo at 3.5 weeks' gestation shows the open anterior neuropore (AN, also referred to as a rostral or cranial neuropore) and an open posterior neuropore (PN, also referred to as a caudal neuropore). The cranial opening closes at 24 days after conception and the caudal opening closes at 26 days. (Reprinted with permission from Hansen PE, Ballesteros MC, Soila K, et al: MR imaging of the developing human brain. RadioGraphics 13:21–36, 1993.)

ninges and cerebrospinal fluid (CSF) extend into the spinal defect, and (2) a myelomeningocele, in which nerve fibers are present as well as meninges and CSF. A potential adverse effect of NTDs is low intelligence. Approximately 27% of people affected by spina bifida have an IQ of less than 50, 50% have a learning disability, and 23% have an IQ greater than 100.[9] Intelligence levels cannot be predicted prenatally, but in general, a better prognosis can be expected when a neural tube defect is isolated and involves only a few lower spinal segments.[10] Ultrasound plays an important role in detecting and characterizing spinal defects in order to help predict the outcome.[11]

Maternal serum alpha-fetoprotein (AFP) screening is used to detect open neural tube defects. AFP is a glycoprotein first made by the yolk sac and subsequently made by the fetal liver. Maternal serum AFP levels are usually low and peak at 28 to 32 weeks. If fetal tissue is not covered by skin, as in open neural tube defects, the AFP concentration in the amniotic fluid is elevated, and AFP subsequently enters the maternal serum. AFP screening programs use radioimmunoassay testing to detect AFP levels between 15 and 20 weeks' menstrual age. Maternal serum AFP levels greater than 2.5 multiples of the median (MoM) for singleton pregnancies (4.5 MoM for multiple gestations) are considered elevated.[1, 11, 12] With this cut-off, elevated maternal serum AFP can detect practically all cases of spina bifida and anencephaly (98% of cases).[13] Maternal serum AFP is often elevated for reasons other than neural tube defects, and potential causes of high AFP levels are summarized in Table 37–1. Ultrasound plays a key role in detecting NTDs, as well as other causes of elevated

Table 37–1. Non-neural Tube Causes for Elevated Maternal Serum Alpha-Fetoprotein Results

Unexplained
Placental etiology:
   Placental insufficiency (may be associated with IUGR, abruption, etc)
   Placental or cord hematomas or tumors
Incorrect menstrual dates
Multiple gestations
Fetal demise
Chromosome abnormalities: Trisomy 13, trisomy 18, Turner's (XO), triploidy
Other anomalies (any anomaly resulting in amniotic fluid contact with internal fetal tissue): Gastroschisis, omphalocele, ectopia cordis, bladder exstrophy, amniotic band syndrome, limb–body wall complex, tumors (cystic adenomatoid malformation, cystic hygroma, intracranial tumor, liver tumor in mother or fetus, sacrococcygeal teratoma), gastrointestinal obstruction, renal anomalies

IUGR, intrauterine growth retardation.

AFP levels; therefore, a patient with an elevated serum AFP level is usually referred immediately for an ultrasound examination.

Ultrasound Diagnosis of Spina Bifida

Sonographic visualization of the fetal spine depends on ossification of the spinal elements, which begins at 8 menstrual weeks. Three ossification centers are present initially. A single ventral ossification center gives rise to the vertebral body, while two paired dorsal centers become the lateral masses and posterior arch of the vertebrae.[14, 15] The paired dorsal ossification centers either may converge in the midline or may be parallel, but they *should never diverge* from each other.[3] Parallel posterior elements are caused by incomplete ossification (seen early in the second trimester) or a lateral recumbent position of the fetus.[3, 16] The spine should always be imaged transverse to its axis as well as in a longitudinal plane (coronal or parasagittal). The transverse view provides the best "look" at the posterior elements, whereas longitudinal views provide the best "overview" of the entire spine. The longitudinal views are best for detecting curvature abnormalities and for showing the extent of spinal dysraphism. The ultrasound features of the normal fetal spine are reviewed in Figure 33–9.

In cases of spina bifida (Fig. 37–2), a coronal view through the posterior elements demonstrates focal widening of the normally parallel line of posterior ossification centers. The transverse view confirms the divergent or U-shaped configuration of the posterior elements, and this is the preferred view for detecting and confirming spina bifida.[10] A longitudinal view through the vertebral bodies (anterior ossification center) and one row of posterior ossification centers is least helpful in detecting spina bifida, although this view is pleasing to the eye and may show the meningocele sac. Careful investigation of the skin helps identify the presence of a meningocele sac projecting posteriorly from the spine/skin defect.[3, 7, 11]

As stated previously, the extent of spinal dysraphism is associated, in a general way, with prognosis; therefore, the sonographer should try to determine the extent of dysraphism. Sonographic landmarks helpful in this respect include the 12th rib, which indicates the T-12 level, and the top of the iliac wing, which indicates the S-1 level.[17] It is interesting that fetal lower extremity movement is not predictive of motor function after birth, but the lower extremity should be evaluated for clubfoot, an associated anomaly.[18]

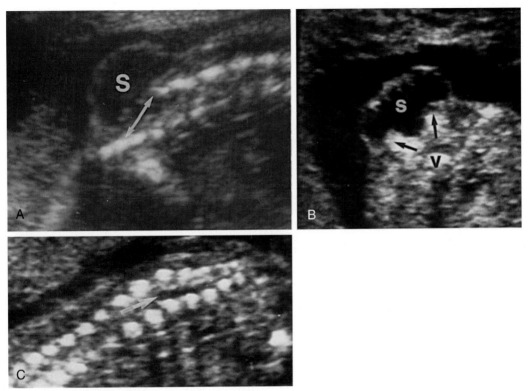

Figure 37-2—Spina Bifida. (A) Coronal view through the spine reveals splaying of the posterior elements (arrows) and a meningocele sac (S). **(B)** Transverse view through another fetus with spina bifida shows divergence of the posterior elements (indicated by direction of arrows) associated with a meningocele sac (S). The vertebral body ossification center (v) is seen anteriorly. **(C)** Longitudinal view of the spine in the same fetus as seen in **B.** In this view, the presence of a meningocele sac is suggested by the hypoechoic linear lesion seen at the sacrum (arrow). Obviously, the transverse view **(B)** is superior to this view of the spine.

Cranial Anomalies Associated with Spina Bifida

Almost all cases of spina bifida fall into the Arnold-Chiari II malformation syndrome,[3,*] and as a result certain cranial features of this syndrome virtually always are present in fetuses with spina bifida. Before 24 weeks, spinal defects are often small and may be difficult to detect with ultrasound, and in such circumstances features of the Chiari II malformation may be easier to see than the spinal defect itself. Ninety-nine percent of fetuses with spina bifida detected before 24 weeks have sonographically visible cranial anomalies.[20] Three findings in the fetal head are most helpful in detecting the presence of an occult spina bifida (Fig. 37–3): (1) obliteration of the cisterna magna, with associated compression of the cerebellum (the banana sign); (2) concavity of the frontal bones (the lemon sign); and (3)

ventricular dilatation. The severity of cranial findings does not reflect the severity of spinal dysraphism, although the presence of hydrocephalus is associated with lower IQ rates.[3]

The cisterna magna is a fluid-filled structure posterior to the cerebellum that should always be visible in the second and third trimesters. The cisterna magna normally measures 3 to 10 mm after 15 weeks[21] (Fig. 37–3). In the presence of open spina bifida, the cerebellum is displaced caudally, and the fluid-filled cisterna magna is small or obliterated.[22–24] If the cerebellum is compressed against the occiput of the skull, it assumes a crescent shape reminiscent of a banana, giving rise to the banana sign.[3, 22, 25] Rather than using this term, we prefer to describe the degree of posterior fossa compression. Furthermore, in my experience with spina bifida, the cisterna magna most often is narrowed or obliterated *without* significant compression of the cerebellum. If only the banana sign is sought, therefore, some cases of spina bifida may be overlooked.

Enlargement of the cerebral ventricles (ventriculomegaly or hydrocephalus) is another clue

---

*Arnold-Chiari II malformation is the term used to describe the classic posterior fossa compressive findings associated with spina bifida.[19] Specifically, the open spinal defect results in a "pull" on the midbrain and cerebellum, resulting in compression of these structures. I will discuss this in depth.

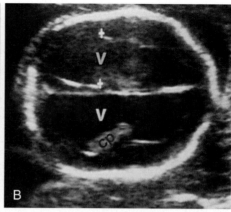

Figure 37-3—Cranial Findings in Spina Bifida. (A) The cerebellum (C) is compressed against the occiput of the skull and assumes a crescent shape (banana sign). The normally seen fluid-filled cisterna magna is absent. Mild concavity of the frontal bones (arrows) is also present (lemon sign). **(B)** The lateral ventricles (V) are dilated (calipers = nearfield ventricular diameter). The gravity-dependent choroid plexus (cp) provides a landmark for the atria of the lateral ventricle. Note how it "dangles" away from the medial wall of the farfield ventricle in this fetus with hydrocephalus.

that a spinal defect may be present. Some investigators reserve the term "hydrocephalus" for cases in which the head is enlarged secondary to ventriculomegaly, and others use the two terms interchangeably. Either way, the most common cause for ventriculomegaly in fetal life is spina bifida, and 75% of fetuses with spina bifida demonstrate some ventricular dilatation by 24 weeks.[25, 26] Ventriculomegaly is best diagnosed by measuring the transverse diameter of either lateral ventricle at the level of the ventricular atrium.* A transverse view of the fetal skull is used for this purpose (Fig. 33–6). At the atrial level, the transverse ventricular diameter should not exceed 10 mm at any gestational age.[27, 28] We will discuss hydrocephalus in greater detail in Chapter 38.

Isolated mild frontal bone concavity can be seen in up to 1% of normal fetuses; however, severe frontal concavity associated with hydrocephalus and/or obliteration of the posterior fossa suggests the presence of spina bifida.[25, 29, 30] The convex frontal deformity gives the skull a "lemon" configuration (Fig. 37–2). As with the banana sign, we prefer to describe the abnormality rather than to use the term "lemon skull." This practice avoids confusion as well as the insensitive use of a "fruit market" description of a potentially serious anomaly. The skull deformity is thought to occur because of low intraspinal pressure (from the open spina bifida), which causes a "pull" on the brain and calvarium. The frontal bones, being soft, are principally affected by this force and "cave in."[25, 30, 31] Eventually,

however, the bones strengthen and the deformity resolves, usually by 32 weeks.[31] The reader is reminded that among the three cranial signs of spina bifida, frontal concavity is the weakest, since isolated frontal concavity can be seen in normal fetuses.

Other Spinal Anomalies

Other anomalies of the fetal spine, such as abnormal spine curvature, sacral anomalies, and sacrococcygeal teratoma, are rare but are worthy of brief discussion. Abnormal spinal curvature is most commonly caused by a neural tube defect, but other causes include primary vertebral structure abnormalities (i.e., hemivertebrae), the amniotic band syndrome, and the limb–body wall complex.[11, 32] Persistent abnormal angulation of the fetal spine (Fig. 37–4) is an important ultrasound finding, for it suggests some type of spinal deformity. Angulation of this type is best seen on coronal or parasagittal views. An absent sacrum is another important finding associated with the caudal regression syndrome or with sirenomelia. The caudal regression syndrome is etiologically related to poorly controlled type 1 diabetes during embryogenesis. Sirenomelia is thought to result from a vascular insult to the developing lower extremities.[33, 34] Ultrasound features of caudal regression include absence of the sacrum, and in some cases the lumbar spine, as well as failure of lower extremity development. Severe renal anomalies (often renal agenesis), two-vessel umbilical cord, and lower extremity fusion are the hallmarks of sirenomelia. The "siren" refers to the mythologic mermaid.

Another rare sacral anomaly is a sacrococcy-

---

*The atrium is the junction of the temporal and the occipital horns with the body of the lateral ventricle.

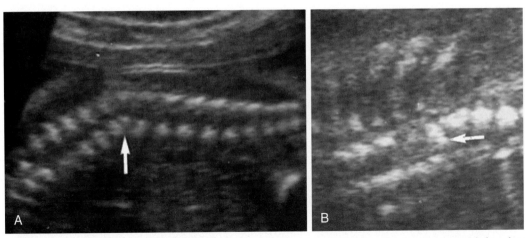

Figure 37-4—Abnormal Spinal Curvature. (A) Acute kyphosis at the thoracolumbar junction (arrow) led to closer investigation of the spine. **(B)** On coronal imaging, a hemivertebra was seen (arrow).

geal teratoma, which is a neoplasm arising from the coccyx and extending posterior to the fetus. A sacrococcygeal teratoma can be solid, a mixture of solid and cystic elements, or, rarely, purely cystic (Fig. 37–5). These tumors are mostly extracorporeal, but every attempt should be made to demonstrate intracorporeal elements (within the pelvic cavity). Rarely, sacrococcygeal teratomas can be malignant; however, sonographic features do not distinguish between the benign and malignant varieties.[11, 35]

Anencephaly and Exencephaly

Anencephaly is a common and uniformly fatal neural tube anomaly that should be 100% detectable with prenatal ultrasound. Female fetuses are affected four times more commonly than male fetuses.[3] In this condition, failure of rostral neuropore closure leads to absence of the cranium above the skull base.[3, 36] The brain is left exposed to amniotic fluid as well as repeated trauma, which eventually leads to destruction of the brain.[37] Midbrain, brain stem, and skull base structures are not affected.

Exencephaly (absent cranium, visualized brain) is probably a precursor of anencephaly (absent cranium, no visualized brain); therefore, exencephaly is seen earlier in gestation than anencephaly. The sonographic hallmark of both anencephaly and exencephaly is absence of a normal cranial vault cephalad to the orbits (Fig. 37–6). Superior to the orbits, there may be no tissue, dysplastic tissue (angiomatous stroma), or tissue resembling brain (exencephaly). Early diagnosis is possible (Fig. 37–7), but care should be taken not to attempt diagnosis of calvarial absence prior to calvarial ossification (about 13 weeks).[38]

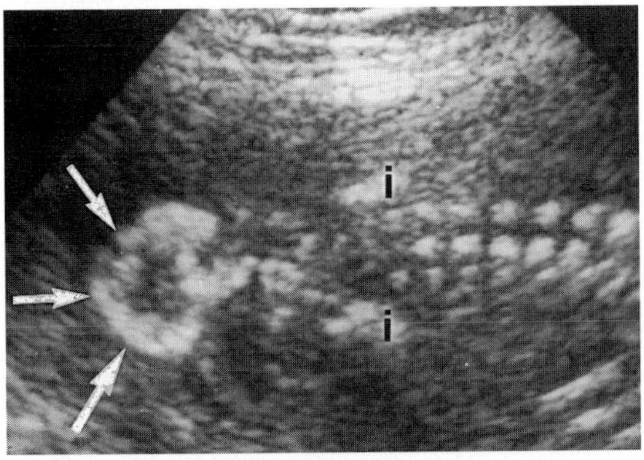

Encephalocele

The rarest neural tube defect, encephalocele, occurs in 1:2000 to 10,000 births. The term encephalocele describes protrusion of brain and/or meninges containing cerebrospinal fluid through a cranial defect.[1, 39] In the United States, encephalocele most commonly occurs in the occipital region (70%), but encephalocele can occur in the parietal (10 to 20%), frontal (10%), or basal (10%) regions as well.[40] Associated CNS anomalies include hydrocephalus (seen in 80% of occipital encephaloceles), spina bifida, and facial clefts.[3, 39] An important syndrome associated with encephalocele is the Meckel-Gruber syndrome, an autosomal recessive disorder characterized by occipital encephalocele, renal cystic dysplasia, and polydactyly.[3, 41]

Figure 37-5—Sacrococcygeal Teratoma. An echogenic mass arising from the caudal tip (coccyx) of the spine in this otherwise normal fetus proved to be a sacrococcygeal teratoma. (i = iliac wings.)

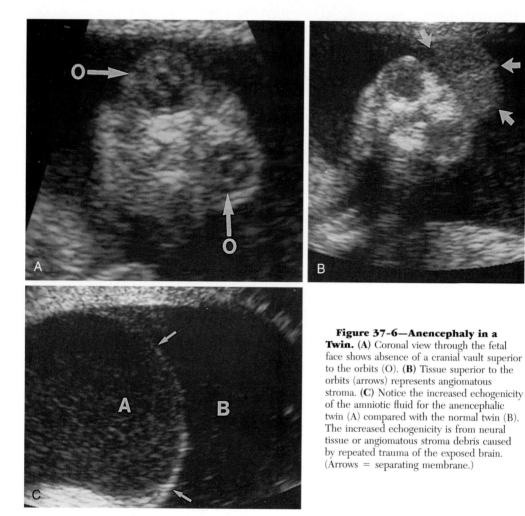

Figure 37-6—Anencephaly in a Twin. (A) Coronal view through the fetal face shows absence of a cranial vault superior to the orbits (O). (B) Tissue superior to the orbits (arrows) represents angiomatous stroma. (C) Notice the increased echogenicity of the amniotic fluid for the anencephalic twin (A) compared with the normal twin (B). The increased echogenicity is from neural tissue or angiomatous stroma debris caused by repeated trauma of the exposed brain. (Arrows = separating membrane.)

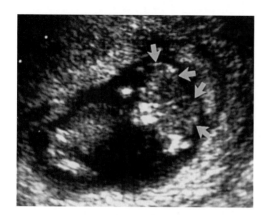

Figure 37-7—First-Trimester Exencephaly. Probably a precursor to anencephaly, exencephaly is absence of the calvarium with presence of brain tissue. In this first-trimester case, brain tissue is present (arrows) but its configuration is abnormal, suggesting absence of a calvarium. Autopsy confirmed the diagnosis of exencephaly/anencephaly. (Reprinted with permission from Sohaey R, Woodward PJ: The spectrum of first-trimester ultrasound findings. Curr Probl Diagn Radiol 25:53–75, 1996.)

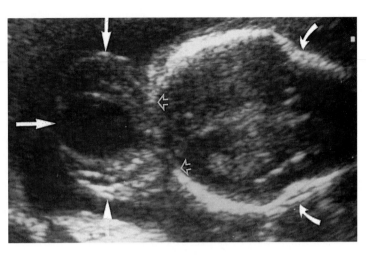

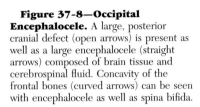

Figure 37-8—Occipital Encephalocele. A large, posterior cranial defect (open arrows) is present as well as a large encephalocele (straight arrows) composed of brain tissue and cerebrospinal fluid. Concavity of the frontal bones (curved arrows) can be seen with encephalocele as well as spina bifida.

Ultrasound features of encephaloceles (Fig. 37–8) depend upon the neural components present. A cranial defect should be visualized (although this sometimes is small). The extracranial mass may be cystic (meningocele), solid (brain parenchyma), or a combination of both.[3]

REFERENCES

1. Main DM, Mennuti MT: Neural tube defects: Issues in prenatal diagnosis and counseling. Obstet Gynecol 67:1–15, 1986.
2. Creasy MR, Albeman ED: Congenital malformations of the central nervous system in spontaneous abortions. J Med Genet 13:9, 1976.
3. Nyberg DA, Mack LA: The spine and neural tube defects. In Nyberg DA, Mahony BS, Pretorius DH (eds): Diagnostic Ultrasound of Fetal Anomalies: Text and Atlas. St. Louis, Mosby–Year Book, 1990, pp 146–202.
4. Lemire RJ: Neural tube defects. JAMA 259:558–562, 1988.
5. Moore KL: The nervous system. In The Developing Human. 3rd ed. Philadelphia, WB Saunders, 1982, pp 375–412.
6. Eskes TK: Possible basis for primary prevention of birth defects with folic acid. Fetal Diagn Ther 9:149–154, 1994.
7. Fiske CE, Fille RA: Ultrasound evaluation of the normal and abnormal fetal neural axis. Radiol Clin North Am 20:285–296, 1982.
8. Ames MD, Schut L: Results of treatment of 171 consecutive myelomeningoceles: 1963–1968. Pediatrics 50:466–470, 1972.
9. Nelson MD Jr, Bracchi M, Naidich TP, et al: The natural history of repaired myelomeningocele. RadioGraphics 8:695–706, 1988.
10. Laurence KM. Effect of early surgery for spina bifida cystica on survival and quality of life. Lancet 1:301–304, 1974.
11. Budorick NE, Pretorius DH, Nelson TR: Sonography of the fetal spine: Technique, imaging findings, and clinical implications. AJR Am J Roentgenol 164:421–428, 1995.
12. Leopold GR: Maternal serum AFP screening. In Nyberg DA, Mahony BS, Pretorius DH (eds): Diagnostic Ultrasound of Fetal Anomalies; Text and Atlas. St. Louis, Mosby–Year Book, 1990, pp 67–82.
13. Wald NJ, Cuckle HS, Brock DJH, et al: Maternal serum alpha-fetoprotein measurement in antenatal screening for anencephaly and spina bifida in early pregnancy. Report of United Kingdom collaborative study of alpha-fetoprotein in relation to neural tube defects. Lancet 1:1323–1332, 1977.
14. Filly RA, Simpson GF, Linkowski G: Fetal spine morphology and maturation during the second trimester. J Ultrasound Med 6:631–636, 1987.
15. Flecker H: Time of appearance and fusion of ossification centers as observed by roentgenographic methods. AJR Am J Roentgenol 47:97–159, 1942.
16. Gray DL, Crane JP, Rudloff MA: Prenatal diagnosis of neural tube defects: Origin of midtrimester vertebral ossification centers as determined by sonographic water bath studies. J Ultrasound Med 7:421–427, 1988.
17. Budorick NE, Pretorius DH, Grafe MR, et al: Ossification of the fetal spine. Radiology 181:561–565, 1991.
18. Warsof SL, Abramowicz JS, Sayegh SK, et al: Lower limb movements and urologic function in fetuses with neural tube and other central nervous system defects. Fetal Diagn Ther 3:129–134, 1988.
19. Funk KC, Siegel MJ: Sonography of congenital midline brain malformations. RadioGraphics 8:11–25, 1988.
20. Watson WJ, Chescheir NC, Katz VL, et al: The role of ultrasound in evaluation of patients with elevated maternal serum alpha-fetoprotein: A review. Obstet Gynecol 78:123–128, 1991.
21. Filly RA, Cardoza JD, Goldstein RB, et al: Detection of fetal central nervous system anomalies: A practical level of effort for a routine sonogram. Radiology 172:403–408, 1989.
22. Benacerraf BR, Stryher J, Figoletto JD Jr, et al: Abnormal US appearance of the cerebellum (banana sign): Indirect sign of spina bifida. Radiology 171:151–153, 1989.
23. Goldstein RB, Podrasky AE, Filly RA, et al: Effacement of the fetal cisterna magna in association with myelomeningocele. Radiology 172:409–413, 1989.
24. Pilu G, Romero R, Reece A, et al: Subnormal cerebellum in fetuses with spina bifida. Am J Obstet Gynecol 158:1052–1056, 1988.
25. Nicolaides KH, Campbell S, Gabbe SG: Ultrasound screening for spina bifida: Cranial and cerebellar signs. Lancet 2:72–74, 1986.
26. Nyberg DA, Mack LA, Hirsch J, et al: Fetal

hydrocephalus: Sonographic detection and clinical significance of associated anomalies. Radiology 163:187–191, 1987.

27. Siedler DE, Filly RA: Relative growth of the higher fetal brain structures. J Ultrasound Med 6:573–576, 1987.

28. Filly RA, Goldstein RB, Callen PW: Fetal ventricle: Importance in routine obstetric sonography. Radiology 181:1–7, 1991.

29. Campbell J, Gilbert WM, Nicolaides KH, et al: Ultrasound screening for spina bifida: Cranial and cerebellar signs in a high-risk population. Obstet Gynecol 70:247–250, 1987.

30. Nyberg DA, Mack LA, Hirsch J, et al: Abnormalities of fetal cranial contour in sonographic detection of spina bifida: Evaluation of the "lemon" sign. Radiology 167:387–392, 1988.

31. Penso C, Redline RW, Benacerraf BR: A sonographic sign which predicts which fetuses with hydrocephalus have an associated neural tube defect. J Ultrasound Med 6:307–311, 1987.

32. Harrison LA, Pretorius DH, Budorick NE: Abnormal spinal curvature in the fetus. J Ultrasound Med 11:473–479, 1992.

33. Stevenson RE, Jones KL, Phelan MC, et al: Vascular steal: The pathogenetic mechanism producing sirenomelia and associated defects of the viscera and soft tissues. Pediatrics 78:451–457, 1986.

34. Twickler D, Budorick NE, Pretorius DH, et al: Caudal regression versus sirenomelia: Sonographic clues. J Ultrasound Med 12:323–330, 1993.

35. Sheth S, Nussbaum AR, Sanders RC, et al: Prenatal diagnosis of sacrococcygeal teratoma: Sonographic-pathologic correlation. Radiology 169:131–136, 1988.

36. Goldstein RB, Filly RA: Prenatal diagnosis of anencephaly: Spectrum of sonographic appearances and distinction from the amniotic band syndrome. AJR Am J Roentgenol 151:547–550, 1988.

37. Cox GG, Rosenthal SJ, Holsapple JW: Exencephaly: Sonographic findings and radiologic-pathologic correlation. Radiology 155:755–756, 1985.

38. Johnson A, Losure TA, Weiner S: Early diagnosis of fetal anencephaly. J Clin Ultrasound 13:503–505, 1985.

39. Fitz CR: Midline anomalies of the brain and spine. Radiol Clin North Am 20:95–104, 1982.

40. Poe LB, Coleman LL, Mahmud F: Congenital central nervous system anomalies. RadioGraphics 9:801–826, 1989.

41. Johnson VP, Holzwarth DR: Prenatal diagnosis of Meckel syndrome: Case reports and review of the literature. Am J Med Genet 18:699–711, 1984.

Chapter 38

The Fetal Head, Neck, and Face

Roya Sohaey

The fetal brain is effectively evaluated with high-resolution ultrasound. More than 95% of central nervous system anomalies can be detected merely by obtaining the three standard views of the cranium described in Chapter 33 (the transthalamic, transventricular, and transcerebellar views).[1] Since most cerebral anomalies are obvious, the ultrasound practitioner generally does not have to struggle with the question, "Is the brain normal?" Instead, the difficult question is, "What is wrong with this brain?" Keys to determining what is wrong include: (1) determining whether the anomaly is global or localized; (2) pinpointing the location of the anomaly; and (3) characterizing the anomaly as cystic or solid. A practical approach to the abnormal fetal brain is outlined in Figure 38–1. Please review this figure before proceeding to the following discussion of major classes of brain anomalies.

GLOBAL CEREBRAL FLUID ANOMALIES

The fluid that fills the ventricles, cisterns, and other structures within the brain is called cerebrospinal fluid (CSF). When there is more CSF than brain parenchyma (in severe anomalies) or just more CSF than normal (in milder anomalies), the sonographer should consider one of three diagnoses: hydrocephalus, holoprosencephaly, or hydranencephaly. A correct diagnosis can usually be suggested by evaluating the brain parenchyma and the morphology of the fluid collection.

Hydrocephalus

Normal ventricular anatomy is presented in Figures 38–2, 38–3, and 38–4. In addition, nor-

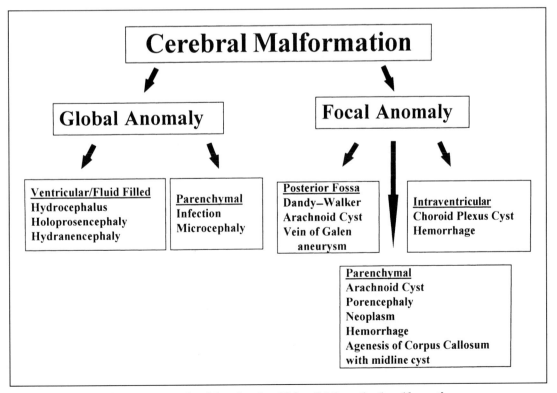

Figure 38-1—Algorithm for classifying fetal cerebral malformations.

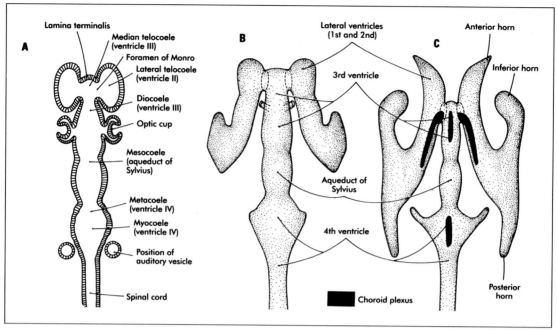

Figure 38-2—Ventricular system embryology. (**A**) Brain vesicles in the early embryo. (**B**) Ventricular system during in utero cerebral hemisphere expansion. (**C**) Postnatal morphology of the ventricular system. Note that the largest and most prominent in utero ventricles are the paired lateral ventricles. The aqueduct of Sylvius connects the third ventricle to the fourth. The choroid plexus fills the bulk of the lateral ventricle in the fetus, but is not present in the ventricular "horns" (anterior or frontal, inferior, and posterior or occipital). The choroid plexus becomes less prominent after birth. (Reprinted with permission from Carlson BJ: The nervous system. *In* Carlson BM (ed): Human Embryology and Developmental Biology. St. Louis, Mosby–Year Book, 1994, pp 204–240.)

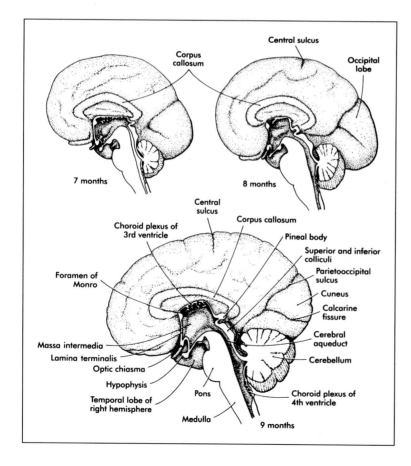

Figure 38-3—Medial views of the brain at 7 months, 8 months, and 9 months gestational age. Note the narrow cerebral aqueduct of Sylvius connecting the third ventricle with the fourth ventricle. The corpus callosum is a prominent conglomeration of deep white matter that joins the cerebral hemispheres. (Reproduced with permission from Carlson BJ: The nervous system. *In* Carlson BM (ed): Human Embryology and Developmental Biology. St. Louis, Mosby–Year Book, 1994, pp 204–240.)

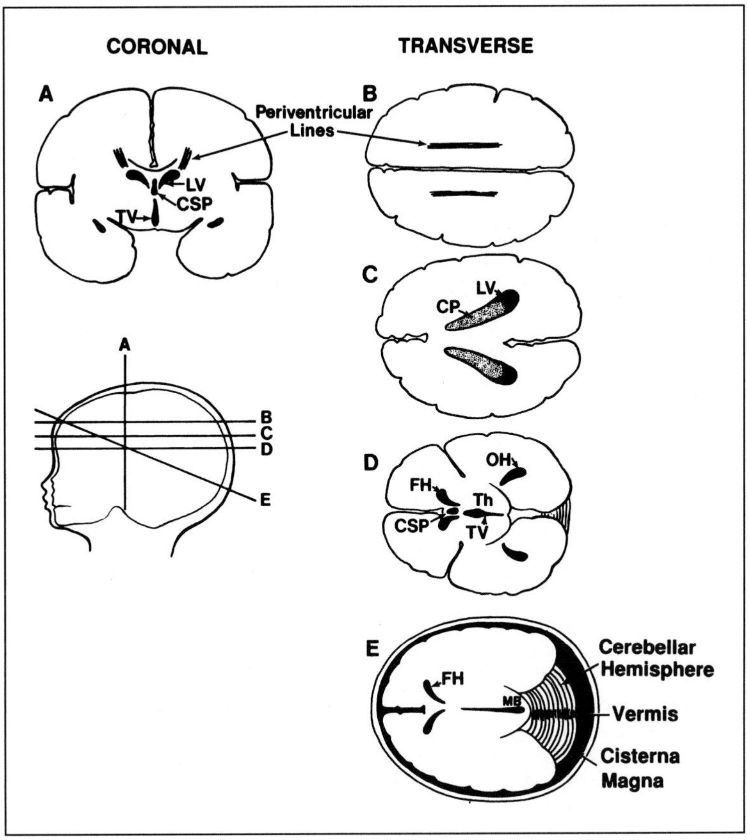

Figure 38-4—Normal ventricular ultrasound anatomy. (A) Coronal plane through the frontal horns of the lateral ventricles (LV), cavum septi pellucidi (CSP), and third ventricle (TV). This plane is often difficult to obtain during ultrasound examination of the fetus. **(B)** Transverse plane superior to the standard axial plane of the lateral ventricles. Thin, echogenic periventricular lines that parallel the falx cerebri seen at this level should not be confused with ventricular walls. **(C)** Axial view through the lateral ventricles is part of the standard recommended views through the fetal brain. Note how the choroid plexus (CP) fills the lateral ventricle (LV). **(D)** Axial view at the level of the thalamus (Th) and cavum septi pellucidi (CSP) is the standard view at which cranial measurements are performed. (FH, frontal horns; OH, occipital horns; TV, third ventricle). **(E)** View of the posterior fossa is obtained by angling the transducer 15 to 20 degrees toward the fetal occiput. This standard view allows for cisterna magna and cerebellar vermis visualization. (Reprinted with permission from Nyberg DA, Pretorius DH: Cerebral malformations. *In* Nyberg DA, Mahony BS, Pretorius DH (eds): Diagnostic Ultrasound of Fetal Anomalies; Text and Atlas. St. Louis, CV Mosby, 1990, pp 83–145.)

mal ultrasound features of the ventricles are presented in Figure 38–5, with expanded figure legends describing the correct techniques for ventricular measurement. As shown in these figures, the normal ventricle measures less than 10 mm at the level of the atria of the lateral ventricle.[2, 3] "Ventriculomegaly" refers to enlargement of the cerebral ventricles; "hydrocephalus" implies enlargement of the cranium, secondary to ventriculomegaly. These terms are often used interchangeably, however, and the term used is not as important as remembering that the fetal head should be measured carefully for signs of macrocephaly when ventriculomegaly is seen.

Ventriculomegaly is diagnosed with ultrasound when the atrium of the lateral ventricle exceeds 10 mm in transverse dimension at any gestational age[2, 3] (Fig. 38–6). An ancillary finding is "droop-

ing" of the choroid plexus to the dependent portion of the lateral ventricles. Normally, the choroid plexus almost completely fills the ventricles and cannot droop.

The most common cause of ventriculomegaly is spina bifida.[4] Therefore, once ventriculomegaly is diagnosed, the sonographer should look at the fetal spine for spina bifida and also the posterior fossa for evidence of cisterna magna obliteration. As discussed in the preceding chapter, spina bifida almost always is part of the Arnold-Chiari spectrum of neural tube defects that includes posterior fossa anomalies. If the posterior fossa and fetal spine appear normal, other causes for ventriculomegaly should be sought, as summarized in Table 38–1. Many of the *cranial* causes of hydrocephalus listed in this table should be evident if the brain parenchyma is examined

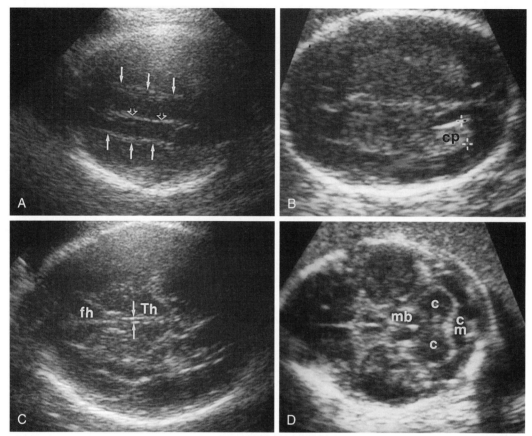

Figure 38-5—Normal ventricular system: Ultrasound findings. Compare these images with corresponding schematic views seen in Figure 38-4, Parts B, C, D, and E. **(A)** Transverse view superior to the lateral ventricles shows the falx cerebrum (open arrows) with bilateral echogenic lines representing periventricular white matter (solid arrows). **(B)** Transverse view at the level of the lateral ventricles shows choroid plexus (cp) filling the majority of the lateral ventricle (calipers). The easiest and most consistent measurement of the lateral ventricle is at the atria of the lateral ventricle (calipers) where the occipital portion of the choroid plexus is found. **(C)** Axial image at the level of the thalamus (Th) shows visualization of a normal third ventricle (arrows) and frontal horns (fh) of the lateral ventricle. Cranial measurements are routinely performed at this level. **(D)** Transverse posterior fossa image shows the bilobed cerebellar hemispheres (c) and a fluid-filled cisterna magna (cm). The cisterna magna measures between 3 and 10 mm during the second and third trimesters. A normal fourth ventricle is not always seen but is located between the midbrain (mb) and the cerebellum.

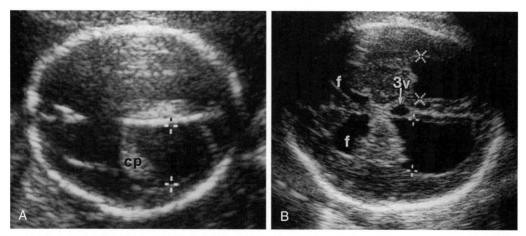

Figure 38-6—Ventriculomegaly. (A) Axial image at the atrium of the lateral ventricles (calipers) shows a "dangling choroid plexus" (cp). The choroid plexus is displaced from the medial ventricular wall and dangles in the dilated lateral ventricle. **(B)** Axial view in another fetus with ventriculomegaly shows dilated lateral ventricles and third ventricles (3v). Calipers mark the atria of the lateral ventricles.

Table 38-1. Causes of Fetal Cerebral Ventriculomegaly

Obstructive Hydrocephalus:
Neural tube defects: Spina bifida, encephalocele
Aqueductal stenosis
Dandy-Walker malformation
Mass lesions: Cystic, solid, or vascular
Intracranial hemorrhage: Rare in utero
Developmental Ventriculomegaly:
Holoprosencephaly
Agenesis of the corpus callosum
Abnormal chromosomes
Idiopathic
Brain Tissue Destruction:
Infection
Vascular insults: Hydranencephaly, porencephaly,
    schizencephaly

carefully. If hydrocephalus is the only *intracranial* abnormality, then the principal considerations are aqueductal stenosis, hydrocephalus associated with other developmental anomalies (e.g., chromosome defects), and idiopathic hydrocephalus.

Aqueductal Stenosis. Stenosis of the aqueduct of Sylvius is a common cause of fetal hydrocephalus (17% of cases in one series).[5] It can be acquired from infection, intraventricular hemorrhage, or a tumor mass, or it may be inherited (X-linked autosomal recessive) or idiopathic.[4, 6] The point of obstruction is the narrow channel that connects the third and fourth ventricles (Fig. 38–3). The stenosis itself is impossible to see with ultrasound prenatally, but severe and progressive dilatation of the lateral *and* third ventricles is seen (Fig. 38–7). Aqueductal stenosis usually becomes apparent in the late second/early third trimester, and the great majority of fetuses with this condition survive. Neurologic outcome varies, however, and is influenced by the cause of

stenosis, as well as the need for postnatal shunting.[7] X-linked aqueductal stenosis has a poorer prognosis than the idiopathic variety.

In up to 35% of cases, hydrocephalus is isolated and idiopathic; however, a careful search for accompanying anomalies is very important because they greatly influence the prognosis.[4, 5] In a large series, 84% of fetuses with hydrocephalus had other anomalies (63% CNS, 49% non-CNS). Among the fetuses with other anomalies, 67% died, compared with 37% for fetuses without other anomalies. All fetuses with multiple extra-CNS anomalies died.[8] Even mild lateral ventricular dilatation can be associated with a poor outcome, as indicated by a mortality rate of 40%.[9] At our institution, the identification of hydrocephalus, even if mild, leads to a careful investigation for other fetal abnormalities as well as recommendation for amniocentesis.

Holoprosencephaly

Holoprosencephaly represents a spectrum of cerebral anomalies resulting from abnormal cleavage (division) of the embryonic forebrain.[10, 11] The result is incomplete or absent division of the cerebral hemispheres and ventricles into right and left halves. Three types of holoprosencephaly have been described,[10] as presented schematically in Figures 38–8 and 38–9.

Alobar holoprosencephaly, the most severe form of this anomaly, results from absence of forebrain cleavage. Instead of two lateral ventricles, two hemispheres, and two thalamic units, the brain consists of a single, midline "monoventricle" surrounded by a mantle of cerebral tissue and subtended by fused thalami. The distinguishing ultrasound findings are a single, featureless monoventricle without evidence for occipital,

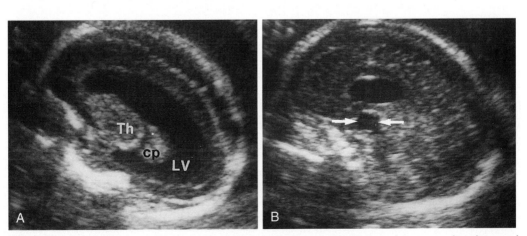

Figure 38-7—Acqueductal stenosis. Parasagittal **(A)** and midline sagittal **(B)** views show massive lateral ventricular (LV) and third ventricular (arrows) dilatation in this second-trimester fetus with a normal posterior fossa and spine. (Th, thalamus; cp, choroid plexus.)

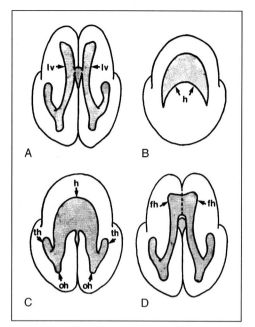

Figure 38-8—Spectrum of ventricular anatomy with holoprosencephaly. (**A**) Normal axial ventricular anatomy (lv, lateral ventricles). (**B**) Alobar holoprosencephaly: Monoventricle of holoprosencephaly (shaded, h) without any cleavage planes—i.e., no "horns." (**C**) Semilobar holoprosencephaly: A variable degree of midline division is present, with partially divided thalami and possible presence of temporal horns (th) and occipital horns (oh). (**D**) Lobar holoprosencephaly: Mildest form of cleavage abnormality, with flattened frontal horns (fh) and cavum septi pellucidi. (Reprinted with permission from Pilu G, Romero R, Rizzo N, et al: Criteria for the prenatal diagnosis of holoprosencephaly. Am J Perinatal 4: 41–49, 1987.)

temporal, and frontal horns; absence of midline structures, including the cavum septi pellucidi and the falx; and midline fusion of the thalami (Fig. 38–10). A particularly confusing feature of

this anomaly is variation in the amount of cerebral tissue that is present. When brain tissue completely surrounds the monoventricle ("ball-shaped" brain), the diagnosis can be made more easily; nonetheless, the unwary may mistake this condition for severe hydrocephalus. Diagnosis is more difficult with the "cup-shaped" variant in which a mantle of brain surrounds only the *anterior portion* of the monoventricle, and the posterior portion of the cranium is occupied solely by the monoventricular fluid sac. The "pancake-shaped" variety is hardest to diagnose. Brain covers only the frontal skull base and is hard to see. The monoventricle presents as a massive dorsal fluid sac that is apt to be mistaken for hydranencephaly (discussed next).[12]

Semilobar holoprosencephaly is similar to alobar holoprosencephaly, but failure of forebrain cleavage is less severe, and some degree of midline division may be apparent. For example, the thalami may be partially separated, and midline structures may be partially formed (Fig. 38–11). The brain mantle findings are similar to those of alobar holoprosencephaly, however.[10, 12]

Lobar holoprosencephaly represents the mildest form of this cleavage abnormality and is the most difficult form to diagnose prenatally. Sonographic features include flattened frontal horns, absent cavum septi pellucidi, and absent corpus callosum.[4, 13] Prenatal diagnosis depends on close scrutiny of brain anatomy, including routine visualization of the cavum septi pellucidi and other midline structures.

The prognosis for fetuses with alobar or semilobar holoprosencephaly is grave, and for that reason prenatal recognition of this condition is important. Most fetuses with the alobar or semilobar varieties die in the neonatal period. Chromosome abnormalities are present in half of

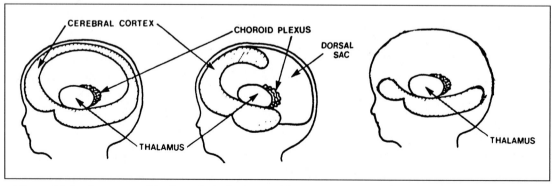

Figure 38-9—Spectrum of brain mantle findings with alobar and semilobar holoprosencephaly. From left to right, the brain mantle can completely surround the monoventricle (ball type), surround only the anterior portion of the monoventricle (cup type with subsequent large dorsal sac), or cover only the base of the skull (pancake type). (Modified and reprinted with permission from McGahan JP, Ellis W, Lindfors KK, et al: Congenital cerebrospinal fluid–containing intracranial abnormalities: A sonographic classification. J Clin Ultrasound 16: 531–544. Copyright © 1988, reprinted by permission of John Wiley & Sons, Inc.)

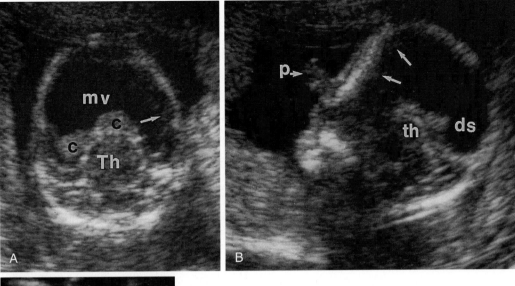

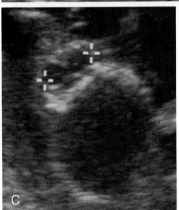

Figure 38-10—Alobar holoprosencephaly in an 18-week fetus. (A) Coronal image shows globular-appearing fused thalami (Th) and a large monoventricle (mv) containing choroid plexus (c). A thin mantle of brain is present (arrow). **(B)** Sagittal view confirms the presence of a thin, anterior mantle of brain (arrows) in a "cup" configuration, as well as a large dorsal sac (ds) posterior to the thalamus (th) (compare with Figure 38–9). The fetal profile is also abnormal with a proboscis (p) present. **(C)** View through the orbits shows marked hypotelorism (calipers measure the outer to outer margins of the bony orbits).

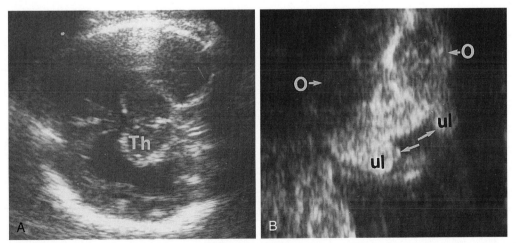

Figure 38-11—Semilobar holoprosencephaly. (A) Coronal image shows partial fusion of the thalamus (Th) and partial separation of the monoventricle. **(B)** Image of the fetal face demonstrates a large midline cleft lip (arrows). (O, orbits; ul, upper lip.)

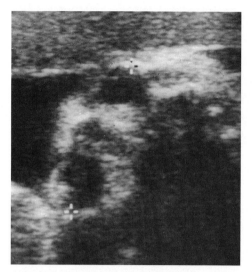

Figure 38-12—Measurement of orbital distance. Axial image at the level of the fetal orbits shows correct caliper placement for measuring binocular distance (BOD), also known as outer orbital distance (OOD).

fetuses with alobar or semilobar holoprosencephaly, the most most common of which is trisomy 13.[14–16]

The human face and brain originate from common embryologic structures, giving rise to the adage, "The face predicts the brain."[17] Because of this relationship, facial anomalies associated with holoprosencephaly are common and predictable (Figs. 38–10, 38–11). The reverse adage, that the brain predicts the face, is not true, and as a consequence, 11% to 17% of fetuses with alobar holoprosencephaly have normal facial features.[17, 18]

Orbital abnormalities in holoprosencephaly vary from hypotelorism to a single central orbit (cyclops).[17, 18] Hypotelorism (close-set eyes) is usually obvious to the experienced sonographer, but whenever the fetal brain appears abnormal, orbital separation should be assessed with the binocular distance (BOD) measurement, which can detect more subtle degrees of hypotelorism than are apparent on gross inspection. The correct technique for measuring the binocular distance is shown in Figure 38–12, and a table of normal BOD values is provided in Figure 38–13.

Nasal anomalies associated with holoprosencephaly range from a single nostril to the formation of a proboscis, which is a bizarre, trunklike, soft tissue protuberance. The proboscis may be located high, between the orbits, or even supraorbital (above a single cyclopic orbit). Lip anomalies associated with holoprosencephaly include median cleft lip, bilateral cleft lip, and premaxillary agenesis.[17, 18]

Hydranencephaly

Hydranencephaly is a rare cause of a fluid-filled calvarium that is thought to result from global cerebral infarction. Hydranencephaly is characterized by absence of the cerebral hemispheres, accompanied by preservation of the skull, meninges, falx, cerebellum, midbrain, thalami, basal ganglia, and choroid plexus.[19, 20] The massive infarction is most likely caused by intracranial cerebral artery obstruction occurring during the second half of pregnancy.[21–23] Ultrasound findings include absence of the cerebral cortex with otherwise normal-appearing brain structures (Fig. 38–14).

Differentiation

The "global" fluid-filled calvarium can be a diagnostic dilemma for the ultrasound practitioner. The best approach is first to try to diagnose or exclude holoprosencephaly with a series of critical observations, as listed in Table 38–2. Please review this material as it is not repeated elsewhere in the text.

GLOBAL BRAIN ANOMALIES

Most diffuse processes that affect brain parenchyma cause brain tissue loss, calcification, or both. The hallmark of global brain abnormalities is microcephaly, which signifies reduced brain mass. Microcephaly is suggested when the fetal biparietal diameter and head circumference are less than 3 standard deviations below the mean.[24, 25] (See Chapter 34 for normal values.)

The numerous causes of microcephaly include environmental etiologies (e.g., infection, anoxia,

Table 38-2. Differential Features of Holoprosencephaly, Hydrocephalus, and Hydranencephaly

Critical Observation	Holoprosencephaly	Hydrocephalus	Hydranencephaly
Is there a falx?	No	Yes	Usually
Are the thalami fused?	Yes	No	No
Is the face normal?	Usually no	Usually yes	Yes
Is there a mantle of cerebral tissue?	Yes	Yes (thin if severe)	No
Intracerebral blood flow?	Yes	Yes	No

BPD	Gestation (wk)	OOD (cm)	BPD	Gestation (wk)	OOD (cm)
1.9	11.6	1.3.	5.8	24.3	4.1
2.0	11.6	1.4	5.9	24.3	4.2
2.1	12.1	1.5	6.0	24.7	4.3
2.2	12.6	1.6	6.1	25.2	4.3
2.3	12.6	1.7	6.2	25.2	4.4
2.4	13.1	1.7	6.3	25.7	4.4
2.5	13.6	1.8	6.4	26.2	4.5
2.6	13.6	1.9	6.5	26.2	4.5
2.7	14.1	2.0	6.6	26.7	4.6
2.8	14.6	2.1	6.7	27.2	4.6
2.9	14.6	2.1	6.8	27.6	4.7
3.0	15.0	2.2	6.9	28.1	4.7
3.1	15.5	2.3	7.0	28.6	4.8
3.2	15.5	2.4	7.1	29.1	4.8
3.3	16.0	2.5	7.3	29.6	4.9
3.4	16.5	2.5	7.4	30.0	5.0
3.5	16.5	2.6	7.5	30.6	5.0
3.6	17.0	2.7	7.6	31.0	5.1
3.7	17.5	2.7	7.7	31.5	5.1
3.8	17.9	2.8	7.8	32.0	5.2
4.0	18.4	3.0	7.9	32.5	5.2
4.2	18.9	3.1	8.0	33.0	5.3
4.3	19.4	3.2	8.2	33.5	5.4
4.4	19.4	3.2	8.3	34.0	5.4
4.5	19.9	3.3	8.4	34.4	5.4
4.6	20.4	3.4	8.5	35.0	5.5
4.7	20.4	3.4	8.6	35.4	5.5
4.8	20.9	3.5	8.8	35.9	5.6
4.9	21.3	3.6	8.9	36.4	5.6
5.0	21.3	3.6	9.0	36.9	5.7
5.1	21.8	3.7	9.1	37.3	5.7
5.2	22.3	3.8	9.2	37.8	5.8
5.3	22.3	3.8	9.3	38.3	5.8
5.4	22.8	3.9	9.4	38.8	5.8
5.5	23.3	4.0	9.6	39.3	5.9
5.6	23.3	4.0	9.7	39.8	5.9
5.7	23.8	4.1			

Figure 38-13—Nomogram of outer orbital diameter (OOD) compared with gestational age and biparietal diameter (BPD). Outer orbital distance is synonymous with binocular distance (BOD). (Reprinted with permission from Mayden KL, Tortoria M, Berkowitz RL, et al: Orbital diameters: A new parameter for prenatal diagnosis and dating. Am J Obstet Gynecol 144: 289–297, 1982.)

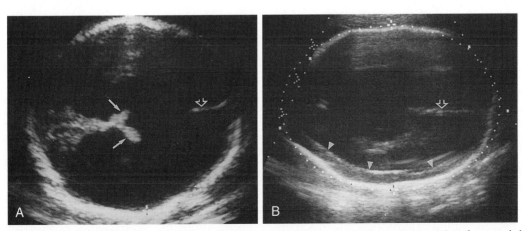

Figure 38-14—The fluid filled calvarium: Hydranencephaly versus hydrocephalus. (A) Hydranencephaly: Although the falx cerebrum (open arrow) and choroid plexus (arrows) are present, a mantle of brain is noticeably absent. **(B)** Severe hydrocephalus: The presence of a mantle of brain (arrowheads) helps differentiate severe hydrocephalus from hydranencephaly. (Open arrow, falx cerebrum.)

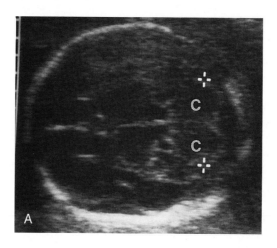

Figure 38-15—Bicerebellar diameter. (A) Axial image through the posterior fossa shows the correct way to measure the maximum bicerebellar diameter (calipers). (C, cerebellar hemispheres.) (B) Nomogram of expected cerebellar diameter (in mm) at different gestational ages. The 10th, 25th, 50th, 75th, and 90th percentile measurements are presented. (Table reprinted with permission from Goldstein I, Reece EA, Pilu G, et al: Cerebellar measurements with ultrasonography in the evaluation of fetal growth and development. Am J Obstet Gynecol 156: 1064–1065, 1987.)

Gestational Age (wk)	Cerebellum Diameter (mm)				
	10	25	50	75	90
15	10	12	14	15	16
16	14	16	16	16	17
17	16	17	17	18	18
18	17	18	18	19	19
19	18	18	19	19	22
20	18	19	20	20	22
21	19	20	22	23	24
22	21	23	23	24	24
23	22	23	24	25	26
24	22	24	25	27	28
25	23	21.5	28	28	29
26	25	28	29	30	32
27	26	28.5	30	31	32
28	27	30	31	32	34
29	29	32	34	36	38
30	31	32	35	37	40
31	32	35	38	39	43
32	33	36	38	40	42
33	32	36	40	43	44
34	33	38	40	41	44
35	31	37	40.5	43	47
36	36	39	43	52	55
37	37	37	45	52	55
38	40	40	48.5	52	55
39	52	52	52	55	55

B

radiation exposure), developmental disorders (e.g., chromosome abnormalities, mendelian syndromes), and rare calvarial abnormalities such as craniosynostosis. Often, it is difficult for the sonographer to differentiate among the causes of microcephaly, but certain clues may suggest a specific diagnosis. Intracranial calcification suggests in utero infection (typically cytomegalovirus or toxoplasmosis).[26, 27] Such calcification usually is periventricular and punctate, but without acoustic shadows.[28] Abnormal cranial shape suggests craniosynostosis (premature closure of skull sutures), as seen with the "clover leaf" skull of thanatophoric dwarfism (Chapter 43). Regardless of cause, the prognosis for microcephaly is poor, with the rate of mental retardation reported as 50% to 99%.[29, 30]

FOCAL INTRACRANIAL ANOMALIES

If an intracranial abnormality does not appear to be global in distribution, the sonographer should try to characterize the anomaly by its appearance (cystic, solid, or mixed) and pinpoint its location. I find it useful to characterize focal anomalies as posterior fossa, cerebral, or interventricular, as this approach assists the diagnostic process.

Focal Posterior Fossa Lesions

The recommended transverse view through the posterior fossa (Chapter 33) demonstrates the normal bilobed shape of the cerebellar hemispheres and the median "wormlike" vermis, which separates the cisterna magna and the fourth ventricle. In normal fetuses, the fourth ventricle often is difficult or impossible to see, and the fourth ventricle and cisterna magna should never communicate after 18 weeks.[31] If the cisterna magna, on a correctly obtained transverse view, measures greater than 10 mm in diameter, a Dandy-Walker malformation may be present. In such cases, the shape and size of the cerebellum should be noted. It usually is obvious to an experienced sonographer that the cerebellum is normal, however, Figure 38–15 provides normal bicerebellar dimensions for cases in which measurement is necessary. The bicerebellar distance also is a good determinant of gestational age.

The *Dandy-Walker malformation (DWM)* is a congenital brain malformation involving the fourth ventricle and the cerebellar vermis that occurs in 1 in 25,000 to 30,000 pregnancies.[32–34] The sonographic hallmark for this malformation is a posterior fossa cyst that represents a communication between the fourth ventricle and the cisterna magna through a defect of the cerebellar vermis.[35, 36] The sonographic findings range in severity from subtle vermian defects to massive cystic dilatation of the fourth ventricle with minimal cerebellar tissue[35] (Fig. 38–16). Secondary obstructive hydrocephalus accompanies 53% of DWM cases.[35] Additional brain abnormalities are often present, but these may not be detectable on prenatal ultrasound examination. These include aqueductal stenosis, gyral anomalies, and agenesis of the corpus callosum (discussed later). The latter anomaly is present in almost 25% of cases and is detectable in utero.[35–37] Associated extracranial anomalies occur in 25% to 60% of cases and include facial, cardiac, genitourinary, gastrointestinal, and skeletal malformation.[35, 37] Obviously, when DWM is seen, the sonographer should carefully investigate the rest of the fetus.

The prognosis in cases of DWM depends on the severity of the defect and the presence of other anomalies. Approximately one third of fetuses with DWM have abnormal chromosomes[35]; therefore, at our institution we recommend amniocentesis in all DWM cases. Mortality rates of 12% to 67% have been reported in the pediatric and sonographic literature.[34, 35, 38] Forty to seventy percent of DWM survivors have subnormal intel-

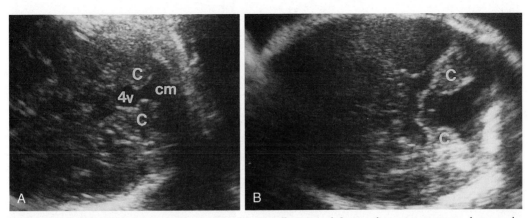

Figure 38-16—Dandy-Walker malformation. (A) A small vermian defect results in communication between the cisterna magna (cm) and the fourth ventricle (4v). Note the "keyhole" appearance of the resulting posterior fossa cyst. (C, cerebellar hemispheres.) **(B)** A larger cerebellar defect results in a larger posterior fossa cyst in this case. (C, cerebellar hemispheres.)

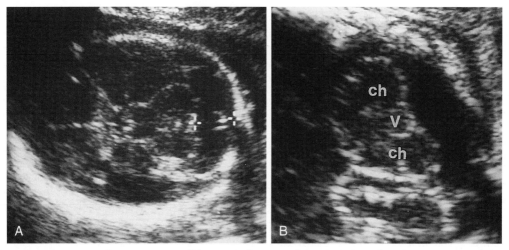

Figure 38-17—Mega cisterna magna. (A) Posterior fossa view demonstrates an enlarged cisterna magna (calipers), and the question of a Dandy-Walker malformation is raised. (B) Attention paid to the morphology of the cerebellum reveals an intact cerebellar vermis (V) and normal cerebellar hemispheres (ch). Therefore, mega cisterna magna, a normal variant, is the correct diagnosis.

ligence, with more severe impairment in cases accompanied by agenesis of the corpus callosum.[4, 34, 38]

A posterior fossa anomaly that mimics the Dandy-Walker malformations is the *mega cisterna magna*.[32, 35] This normal anatomic variant (Fig. 38–17) is not associated with other anomalies and consists of enlargement of the cisterna magna *without* a vermian defect or cisterna magna–fourth ventricle communication (the hallmarks of DWM).[4, 35]

Another posterior fossa cystic abnormality that mimics the Dandy-Walker malformation is an *arachnoid cyst*. These benign developmental cysts of the arachnoid membranes (covering the brain) lie adjacent to the brain but do not communicate with the ventricular system.[39] Detection of a normal cerebellar vermis excludes DWM. Arachnoid cysts may cause hydrocephalus by compressing the ventricular system.[39, 40] Otherwise, like mega cisterna magna, they are not associated with cerebral or extracerebral anomalies.

The *vein of Galen aneurysm* is not in the posterior fossa per se, but its midline-posterior location often mimics a posterior fossa cyst (Fig. 38–18). This anomaly is actually an arteriovenous malformation (AVM) resulting in massive dilatation of the primitive vein of Galen.[41] Doppler investigation, showing blood flow, is often the only way to differentiate this cystic structure from an arachnoid cyst.[42]

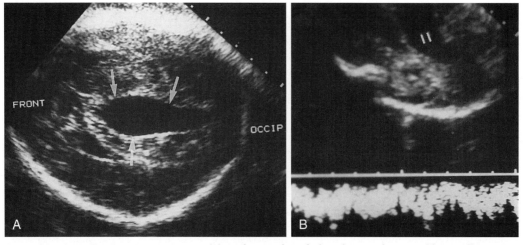

Figure 38-18—Vein of Galen aneurysm. (A) Axial image through the calvarium shows an oblong midline cystic structure (arrows) extending toward the posterior fossa. (B) Pulsed Doppler interrogation reveals high-velocity venous flow.

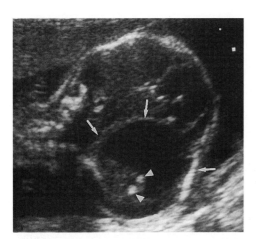

Figure 38-19—Cerebral teratoma. Coronal image through the cranium shows a large cranial mass (arrows) that distorts the shape of the calvarium. This teratoma contains fluid as well as solid and calcific (arrowheads) components.

Focal Cerebral Lesions

Focal intracranial abnormalities that principally involve cerebral structures are listed in Figure 38–1 under the "Parenchymal" heading. Among these, we will briefly consider cerebral neoplasms, porencephaly, and agenesis of the corpus callosum.

Fetal *cerebral neoplasms* are rare, but the most common cell type is the teratoma.[43] Teratomas usually are large and are bizarre in appearance, typically with mixed solid and cystic components and occasional calcification (Fig. 38–19).[4, 43] Serial examinations show rapid enlargement of the mass and the cranium, with possible extracranial extension. The prognosis is dismal, and in a large published series, all fetuses with cranial

teratomas died during the prenatal or neonatal period.[44]

Porencephaly refers to *focal* loss of brain parenchyma, which usually occurs in utero because of a vascular insult. The focal destruction of brain tissue leaves a cystic space (where brain should be) that communicates with the subarachnoid space or ventricular system.[4, 45] Because of the reduction of brain tissue, the ipsilateral ventricle is often enlarged. This finding helps distinguish porencephaly from arachnoid cysts (Fig. 38–20), which cause mass effect on brain parenchyma and are usually separate from the ventricle.[4]

Agenesis of the corpus callosum is an uncommon but important focal brain anomaly that can be detected sonographically in utero. The corpus callosum is a conglomeration of deep white matter that joins the cerebral hemispheres (see Fig. 38–2). Agenesis of the corpus callosum (ACC) may be complete or partial (involving only the posterior corpus callosum).[46] The most characteristic sonographic finding of this anomaly is a midline interhemispheric cyst that represents a dilated, "unroofed" third ventricle. This cyst separates the lateral ventricles. Other findings include nonvisualization of the corpus callosum, dilatation of the occipital horns of the lateral ventricles, and abnormal radial orientation of the medial cerebral gyri[4, 47] (Fig. 38–21). The prognosis for ACC depends on whether or not it is associated with other anomalies (as often it is). Isolated ACC can be asymptomatic; however, most children exhibit some intelligence impairment and seizures.[48]

Focal Intraventricular Abnormalities

The lateral ventricles are filled by the echogenic choroid plexus during fetal life (see Fig.

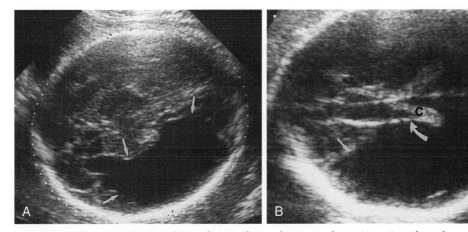

Figure 38-20—Arachnoid cyst. (**A**) Axial image shows a large cystic lesion (arrows) involving the parietal lobe. (**B**) Axial view obtained slightly superior to that in (**A**) shows that the mass is extraventricular (curved arrow shows ventricular wall) and therefore is more likely to be an arachnoid cyst than a porencephalic cyst.

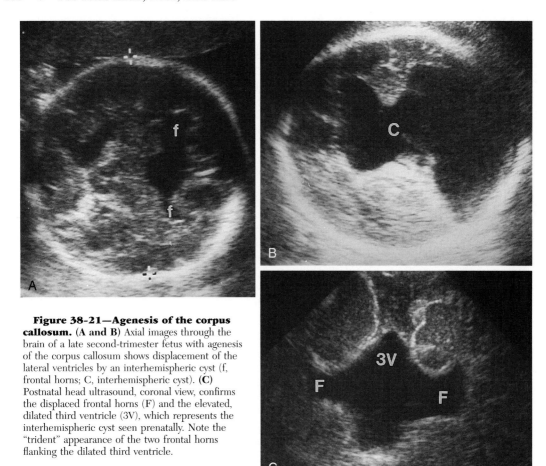

Figure 38-21—Agenesis of the corpus callosum. (A and B) Axial images through the brain of a late second-trimester fetus with agenesis of the corpus callosum shows displacement of the lateral ventricles by an interhemispheric cyst (f, frontal horns; C, interhemispheric cyst). **(C)** Postnatal head ultrasound, coronal view, confirms the displaced frontal horns (F) and the elevated, dilated third ventricle (3V), which represents the interhemispheric cyst seen prenatally. Note the "trident" appearance of the two frontal horns flanking the dilated third ventricle.

38–5B). The most common and most interesting intraventricular lesions during fetal life are *choroid plexus cysts* (CPCs). These cysts present as anechoic or hypoechoic lesions within the choroid plexus that are easily seen on the transventricular view (Fig. 38–22). CPCs are not rare, occurring in 0.2% to 3.6% of second-trimester fetuses.[49–51] They disappear, usually during fetal life, and do not cause neurologic sequelae.[49] However, an association has been shown between CPCs and chromosome abnormalities, particularly trisomy 18. Basically, while up to 4% of normal fetuses may have CPCs, almost half of fetuses with trisomy 18 will have CPCs.[52] Controversy exists regarding performing amniocentesis in all pregnancies with CPCs. Chinn and colleagues[49] combined their data with 10 recent large series of fetuses with CPCs and concluded that an isolated CPC seen in utero (no other anomalies seen in the fetus) does not warrant amniocentesis. At our institution, when a CPC is seen in a low-risk patient, a detailed examination of the fetus is performed with careful attention to the fetal hands (overlapping fingers are a hall-

mark of trisomy 18) and heart. We recommend chromosome analysis only if a sonographic abnormality is seen in addition to the CPC.

Intraventricular hemorrhage in fetal life is rare (Fig. 38–23) but is worthy of mention as it is detectable with ultrasound.[53] The hemorrhage originates in the germinal matrix, which is located in the region of the superior thalamus, and hemorrhage may extend into the ventricular system or brain parenchyma. Intracranial hemorrhage probably results from fetal anoxia, maternal hypertension or hypotensive episodes, and alloimmune thrombocytopenia (from maternal antiplatelet antibodies).[54]

THE FETAL FACE

Visualization of the fetal face is emotionally desirable for patients and in addition gives the sonographer an opportunity to diagnose important malformations. We routinely obtain coronal and profile images of the fetal face, even though these are not required in standards issued by professional organizations. These two planes,

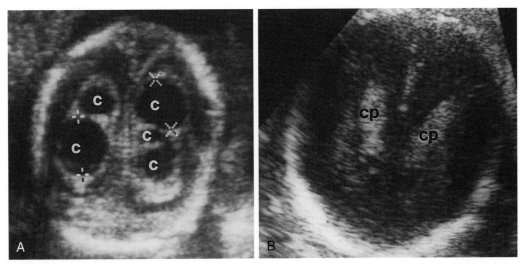

Figure 38-22—Choroid plexus cysts. (A) Axial image through the lateral ventricles shows multiple choroid plexus cysts (c) in this 18-week fetus. No other fetal anomalies were seen, and fetal karyotype was normal. **(B)** Six weeks later, the cysts resolved. (cp, choroid plexus filling the lateral ventricles.)

which are illustrated in Chapter 33, permit examination of the fetal orbits, nose, mouth, and chin. The face is a complex structure, however, that does not lend itself easily to two-dimensional visualization. As three-dimensional ultrasound becomes more widely available, fetal face evaluation will become easier technically, and it will be more rewarding for patients, sonographers, and referring physicians.[55] Detailed discussion of dysmorphic facies is beyond the scope of this book, but we will discuss the most common anomalies—cleft lip and cleft palate.

The most common anomaly affecting the fetal face is the cleft lip. Cleft lip, with or without cleft palate, affects 1:1000 live births in the white population and is the most common facial anomaly. A higher incidence of cleft lip is seen in native American and Asian populations, and a lower incidence is reported in African-Americans.[55] An ultrasound classification system that resembles the surgical classification system has been proposed by Nyberg and colleagues[56] (Fig. 38–24). It is very important to define (as well as possible) the extent and type of facial cleft, using coronal and profile images. Unilateral cleft lip (Fig. 38–25), with or without cleft palate (types 1 or 2), carries a better prognosis than the other types of facial clefts. Sixteen to thirty-one percent of facial clefts are accompanied by chromosome abnormalities,[56, 57] and for that reason we offer amniocentesis for all cases of facial cleft. We also offer amniocentesis because cleft palate frequently is difficult to detect and, if cleft palate is present, it increases the chance for aneuploidy.

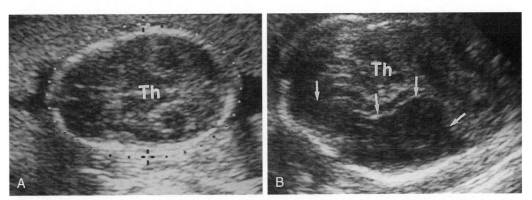

Figure 38-23—Intracranial hemorrhage. (A) At 18 weeks menstrual age, this fetus first presented with oligohydramnios and echogenic bowel. Although the fetal head is dolichocephalic, no intracranial abnormalities were seen. (Th, thalamus.) **(B)** Two weeks later, a large parietal hypoechoic mass (arrows) was present. Note displacement of the thalamus (Th). Subsequently, the fetus suffered in utero demise, and autopsy findings confirmed intracranial hemorrhage and fetal sepsis from cytomegalovirus (CMV).

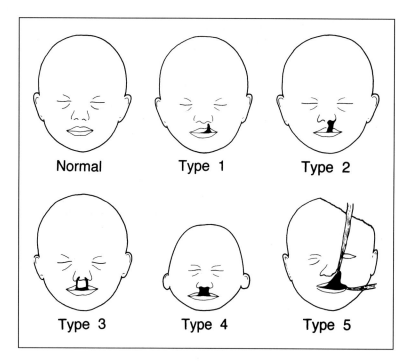

Figure 38-24—Ultrasound classification of facial clefts. Type 1 represents isolated unilateral cleft lip, without cleft palate. Type 2 represents unilateral cleft lip and palate. Type 3 represents bilateral cleft lip and palate. Type 4 represents midline cleft lip and palate. Type 5 represents lip and/or palate clefts associated with amniotic bands or limb-body-wall complex. (Reprinted with permission from Nyberg DA, Sickler GK, Hegge FN, et al: Fetal cleft lip with and without cleft palate: US classification and correlation with outcome. Radiology 195: 677–684, 1995.)

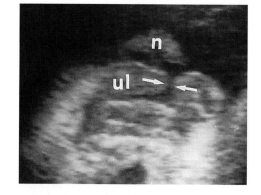

Figure 38-25—Isolated cleft lip, type 1. Coronal image through the fetal nose (n) and lips shows an upper lip (ul) cleft (arrows).

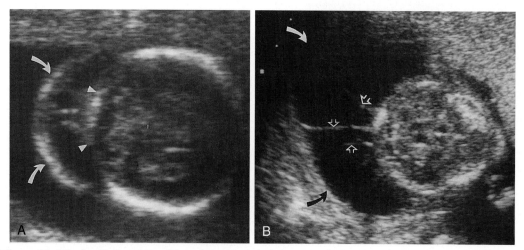

Figure 38-26—Cystic hygroma. (A) Axial view through the posterior fossa of an early second-trimester fetus shows a small, complex cystic area along the back of the neck (curved arrows). Demonstration of an intact occipital calvarium (arrowheads) helps differentiate the cystic hygroma from an occipital encephalocele. **(B)** This large cystic hygroma (curved arrows show outer perimeter) contains many internal septations (open arrows).

As implied in the preceding discussion of holoprosencephaly, a *midline* cleft lip and palate (type 4) is highly associated with trisomy 13 (see Fig. 38–11).[4]

Fetal Neck

Portions of the fetal neck are seen routinely as the sonographer visualizes the posterior fossa of the cranium and the cervical spine. Neck masses tend to be large and *hard to miss*. The most common fetal neck mass is a cystic hygroma. Rarer mass lesions include cervical teratomas and goiters.

Cystic hygromas (CH) are thought to form because of lymphatic obstruction or lack of normal communication between cervical lymphatics and the jugular veins. As seen with ultrasound, a cystic hygroma is a lucent area along the back of the neck (Fig. 38–26) that may be quite large. The lucency may be unilocular and anechoic, or it may be septate. Cystic hygroma implies a grave prognosis when seen in the second trimester, for it is often associated with hydrops fetalis and other anomalies. In our experience, *second-trimester* CH is associated with an 80% fetal mortality rate and a 70% aneuploidy rate.[58] The most common chromosome abnormality associated with second-trimester CH is Turner syndrome (XO).[4, 58]

The implications of nuchal lucency detected in the first trimester are quite different from those seen in the second trimester (Fig. 38–27). The normal first-trimester fetus has an area of posterior nuchal lucency measuring less than 3 mm in thickness (anteroposterior). A large series has shown that 46% of fetuses with nuchal trans-

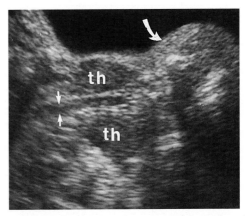

Figure 38-28—Fetal goiter. Coronal image through persistently extended neck (curved arrow, chin) of a 34-week fetus shows a prominent thyroid gland (th). The trachea (small arrows) was not displaced. This fetus was exposed to thyroid hormone blocking agents throughout the pregnancy because of maternal hyperthyroidism and was subsequently hypothyroid at birth.

lucency *greater than 3 mm* have an abnormal karyotype.[59] Unlike the second-trimester association between CH and Turner syndrome, first-trimester nuchal lucency is more often associated with Down syndrome (trisomy 21). It is postulated that a prominent first-trimester nuchal lucency is the precursor of the second-trimester nuchal skin thickening shown to be associated with trisomy 21.[59, 60] We routinely evaluate the skin behind the neck in all first- and second-trimester fetuses, as shown in Chapter 33. Normal anteroposterior values are less than 3 mm in the first trimester and less than 6 mm between 16 and 20 weeks.

Other masses affecting the fetal neck are rare. Solid anterior lesions include teratomas and fetal goiter, which typically are easy to see since they cause hyperextension of the fetal head. Teratomas are isolated benign masses that contain solid, cystic, and calcified components and resemble teratomas elsewhere in the body. The prognosis is related to the size of the lesion, and most fetuses need prompt surgical resection to avoid respiratory obstruction.[60] A fetus may develop a goiter (thyromegaly) in utero, either because of hypothyroidism or hyperthyroidism. The usual cause is maternal use of thyroid-blocking agents that cross the placenta and cause fetal hypothyroidism. The enlarged thyroid presents sonographically as a bilobed, anterior neck mass that displaces the neck vessels laterally (Fig. 38–28).[60]

REFERENCES

1. Filly RA, Cardoza JD, Goldstein RB, et al: Detection of fetal central nervous system anomalies:

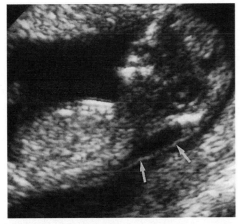

Figure 38-27—First-trimester nuchal lucency. Sagittal view of a 12-week fetus shows an abnormally increased nuchal lucency (arrows) measuring greater than 3 mm. Based solely on this finding, amniocentesis was suggested, and revealed an unbalanced translocation.

A practical level of effort for a routine sonogram. Radiology 172:403–408, 1989.

2. Filly RA, Goldstein RB, Callen PW: Fetal ventricle: Importance in routine obstetric sonography. Radiology 181:1–7, 1991.

3. Cordoza JD, Goldstein RB, Filly RA: Exclusion of fetal ventriculomegaly with a single measurement: The width of the lateral ventricular atrium. Radiology 169:711–714, 1988.

4. Nyberg DA, Pretorius DH: Cerebral malformation. *In* Nyberg DA, Mahony BS, Pretorius DH (eds): Diagnostic Ultrasound of Fetal Anomalies: Text and Atlas. St. Louis, CV Mosby, 1990, pp 83–145.

5. Pretorius D, Davis K, Manco-Johnson M, et al: Clinical course of fetal hydrocephalus: 40 cases. AJNR Am J Neuroradiol 6:23–27, 1985.

6. Halliday J, Chow CW, Wallace D, et al: X-linked hydrocephalus: A survey of a 20 year period in Victoria, Australia. J Med Genet 23:23–31, 1986.

7. Vintzileos AM, Ingardia CJ, Nochimson DJ: Congenital hydrocephalus: A review and protocol for perinatal management. Obstet Gynecol 62:539–549, 1983.

8. Nyberg DA, Mack LA, Hirsch J, et al: Fetal hydrocephalus: Sonographic detection and clinical significance of associated anomalies. Radiology 163:187–191, 1987.

9. Mahony BS, Nyberg DA, Hirsch JH, et al: Mild idiopathic lateral cerebral ventricular dilatation in utero: Sonographic evaluation. Radiology 169:715–721, 1988.

10. DeMeyer W: Classification of cerebral malformations. Birth Defects 7:78–93, 1971.

11. Fitz CR: Holoprosencephaly and related entities. Neuroradiology 25:225–238, 1983.

12. McGahan JP, Ellis W, Lindfors KK, et al: Congenital cerebrospinal fluid–containing intracranial abnormalities: A sonographic classification. J Clin Ultrasound 16:531–544, 1988.

13. Hoffman-Tietin JC, Horoupian DS, Koenigsberg M, et al: Lobar holoprosencephaly with hydrocephalus: Antenatal demonstration and differential diagnosis. J Ultrasound Med 5:691–697, 1986.

14. Chervenak FA, Isaacson G, Hobbins JC, et al: Diagnosis and management of fetal holoprosencephaly. Obstet Gynecol 60:322–326, 1985.

15. Green MF, Benacerraf BR, Frigoletto FD Jr: Reliable criteria for the prenatal diagnosis of alobar holoprosencephaly. Am J Obstet Gynecol 156:687–689, 1987.

16. Nyberg DA, Mack LA, Bronstein A, et al: Holoprosencephaly: Prenatal sonographic diagnosis. AJR Am J Roentgenol 149:1050–1058, 1987.

17. DeMeyer W, Zeman W, Palmer C: The face predicts the brain: Diagnostic significance of median facial anomalies for holoprosencephaly. Pediatrics 34:256–263, 1964.

18. McGahan JP, Nyberg DA, Mack LA: Sonography of facial features of alobar and semilobar holoprosencephaly. AJR Am J Roentgenol 154:143–148, 1990.

19. Fiske CE, Filly RA: Ultrasound of the normal and abnormal fetal neural axis. Radiol Clin North Am 20:285–296, 1982.

20. Raybaud C: Destructive lesions of the brain. Neuroradiology 25:265–291, 1983.

21. Dublin A, French B: Diagnostic image evaluation of hydranencephaly and pictorially similar entities, with emphasis on computed tomography. Radiology 137:81–91, 1980.

22. Greene MF, Benacerraf BR, Crawford JM: Hydranencephaly: US appearance during in utero evolution. Radiology 156:779–780, 1985.

23. Pretorius D, Russ P, Rumack C, et al: Diagnosis of brain neuropathology in utero. Neuroradiology 28:386–397, 1986.

24. Kurtz A, Wapner R, Rubin C, et al: Ultrasound criteria for in utero diagnosis of microcephaly. J Clin Ultrasound 8:11–16, 1980.

25. Bromley B, Benacerraf BR: Difficulties in the prenatal diagnosis of microcephaly. J Ultrasound Med 14:303–305, 1995.

26. Graham D, Guidi SM, Sanders RC: Sonographic features of in utero periventricular calcifications due to cytomegalovirus infection. J Ultrasound Med 1:171–173, 1982.

27. Ghidini A, Sirtori M, Vergani P, et al: Fetal intracranial calcifications. Am J Obstet Gynecol 160:86–87, 1989.

28. Fakhry J, Khoury A, et al: Fetal intracranial calcifications: The importance of periventricular hyperechoic foci without shadowing. J Ultrasound Med 10:51–54, 1991.

29. Grannum P, Pilu G: In utero neurosonography: The normal fetus and variations in cranial size. Semin Perinatol 11:85–97, 1987.

30. Martin H: Microcephaly and mental retardation. Am J Dis Child 119:128–131, 1970.

31. Bromley B, Nadel AS, Pauker S, et al: Closure of the cerebellar vermis: Evaluation with second trimester US. Radiology 193:761–763, 1991.

32. Dempsey PJ, Koch HJ: In utero diagnosis of the Dandy-Walker syndrome: Differentiation from extra-axial posterior fossa cyst. J Clin Ultrasound 9:403–405, 1981.

33. Newman GC, Buschi AI, Sugg NK, et al: Dandy-Walker syndrome diagnosed in utero by ultrasonography. Neurology 32:180–184, 1982.

34. Hirsch JF, Pierre-Kahn A, Renier D, et al: The Dandy-Walker malformation: A review of 40 cases. J Neurosurg 61:515–522, 1984.

35. Russ PD, Pretorius DH, Johnson MJ: Dandy-Walker syndrome: A review of fifteen cases evaluated by prenatal sonography. Am J Obstet Gynecol 161:401–406, 1989.

36. Pilu G, Romero R, De Palma L, et al: Antenatal diagnosis and obstetric management of Dandy-Walker syndrome. J Reprod Med 31:1017–1022, 1986.

37. Hart MN, Malamud N, Ellis WG: The Dandy-Walker syndrome: A clinico-pathological study based on 28 cases. Neurology 22:771–780, 1972.

38. Nyberg DA, Cyr DR, Mack LA, et al: The Dandy-Walker malformation: Prenatal sonographic diagnosis and its clinical significance. J Ultrasound Med 7:65–71, 1988.

39. Rengachary SS: Intracranial arachnoid and ependymal cyst. *In* Wilkins RH, Rengachary SS (eds): Neurosurgery. New York, McGraw-Hill, 1985, pp 2160–2171.

40. Anderson FM, Landeng BH: Cerebral arachnoid cysts in infants. J Paediatr 69:88–90, 1966.

41. O'Brien J, Schechter MM: Arteriovenous malformations involving the Galenic system. AJR Am J Roentgenol 110:50–55, 1970.

42. Rizzo G, Arduini D, Colosimo C Jr, et al: Abnormal fetal cerebral blood flow velocity waveforms as a sign of an aneurysm of the vein of Galen. Fetal Ther 2:75–79, 1987.

43. Lipman S, Pretorius D, Rumack C, et al: Fetal intracranial teratoma: US diagnosis of three cases

and a review of the literature. Radiology 157:491–494, 1985.

44. Takaku A, Kodama N, Ohara H, et al: Brain tumor in newborn babies. Child's Brain 4:365–375, 1973.

45. Berg R, Aleck K, Kaplan A: Familial porencephaly. Arch Neurol 40:567–569, 1983.

46. Warkany J, Lemore RJ, Cohen MM. Agenesis of the corpus callosum. *In* Mental Retardation in Congenital Malformation of the Central Nervous System. Chicago, Year Book Medical Publishers, Inc, 1981, pp 224–241.

47. Babcock D: The normal absent and abnormal corpus callosum: Sonographic findings. Radiology 151:449–453, 1984.

48. Loeser J, Alvord E: Clinicopathological correlations in agenesis of the corpus callosum. Neurology 18:745–756, 1987.

49. Chinn DH, Miller EI, Worthy LM, et al: Sonographically detected fetal choroid plexus cysts: Frequency and association with aneuploidy. J Ultrasound Med 10:255–258, 1991.

50. Chitkara U, Cogswell C, Norton K, et al: Choroid plexus cysts in the fetus: A benign anatomic variant or pathologic entity? Report of 41 cases and review of the literature. Obstet Gynecol 72:185–189, 1988.

51. Chan L, Hixon JL, Laifer SA, et al: A sonographic and karyotypic study of second trimester fetal choroid plexus cysts. Obstet Gynecol 73:703–706, 1989.

52. Benacerraf BR, Nadel A, Bromley B: Identification of second trimester fetuses with autosomal trisomy by use of a sonographic scoring index. Radiology 193:135–140, 1994.

53. Johnson M, Rumack C, Mannes E, et al: Detection of neonatal intracranial hemorrhage utilizing real time and static ultrasound. J Clin Ultrasound 9:427–433, 1981.

54. Pretorius DH, Nelson TR: Fetal face visualization using three-dimensional ultrasonography. J Ultrasound Med 14:349–356, 1995.

55. Melnick M: Cleft lip and cleft palate: Etiology and pathogenesis. *In* Kernahan DA, Rosenstein SW, Dado DV (eds): Cleft Lip and Palate: A System of Management. Baltimore, Williams & Wilkins, 1990, pp 3–12.

56. Nyberg DA, Sickler GK, Hegge FN, et al: Fetal cleft lip with and without cleft palate: US classification and correlation with outcome. Radiology 195:677–684, 1995.

57. Benacerraf BR, Mulliken JB: Fetal cleft lip and palate: Sonographic diagnosis and postnatal outcome. Plast Reconstr Surg 92:1045–1049, 1993.

58. Sohaey RS, Fillmore DJ, Woodward PJ, et al: Cystic hygroma: How poor is the prognosis? Presentation at 38th Annual Convention of American Ultrasound in Medicine, Baltimore, March, 1994.

59. van Vugt JMG, van Zalen-Sprock RM, Kostense PJ: First trimester nuchal translucency: A risk analysis on fetal chromosome abnormality. Radiology 200:537–540, 1996.

60. Mahony BS, Hegge FN: The face and neck. *In* Nyberg DA, Mahony BS, Pretorius DH (eds): Diagnostic Ultrasound of Fetal Anomalies: Text and Atlas. St. Louis, CV Mosby, 1990, pp 203–261.

Chapter 39

The Fetal Thorax

Roya Sohaey

The majority of fetal chest anomalies are visible with ultrasound on routinely obtained transverse images at the level of the four-chamber heart. In this chapter, normal lung development, pulmonary hypoplasia, and common fetal chest masses are considered. A practical approach for sonographic differentiation of chest masses is stressed.

LUNG DEVELOPMENT

Lung development begins at 5 weeks' menstrual age and continues through the eighth year of life. Four stages of lung development have been described, as summarized in Table 39–1.[1] These stages are significant with respect to the pathogenesis of anomalies described in this chapter.

The longest period of lung development is the alveolar period, during which type 1 alveolar cells develop, which are thin and allow for easier gas exchange. At birth, the primitive alveoli expand slightly, and the lungs subsequently expand as well. Surfactant, a substance formed by type 2 alveolar epithelial cells during the 23rd to 24th weeks of gestation, is rapidly expelled during the first breaths that a newborn infant takes. Surfactant lowers the surface tension at the air/alveolar interface, maintaining patency of the alveoli and preventing atelectasis (collapse of the lung). Further increase in lung size after birth occurs not from an increase in alveolar size but rather from an increase in the number of alveoli. Immature alveoli form additional primitive alveoli, which grow and mature. The neonate has only one eighth to one sixth of the adult number of alveoli. Alveolar production progresses to approximately 8 years of age. By 25 to 28 weeks, and coinciding with a fetal weight near 1000 gm, alveolar development may permit enough gas exchange for survival of a prematurely born infant.[1]

Four factors must be present if normal lung development is to occur: adequate gestational age, adequate amniotic fluid, adequate space, and adequate in utero "breathing."[2] In addition, pulmonary fluid dynamics and hormonal effects are important for lung development.[3]

The fetal lungs are seen well with ultrasound and normally are homogeneous and medium in echogenicity. The echo level of the lungs either equals or slightly exceeds that of the fetal liver[4] (Fig. 39–1). Fetal lungs extend in the coronal plane from the clavicle to the diaphragm, which is visible as an echolucent band between the lungs and the liver or spleen (Fig. 39–2). Ultrasound, unfortunately, is a poor predictor of lung maturity. Attempts at predicting lung maturity based on pulmonary echogenicity, coarsening of echotexture, and progressive increase in sound transmission have been unsuccessful.[2, 4, 5]

PULMONARY HYPOPLASIA

Pulmonary hypoplasia, defined as an absolute decrease in lung volume or weight when compared with gestational age,[6, 7] occurs for two principal reasons: primary failure of lung development or compression of the lungs, which restricts lung growth. Pulmonary hypoplasia is the cause of death in 10% to 15% of all neonatal autopsies, and is the most common cause of death in fetuses with chest masses.[8–10] When pulmonary hypoplasia is diagnosed in utero, the mortality rate is 80%.[11] Parenchymal abnormalities, such as cys-

Table 39-1. Embryology of Lung Development

Period	Menstrual Age	Embryologic Events
Pseudoglandular	5–17 wk	Laryngotracheal tube Two lung buds Terminal bronchioles (TB) (blind-ending tubes) TB branching
Canalicular	13–25 wk	Respiratory bronchioles Primitive alveoli
Terminal sac	24 wk–term	Alveoli thin Capillary proliferation Gas exchange possible (fetus near 1000 gm)
Alveolar	Birth–age 8 yr	Alveoli thin further (type 1 cells) Increase in the number of alveoli 6- to 8-fold

From Sohaey R, Zwiebel WJ: The fetal thorax: Noncardiac chest anomalies. Semin Ultrasound CT MRI 17:34–50, 1996.

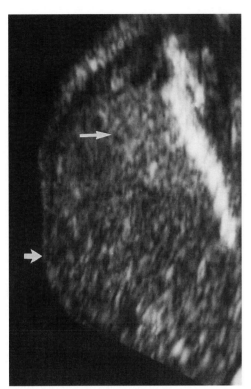

Figure 39-1—Normal fetal lung. Sagittal image throughout the fetal chest shows that the lung (long arrow) is slightly more echogenic than the fetal liver (short arrow). (Reprinted with permission from Sohaey R, Zwiebel WJ: The fetal thorax: Noncardiac chest anomalies. Semin Ultrasound CT MRI 17:34–50, 1996.)

tic adenomatoid malformation, pulmonary sequestration, and bronchial atresia, may cause pulmonary hypoplasia by replacing normal lung with nonfunctioning tissue. Compression of the lungs, however, is the most important cause of pulmonary hypoplasia, as seen in prolonged oligohydramnios, which compresses the chest, or a small thorax secondary to a structural or chromosomal abnormality.[11] Chest masses, including diaphragmatic hernia, also cause lung compression and account for numerous cases of hypoplasia. Skeletal cage or neural abnormalities that reduce fetal breathing are additional rare causes of hypoplasia.[8, 12–14]

Prenatal prediction of pulmonary hypoplasia is possible with ultrasound, by comparing chest size with gestational age.[15] A recent study of singleton pregnancies showed a high positive predictive value for pulmonary hypoplasia using fetal chest circumference measurements.[16] After 16 weeks' menstrual age, chest circumference growth is linear, and after 20 weeks', the ratio of chest circumference to abdominal circumference is greater than 0.8 in nearly all normal pregnancies.[15] The thoracic circumference is measured

at the level of the four-chamber cardiac view, excluding the skin and subcutaneous tissues[11] (Fig. 39–3). Normal thoracic circumference measurements are provided in Table 39–2. Circumference values less than the fifth percentile for gestational age are considered abnormal.[17] Fetal thoracic length (Table 39–3) may be superior to chest circumference measurements in identifying pulmonary hypoplasia.[18] Reduced lung or thoracic length is best appreciated on coronal or sagittal images from which the chest and abdomen sizes can be compared easily (Fig. 39–4). On such images, pulmonary hypoplasia usually is obvious to an experienced sonologist. Idiopathic pulmonary hypoplasia or hypoplasia from masses can be overlooked sonographically, however. The chest size commonly is normal in these cases, even though the lung volume may be very small.

PLEURAL EFFUSION

The most common cause for a fetal pleural effusion is hydrops fetalis. Once a pleural effusion is seen, a careful search should ensue for associated manifestations of hydrops, including skin edema, ascites, polyhydramnios, and placentamegaly.[19] Many immune and nonimmune causes

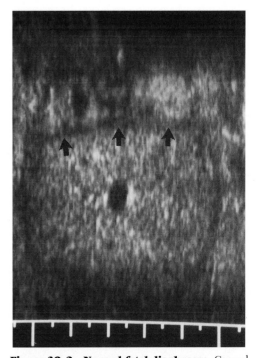

Figure 39-2—Normal fetal diaphragm. Coronal image through the abdomen and chest shows a hypoechoic band (arrows) representing the intact fetal diaphragm. (Reprinted with permission from Sohaey R, Zwiebel WJ: The fetal thorax: Noncardiac chest anomalies. Semin Ultrasound CT MRI 17:34–50, 1996.)

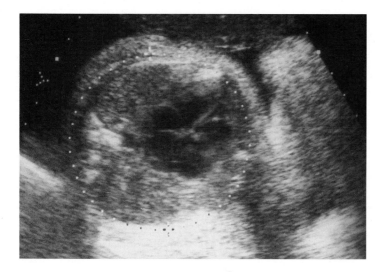

Figure 39-3—Thoracic circumference. Correct technique for measuring the thoracic circumference at the level of the four-chamber view of the heart. Note that subcutaneous tissues are excluded. (Reprinted with permission from Sohaey R, Zwiebel WJ: The fetal thorax: Noncardiac chest anomalies. Semin Ultrasound CT MRI 17:34–50, 1996.)

for hydrops exist, and pleural effusions, usually bilateral, can be an early sign for hydrops. The pleural effusion in these cases is a hydrothorax.

A unilateral pleural effusion, on the other hand, is most likely a chylothorax, which is caused by fetal thoracic duct malformations. Chylothorax tends to involve the right chest and is more common in males than in females.[20] Although chylothorax fluid is white and milky in a neonate that has been milk fed, fetal and newborn chylothorax fluid is clear. If intrauterine fluid aspiration is performed to diagnose a chylothorax, therefore, the fluid should be analyzed by lipoprotein electrophoresis to detect the predominance of high-density lipoprotein.[21] A chylothorax can be idiopathic or associated with trisomy 21, monosomy X (Turner syndrome), pulmonary lymphangiectasia, or other syndromes.[11]

Table 39-2. Fetal Thoracic Circumference Measurements

Gestational Age (wk)	No.	Predictive Percentiles								
		2.5	5	10	25	50	75	90	95	97.5
16	6	5.9	6.4	7.0	8.0	9.1	10.3	11.3	11.9	12.4
17	22	6.8	7.3	7.9	8.9	10.0	11.2	12.2	12.8	13.3
18	31	7.7	8.2	8.8	9.8	11.0	12.1	13.1	13.7	14.2
19	21	8.6	9.1	9.7	10.7	11.9	13.0	14.0	14.6	15.1
20	20	9.5	10.0	10.6	11.7	12.8	13.9	15.0	15.5	16.0
21	30	10.4	11.0	11.6	12.6	13.7	14.8	15.8	16.4	16.9
22	18	11.3	11.9	12.5	13.5	14.6	15.7	16.7	17.3	17.8
23	21	12.2	12.8	13.4	14.4	15.5	16.6	17.6	18.2	18.8
24	27	13.2	13.7	14.3	15.3	16.4	17.5	18.5	19.1	19.7
25	20	14.1	14.6	15.2	16.2	17.3	18.4	19.4	20.0	20.6
26	25	15.0	15.5	16.1	17.1	18.2	19.3	20.3	21.0	21.5
27	24	15.9	16.4	17.0	18.0	19.1	20.2	21.3	21.9	22.4
28	24	16.8	17.3	17.9	18.9	20.0	21.2	22.2	22.8	23.3
29	24	17.7	18.2	18.8	19.8	21.0	22.1	23.1	23.7	24.2
30	27	18.6	19.1	19.7	20.7	21.9	23.0	24.0	24.6	25.1
31	24	19.5	20.0	20.6	21.6	22.8	23.9	24.9	25.5	26.0
32	28	20.4	20.9	21.5	22.6	23.7	24.8	25.8	26.4	26.9
33	27	21.3	21.8	22.5	23.5	24.6	25.7	26.7	27.3	27.8
34	25	22.2	22.8	23.4	24.4	25.5	26.6	27.6	28.2	28.7
35	20	23.1	23.7	24.3	25.3	26.4	27.5	28.5	29.1	29.6
36	23	24.0	24.6	25.2	26.2	27.3	28.4	29.4	30.0	30.6
37	22	24.9	25.5	26.1	27.1	28.2	29.3	30.3	30.9	31.5
38	21	25.9	26.4	27.0	28.0	29.1	30.2	31.2	31.9	32.4
39	7	26.8	27.3	27.9	28.9	30.0	31.1	32.2	32.8	33.3
40	6	27.7	28.2	28.8	29.8	30.9	32.1	33.1	33.7	34.2

NOTE: Measurements in centimeters.

Reprinted with permission from Chitkara U, Rosenberg J, Chervenak FA, et al: Prenatal sonographic assessment of the fetal thorax: Normal values. Am J Obstet Gynecol 156:1069–1074, 1987.

Table 39-3. Fetal Thoracic Length Measurements

Gestational Age (wk)	No.	Predictive Percentiles								
		2.5	5	10	25	50	75	90	95	97.5
16	6	0.9	1.1	1.3	1.6	2.0	2.4	2.8	3.0	3.2
17	22	1.1	1.3	1.5	1.8	2.2	2.6	3.0	3.2	3.4
18	31	1.3	1.4	1.7	2.0	2.4	2.8	3.2	3.4	3.6
19	21	1.4	1.6	1.8	2.2	2.7	3.0	3.4	3.6	3.8
20	20	1.6	1.8	2.0	2.4	2.8	3.2	3.6	3.8	4.0
21	30	1.8	2.0	2.2	2.6	3.0	3.4	3.7	4.0	4.1
22	18	2.0	2.2	2.4	2.8	3.2	3.6	3.9	4.1	4.3
23	21	2.2	2.4	2.6	3.0	3.4	3.8	4.1	4.3	4.5
24	27	2.4	2.6	2.8	3.1	3.5	3.9	4.3	4.5	4.7
25	20	2.6	2.8	3.0	3.3	3.7	4.1	4.5	4.7	4.9
26	25	2.8	2.9	3.2	3.5	3.9	4.3	4.7	4.9	5.1
27	24	2.9	3.1	3.3	3.7	4.1	4.5	4.9	5.1	5.3
28	24	3.1	3.3	3.5	3.9	4.3	4.7	5.0	5.4	5.4
29	24	3.3	3.5	3.7	4.1	4.5	4.9	5.2	5.5	5.6
30	27	3.5	3.7	3.9	4.3	4.7	5.1	5.4	5.6	5.8
31	24	3.7	3.9	4.1	4.5	4.9	5.3	5.6	5.8	6.0
32	28	3.9	4.1	4.3	4.6	5.0	5.4	5.8	6.0	6.2
33	27	4.1	4.3	4.5	4.8	5.2	5.6	6.0	6.2	6.4
34	25	4.2	4.4	4.7	5.0	5.4	5.8	6.2	6.4	6.6
35	20	4.4	4.6	4.8	5.2	5.6	6.0	6.4	6.6	6.8
36	23	4.6	4.8	5.0	5.4	5.8	6.2	6.5	6.8	7.0
37	22	4.8	5.0	5.2	5.6	6.0	6.4	6.7	7.0	7.1
38	21	5.0	5.2	5.4	5.8	6.2	6.6	6.9	7.1	7.3
39	7	5.2	5.4	5.6	6.0	6.4	6.8	7.1	7.3	7.5
40	6	5.4	5.6	5.8	6.1	6.5	6.9	7.3	7.5	7.7

NOTE: Measurements in centimeters.
Reprinted with permission from Roberts AB, Mitchell JM: Direct ultrasonographic measurement of fetal lung length in normal pregnancies and pregnancies complicated by prolonged rupture of membranes. Am J Obstet Gynecol 163:1560–1566, 1990.

Ultrasound Findings

Pleural fluid appears as an anechoic collection surrounding the fetal lungs. Pleural fluid often is first seen on the transverse chest images, but fluid is best appreciated on coronal images. When pleural fluid is bilateral and large in volume, the fluid is seen to surround small, "winglike" lungs (Fig. 39–5). The sonographer should look carefully for other fluid collections if pleural fluid is seen. Sonographic findings more indicative of a chylothorax include a unilateral collection or asymmetric bilateral collections (Fig. 39–6).

Prognosis and Treatment

The prognosis for a fetus with pleural effusion depends on the presence or absence of hydrops. Overall mortality is greater than 50% for all fetuses with hydrothorax. Even a benign-appearing, uni-

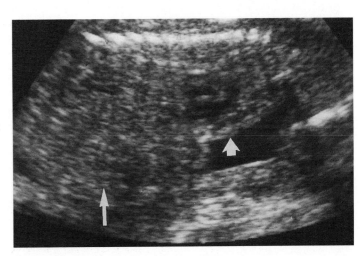

Figure 39-4—Pulmonary hypoplasia secondary to a small chest (short ribs). Sagittal image (spine toward transducer) shows a very small chest (short arrow) compared with the abdomen (long arrow). (Reprinted with permission from Sohaey R, Zwiebel WJ: The fetal thorax: Noncardiac chest anomalies. Semin Ultrasound CT MRI 17:34–50, 1996.)

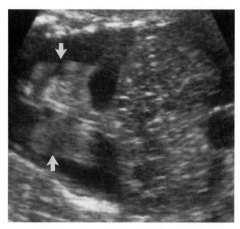

Figure 39-5—Bilateral pleural effusions. Coronal view through the chest and upper abdomen in a fetus with hydrops fetalis shows small "winglike" lungs (arrows) surrounded by large bilateral pleural effusions (anechoic region completely surrounding the lungs). (Reprinted with permission from Sohaey R, Zwiebel WJ: The fetal thorax: Noncardiac chest anomalies. Semin Ultrasound CT MRI 17:34–50, 1996.)

lateral effusion is associated with 15% to 25% mortality.[22] Prenatal thoracentesis can be performed with ultrasound guidance. In the second trimester, fetal thoracentesis may be performed to enable further lung development, but reaccumulation of fluid is a problem (Fig. 39–7). Thoracoamniotic shunts also can be placed in utero for long-term drainage purposes. Fetal thoracentesis performed in the third trimester (usually immediately prior to delivery) facilitates resuscitation efforts in the compromised newborn infant.[23]

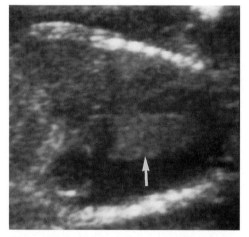

Figure 39-6—Unilateral pleural effusion. Fluid completely surrounds only one lung (arrow) in this fetus with congenital chylothorax. (Reprinted with permission from Sohaey R, Zwiebel WJ: The fetal thorax: Noncardiac chest anomalies. Semin Ultrasound CT MRI 17:34–50, 1996.)

CHEST MASSES

A fetal chest mass should be suspected when ultrasound shows deviation of the fetal heart from its expected position, as seen on the four-chamber view. The chest mass may be cystic, solid, or a combination of both. The most common fetal chest mass is displaced abdominal viscera resulting from a diaphragmatic hernia.[8, 12, 13] The second most common fetal chest mass is a cystic adenomatoid malformation, followed by pulmonary sequestration, bronchogenic cyst, and bronchial atresia.[2, 11] Asymmetric pleural effusions are additional causes of mass effect. Mass-creating intrathoracic entities often can be differentiated on the basis of sonographic findings, as outlined later for the more common chest masses.

CONGENITAL DIAPHRAGMATIC HERNIA

Congenital diaphragmatic hernias (CDHs) occur in 1:2000 to 3000 births.[24-26] They are left sided in 85% to 90% of cases and unilateral in 97% of cases.[2, 11] A high proportion of fetuses with diaphragmatic hernias have other structural malformations, as discussed later.[11]

A variety of diaphragmatic hernias can occur, reflecting the complexity of diaphragmatic embryology.[1] Bochdalek hernias account for 90% of CDHs and are caused by failed or incomplete closure of the posterior pleuroperitoneal reflection. These embryologic reflections are lateral structures that normally fuse posteriorly; therefore, Bochdalek hernias classically are posterolateral in location. Bochdalek hernias also are classically left sided. Foramen of Morgagni (FM) hernias are the second most common CDH type. They occur in the anteromedial, retrosternal portion of the diaphragm, consistent with maldevelopment of the septum transversum, which is the most anterior diaphragmatic tissue, from an embryologic perspective.[1, 11] One can remember the location of these hernias by a simple mnemonic: *BochdaLek's is Back Lateral* and *Foramen of Morgagni is Forward Medial.*

Ultrasound Findings

Since the great majority of CDHs are left sided, the most common ultrasound finding is displacement of the fetal heart and mediastinum toward the right.[27, 28] Four classic findings are present with left sided CDH: (1) a cystic mass (displaced bowel) in the left side of the chest; (2) displacement or deviation of the heart toward the right; (3) absence of the fluid-filled stomach

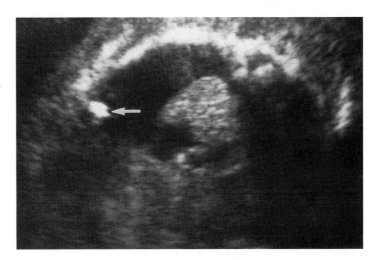

Figure 39-7—In utero thoracentesis. Ultrasound guidance was provided for in utero thoracentesis. The needle tip (arrow) is seen within the pleural fluid. Unfortunately, the fluid quickly reaccumulated, the fetus developed hydrops fetalis, and died shortly after birth. (Reprinted with permission from Sohaey R, Zwiebel WJ: The fetal thorax: Noncardiac chest anomalies. Semin Ultrasound CT MRI 17:34–50, 1996.)

fundus in the abdomen; and (4) polyhydramnios (Fig. 39–8). Smaller-than-expected abdominal circumference is an additional sign of CDH (the abdomen may be scaphoid in severe cases).[27, 28] The visualization of peristalsis within the cystic chest mass is pathognomonic![29] Large diaphragmatic defects can permit the spleen, left kidney, and left lobe of the liver to enter the chest.

Right-sided diaphragmatic defects may be more difficult to visualize than left-sided defects, since the echogenicity of the displaced liver is similar to that of the lung.[30] An intact portion of the diaphragm or a hepatic interlobar fissure

that mimics the diaphragm may cause confusion diagnostically.[31] In any case, ultrasound visualization of an apparently intact diaphragm does not exclude a diaphragmatic hernia (Fig. 39–9). Sonographic findings associated with a bad prognosis in CDH include a dilated intrathoracic stomach, diagnosis of CDH before 25 weeks, liver herniation, hydrops, and associated anomalies.[2, 11]

Associated Anomalies

Survival in fetuses with CDH is greatly influenced by the presence of associated anomalies.

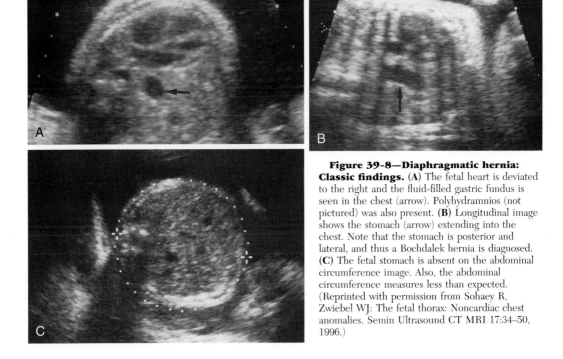

Figure 39-8—Diaphragmatic hernia: Classic findings. (A) The fetal heart is deviated to the right and the fluid-filled gastric fundus is seen in the chest (arrow). Polyhydramnios (not pictured) was also present. **(B)** Longitudinal image shows the stomach (arrow) extending into the chest. Note that the stomach is posterior and lateral, and thus a Bochdalek hernia is diagnosed. **(C)** The fetal stomach is absent on the abdominal circumference image. Also, the abdominal circumference measures less than expected. (Reprinted with permission from Sohaey R, Zwiebel WJ: The fetal thorax: Noncardiac chest anomalies. Semin Ultrasound CT MRI 17:34–50, 1996.)

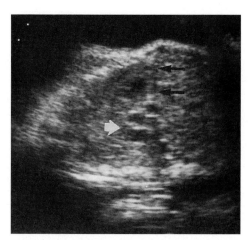

Figure 39-9—Diaphragmatic hernia. Although the diaphragm is visible (black arrows), a posterior diaphragmatic hernia is present. Bowel (white arrow) is seen extending into the chest. (Cephalad is left and caudal is right in this coronal view through the chest and abdomen.) (Reprinted with permission from Sohaey R, Zwiebel WJ: The fetal thorax: Noncardiac chest anomalies. Semin Ultrasound CT MRI 17:34–50, 1996.)

More than 50% of fetuses with CDH have other structural or chromosomal abnormalities,[26] and the likelihood of anomalies is particularly high if the fetus is growth retarded.[24, 28] Cardiac malformations are seen in 9% to 23% of CDH cases[11, 24] and neural tube defects in 28%.[2, 11] In our experience, the combination of cardiac malformation and diaphragmatic hernia is lethal.[32] In addition, 4% of CDH cases are associated with trisomy 18 and trisomy 21.[33] At our institution, therefore, amniocentesis is recommended for all pregnancies with CDH. Finally, diaphragmatic hernia can be a component of several syndromes.[34]

Prognosis and Treatment

The mechanical effects of intrathoracic bowel lead to pulmonary hypoplasia and an associated deficiency of surfactant.[35] Therefore, pulmonary hypoplasia and resultant persistence of the fetal circulation (Chapter 40) are the leading causes of perinatal death in CDH cases.[2, 11] Overall mortality from CDH is reported as 70% to 75%,[24, 33, 36] but survival odds may be better if the CDH is localized and the patient delivers at a tertiary center with extracorporeal membrane oxygenation capability.[37] A 50% rate of intrauterine fetal demise and an overall survival rate of only 7% has been reported when CDH is associated with other structural anomalies![24, 33, 38]

Immediate postpartum surgical correction of CDH is the mainstay of treatment.[37] Despite technical improvements, the results of in utero surgery for CDH have been disappointing.[39-41]

CYSTIC ADENOMATOID MALFORMATION

Cystic adenomatoid malformations (CAMs) comprise 25% of congenital chest lesions. The insult to lung development that leads to a CAM occurs very early, at probably less than 10 weeks' menstrual age.[42] Some investigators believe CAMs are hamartomas,[43, 44] but others believe CAMs result from bronchial atresia and that histologic differences among CAMs reflect differing degrees of dysplastic lung development beyond atretic segments.[45] Three types of CAM have been described by Stocker and colleagues,[46] and this pathologic categorization correlates well with sonographic findings. Type I CAMs contain large cysts that measure greater than 2 cm in diameter. The cysts are clustered, with one or more large cyst of 2 to 10 cm in diameter surrounded by multiple smaller cysts. The large cysts contain respiratory epithelium whereas the smaller ones resemble dilated bronchioles.[42] Type II CAMs are characterized by uniform, medium-sized cysts usually not greater than 2 cm in diameter. Type III CAMs contain small cysts, not greater than 0.3 to 0.5 cm in diameter, which may involve an entire lobe or lung.[42]

Ultrasound Findings

The ultrasound appearance of a CAM is directly related to the histologic structure of the

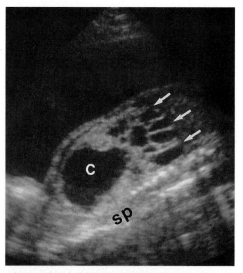

Figure 39-10—Cystic adenomatoid malformation (CAM), type I. Sagittal image through the fetal chest shows a large mass containing multiple cysts. The chest mass fills the right chest and impresses upon the diaphragm (arrows). The largest cyst (c) measures greater than 2.0 cm. The morphology of the mass allows for the correct diagnosis of a type I CAM. (Fetal position is spine (sp) down; cranial is left and caudad is right.)

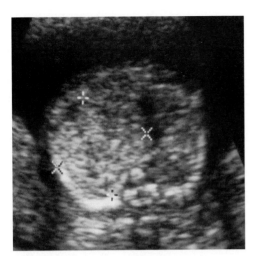

Figure 39-11—Cystic adenomatoid malformation (CAM), type III. A large echogenic mass (calipers) displaces the heart. No discrete cysts are seen (CAM III cysts are too small to resolve; instead, the many interfaces they cause result in a diffusely echogenic mass). (Reprinted with permission from Sohaey R, Zwiebel WJ: The fetal thorax: Noncardiac chest anomalies. Semin Ultrasound CT MRI 17:34–50, 1996.)

lesion. A multicystic lung mass with cysts of varying sizes, some greater than 2 cm, is typical for the Type I CAM (Fig. 39–10). A lung mass with multiple cysts of uniform size, none greater than 2 cm, is most likely a Type II CAM. The Type III CAM presents as a solid-appearing, bulky, echogenic lung mass (Fig. 39–11). The mass appears solid because the sound beam traverses multiple interfaces caused by the walls of myriad tiny cysts.[47] The appearance of Type III CAM in the lung is reminiscent of autosomal recessive polycystic kidney disease in the abdomen. CAM

can regress in size or disappear during fetal life, although this occurs uncommonly[48] (Fig. 39–12).

CAMs are often associated with additional significant anomalies. Type II CAM, in particular, is associated with severe fetal malformations (usually cardiac or renal), as well as chromosome abnormalities.[11, 44] Pulmonary hypoplasia may result from the mass effect of the lesion. Hydrops fetalis, seen in 62% of CAM cases,[11] is caused by mass effect on the heart and inferior vena cava. The principal hemodynamic mechanism here is poor venous return, which results in impaired cardiac function.[49, 50] Polyhydramnios is seen in the majority of fetuses with CAM and most likely results either from decreased fetal swallowing or increased fluid production by the mass. Serial ultrasound examinations are recommended for fetuses identified with CAMs in order to follow the severity of polyhydramnios and hydrops.

Prognosis and Treatment

CAM is rarely asymptomatic in the neonate, and prompt postnatal intervention is necessary in most cases.[42, 51] Neonates with CAM often develop acute, progressive respiratory distress that begins immediately after birth. The prognosis in such cases is related to the size rather than the type of the lung lesion,[42] as well as the presence of pulmonary hypoplasia, hydrops, and other anomalies. In fetuses with uncomplicated, localized CAM, however, immediate respiratory support and surgery tend to produce a good outcome.[50] Neonates tolerate lobectomy well, and re-expansion of residual lung tissue results in near-normal clinical function.[52] Case reports indicate that intrauterine therapy is successful in

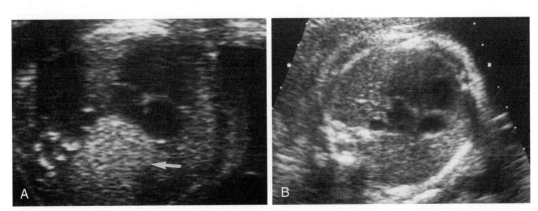

Figure 39-12—Disappearing lung mass, probably CAM. (A) An echogenic mass (arrow) impresses upon the atria of the heart. Fetus is 20 weeks' gestational age. **(B)** Six weeks later, the mass is gone; it probably represented a small, type III CAM. (Reprinted with permission from Sohaey R, Zwiebel WJ: The fetal thorax: Noncardiac chest anomalies. Semin Ultrasound CT MRI 17:34–50, 1996.)

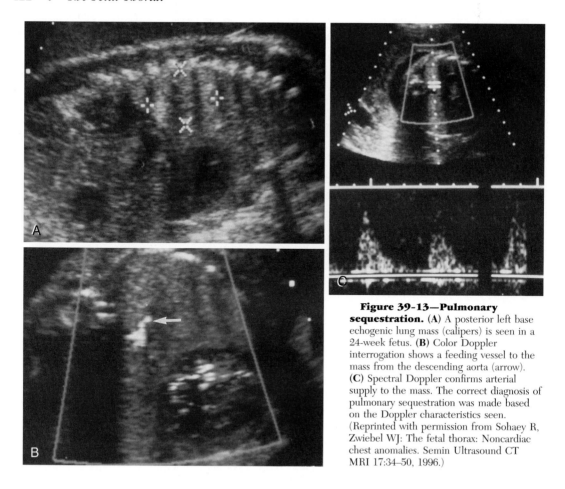

Figure 39-13—Pulmonary sequestration. (A) A posterior left base echogenic lung mass (calipers) is seen in a 24-week fetus. **(B)** Color Doppler interrogation shows a feeding vessel to the mass from the descending aorta (arrow). **(C)** Spectral Doppler confirms arterial supply to the mass. The correct diagnosis of pulmonary sequestration was made based on the Doppler characteristics seen. (Reprinted with permission from Sohaey R, Zwiebel WJ: The fetal thorax: Noncardiac chest anomalies. Semin Ultrasound CT MRI 17:34–50, 1996.)

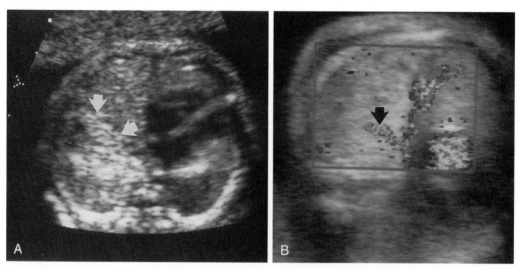

Figure 39-14—Doppler investigation of cystic adenomatoid malformation. (A) Echogenic posterior chest mass (arrows) displaces the heart. **(B)** Color Doppler examination shows pulmonary arterial (not systemic arterial) supply to the mass (arrow). Therefore, the correct diagnosis of CAM (not pulmonary sequestration) was made. (Reprinted with permission from Sohaey R, Zwiebel WJ: The fetal thorax: Noncardiac chest anomalies. Semin Ultrasound CT MRI 17:34–50, 1996.)

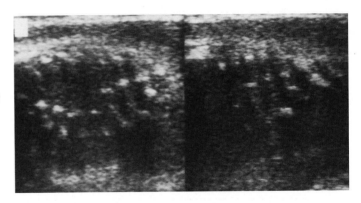

Figure 39-15—Osteogenesis imperfecta with rib fractures. Longitudinal views through the fetal ribs show multiple focal echogenic regions (bright areas) representing many rib fractures. (Reprinted with permission from Sohaey R, Zwiebel WJ: The fetal thorax: Noncardiac chest anomalies. Semin Ultrasound CT MRI 17:34–50, 1996.)

some cases, including draining the larger cysts associated with Types I and II CAM.[53, 54]

PULMONARY SEQUESTRATION

Pulmonary sequestration, defined as a bronchopulmonary mass separate from the normal bronchial system and supplied by an anomalous *systemic* artery,[55] is the third most common cause for a fetal chest mass (after diaphragmatic hernia and cystic adenomatoid malformation). There are two types of pulmonary sequestrations. The first is an extralobar sequestration (ELS), which has its own pleural investment and is separate, therefore, from the rest of the lung. The venous drainage for an ELS is systemic, and the vascularity of an ELS leads to a left-to-right shunt. The second type is the intralobar pulmonary sequestration (ILS), which shares pleura with the lung. Venous drainage usually is through a pulmonary vein, and the vascularity of ILS leads to a left-to-left shunt. The majority of pulmonary sequestrations detected in fetuses are ELS, but symptomatic pulmonary sequestrations diagnosed in children or adults tend to be ILS.[11, 56]

Ultrasound Findings

Pulmonary sequestrations seen in the fetus typically are echogenic, homogeneous, well-defined masses (Fig. 39–13), located in the posterior basilar segment of the left lung (60% of ILS and 90% of ELS are left-sided).[56, 57] Subdiaphragmatic sequestrations are rare and occur in only 5% of cases.[56] ILS is usually spherical in shape whereas ELS is triangular.[58, 59] This difference in appearance most likely is due to the separate pleural covering of the ELS.

Doppler Differentiation of Sequestration and CAM

Pulmonary sequestration and cystic adenomatoid malformation Type III may resemble each other. Rarely, a pulmonary sequestration may contain cysts and may resemble CAM I, CAM II, or even diaphragmatic hernias.[60] Doppler examination of the lung lesion may demonstrate the vascular characteristics of these lesions and allow for correct prenatal diagnosis,[61] as illustrated in Figures 39–13 and 39–14. Mapping the venous drainage of pulmonary sequestrations can differ-

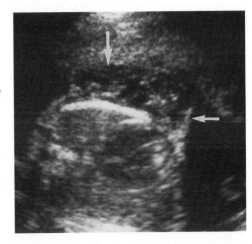

Figure 39-16—Chest wall lymphangioma. Transverse view through the fetal chest shows a complex cystic mass (arrows) external to the ribs (echogenic horizontal structure). This large lymphangioma was centered in the axilla and extended down the chest wall. (Reprinted with permission from Sohaey R, Zwiebel WJ: The fetal thorax: Noncardiac chest anomalies. Semin Ultrasound CT MRI 17:34–50, 1996.)

Table 39-4. Chest Mass with Multiple Cysts

Diagnosis	Sonographic Characteristics
Diaphragmatic hernia	Left-sided, absent stomach fundus in abdomen, peristaltic bowel in chest
CAM I	Multiple cysts of varying sizes, some > 2 cm, normal stomach fundus
CAM II	Multiple uniform cysts < 2 cm, normal stomach
Bronchial atresia	Echogenic mass with dilated bronchi; look for branching, normal stomach

From Sohaey R, Zwiebel WJ: The fetal thorax: Noncardiac chest anomalies. Semin Ultrasound CT MRI 17:34–50, 1996.

Table 39-6. Chest Mass with Single Cyst

Diagnosis	Sonographic Characteristics
Diaphragmatic hernia	Left-sided, only stomach fundus seen in chest; look for absent stomach fundus in abdomen
Bronchogenic cyst	Midline or within lung parenchyma
Neurenteric cyst	Associated with vertebral anomalies
Gastric duplication cyst	Right-sided, involving mid or lower esophagus
CAM I or II	May be a rare variety with only one cyst; CAM I if cyst > 2 cm

From Sohaey R, Zwiebel WJ: The fetal thorax: Noncardiac chest anomalies. Semin Ultrasound CT MRI 17:34–50, 1996.

entiate ILS from ELS.[61] This can be important, since ELS is more commonly associated with other anomalies (60% of ELS cases versus 14% of ILS cases).[56] The prognosis for pulmonary sequestration generally is good in the absence of other anomalies. Symptoms usually do not occur in neonatal life, and some people remain asymptomatic indefinitely. Excellent results can be expected when sequestration is treated with resection.[56]

BRONCHOPULMONARY FOREGUT MALFORMATIONS

During embryonic life, the bronchial tree forms as a ventral outpouching from the foregut.[1] Malformations involving both the tracheobronchial tree and esophagus are called bronchopulmonary foregut malformations, and these include bronchogenic cysts, neurenteric cysts, gastroenteric duplication cysts, and bronchial atresia. These malformations usually generate cystic chest lesions that are solitary and midline. Bronchogenic cysts typically are located near the ca-

Table 39-5. Solid-Appearing Chest Mass

Diagnosis	Sonographic Characteristics
CAM III	Left side = right side; can be lobar or involve whole lung
Extralobar PS	Left lower lobe, triangular in shape, systemic arterial supply, 5% subdiaphragm in location
Intralobar PS	Lower lobe, circular in shape, systemic arterial supply
Bronchial atresia	Segmental without dilated distal bronchi
Diaphragmatic hernia	Containing liver, spleen, kidney, or decompressed bowel

From Sohaey R, Zwiebel WJ: The fetal thorax: Noncardiac chest anomalies. Semin Ultrasound CT MRI 17:34–50, 1996.

rina, but they may be located within the lung parenchyma or below the diaphragm. Neurenteric cysts originate from the notochord and are associated with vertebral body anomalies. Gastroenteric duplication cysts result from failure of vacuolation of the primitive solid esophagus. These cysts usually are located to the right of the midline and tend to involve the middle or posterior portion of the esophagus.[11, 62] Finally, bronchial atresia appears as an echogenic mass that contains anechoic or hypoechoic areas. A segment, a lobe, or an entire lung may be involved in this anomaly, which is thought to result from an early vascular insult to the developing bronchus.[63] The lung distal to the atretic segment is dilated and mucus filled.[62]

CHEST WALL ABNORMALITIES

The thoracic cage should also be evaluated for anomalies. Rib fractures can be seen with prenatal ultrasound and are usually from osteogenesis imperfecta (Fig. 39–15). Chest wall anomalies and masses are usually easy to visualize with ultrasound in the fetus (Fig. 39–16).

The scope of this chapter does not permit detailed discussion of all chest masses. However, Tables 39–4, 39–5, and 39–6 will help the ultrasound practitioner differentiate among chest masses. The diagnoses in these tables are listed in order, from most common to least common.

REFERENCES

1. Moore KL: The respiratory system. *In* Moore KL, Persaud TVN (eds): The Developing Human: Clinically Oriented Embryology. 5th ed. Philadelphia, WB Saunders, 1993.
2. Goldstein RB: Fetal chest masses. Presentation at Fifth Annual Pacific Northwest Diagnostic Ultrasound:OB/GYN Symposium. Seattle, September 8–10, 1995.
3. Hislop A, Hey E, Reid L: The lungs in congenital

bilateral renal agenesis and aplasia. Arch Dis Child 54:32–38, 1979.

4. Fried AM, Loh RK, Umer MA, et al: Echogenicity of fetal lung: Relation to fetal age and maturity. AJR Am J Roentgenol 145:591–594, 1985.

5. Cayea PD, Grant DC, Coublet PM, et al: Prediction of fetal lung maturity: Inaccuracy of study using conventional ultrasound instruments. Radiology 155:473–475, 1985.

6. Schinzel A, Savodelli G, Briner J, et al: Prenatal sonographic diagnosis of Jeune syndrome. Radiology 154:777–778, 1985.

7. Swischuk LE, Richardson CJ, Nichols MM, et al: Primary pulmonary hypoplasia in the neonate. J Pediatr 95:573–577, 1979.

8. Knox WF, Barson AJ: Pulmonary hypoplasia in a regional perinatal unit. Early Hum Dev 14:33–42, 1986.

9. Reale FR, Esterly JR: Pulmonary hypoplasia: A morphometric study of the lungs of infants with diaphragmatic hernia, anencephaly, and renal malformations. Pediatrics 51:91–96, 1973.

10. Wigglesworth JS, Desia R: Use of DNA estimation for growth assessment in normal and hypoplastic fetal lungs. Arch Dis Child 56:601–605, 1981.

11. Hilpert PL, Pretorius DH: The thorax. *In* Nyberg DA (ed): Diagnostic Ultrasound of Fetal Anomalies. St. Louis, Mosby–Year Book, 1990; pp 262–299.

12. Nimrod C, Varela-Gittings F, Machin G, et al: The effect of very prolonged membrane rupture on fetal development. Am J Obstet Gynecol 148:540–543, 1984.

13. Page DV, Stocker JT: Anomalies associated with pulmonary hypoplasia. Am Rev Respir Dis 125:216–221, 1982.

14. Wigglesworth JS, Desia R: Is fetal respiratory function a major determinant of perinatal survival? Lancet 1:264–267, 1982.

15. D'Alton M, Mercer B, Riddick E, et al: Serial thoracic versus abdominal circumference ratios for the prediction of pulmonary hypoplasia in premature rupture of the membranes remote from term. Am J Obstet Gynecol 166:658–663, 1992.

16. Ohlsson A, Fong K, Rose T, et al: Prenatal ultrasonic prediction of autopsy proven pulmonary hypoplasia. Am J Perinatol 9:334–337, 1992.

17. Chitkara U, Rosenberg J, Chervenak FA, et al: Prenatal sonographic assessment of the fetal thorax: Normal values. Am J Obstet Gynecol 156:1069–1074, 1987.

18. Roberts AB, Mitchell JM: Direct ultrasonographic measurement of fetal lung length in normal pregnancies and pregnancies complicated by prolonged rupture of membranes. Am J Obstet Gynecol 163:1560–1566, 1990.

19. Mahony BS, Filly RA, Callen PW, et al: Severe nonimmune hydrops fetalis: Sonographic evaluation. Radiology 151:757–761, 1984.

20. Randolph JG, Gross RE: Congenital chylothorax. AMA Arch Surg 74:405–419, 1987.

21. Meizner I, Carmi R, Bar-Ziv J: Congenital chylothorax: Prenatal ultrasonic diagnosis and successful postpartum management. Prenat Diagn 6:217–221, 1986.

22. Longaker MT, Laberge JM, Dansereau J, et al: Primary fetal hydrothorax: Natural history and management. J Pediatr Surg 24:573, 1989.

23. Schmidt W, Harms E, Wolf D: Successful prenatal treatment of nonimmune hydrops fetalis due to congenital chylothorax. Br J Obstet Gynecol 92:685–687, 1985.

24. David TJ, Illinsworth CA: Diaphragmatic hernia in the southwest of England. J Med Genet 13:253–262, 1976.

25. Harrison MR, deLorimier AA: Congenital diaphragmatic hernia. Surg Clin North Am 61:1023–1035, 1981.

26. Puri P, Gorman F: Lethal nonpulmonary anomalies associated with congenital diaphragmatic hernia: Implications for early intrauterine surgery. J Pediatr Surg 19:29–32, 1984.

27. Chinn DH, Filly RA, Callen PW, et al: Congenital diaphragmatic hernia diagnosed prenatally by ultrasound. Radiology 148:119–123, 1983.

28. Comstock CH: The antenatal diagnosis of diaphragmatic anomalies. J Ultrasound Med 5:391–396, 1986.

29. Comstock CH: Normal fetal heart axis and position. Obstet Gynecol 70:255–259, 1987.

30. Whittle MJ, Gilmore DH, McNay MB, et al: Diaphragmatic hernia presenting in utero as a unilateral hydrothorax. Prenat Diag 9:115–118, 1989.

31. Sherer DM, Abramowicz JS, D'Angio C, et al: Hepatic interlobar fissure sonographically mimicking the diaphragm in a fetus with right congenital diaphragmatic hernia. Am J Perinatol 10:319–322, 1993.

32. Kennedy AM, Sohaey R, Woodward PJ: Cardiac evaluation in fetuses with diaphragmatic hernia: How accurate is the prenatal diagnosis? Presentation at 38th Annual Meeting of American Ultrasound in Medicine, Baltimore, March 20–23, 1994.

33. Adzick NS, Harrison MR, Glick PL, et al: Diaphragmatic hernia in the fetus: Prenatal diagnosis and outcome in 94 cases. J Pediatr Surg 20:357–361, 1985.

34. Cunniff C, Jones KL, Saal HM, et al: Fryns syndrome: An autosomal recessive disorder associated with craniofacial anomalies, diaphragmatic hernia, and distal digital hypoplasia. Pediatrics 85:499–504, 1990.

35. Wilcox DT, Glick PL, Karamanoukian HL, et al: Pathophysiology of congenital diaphragmatic hernia. IX. Correlation of surfactant maturation with fetal cortisol and triiodothyronine concentration. J Pediatr Surg 29:825–827, 1994.

36. Nakayama DK, Harrison MR, Chinn DH, et al: Prenatal diagnosis and natural history of the fetus with a congenital diaphragmatic hernia: Initial clinical experience. J Pediatr Surg 20:118–124, 1985.

37. Harrison MR, Adzick NS, Estes JM, et al: A prospective study of the outcome for fetuses with diaphragmatic hernia. JAMA 271:382–384, 1994.

38. Benacerraf BR, Greene MF: Congenital diaphragmatic hernia: Ultrasound diagnosis and clinical outcome in 19 cases. Am J Obstet Gynecol 156:573–576, 1987.

39. Ford WD: Fetal intervention for congenital diaphragmatic hernia. Fetal Diagn Ther 9:398–408, 1994.

40. Harrison MR, Adzick NS, Flake AW, et al: Correction of congenital diaphragmatic hernia in utero: VI. Hard-earned lessons. J Pediatr Surg 28:1411–1418, 1993.

41. Hedrick MH, Estes JM, Sullivan KM, et al: Plug the lung until it grows (PLUG): A new method to treat congenital diaphragmatic hernia in utero. J Pediatr Surg 29:612–617, 1994.

42. Rosado-de-Christenson ML, Stocker JT: Congenital cystic adenomatoid malformation. RadioGraphics 11:865–886, 1991.

43. Johnson JA, Rumack CM, Johnson ML, et al: Cystic adenomatoid malformation: Antenatal diagnosis. AJR Am J Roentgenol 142:483–484, 1984.

44. Miller RK, Sieber WK, Yunis EJ: Congenital cystic adenomatoid malformation of the lung: A report of 17 cases and a review of the literature. Pathol Annu 1:387–407, 1980.

45. Moerman P, Fryns JP, Vandenberghe K, et al: Pathogenesis of congenital cystic adenomatoid malformation of the lung. Histopathology 21:315–321, 1992.

46. Stocker JT, Madewell JE, Drake RM: Congenital cystic adenomatoid malformation of the lung: Classification and morphologic spectrum. Hum Pathol 8:155–171, 1977.

47. Diwan RV, Brennan JN, Philipson EH, et al: Ultrasonic prenatal diagnosis of type III congenital cystic adenomatoid malformation of lung. J Clin Ultrasound 11:218–221, 1983.

48. Fine C, Adzick NS, Doubilet PM: Decreasing size of a cystic adenomatoid malformation in utero. J Ultrasound Med 7:405–408, 1988.

49. Moerman P, Fryns J, Goddeeris P, et al: Nonimmunologic hydrops fetalis: A study of ten cases. Arch Pathol Lab Med 106:635–640, 1982.

50. Adzick NS, Harrison MR, Glick PL, et al: Fetal cystic adenomatoid malformation: Prenatal diagnosis and natural history. J Pediatr Surg 20:483–488, 1985.

51. Harrison MR, Adzick NS, Jennings RW, et al: Antenatal intervention for congenital cystic adenomatoid malformation. Lancet 336:965–967, 1990.

52. Walker J, Cudmore RE: Respiratory problems and cystic adenomatoid malformation of lung (letter). Arch Dis Child 65:649–650, 1990.

53. Kyle PM, Lange IR, Menticoglou SM, et al: Intrauterine thoracentesis of fetal cystic lung malformations. Fetal Diagn Ther 9:84–87, 1994.

54. Revillon Y, Jan D, Plattner V, et al: Congenital cystic adenomatoid malformation of the lung: Prenatal management and prognosis. J Pediatr Surg 28:1009–1011, 1993.

55. Clements BS, Warner JO, Shinebourne EA: Congenital bronchopulmonary vascular malformations: Clinical application of a simple anatomic approach in 25 cases. Thorax 42:409–416, 1987.

56. Savic B, Britel FJ, Tholen W, et al: Lung sequestration: Report of seven cases and review of 540 published cases. Thorax 34:96–101, 1979.

57. West MS, Donaldson JS, Shkolnik A: Pulmonary sequestration: Diagnosis by ultrasound. J Ultrasound Med 8:125–129, 1989.

58. Davies RP, Ford WDA, Lequesne GW, et al: Ultrasonic detection of subdiaphragmatic pulmonary sequestration in utero and postnatal diagnosis by fine needle aspiration biopsy. J Ultrasound Med 8:47–49, 1989.

59. Romero R, Chervenak FA, Kotzen J, et al: Antenatal sonographic findings of extralobar pulmonary sequestration. J Ultrasound Med 1:131–132, 1982.

60. Benya EC, Bulas DI, Selby DM, et al: Cystic sonographic appearance of extralobar pulmonary sequestration. Pediatr Radiol 23:605–607, 1993.

61. Sauerbrei E: Lung sequestration: Duplex Doppler diagnosis at 19 weeks' gestation. J Ultrasound Med 10:101–105, 1991.

62. Siffring PA, Forrest TS, Hill WC, et al: Prenatal sonographic diagnosis of bronchopulmonary foregut malformation. J Ultrasound Med 8:277–280, 1989.

63. McAlister WH, Wright JR, Crane JP: Main stem bronchial atresia: Intrauterine sonographic diagnosis. AJR Am J Roentgenol 148:364–366, 1987.

Chapter 40
The Fetal Heart

Roya Sohaey

Fetal cardiac evaluation is challenging to most ultrasound practitioners; nevertheless, it is essential for sonographers to conduct the cardiac examination well, because cardiovascular anomalies are not rare. The reported incidence of congenital heart defects (CHDs) in fetuses is 0.8% to 2.4%,[1–4] and this risk increases to 4% and 12%, respectively, if a sibling or parent was affected with CHD.[5] Structural abnormalities of the heart and great vessels occur in more than 8 per 1000 live births,[1, 2] and they represent the most common severe congenital anomalies seen in neonates.[3]

This chapter reviews cardiac embryology, the fetal circulation, routine sonographic cardiac evaluation, selected (more common) heart anomalies, and common cardiac arrhythmias. Certain pitfalls of cardiac sonography are also considered.

EMBRYOLOGY

The cardiovascular system is the first system to function in an embryo. Heart development begins 18 to 19 days postfertilization. From the embryonic "cardiogenic area," two thin-walled tubes form and eventually fuse to become the endocardial tube. As the embryo assumes a "C" shape, the heart comes to lie ventral to the foregut and caudal to the oral pharyngeal membrane. The single tubular heart elongates and develops alternating areas of dilatation and constriction. The superior dilatation, the bulbus cordis, eventually becomes the aorta and pulmonary artery. The atrial constriction is initially caudal to the ventricular bulge, but at 22 to 24 days the heart bends, and the atria come to lie superior to the ventricles. The four chambers of the heart form between the fourth and seventh weeks. The endocardial cushion is a key element in cardiac development. This centrally located structure affects the formation of the atrial septum, the ventricular septum, and the valves.[6] The embryology of the atrial septum is illustrated schematically in Figure 40–1. Please review this material before proceeding with the text.

Partition of the cardiac ventricles (into the right and left ventricles) first occurs when the interventricular septum grows cranially from the cardiac apex. The muscular portion of the interventricular septum forms prior to the more cranial, membranous portion, which is derived from the endocardial cushion. The interventricular foramen closes near the end of the seventh week of gestation. Therefore, the normal fetal heart, as seen with ultrasound, always demonstrates an intact ventricular septum, whereas the atrial septum normally contains a patent foramen ovale throughout fetal life.

The great vessels are derived from the fetal branchial arches during the fourth week. A total of six pairs of aortic arches is present initially, but some of the arches contribute little to the final cardiovascular system. The final disposition of the aortic arches is outlined in Table 40–1. Please review this material before proceeding.[6]

Fetal Circulation

Since prenatal life is "aquatic," the prenatal circulation differs vastly from the postnatal circulation. The unique characteristics of fetal circulation are demonstrated in schematic form in Figure 40–2 and by ultrasound in Figures 40–3 and 40–4. Please review this material, which is not repeated in the text, and note in particular that the foramen ovale and ductus arteriosus shunt blood from the pulmonary circulation to the systemic circulation.

The pulmonary circulation, in a sense, is not needed in fetal life. At birth, however, the pulmonary circulation is abruptly called into service. Aeration of the lungs leads to a fall in pulmonary vascular resistance and an increase in left atrial

Table 40-1. Branchial Arch Derivation

Branchial Arch Pair	Final Anatomy
1	Portion of maxillary arteries
2	Foramina in stapes of the ears
3	Proximal: Common carotid arteries
	Distal: Internal carotid arteries
4	Right: Proximal right subclavian artery
	Left: Part of aortic arch
5	No derivatives
6	Right: Proximal right pulmonary artery
	Left: Proximal left pulmonary artery, ductus arteriosus

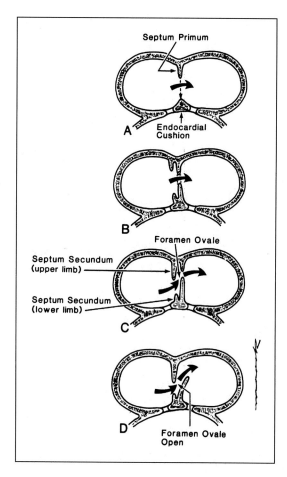

Figure 40-1—Atrial Septal Embryology.
(**A**) Initially, the septum primum develops and begins to elongate. The right and left atria communicate through the foramen primum (arrow). (**B**) Perforations develop in the septum primum, creating the foramen secundum (arrow) and the septum primum closes. (**C**) Concurrently, the septum secundum elongates (upper limb and lower limb) parallel to the septum primum. At this stage, the foramen secundum becomes the foramen ovale, which is seen routinely with ultrasound. (**D**) In its final form, the foramen ovale is composed principally of the septum secundum superiorly and the septum primum inferiorly. The foramen ovale valve opens from the right atrium into the left atrium. (Reprinted with permission from Sohaey R, Zwiebel WJ: The fetal heart: A practical sonographic approach. Semin Ultrasound CT MRI 17:15–33, 1996.)

Figure 40-2—Fetal Circulation. Oxygenated blood from the placenta enters the fetus through the umbilical vein. Half of the blood passes through the hepatic sinusoids. The remainder bypasses the liver, through the ductus venosus, and goes into the inferior vena cava. This oxygenated blood enters the right atrium and mixes with deoxygenated blood from the fetal lower limbs, abdomen, and pelvis. The majority of the blood is directed from the right atrium through the foramen ovale and into the left atrium where it mixes with a small amount of deoxygenated blood returning from the fetal lungs via the pulmonary veins. The blood then passes through the mitral valve, into the left ventricle, and into the ascending aorta.

A small stream of oxygenated blood from the ductus venosus reaches the right ventricle and is pumped into the pulmonary trunk, but most of this passes through the ductus arteriosus into the aorta. Pulmonary vascular resistance is high, resulting in low pulmonary blood flow. Not more than 10% of the blood reaches the fetal lungs, yet this is enough for oxygenating the tissue. Most of the blood in the descending aorta passes into the umbilical arteries and returns to the placenta, while a small amount circulates through the lower part of the body. (Reprinted with permission from Sohaey R, Zwiebel WJ: The fetal heart: A practical sonographic approach. Semin Ultrasound CT MRI 17:15–33, 1996.)

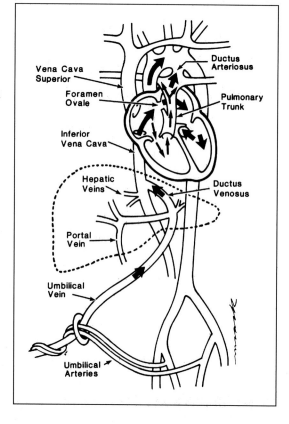

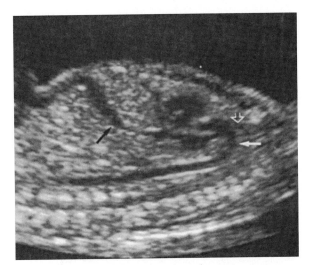

Figure 40-3—Ultrasound of the Fetal Circulation. A sagittal image demonstrates the ductus venosus (black arrow) and the aortic arch (white arrow). The great vessels arise from the aortic arch (open arrow). (Reprinted with permission from Sohaey R, Zwiebel WJ: The fetal heart: A practical sonographic approach. Semin Ultrasound CT MRI 17:15–33, 1996.)

pressure, which closes the foramen ovale. The ductus arteriosus (between the pulmonary artery and aorta) usually remains patent for a few days but eventually constricts. Initially, the closure of this vessel and the foramen ovale is a functional change, but closure later becomes anatomic as endothelial and fibrous tissues proliferate.[6]

Routine Cardiac Examination

The recommended screening test for the fetal heart is the four-chamber view, which can be obtained in 95% of fetuses between 18 and 40 weeks.[7–9] It is essential to note the cardiac axis on the four-chamber view, by drawing an imaginary line through the interventricular septum and a second imaginary line through the spine and sternum (Fig. 40–5). The angle subtended by these lines is the cardiac axis, which usually is *45° to the left* (range 22°–75°).[10] It also is important to note that the right ventricle of the properly oriented heart contacts the anterior chest wall. To assess the heart properly, of course, the sonographer must know the fetal position; otherwise, there is no way of knowing which side is right and which is left on the four-chamber view. For a quick frame of reference, however, the sonographer can glance below the heart and confirm that the cardiac apex is on the same side of the fetus as the gastric fundus (which normally is on the left).

Once cardiac situs and orientation are confirmed, intracardiac anatomy should be assessed. The right and left ventricles tend to be the same size (RV:LV ratio of 1:1),[11] and it is not necessary to measure the ventricles routinely if they are symmetric. Where the ventricles appear asym-

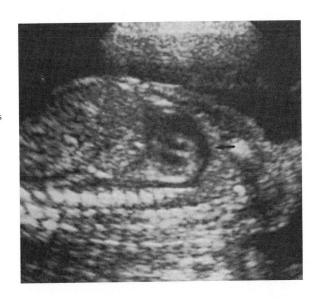

Figure 40-4—Ductal Arch. The ductus arteriosus connects the pulmonary artery with the descending aorta, and a "ductal arch" is formed (black arrow). Notice the difference in configuration between the aortic arch (Fig. 40–3) and the ductal arch. (Reprinted with permission from Sohaey R, Zwiebel WJ: The fetal heart: A practical sonographic approach. Semin Ultrasound CT MRI 17:15–33, 1996.)

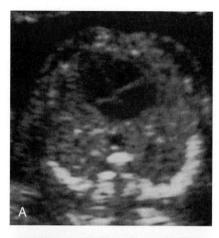

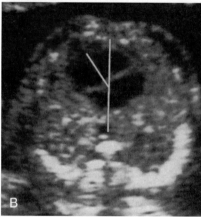

Figure 40-5—Normal Heart. (A) Normal four-chamber view. (B) Normal cardiac axis. The line drawn from the spine to the sternum forms a 45-degree angle with the line drawn through the intraventricular septum. (Reprinted with permission from Sohaey R, Zwiebel WJ: The fetal heart: A practical sonographic approach. Semin Ultrasound CT MRI 17:15–33, 1996.)

metric, however, they should be measured at their maximum transverse diameter. It is important to document *which* ventricle is large or small as this often cannot be determined through visual inspection. Figure 40–6 is a standardized list of ventricular measurements, related to biparietal diameter, which may be used in cases that appear abnormal.[11]

An intact ventricular septum should be seen at all times. If the ventricular septum appears interrupted, care should be taken that this is not an artifact from echo "drop out," which occurs if the image is aligned parallel to the long axis of the septum. In such cases, a change of transducer angle (perpendicular to the septum) usually shows that the septum is intact (Fig. 40–7). The right ventricle contains a prominent muscular band, called the "moderator band," near the apex (Fig. 40–8). In certain image planes, this band of

muscle may artifactually cause the right ventricle to appear small. The left ventricle may contain an echogenic focus within its lumen that probably represents the papillary muscle.[12] This and other "bright spots" in the heart are discussed later.

The atria also should be symmetric in size, and the foramen ovale should be seen routinely (Fig. 40–9). The flap or "valve" covering the foramen ovale extends into the *left* atrium, since the route of fetal blood flow is from right to left. The foramen ovale valve is a complex, three-dimensional structure[13] that can have a variety of appearances, which will be discussed in the "Pitfalls" section of this chapter.

The tricuspid valve is located between the right atrium and the right ventricle, and the mitral valve is located between the left atrium and left ventricle. The "valve ring" is an echogenic structure to which the valve leaflets attach. The ring of the tricuspid valve is positioned slightly *inferior* to the mitral valve ring[14] (Fig. 40–10). The motion of the mitral and tricuspid valves should be synchronous and regular.

The normal elements of the four-chamber view are summarized in Table 40–2. Most cardiac anomalies can be identified with the four-chamber view, although the sensitivity of this view for detecting congenital heart disease (CHD) is debatable. Some investigators quote 96% sensitivity for CHD,[8] whereas others report only 63% sensitivity.[15] To insure a high level of sensitivity for CHD, therefore, many ultrasound departments routinely obtain ventricular outflow tract images, in addition to the four-chamber view. The outflow tract views show additional normal anatomy, including the connection of the ventricles with the great vessels. Obtaining these views is more challenging than obtaining the four-chamber view, but with practice the output tracts can be examined routinely. In a recent study, 83% of fetuses with cardiac anomalies were identified prenatally when both the four-chamber and outflow tract views were utilized. Only 63% of anomalies were recognized, however, with the four-chamber view used alone.[15]

Table 40–2. Characteristics of the Normal Four-Chamber View of the Heart

Cardiac axis to the left (45°)
Cardiac axis and stomach on the same side
RV contacts the anterior chest wall
RV identified by the moderator band
RV:LV size 1:1
Right atrium:left atrium size 1:1
Ventricular septum intact
Foramen ovale flap moves from right to left
Tricuspid valve slightly inferior to the mitral valve

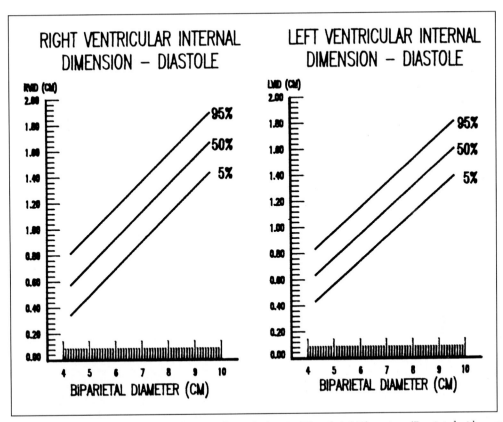

Figure 40-6—Diastolic RV and LV Diameter in Relation to Biparietal Diameter. (Reprinted with permission from DeVore GR: Fetal echocardiography: The challenge of the 1980s. Semin Ultrasound CT MRI 5:229–248, 1984.)

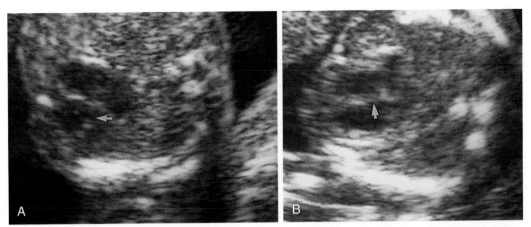

Figure 40-7—Pseudoventricular Septal Defect. (A) The ventricular septum appears interrupted (arrow) because the sound beam is parallel to the thin, membranous portion of the septum. **(B)** A change in the angle of the beam shows an intact ventricular septum (arrow). (Reprinted with permission from Sohaey R, Zwiebel WJ: The fetal heart: A practical sonographic approach. Semin Ultrasound CT MRI 17:15–33, 1996.)

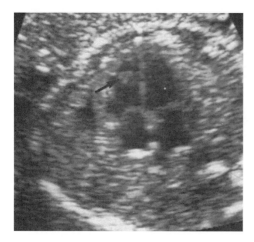

Figure 40-8—Moderator Band. The right ventricle contains a moderator band (black arrow) near the apex. This band identifies the ventricle as the anatomic right ventricle. (Reprinted with permission from Sohaey R, Zwiebel WJ: The fetal heart: A practical sonographic approach. Semin Ultrasound CT MRI 17:15–33, 1996.)

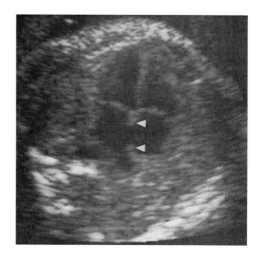

Figure 40-9—Normal Atria and Foramen Ovale. The atria are symmetric in size and the normal atrial septum (arrowheads) bows into the left atrium because the flow of blood is from the right atrium into the left atrium. The foramen ovale is clearly seen. (Reprinted with permission from Sohaey R, Zwiebel WJ: The fetal heart: A practical sonographic approach. Semin Ultrasound CT MRI 17:15–33, 1996.)

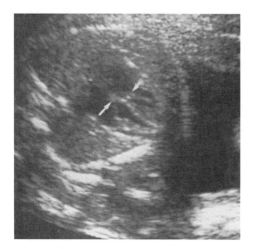

Figure 40-10—Tricuspid Valve Position. The normal tricuspid valve (short arrow) is attached slightly more toward the cardiac apex than the mitral valve (long arrow). (Reprinted with permission from Sohaey R, Zwiebel WJ: The fetal heart: A practical sonographic approach. Semin Ultrasound CT MRI 17:15–33, 1996.)

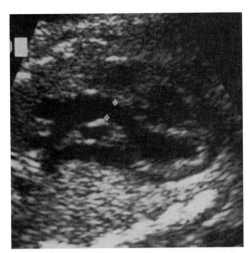

Figure 40-11—Left Ventricular Outflow Tract (Long Axis View). A normal aorta (calipers) is seen attached to the left ventricle. (Reprinted with permission from Sohaey R, Zwiebel WJ: The fetal heart: A practical sonographic approach. Semin Ultrasound CT MRI 17:15–33, 1996.)

To visualize the aortic outflow tract, begin with the four-chamber view and rotate the transducer a quarter turn (either clockwise or counterclockwise, depending on fetal position). The left atrium will disappear from view and the left ventricular outflow tract will appear in its place, as shown in Figure 40–11. A view of the pulmonary outflow tract (Fig. 40–12) is achieved by returning to the four-chamber view and then rotating the transducer sharply in the direction opposite that used for the aortic view. At the same time, the ultra-

sound beam is angled toward the fetal head. From this perspective, the pulmonary artery always is seen anterior to the aortic root, and the patent ductus arteriosus extends posteriorly toward the aorta. The ductus forms the so-called "ductal arch" shown in Figure 40–4. If the pulmonary artery is not clearly anterior to the aorta, then transposition of the great vessels should be suspected. In addition, the diameters of the aortic root and pulmonary artery should be about the same. The graphs shown in Figure 40–13 can be used if measurements of the aorta and pulmonary artery are needed in cases of apparent abnormalities.[16] These reference diameters are particularly useful in deciding which outflow tract is normal and which is abnormal in size.

The Abnormal Four-Chamber View

When a cardiac abnormality is detected, the sonologist must attempt to diagnose the problem in as much detail as possible. McGahan[17] has described a six-step approach to the abnormal four chamber view that helps characterize the vast majority of cardiac defects. The approach asks six questions about the abnormal-appearing heart:

1. Is the heart in a normal position?

   Overall, an abnormal cardiac axis is associated with a 50% to 81% fetal mortality rate.[10] As noted previously, the heart axis should be about 45° to the left of midline, and the anterior aspect of the heart (right ventricle) should touch the anterior chest wall (see Fig. 40–5).

   Dextrocardia is defined as malposition of the cardiac apex toward the right. This position can be caused by either inversion of the normal ventricular relationship (right and left are switched) or simple rotation of the heart (dextroversion). The moderator band (see Fig. 40–8) may help differentiate between these types of dextrocardia by identifying the anatomic right ventricle. Levoversion is defined as a cardiac axis that is more to the left than normal. Mesocardia is a midline-appearing heart, often associated with midline anatomic defects, and possibly with transposition of the great vessels.

   In some cases, the heart may be intrinsically normal but displaced from its normal position, in which case a thoracic mass or diaphragmatic hernia should be sought diligently (Fig. 40–14). The most common cause of cardiac malposition is a diaphragmatic hernia,[10] as discussed in Chapter 39.

   The heart also may be located outside the

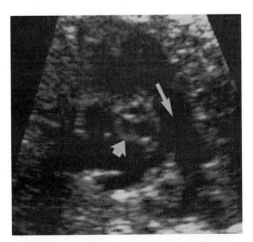

Figure 40-12—Right Ventricular Outflow Tract (Short Axis View). The pulmonary artery (long arrow) is anterior to the aorta (short arrow). (Reprinted with permission from Sohaey R, Zwiebel WJ: The fetal heart: A practical sonographic approach. Semin Ultrasound CT MRI 17:15–33, 1996.)

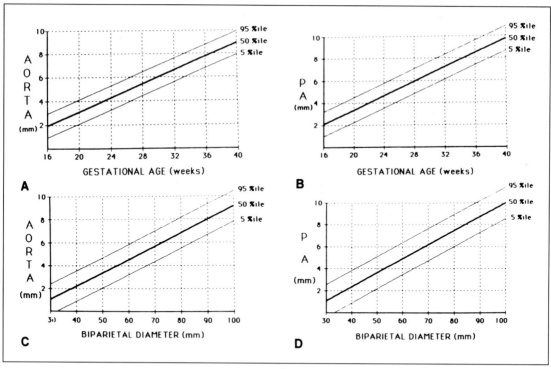

Figure 40-13—Aorta and Pulmonary Artery (PA) Size in Relation to Biparietal Diameter. (Reprinted with permission from Cartier MS, Davidoff A, Warneke LA, et al: The normal diameter of the fetal aorta and pulmonary artery. Am J Roentgenol AJR 149:1003–1007, 1987.)

chest (ectopia cordis), and this is a fatal anomaly.[18] If ectopia cordis is associated with a large upper abdominal omphalocele, then an anomaly complex called the pentalogy of Cantrel should be suspected (Fig. 40–15). This anomaly complex consists of an omphalocele (midline abdominal wall defect), a sternal cleft, a diaphragmatic hernia, and a variety of cardiovascular malformations.[19]

2. Is the heart size normal?

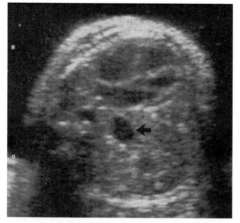

Figure 40-14—Diaphragmatic Hernia. The heart is displaced into the right chest by a left-sided diaphragmatic hernia. The fluid-filled stomach fundus is seen in the chest (arrow). (Reprinted with permission from Sohaey R, Zwiebel WJ: The fetal heart: A practical sonographic approach. Semin Ultrasound CT MRI 17:15–33, 1996.)

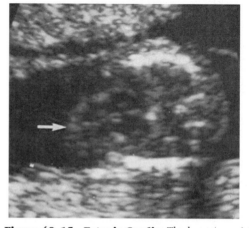

Figure 40-15—Ectopia Cordis. The heart (arrow) is clearly outside the confines of the thoracic cage. This fetus also had an omphalocele and was diagnosed with pentalogy of Cantrel. (Reprinted with permission from Sohaey R, Zwiebel WJ: The fetal heart: A practical sonographic approach. Semin Ultrasound CT MRI 17:15–33, 1996.)

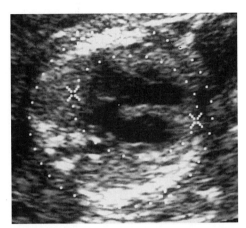

Figure 40-16—Cardiomegaly. The fetal heart is enlarged, filling more than 50% of the thoracic cage. In this case, cardiomegaly was caused by fetal anemia, secondary to alpha-thalassemia. X, ellipse around the heart; +, ellipse around the chest.

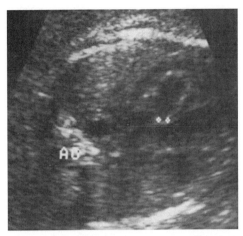

Figure 40-18—Hypoplastic Aorta. A less severe case of hypoplastic left heart is shown with a smaller than expected aortic diameter (calipers). (Reprinted with permission from Sohaey R, Zwiebel WJ: The fetal heart: A practical sonographic approach. Semin Ultrasound CT MRI 17:15–33, 1996.)

Cardiac size can be assessed by comparing the cardiac circumference with the chest circumference on the standard four-chamber view.[20] Overall, the fetal heart, as seen on the four-chamber view, should not take up more than 50% of the area of the thorax. An abnormal cardiothoracic ratio may result from cardiomegaly (Fig. 40–16), a small chest (pulmonary hypoplasia), or a combination of both. Comparison with standard tables usually differentiates between an abnormally small chest and an abnormally enlarged heart. A full discussion of the small thorax and its usual cause,

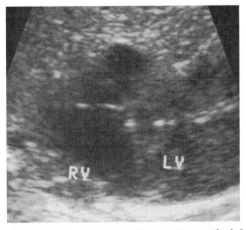

Figure 40-17—Hypoplastic Left Heart. The left ventricle (LV) and left atrium are small and echogenic as compared with the right atrium and right ventricle (RV) in this case of severe hypoplastic left heart. On Doppler examination, no blood flow was seen in the left side of the heart. (Reprinted with permission from Sohaey R, Zwiebel WJ: The fetal heart: A practical sonographic approach. Semin Ultrasound CT MRI 17:15–33, 1996.)

pulmonary hypoplasia, is included in Chapter 39.

3. Are the ventricles equal in size?

As stated previously, the right and left ventricles should be equal in size throughout pregnancy. If the left ventricle is smaller than expected, the fetus may have one of a variety of hypoplastic left heart syndromes[21] (Fig. 40–17), or the small left ventricle may be a secondary sign of coarctation of the aorta.[22] A hypoplastic aorta is almost always seen in association with a hypoplastic left ventricle (Fig. 40–18). If the right ventricle is small, the fetus may have a hypoplastic right heart, which is a more complex anomaly. Hypoplastic right heart can be associated with pulmonary artery atresia in company with an intact ventricular septum, or tricuspid atresia with associated ventricular septal defect.[17, 23] Finally, either the right or left side of the heart may be atretic and the fetus may appear to have a single ventricle.[24]

4. Is there a septal defect?

The normal atrial septum contains the foramen ovale and its valve. If the valve is not seen within the left atrium, then an atrial septal defect may be present, but sonographic confirmation of such a defect is difficult (Fig. 40–19).[25] It is easier to confirm that the interventricular septum is intact on the four-chamber view. Large ventricular septal defects (VSDs) may be detected with ultrasound (Fig. 40–20); however, small and even moderate-sized VSDs can be overlooked.[8, 26, 27] VSDs are often associated with complex cardiac abnormalities, such as tetralogy of Fallot (Fig. 40–

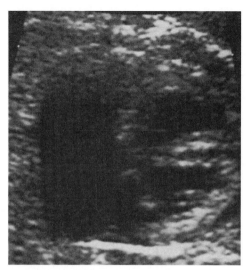

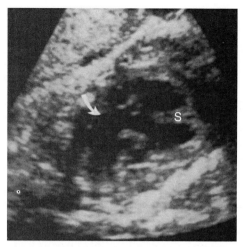

Figure 40-19—Atrial Septal Defect. There is a complete absence of septal tissue between the right and left atria. The ventricular septum is intact. (Reprinted with permission from Sohaey R, Zwiebel WJ: The fetal heart: A practical sonographic approach. Semin Ultrasound CT MRI 17:15–33, 1996.)

Figure 40-21—Tetralogy of Fallot. The aorta (arrow) overrides a ventricular septal defect. Great vessel anomalies, such as this, are best seen on outflow tract images. S, interventricular septum. (Reprinted with permission from Sohaey R, Zwiebel WJ: The fetal heart: A practical sonographic approach. Semin Ultrasound CT MRI 17:15–33, 1996.)

21); therefore, the initial detection of a VSD necessitates a more careful examination of the fetal heart. Complete atrioventricular septal defect (endocardial cushion defect) is almost always detected with the four-chamber view (Fig. 40–22).[8] Fetuses with this defect are at an increased risk for chromosome abnormalities, commonly trisomy 21.[25, 26]

5. Are the atrioventricular valves in a normal position?

   In general, tricuspid valve malformations

occur more commonly than mitral valve malformations and usually are heralded by dilatation of the right atrium. As noted previously, the tricuspid valve normally is located slightly inferior to the mitral valve (see Fig. 40–10).[14] Abnormal inferior displacement of the septal leaflet of the tricuspid valve into the right ventricle is a feature of Ebstein anomaly (Fig. 40–23). In this condition, the right ventricle

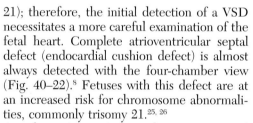

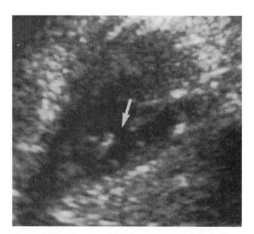

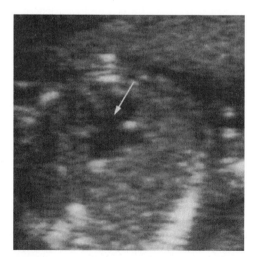

Figure 40-20—Ventricular Septal Defect. An oblique image showing only the ventricles demonstrates a moderate-sized membranous ventricular septal defect (arrow). (Reprinted with permission from Sohaey R, Zwiebel WJ: The fetal heart: A practical sonographic approach. Semin Ultrasound CT MRI 17:15–33, 1996.)

Figure 40-22—Endocardial Cushion Defect. A complete atrioventricular septal defect (arrow) is seen in this fetus with trisomy 21. (Reprinted with permission from Sohaey R, Zwiebel WJ: The fetal heart: A practical sonographic approach. Semin Ultrasound CT MRI 17:15–33, 1996.)

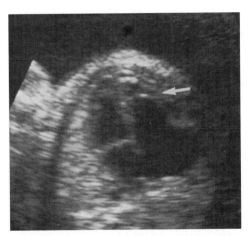

Figure 40-23—Ebstein Anomaly. The tricuspid valve is displaced inferiorly (arrow), and the right atrium is enlarged. (Reprinted with permission from Sohaey R, Zwiebel WJ: The fetal heart: A practical sonographic approach. Semin Ultrasound CT MRI 17:15–33, 1996.)

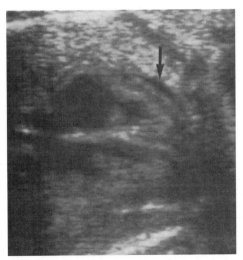

Figure 40-25—Normal Pericardial Fluid. A small amount of pericardial fluid (arrow) can normally be seen and usually measures less than 2 mm in "thickness." (Reprinted with permission from Sohaey R, Zwiebel WJ: The fetal heart: A practical sonographic approach. Semin Ultrasound CT MRI 17:15–33, 1996.)

is small functionally, and the tricuspid valve is insufficient. The result is massive right atrial dilation, as seen on the four-chamber view.[8] Right atrial dilation can also result from tricuspid dysplasia and regurgitation; however, in these cases the tricuspid valve attachment is not displaced inferiorly.[14]

6. Is there any abnormality of the endocardium, myocardium, or pericardium?

Increased thickness and abnormal echogenicity of the endocardium may be caused by a cardiomyopathy, such as endocardial fibroelastosis. In this condition, the heart is dilated and contracts poorly, and the endocardium is

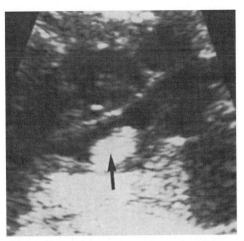

Figure 40-24—Rhabdomyoma. This echogenic left ventricular mass (arrow) proved to be a rhabdomyoma. (Reprinted with permission from Sohaey R, Zwiebel WJ: The fetal heart: A practical sonographic approach. Semin Ultrasound CT MRI 17:15–33, 1996.)

diffusely thickened and echogenic.[28] Focally increased echogenicity within the ventricles may be caused by a tumor, the most common being rhabdomyoma (Fig. 40–24). Tuberous sclerosis should be suspected when multiple rhabdomyomas are seen.[29, 30] Focal echogenicities can occur normally in the ventricles, as discussed later.

A small amount of fluid within the pericardial sac also can be a normal finding (Fig. 40–25). Pericardial effusions appear as an anechoic region separating the two layers of the pericardium. A pericardial fluid collection measuring greater than 2 mm in width is probably abnormal (Fig. 40–26).[31] Depending on the cause for the fluid collection, pericardial effusions can be transient or lethal.[32] When pericardial effusion is identified, further clinical evaluation is indicated as the effusion may be a clue to a systemic disorder that may lead ultimately to fetal hydrops.[17, 32]

THE DEDICATED CARDIAC EXAMINATION

Any abnormality observed on the four-chamber view that cannot be explained easily should be investigated with a complete fetal echocardiogram, performed and interpreted by an experienced sonologist. With respect to complicated cardiac anomalies, we have found that diagnostic accuracy is enhanced when the sonologist with the most echocardiography experience performs

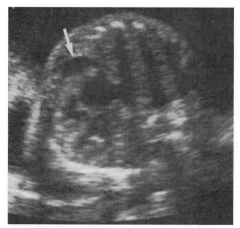

Figure 40-26—Pericardial Effusion. This monochorionic twin fetus involved with twin-twin transfusion developed a pericardial effusion (arrow) and subsequently developed hydrops fetalis. (Reprinted with permission from Sohaey R, Zwiebel WJ: The fetal heart: A practical sonographic approach. Semin Ultrasound CT MRI 17:15–33, 1996.)

the examination at a scheduled time that is different from the initial obstetric examination.[33] An attempt to diagnose a complex anomaly "on the spur of the moment" is not recommended.

A detailed discussion of fetal echocardiography is beyond the scope of this work, but we would like to provide some guidance about what anomaly should be considered when the heart appears abnormal in one way or another. To this end,

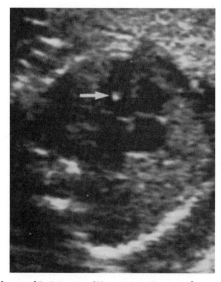

Figure 40-27—Papillary Muscle. An echogenic focus within the lumen of the left ventricle represents a normal papillary muscle (arrow). (Reprinted with permission from Sohaey R, Zwiebel WJ: The fetal heart: A practical sonographic approach. Semin Ultrasound CT MRI 17:15–33, 1996.)

a guideline to differential diagnosis is listed in Table 40–3.

NORMAL VARIANTS AND PITFALLS

Occasionally, normal structures associated with the fetal heart or chest may mimic pathology. Familiarity with these normal variants and certain other pitfalls helps prevent diagnostic error.[34]

Echogenic foci are sometimes seen within the lumen of the ventricles (Fig. 40–27). In almost all cases, these foci are of no clinical significance, and they most likely represent normal papillary muscles or chordae tendineae. Up to 20% of normal fetuses may have an echogenic focus within the left ventricle, and such foci also may be seen in the right ventricle.[12]

An anterior rib end or part of the sternum can produce an echogenic focus located in or at the periphery of the ventricular myocardium (Fig. 40–28). This echogenic focus should not be mistaken for a tumor or pericardial calcification. By changing the image plane, the focus may readily be identified as a rib or the sternum.[34]

Table 40-3. Cardiovascular Chamber Abnormalities: Differential Considerations

Large RV
Ventricular failure
Cardiomyopathy
Aortic interruption or coarctation
Total anomalous pulmonary venous return

Small RV
Hypoplastic right heart
Ebstein anomaly
Single ventricle

Small LV
Hypoplastic left heart
Single ventricle
Aortic coarctation

Large Right Atrium
Ebstein anomaly
Tricuspid dysplasia with regurgitation
Pulmonary stenosis

Small Aorta
Hypoplastic left heart
Supravalvular aortic stenosis
Aortic atresia
Aortic coarctation or interruption

Small Pulmonary Artery
Pulmonary stenosis
Pulmonary atresia
Tetralogy of Fallot

Incorrect Great Vessel Orientation
Transposition
Tetralogy of Fallot
Truncus arteriosus
Double outlet RV

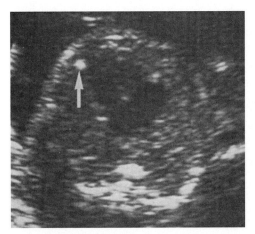

Figure 40-28—Rib End. An echogenic focus adjacent to the RV myocardium (arrow) proved to be the end of a rib on oblique imaging. (Reprinted with permission from Sohaey R, Zwiebel WJ: The fetal heart: A practical sonographic approach. Semin Ultrasound CT MRI 17:15–33, 1996.)

A ventricular septal defect may be wrongly identified if the ultrasound beam is parallel to the membranous portion of the septum (see Fig. 40–7). Since the membranous portion is very thin, it may not reflect ultrasound sufficiently for visualization when viewed "on end." When a VSD is suspected, therefore, the sonographer should confirm its presence by demonstrating the defect in orthogonal planes.

As described previously, the foramen ovale is a complex, three-dimensional structure that can have a variety of appearances. The redundant flap can appear circular and mimic an atrial septal aneurysm or the aortic root (Fig. 40–29).[13] The flap should always project into the left atrium.

Although a small amount of pericardial fluid can be seen in normal second- and third-trimester fetuses (Fig. 40–25), pericardial fluid measuring greater than 2 mm is abnormal (Fig. 40–26).[31] A pitfall leading to overdiagnosis of pericardial effusion is the peripheral hypoechoic part of the myocardium (Fig. 40–30). This hypoechoic rim measures 0.6 to 6.0 mm and can be seen in 94% of fetal hearts when sought diligently.[35] The hypoechoic layer most likely results from differences in orientation of muscle fibers within the ventricle. The longitudinal fibers are closer to the ventricular lumen, whereas the more circular fibers are located peripherally. The latter most likely cause the hypoechoic appearance seen with ultrasound.[35]

A final diagnostic pitfall relates to misinterpretation of cardiac chamber size discrepancies. For instance, in Figure 40–31 it appears that the left atrium and ventricle are small. In fact, the right atrium and right ventricle are dilated and the left chambers are normal in size. Misinterpretation of this sort can be avoided by measuring the chambers and referring the measurements to standard tables such as those presented herein.

CARDIAC ARRHYTHMIAS

The normal fetal heart rate varies according to gestational age. At 20 weeks, the fetal heart rate

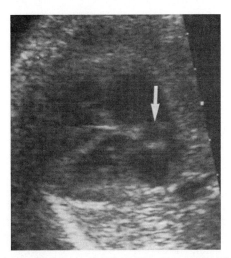

Figure 40-29—Redundant Foramen Ovale Flap. The anatomy of the foramen ovale is complex, and a normal flap may appear circular (arrow). (Reprinted with permission from Sohaey R, Zwiebel WJ: The fetal heart: A practical sonographic approach. Semin Ultrasound CT MRI 17:15–33, 1996.)

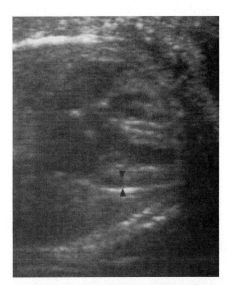

Figure 40-30—Normal Myocardium. The peripheral rim of the myocardium may appear hypoechoic (arrowheads) compared with the inner portion of the myocardium. This should not be confused with a pericardial effusion. (Reprinted with permission from Sohaey R, Zwiebel WJ: The fetal heart: A practical sonographic approach. Semin Ultrasound CT MRI 17:15–33, 1996.)

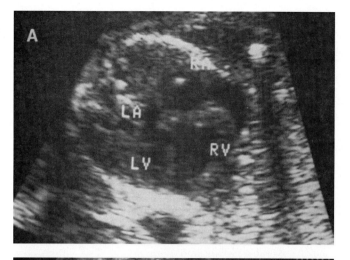

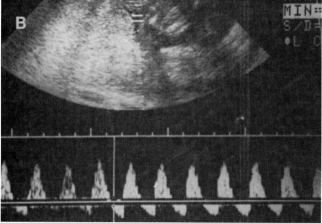

Figure 40-31—Heart Failure in the Donor Twin with Twin-Twin Transfusion. (A) The right atrium (RA) and (RV) are larger than the left atrium (LA) and (LV), and a pericardial effusion is present. It appears that the left chambers are small, but end-diastolic ventricular measurements showed the left ventricle normal in size, and the right heart is enlarged. **(B)** Doppler examination of the umbilical cord in the compromised twin showed reversal of diastolic flow. This twin was in heart failure and died 5 days after this examination despite reduction amniocentesis of the polyhydramnios twin. (Reprinted with permission from Sohaey R, Zwiebel WJ: The fetal heart: A practical sonographic approach. Semin Ultrasound CT MRI 17:15–33, 1996.)

is 140 (±20) beats per minute and falls to 130 (±20) bpm near term. Arrhythmias are defined as sustained fetal heart rates that are too slow, too fast, or irregular.[14] In general, a rate greater than 180 bpm is considered to be tachycardia and a rate less than 100 bpm is bradycardia.[36, 37] An irregular heart rate may be detected during routine office fetal monitoring, and prenatal ultrasound is then required to better define the nature of the irregularity. A complete discussion of arrhythmias is beyond the scope of this book. We will, however, discuss common arrhythmias, since the sonographer should be able to recognize which arrhythmias are "benign" and which require further detailed investigation.

When an arrhythmia is suspected, the sonographer should first evaluate the heart for morphologic abnormalities. After this is accomplished, M-mode Doppler examination of the heart is most useful in characterizing an arrhythmia. Since most arrhythmias originate from the supraventricular region and affect both sides of the heart symmetrically, the M-mode cursor opti-

mally should be placed through an atrium (right or left), the corresponding atrioventricular valve, and the corresponding ventricle (Fig. 40–32). If this positioning is not possible, the sonographer may need to obtain biatrial and biventricular M-mode Doppler tracings, which are less optimal but often diagnostic.

Irregular Rhythms: Premature Atrial Contraction and Premature Ventricular Contraction

The most common arrhythmia seen in fetal life is an occasional ectopic beat. These ectopic beats are sometimes frequent enough to produce a clinically detectable irregular rhythm.[14] The great majority of these ectopic beats originate in the atria and are called premature atrial contractions (PACs). Less commonly, these ectopic beats originate in the ventricle and are called premature ventricular contractions (PVCs). M-mode

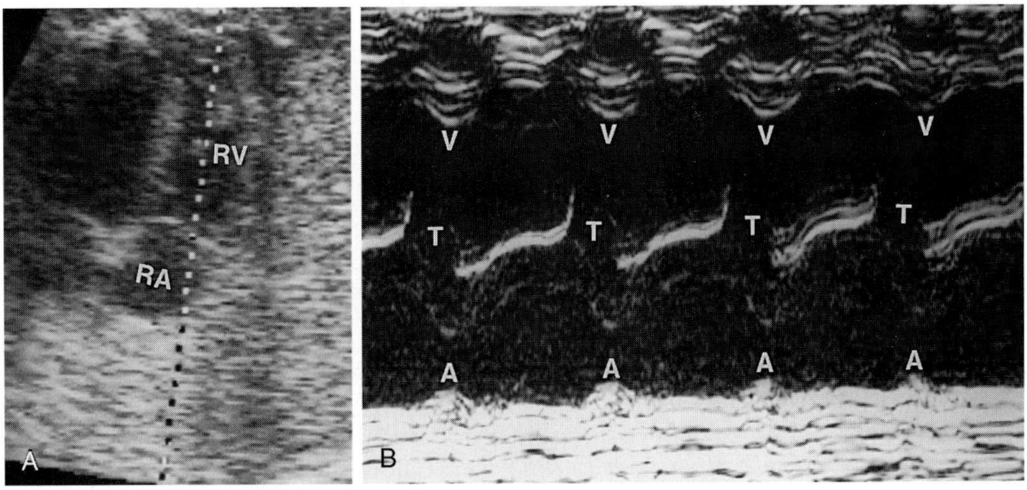

Figure 40-32—Arrhythmia Assessment. (A) Optimal positioning of the M-mode Doppler cursor (dotted line) through the right ventricle (RV), tricuspid valve, and right atrium (RA). The left side of the heart can be equally adequate for M-mode sampling since most arrhythmias affect the heart symmetrically. **(B)** Normal M-mode tracing. Regular normal rhythm of the atria (A), tricuspid valve (T), and ventricles (V) is seen. Unfortunately, the atrial contractions are usually the most difficult to see. Fetal heart rate was normal at 135 beats per minute.

tracings can determine whether the origin of the ectopic beats is atrial or ventricular by showing an "early" contraction of either chamber followed by either a "reset time" or a "compensatory pause." After a PAC, the sinoatrial node resets and normal rhythm usually ensues (Fig. 40–33). This reset time usually corresponds to the time interval between normal atrial contractions (sometimes slightly longer). Rarely, PACs can cause a compensatory pause. A compensatory pause is relatively long, lasting the time normally taken for two heart beats. The less common PVCs are more likely to demonstrate a compensatory pause. PACs may be conducted to the ventricles, and an M-mode tracing through both an atrium and a ventricle will show whether the PACs are conducted or not.

Isolated PACs and PVCs rarely result in fetal morbidity or mortality. They are not associated with morphologic abnormalities of the heart and tend to resolve either in utero or shortly after birth. Since they may be induced by maternal use of caffeine, cigarettes, or alcohol,[14] we advise our patients against the use of these materials if frequent premature contractions are seen. Rarely, PACs may progress to sustained supraventricular tachycardia requiring therapy. At our institution, we recommend weekly or biweekly heart rate monitoring by the referring primary care physician when PACs are frequent (25% or more of all observed atrial beats).

Tachycardia

As noted previously, tachycardia is defined as a sustained fetal heart rate greater than 180 bpm.

Figure 40-33—Premature Atrial Contraction. The M-mode tracing demonstrates a premature atrial contraction (PAC). The PAC is followed by a period of time equivalent to one normal cardiac cycle interval (arrows), representing a "reset" of the sinoatrial node. This PAC was not conducted to the ventricles.

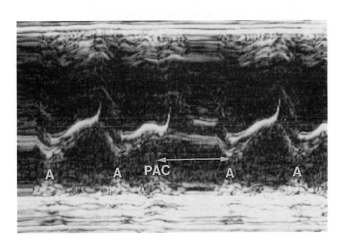

Tachycardia can originate from the ventricle or the supraventricular region. Supraventricular tachycardia is most common in fetal life and can lead to significant fetal morbidity, including congestive heart failure, hydrops, and death.[38] Less common subsets of supraventricular tachycardia include atrial flutter and atrial fibrillation.[14, 38]

M-mode Doppler helps differentiate between the different types of tachyarrhythmia. Atrial rates of 180 to 300 bpm are typical of supraventricular tachycardia, atrial rates of 300 to 400 bpm are typical for atrial flutter, and rates of 400 to 700 bpm are seen with atrial fibrillation. The ventricular rates are considerably slower than the atrial rates in supraventricular tachycardia, and they vary from 60 to 200 bpm. The ventricular rate is slower because atrioventricular block is usually present and every atrial beat is not conducted to the ventricle (Fig. 40–34).[14, 38]

Tachyarrhythmia may be associated with redundancy of the foramen ovale flap (often called an "aneurysm of the foramen ovale"),[39, 40] Ebstein anomaly,[41] cardiac tumors, or the Wolff-Parkinson-White syndrome (from an anomalous atrioventricular connection).[14, 42] Regardless of the cause, the fetus with tachycardia is at risk for hydrops and death. Aggressive treatment of tachycardia is recommended to avoid complications of hydrops. Intravenous administration of digoxin to the mother is usually the initial therapy of choice.[42] Other treatment choices include transplacental administration of antiarrhythmic drugs such as digoxin, flecainide, verapamil, procainamide, quinidine, or propranolol.[43]

Bradycardia

Bradycardia may be transient (temporary) or sustained. Transient bradycardia is probably induced by transducer pressure upon the fetus during the ultrasound examination, which causes a vasovagal response.[14, 36] Therefore, the easiest treatment is to reduce pressure or take a break in scanning before re-evaluating the heart rate. Sustained bradycardia, on the other hand, is a significant finding.

Complete heart block (dissociation between the atria and the ventricles) is the commonest and most important cause for sustained bradycardia.[38, 43] M-mode tracings show atrial rates of 120 to 140 bpm while ventricular rates are only 40 to 60 bpm.[14] Complete heart block is commonly associated with structural abnormalities of the heart (50% of cases), as well as maternal collagen vascular disease (most commonly systemic lupus erythematosus).[14, 44] Additional types of sustained bradycardia include sinus bradycardia (in which the atria and ventricles are synchronous), nonconducted frequent premature atrial contractions, and incomplete heart block of the Wenckebach type.[14] Sinus bradycardia may occur secondary to fetal distress and should be differentiated from other types of heart block. The prognosis for bradycardia depends on the presence of associated anomalies and whether or not the slow heart rate causes hydrops. The prognosis is quite poor if associated cardiac malformations are present.

Approach to Arrhythmias

The great majority of observed arrhythmias during the course of a routine obstetric examination are harmless and self-limited in nature. If bradycardia is observed during routine scanning, the sonographer should reduce transducer pressure or stop scanning for 15 to 30 seconds and then re-observe the heart. Usually bradycardia is transient and of no clinical significance. If an irregular rhythm is noticed, M-mode examination, should document the nature of the arrhythmia. Premature atrial contractions comprise the majority of observed arrhythmias. The patient can be questioned with regard to caffeine, tobacco, and alcohol use. The referring physician should be contacted about office surveillance of the fetal heart rate, since PACs can rarely progress to tachycardia. A careful examination of car-

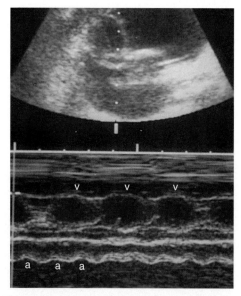

Figure 40-34—Supraventricular Tachycardia with Atrioventricular Block. The M-mode tracing shows an atrial rate (a) of 271 beats per minute. The ventricular rate (v) is only 132 beats per minute and therefore a 2:1 AV block is present. The fetus was successfully treated with digoxin.

diac morphology is important in all cases of sustained or recurrent arrhythmia. It is our belief that any arrhythmia other than transient bradycardia or PACs should be referred for formal fetal echocardiography.

REFERENCES

1. Hoffman JIE, Christianson R: Congenital heart disease in a cohort of 19,502 births with long-term follow-up. Am J Cardiol 42:641–647, 1978.
2. Mitchell SC, Korones SB, Berendes HW: Congenital heart disease in 56,109 births: Incidence and natural history. Circulation 43:323–332, 1971.
3. Allan LD, Crawford DC, Chita SK, et al: Prenatal screening for congenital heart disease. Br Med J 292:1717–1719, 1986.
4. Moller JH, Neal WA: Heart Disease in Infancy. New York, Appleton-Century-Crofts, 1981.
5. Benacerraf BR, Sanders SP: Fetal echocardiography. Radiol Clin North Am 28:131–147, 1990.
6. Moore KL: The circulatory system. *In* Moore KL (ed): The Developing Human: Clinically Oriented Embryology. 2nd ed. Philadelphia, WB Saunders, 1977, pp 259–300.
7. Cyre DR, Guntheroth WG, Mack LA, et al: A systematic approach to fetal echocardiography using real time/two dimensional sonography. J Ultrasound Med 5:343–350, 1985.
8. Copel JA, Pilu G, Green J, et al: Fetal echocardiographic screening for congenital heart disease: The importance of the four-chamber view. Am J Obstet Gynecol 157:648–655, 1987.
9. Lange LW, Sahn DJ, Allen HD, et al: Qualitative real time cross-sectional echocardiographic imaging of the human fetus during the second half of pregnancy. Circulation 62:799–806, 1980.
10. Comstock CH: Normal fetal heart axis and position. Obstet Gynecol 70:255–259, 1987.
11. DeVore GR: Fetal echocardiography: The challenge of the 1980s. Semin Ultrasound CT MR 5:229–248, 1984.
12. Levy DW, Mintz MC: The left ventricular echogenic focus: A normal finding. Am J Roentgenol AJR 150:85–86, 1988.
13. Kachalia P, Bowie JD, Adams DB, et al: In utero sonographic appearance of the atrial septum primum and septum secundum. J Ultrasound Med 10:423–426, 1991.
14. Nyberg DA, Emerson DS: Cardiac malformations. *In* Nyberg DA (ed): Diagnostic Ultrasound of Fetal Anomalies. St. Louis, Mosby–Year Book, 1990, pp 300–341.
15. Bromley B, Estroff JA, Sanders SP: Fetal echocardiography: Accuracy and limitations in a population at high and low risk for heart defects. Am J Obstet Gynecol 166:1473–1481, 1992.
16. Cartier MS, Davidoff A, Warneke LA, et al: The normal diameter of the fetal aorta and pulmonary artery: Echocardiographic evaluation in utero. Am J Roentgenol AJR 149:1003–1007, 1987.
17. McGahan JP: Sonography of the fetal heart: Findings on the four chamber view. Am J Roentgenol AJR 156:547–553, 1991.
18. Klinensmith WC III, Cioffi-Ragan DT, Harvey DE: Diagnosis of ectopia cordis in the second trimester. J Clin Ultrasound 16:204–206, 1988.
19. Nyberg DA, Mack LA: Abdominal wall defects. *In* Nyberg DA (ed): Diagnostic Ultrasound of Fetal Anomalies. St. Louis, Mosby–Year Book, 1990, pp 395–432.
20. DeVore GR, Siassi B, Platt LD: Fetal echocardiography. IV: M-mode assessment of ventricular size and contractility during the second and third trimesters of pregnancy in the normal fetus. Am J Obstet Gynecol 150:981–988, 1984.
21. Yagel S, Mandelberg A, Hurwitz A, et al: Prenatal diagnosis of hypoplastic left ventricle. Am J Perinatol 3:6–8, 1986.
22. Benacerraf BR, Saltzman DH, Sanders SP: Sonographic sign suggesting the prenatal diagnosis of coarctation of the aorta. J Ultrasound Med 8:65–69, 1989.
23. Marvin WJ Jr, Mahoney LT: Pulmonary atresia with intact ventricular septum. *In* Adams FH, Emmanouilides GC, Riemenschneider TA (eds): Moss' Heart Disease in Infants, Children and Adolescents. 4th ed. Baltimore, Williams and Wilkins, 1989, pp 485–503.
24. Elliot LP, Anderson RH, Bargerron LM Jr, et al: Single ventricle or univentricular heart. *In* Adams FH, Emmanouilides GC, Riemenschneider TA (eds): Moss' Heart Disease in Infants, Children and Adolescents. 4th ed. Baltimore, Williams and Wilkins, 1989, pp 485–503.
25. Machado MVL, Crawford DC, Anderson RH, et al: Atrioventricular septal defect in prenatal life. Br Heart J 59:352–355, 1988.
26. Ferencz C, Rubin JD, McCarte RJ, et al: Cardiac and non-cardiac malformations: Observations in a population-based study. Teratology 35:367–378, 1987.
27. Benacerraf BR, Pober BR, Sanders SP: Accuracy of fetal echocardiography. Radiology 165:847–849, 1987.
28. Achiron R, Malinger G, Zaidel L, Zakut H: Prenatal sonographic diagnosis of endocardial fibroelastosis secondary to aortic stenosis. Prenat Diagn 8:73–77, 1988.
29. Schaffer RM, Cabbad J, Minkoff H, et al: Sonographic diagnosis of fetal cardiac rhabdomyoma. J Ultrasound Med 5:531–533, 1986.
30. Green KW, Bors-Koefoed R, Pollack P, et al: Antepartum diagnosis and management of multiple fetal cardiac tumors. J Ultrasound Med 10:697–699, 1991.
31. Jeanty P, Romero R, Hobbins JC: Fetal pericardial fluid: A normal finding of the second half of gestation. Am J Obstet Gynecol 149:529–531, 1984.
32. Shenker L, Reed KL, Anderson CF, et al: Fetal pericardial effusion. Am J Obstet Gynecol 160:1505–1508, 1989.
33. Kennedy AM, Sohaey R, Woodward PJ: Cardiac evaluation in fetuses with diaphragmatic hernia: How accurate is the prenatal diagnosis? Presentation at American Institute of Ultrasound in Medicine, 38th Annual Meeting, Baltimore, March 20–23, 1994.
34. Brown DL, DiSalvo DN, Frates MC, et al: Sonography of the fetal heart: Normal variants and pitfalls. Am J Roentgenol AJR 160:1251–1255, 1993.
35. Brown DL, Cartier MS, Emerson DS, et al: The peripheral hypoechoic rim of the fetal heart. J Ultrasound Med 8:603–608, 1989.
36. Allan LD, Anderson RH, Sullivan ID, et al: Evaluation of fetal arrhythmias by echocardiography. Br Heart J 50:240–245, 1983.
37. Silverman NH, Enderlein MA, Stranger P, et al: Recognition of fetal arrhythmias by

echocardiography. J Clin Ultrasound 13:255–263, 1985.

38. Silverman NH, Schmidt KG: Ultrasound evaluation of the fetal heart. *In* Callen PW (ed): Ultrasonography in Obstetrics and Gynecology. 3rd ed. Philadelphia, WB Saunders, 1994, pp 291–332.

39. Rice MJ, McDonald RW, Reller MD: Fetal atrial septal aneurysm: A cause of fetal arrhythmias. J Am Coll Cardiol 12:1292–1297, 1988.

40. Toro L, Weintraub RG, Shiota T, et al: Relation between persistent atrial arrhythmias and redundant septum primum flap (atrial septal aneurysm) in fetuses. Am J Cardiol 73:711–713, 1994.

41. Westaby S, Karp RB, Kirklin JW, et al: Surgical treatment in Ebstein's malformation. Ann Thorac Surg 34:338–395, 1982.

42. Kleinman CS, Copel JA, Weinstein EM, et al: In utero diagnosis and treatment of supraventricular tachycardia. Semin Perinatol 9:113–129, 1985.

43. Crawford D, Chapman M, Allan LD: The assessment of persistent bradycardia in prenatal life. Br J Obstet Gynecol 92:941–944, 1985.

44. McCue CM, Mantakas ME, Tinglestad JB, et al: Congenital heart block in newborns of mothers with connective tissue disease. Circulation 56:82–89, 1977.

Chapter 41

The Fetal Gastrointestinal Tract

Roya Sohaey

Prenatal ultrasound can detect the majority of significant anomalies that involve the fetal gastrointestinal (GI) tract. These anomalies are somewhat difficult to evaluate, since the abdomen contains many different organs, bowel anatomy is complex, and the sonographic findings are inconstant. To further complicate matters, the normal fetal bowel varies in appearance at different gestational ages. The goal in this chapter is to present a practical approach to the abnormal fetal abdominal examination. I first review the recommended imaging technique for the fetal abdomen and then discuss fetal abdominal disorders, with emphasis on common bowel abnormalities and abdominal wall defects. Other fetal abdominal pathology is rare and is mentioned only briefly.

EMBRYOLOGY

An understanding of the basic embryology of the gastrointestinal system is important for appreciation of GI anomalies. Key embryologic features of GI tract development, with theories on the causes of some common anomalies, are presented in Tables 41–1 and 41–2.[1] Please review

this material before proceeding, as the contents of these tables are not repeated in the text.

THE FETAL ABDOMINAL EXAMINATION

The American Institute of Ultrasound in Medicine (AIUM) and the American College of Radiology (ACR) have published guidelines for fetal abdominal evaluation.[2, 3] All ultrasound examinations should document five features of the fetal abdomen: (1) the abdominal circumference; (2) the fluid-filled stomach; (3) the cord insertion and the adjacent abdominal wall; (4) the kidneys and surrounding structures; and (5) the urinary bladder. Taken together, the recommended abdominal views demonstrate abnormalities of both the viscera and the abdominal wall, from high in the epigastrium to low in the pelvis. A recent study has shown that 96% of abdominal disorders are detected if these five features are evaluated.[4]

Normal Findings

The abdominal circumference (AC) is the key image for identifying upper abdominal disorders, including gastric and liver anomalies.[5, 6] As shown in Figure 41–1, the correctly obtained AC is round (not ovoid), demonstrates a fluid-filled stomach fundus, and *includes* the subcutaneous tissues.[7] The sonographic characteristics of the normal AC image are summarized in Table 41–3. The fetal stomach can be seen on the AC view as early as 9 weeks and is almost always seen by 14 weeks.[4, 8–11] The stomach is considered abnormal if it is on the right side or if it is unusually large, small, or absent. The size of the fetal stomach varies with normal filling and emptying; nonetheless, a small or absent stomach during 45 minutes of observation is an abnormal finding.[8]

The umbilical cord insertion is evaluated on a transverse view of the mid-abdomen, obtained caudal to the AC view (Fig. 41–2). Care should be taken to visualize both the right and left margins of the cord, since a gastroschisis defect (located lateral to the cord) can be subtle, as discussed later.

The fetal bowel is evaluated on images ob-

Table 41-1. Gastrointestinal Tract Embryology

Embryologic Structure	Derivative
Foregut	Pharynx
	Lower respiratory tract
	Esophagus
	Stomach
	Proximal duodenum—to common bile duct entrance
	Liver, pancreas, biliary system
Midgut	Distal duodenum—from common bile duct entrance
	Small intestines
	Cecum and appendix
	Ascending colon
	Proximal transverse colon
Hindgut	Distal transverse colon
	Descending colon
	Sigmoid colon
	Rectum
	Upper anal canal
	Bladder and urethra

Table 41-2. Important Embryologic Events and Subsequent Anomalies

Embryology	Anomaly
Esophagus	
Tracheoesophageal septum divides the foregut into a laryngotracheal tube and an esophagus	Tracheoesophageal fistula results from a defective septum
Duodenum	
The foregut and midgut meet at the level of the duodenal C loop. The duodenal lumen may close with subsequent recanalization	Duodenal atresia or stenosis from failure to recanalize or in utero vascular insult at the point of foregut/midgut junction
Pancreas	
Complex fusion and rotation of the ventral and dorsal pancreas buds	Annular pancreas from a bifid ventral bud encircles the duodenum and may cause obstruction
Midgut	
Midgut grows faster than embryo. Midgut herniates into the base of the cord at 6 wk, rotates 90° clockwise (viewed ventrally), returns to abdomen at 12 wk, and rotates 180° counterclockwise	Omphalocele forms if the gut fails to internalize. Liver involved if lateral body folds do not fuse
Lateral body folds fuse	Bowel nonrotation occurs if the bowel fails to rotate once it internalizes
	Bowel malrotation occurs if the bowel fails to rotate the last 90°. Ladd bands form in the mesentery and may cause duodenal obstruction
Rectum and Anus	
The terminal part of the hindgut is initially a cloaca. The urorectal septum is a coronal sheet of mesenchyme that divides the cloaca into the rectum and upper anal canal dorsally and the urogenital sinus ventrally. The cloacal membrane separates the rectum and anal invagination and is absorbed by the 8th week	Imperforate anus occurs if the distal cloacal membrane does not resorb
	Fistula between the rectum and the urogenital sinus may be present if the urorectal septum does not form well

tained in the area of the cord insertion, kidneys, and bladder. The bowel should be examined for abnormal echogenicity, dilatation, or other abnormalities, to be discussed later. The appearance of the normal fetal bowel and colon vary at different menstrual ages.[12] Physiologic small bowel herniation (as detailed in Table 41–2) is visualized normally with ultrasound at about 11 to 12 weeks' menstrual age (Fig. 41–3) and should not be mistaken for an abdominal wall defect.[12] The herniated bowel does not measure greater than 10 mm in diameter.[13] Some investigators recommend that an abdominal wall defect should not be diagnosed before 14 weeks.[13]

The diameter of small bowel loops increases with gestational age but rarely exceeds 6 mm. Peristalsis is seen with increasing menstrual age. Between 10 and 20 weeks, the small bowel lumen is difficult to see, and bowel is isoechoic or mildly echogenic relative to the fetal liver.[12, 14] It is postulated that the mildly increased echogenicity of small bowel in some fetuses at this stage is from the reflection of sound as it passes through multiple collapsed bowel loops or mesenteric

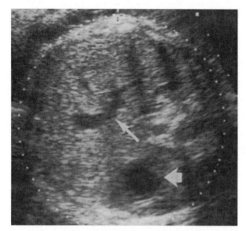

Figure 41-1—Normal abdominal circumference (AC). The AC should be round, and it should include a fluid-filled gastric fundus (short arrow). Note the C-shaped portal venous connection (long arrow) seen in the liver. This represents the junction of the left portal vein with the right portal vein via the pars transversa (tip of long arrow). (Reprinted with permission from Sohaey R, Woodward P, Zwiebel WJ: Fetal gastrointestinal anomalies. Semin Ultrasound CT MRI 17:51–65, 1996.)

Table 41-3. Features of the Normal Abdominal Circumference Image

Round transverse upper abdominal image
Gastric fundus on left
Include subcutaneous tissue in measurement
Liver seen at the level of left portal vein junction with pars transversa
Spine seen in cross-section

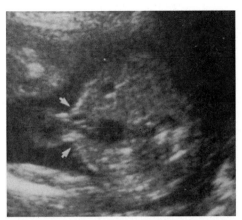

Figure 41-2—Normal umbilical cord insertion site. Both margins of the umbilical cord are seen on this transverse view (arrows). (Reprinted with permission from Sohaey R, Woodward P, Zwiebel WJ: Fetal gastrointestinal anomalies. Semin Ultrasound CT MRI 17:51-65, 1996.)

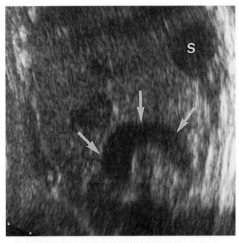

Figure 41-4—Normal fetal colon. Coronal image of the lower abdomen in a third-trimester fetus shows normal meconium-filled sigmoid colon (arrows). (S, fluid-filled stomach.)(Reprinted with permission from Sohaey R, Woodward P, Zwiebel WJ: Fetal gastrointestinal anomalies. Semin Ultrasound CT MRI 17:51-65, 1996.)

fat.[12] Hyperechoic bowel may be pathologic when seen in the second and third trimesters, as discussed later.

The fetal colon is recognized by its peripheral location within the abdomen. As the fetus matures, the colon increases in diameter but rarely exceeds 23 mm.[12] Colonic peristalsis is not seen in utero; however, haustral folds can be seen. Later in pregnancy, the colon contains meconium that is hypoechoic with respect to the liver and the bowel wall (Fig. 41-4). The meconium-filled fetal colon should not be mistaken for a mass. In 6% of third-trimester fetuses, the meconium-filled rectum may appear as a presacral hypo-echoic mass measuring 15 to 30 mm. The diagnosis of a normal rectum in such a case should be favored over the diagnosis of a presacral teratoma (the incidence of the latter is 0.0025%).[15]

HYPERECHOIC BOWEL

As noted earlier, the normal fetal bowel is isoechoic or mildly echogenic when compared to the fetal liver.[12, 14] Hyperechoic bowel (Fig. 41-5) sometimes is seen in the second trimester and is associated with a significant risk of adverse pregnancy outcome. Nyberg and colleagues[14] prospectively studied 95 fetuses with hyper-echoic bowel and found an associated increased incidence of chromosomal abnormalities (25%),

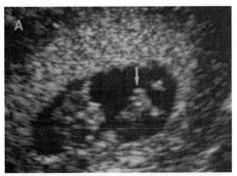
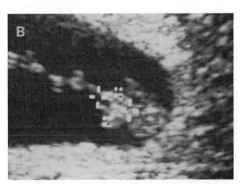

Figure 41-3—Physiologic small bowel herniation. (**A**) First-trimester fetus seen in a sagittal view. Note the echogenic focus of normally herniated small bowel (arrow). This should not be confused with an abdominal wall defect. (**B**) First-trimester abdomen seen in a transverse view. The physiologic bowel herniation is small (less than 10 mm), echogenic, and seen at the base of the umbilical cord insertion site (calipers delineate herniated bowel). (Reprinted with permission from Sohaey R, Woodward P, Zwiebel WJ: Fetal gastrointestinal anomalies. Semin Ultrasound CT MRI 17:51-65, 1996.)

intrauterine growth retardation (10%), fetal demise (6%), and other anomalies (5%). These investigators graded bowel echogenicity as follows:

- Grade 0, isoechoic with liver;
- Grade 1, mildly echogenic when compared with liver;
- Grade 2, moderately echogenic;
- Grade 3, markedly echogenic (as echogenic as bone).

In the Nyberg series, Grade 2 or 3 echogenic bowel was associated with a 62% chance for an adverse pregnancy outcome.[14] Echogenic bowel has also been found in association with cystic fibrosis.[16, 17] We consider grade 1, or mildly echogenic bowel, to be normal, but we recommend genetic counseling and amniocentesis when markedly echogenic (grade 3) bowel is seen.

THE SMALL FETAL STOMACH

As noted, the fluid-filled gastric fundus is seen routinely after 14 weeks' menstrual age.[10, 11] Basically, any anomaly that impairs fetal swallowing, obstructs the flow of amniotic fluid into the stomach, or decreases the overall availability of amniotic fluid may cause a small or absent fetal stomach. Esophageal atresia is the diagnosis most commonly entertained when the fetal stomach is not seen. However, most cases of esophageal atresia are accompanied by tracheoesophageal fistula, which transmits enough amniotic fluid for

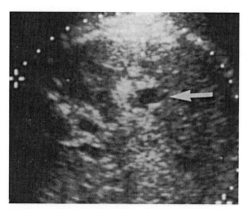

Figure 41-6—Small stomach. The fetal gastric fundus contains little amniotic fluid (arrow). A diagnosis of esophageal atresia with distal tracheoesophageal fistula was made after birth. (Reprinted with permission from Sohaey R, Woodward P, Zwiebel WJ: Fetal gastrointestinal anomalies. Semin Ultrasound CT MRI 17:51-65, 1996.)

visualization of the gastric fundus (Fig. 41–6).[18, 19] Therefore, the *presence* of the fluid-filled stomach does not exclude esophageal atresia. Other conditions that cause a small or absent stomach include diaphragmatic hernia,[20] cleft palate,[21] oligohydramnios, intrauterine growth retardation, and central nervous system disorders.[10]

Nonvisualization of the stomach occurred in only 0.4% of all fetal examinations in a large reported series.[22] Almost half (48%) the fetuses with nonvisualized stomachs were abnormal, and in 20% of cases, an absent stomach was the only anomaly seen. The risk of abnormality was not eliminated even if a normal stomach was seen on a subsequent examination. Some pregnancies were normal, however, in spite of consistent nonvisualization of the stomach. In summary, fetuses with a small or absent stomach should be carefully evaluated for further anomalies, and even if a normal stomach is seen on a subsequent examination, the prognosis remains guarded.

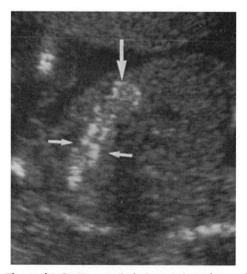

Figure 41-5—Hyperechoic bowel. Sagittal view of the abdomen shows markedly echogenic bowel (arrows). The bowel is as echogenic as bone. (Reprinted with permission from Sohaey R, Woodward P, Zwiebel WJ: Fetal gastrointestinal anomalies. Semin Ultrasound CT MRI 17:51-65, 1996.)

THE DISTENDED FETAL STOMACH AND DUODENUM

An enlarged or distended fetal stomach is also abnormal, and it is usually associated with polyhydramnios. A pyloric web can cause gastric outlet obstruction, but this is a rare anomaly accounting for approximately 1% of gastrointestinal atresia.[23] More commonly, gastric dilatation results from duodenal obstruction. Once the dilated stomach is seen, the dilated duodenum is not difficult to find. The term "double bubble" is used for the radiographic appearance of duodenal obstruction, since the air-filled duodenum and stomach appear as two gas bubbles on a

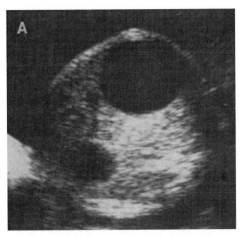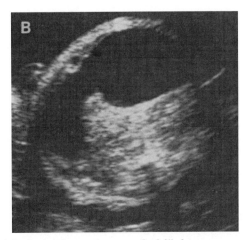

Figure 41-7—Duodenal atresia. (A) Transverse image of the fetal abdomen shows two fluid-filled structures ("sonographic double bubble"). (B) By changing the scanning plane, the sonographer demonstrates the connection between the dilated gastric fundus and the dilated duodenum in this case of duodenal atresia. (Reprinted with permission from Sohaey R, Woodward P, Zwiebel WJ: Fetal gastrointestinal anomalies. Semin Ultrasound CT MRI 17:51-65, 1996.)

radiograph. The fluid-filled double bubble equivalent is seen with ultrasound (Fig. 41–7). By maneuvering the image plane, the sonographer can show the gastric-duodenal connection and correctly diagnose duodenal obstruction. Duodenal obstruction can be seen as early as 14 weeks,[24] but most cases are not diagnosed until polyhydramnios causes clinically apparent uterine enlargement (after 26 weeks). Polyhydramnios occurs because small bowel resorption of amniotic fluid is prevented (Chapter 35).

The most common cause of duodenal obstruction is duodenal atresia, which occurs in 1 per 10,000 live births.[25] As stated in Table 41–2, atresia at this location is thought to result from failure of recanalization of the duodenum at the junction of the foregut and midgut. This junction corresponds to the area of the ampulla of Vater, within the descending duodenum.[1] The duodenum also may be obstructed by an annular pancreas, peritoneal band, volvulus, intestinal duplication, or duodenal stenosis.

Additional structural anomalies and karyotype abnormalities have been found in 52% of fetuses with duodenal obstruction, including cardiac defects in 34% of cases, and trisomy 21 in 30%.[26] Overall, duodenal atresia is associated with a 36% mortality rate. Associated anomalies, and particularly cardiac defects, account for most deaths.[27] Isolated duodenal obstruction is a relatively innocuous anomaly associated with an operative survival rate of 95%.[26]

NONDUODENAL BOWEL OBSTRUCTION

As described previously, the diameter of the normal small bowel lumen rarely exceeds 6 mm,

and the colon diameter rarely exceeds 23 mm.[12] Fetal bowel obstruction should be suspected when one or more dilated loops of bowel are seen in the fetal abdomen (Fig. 41–8). In the third trimester, polyhydramnios is usually seen in association with bowel obstruction, because of decreased fetal absorption of ingested amniotic fluid.

Malrotation, volvulus, peritoneal bands, and cystic fibrosis may cause in utero small bowel obstruction, but the most common cause is jejunoileal atresia.[28] The latter condition is so named because either the proximal jejunum or the distal ileum is commonly involved. Atresia, in these cases, probably occurs as a result of a vascular insult to the bowel.[29] The exact point of obstruction is usually impossible to determine by prenatal sonography.

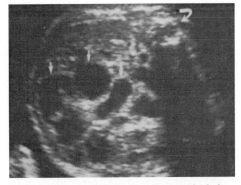

Figure 41-8—Bowel obstruction. Multiple loops of dilated bowel (small arrows) are present on this transverse image. Neonatal surgery showed multiple distal small bowel atresias. (Curved arrow, spine with shadowing.) (Reprinted with permission from Sohaey R, Woodward P, Zwiebel WJ: Fetal gastrointestinal anomalies. Semin Ultrasound CT MRI 17:51-65, 1996.)

Nonduodenal bowel atresia is a sporadic event unassociated with chromosome or other anomalies,[28] with one exception: meconium ileus. Meconium ileus is seen most often in neonates with cystic fibrosis, and it is difficult to diagnose in utero because the meconium-obstructed distal ileum does not dilate until late in pregnancy.[30] Fetuses with cystic fibrosis have an elevated incidence of bowel atresia, even in the absence of meconium ileus. Therefore, the diagnosis of cystic fibrosis should be considered in any fetus with a nonduodenal bowel obstruction.

ANORECTAL MALFORMATIONS

A spectrum of anal and rectal anomalies exists that can lead to colonic obstruction. Anorectal anomalies occur in 1 in 5000 live births and range in severity from a persistent cloaca to anal atresia.[31, 32] The so-called VATER association consists of *v*ertebral anomalies, *a*nal atresia, *t*racheoesophageal fistula, and *r*adial and *r*enal dysplasia.[31] Anal atresia can be located "high" (above the levator ani) or "low" (below the levator ani), but the exact level is difficult to discern with fetal ultrasound.[32] High anal atresia is more frequently associated with genitourinary anomalies such as vesicoenteric fistulas.[33]

Studies show that the fetus may normally pass small amounts of meconium in utero,[34, 35] preventing colonic dilatation. Anal atresia, therefore, can result in colonic dilatation, but this usually is apparent only in the late third trimester. The sonographic finding of a dilated fetal colon *with* intraluminal calcification is specific for anal atresia with associated vesicoenteric fistula. The rectourinary fistula, in such cases, allows intraluminal mixing of meconium and urine, which promotes the development of calcification (Fig. 41–9).[36, 37]

MECONIUM PERITONITIS

Small bowel perforation leads to meconium peritonitis, which occurs in 1:35,000 live births. Meconium peritonitis can occur in fetuses with underlying bowel abnormalities such as jejunoileal atresia, or it can be idiopathic and potentially without sequelae.[38, 39] When leaked from the bowel, digestive enzymes and meconium cause an intense sterile chemical peritonitis. An inflammatory response is mounted, giant cells and histiocytes surround the meconium, foreign body granulomas form, and these quickly calcify. The inflammatory response actually may seal a bowel perforation.[40] Meconium peritonitis can be associated with cystic fibrosis,[41, 42] but it is interesting to note that calcification generally does not occur in these cases. One explanation for the absence of calcification is that chemical peritonitis is less severe with cystic fibrosis because of pancreatic enzyme deficiency.[42]

The sonographic findings of meconium peritonitis include (1) sudden decompression of previously visualized dilated bowel, associated with interval development of ascites (Fig. 41–10); (2) an intraperitoneal mass; or (3) increased bowel echogenicity associated with peritoneal calcification.[39] The calcifications may be linear or clumped. Sometimes peritoneal calcifications are the only visible signs of meconium peritonitis[39] (Fig. 41–11) and are seen incidentally during prenatal sonography or on radiographs of the neonatal abdomen. Rarely, meconium peritonitis can present as an abdominal "pseudocyst." The cyst, in such cases, is a loculated collection of bowel contents that is called a pseudocyst be-

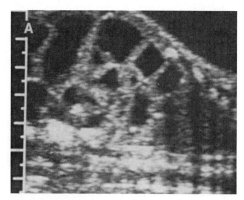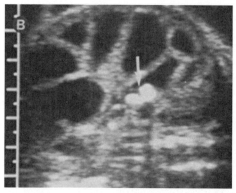

Figure 41-9—Anal atresia. (A) Coronal view of the lower chest and upper abdomen shows abdominal distention and bowel dilatation. **(B)** Some of the dilated loops of bowel contain intraluminal calcifications (arrow). This observation allowed for the correct diagnosis of anal atresia with rectourinary fistula. Meconium may calcify in the presence of urine, whereas intraluminal meconium, alone, does not calcify. (Reprinted with permission from Sohaey R, Woodward P, Zwiebel WJ: Fetal gastrointestinal anomalies. Semin Ultrasound CT MRI 17:51-65, 1996.)

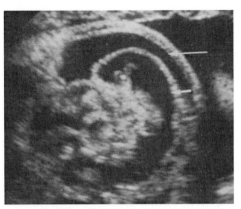

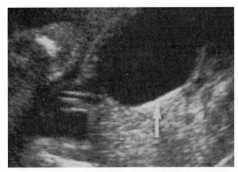

Figure 41-12—Atypical meconium pseudocyst.
A large, featureless abdominal cyst is seen (arrow). The fetus subsequently developed bowel obstruction and this cyst resolved. Pseudocysts are usually hypoechoic, not anechoic, and are seen in conjunction with bowel obstruction. (Reprinted with permission from Sohaey R, Woodward P, Zwiebel WJ: Fetal gastrointestinal anomalies. Semin Ultrasound CT MRI 17:51-65, 1996.)

Figure 41-10—Meconium peritonitis. Fetus with bowel obstruction and perforation. Note the dilated bowel (short arrow) and ascites (long arrow) (Reprinted with permission from Sohaey R, Woodward P, Zwiebel WJ: Fetal gastrointestinal anomalies. Semin Ultrasound CT MRI 17:51-65, 1996.)

cause it does not have an epithelial wall.[43] A meconium pseudocyst may have a variety of ultrasound appearances, but usually it presents as a hypoechoic mass surrounded by an echogenic calcified wall. The evolving pseudocyst may be difficult to differentiate from other intra-abdominal cysts[28] (Fig. 41–12). The differential diagnosis of an abdominal cyst seen in utero includes urinary tract dilatation and related cysts, bowel dilatation, ovarian cysts, meconium pseudocysts, bowel duplication cysts, cystic neoplasms, and lymphangioma.[28]

FETAL GALLBLADDER DISORDERS

Fetal cholelithiasis can be seen with prenatal ultrasound (Fig. 41–13) and is probably of no

clinical significance.[44, 45] Echogenic material in the fetal gallbladder may cause an acoustic shadow or a comet tail artifact, or it may simply appear echogenic. The echogenic material tends to resolve, sometimes in weeks to months. Usually the fetus remains asymptomatic, even if the stones or echogenic material persists throughout the pregnancy.[45]

FETAL LIVER LESIONS

Fetal liver lesions occur rarely. Punctate liver calcifications can be seen with viral infections (Fig. 41–14), and may be a significant finding in a patient exposed to a virus that might adversely affect fetal development.[46] Liver tumors are exceedingly rare. Hemangiomas represent congenital vascular malformations composed of capillary

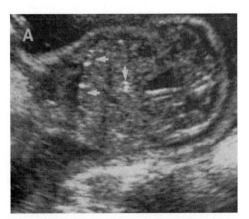

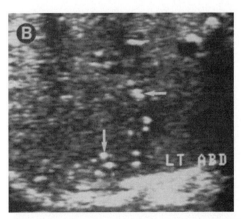

Figure 41-11—Meconium peritonitis. (A) Multiple tiny calcifications surround the fetal liver (arrows). **(B)** Later in gestation, peritoneal calcifications are also seen surrounding bowel (arrows). No adverse effects of meconium peritonitis occurred in fetal or neonatal life. (Reprinted with permission from Sohaey R, Woodward P, Zwiebel WJ: Fetal gastrointestinal anomalies. Semin Ultrasound CT MRI 17:51-65, 1996.)

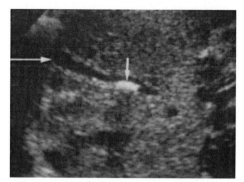

Figure 41-13—Fetal gallstones. The fetal gallbladder (long arrow) contains a shadowing echogenic focus (short arrow). This neonate had gallstones but remains asymptomatic. (Reprinted with permission from Sohaey R, Woodward P, Zwiebel WJ: Fetal gastrointestinal anomalies. Semin Ultrasound CT MRI 17:51-65, 1996.)

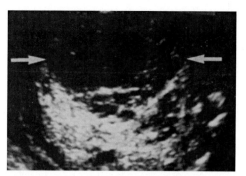

Figure 41-15—Hemangioendothelioma. A large, multicystic liver lesion (arrows) practically replaces the fetal liver. (Reprinted with permission from Sohaey R, Woodward P, Zwiebel WJ: Fetal gastrointestinal anomalies. Semin Ultrasound CT MRI 17:51-65, 1996.)

channels. Although histologically benign, they can cause high-output failure. With ultrasound, they can be hypoechoic, hyperechoic, or mixed in appearance. They rarely contain calcium.[47] Hemangioendothelioma (Fig. 41–15) and mesenchymal hamartoma are other benign liver tumors that can occur in fetuses.[28] Hepatoblastoma (Fig. 41–16) is the most common malignant tumor seen in the fetal liver. It is vascular, solid, and echogenic and may contain calcium.[28]

FETAL ASCITES

Fetal ascites is most commonly seen in cases of fetal hydrops[48] (Fig. 41–14). Fetal ascites not associated with hydrops can result from many different etiologies, including chromosome abnormality, intrauterine infection, and gastrointestinal and genitourinary anomalies. Isolated fetal ascites also may be idiopathic.[49]

ABDOMINAL WALL DEFECTS

If the standard abdominal views are obtained routinely, as recommended previously, fetal abdominal wall defects should be detected consistently with ultrasound. Once a defect is seen, it is important to identify correctly the type of defect present. Key differential features are the position of the defect relative to the cord insertion, the size of the defect, and the organs involved. Common abdominal wall defects include

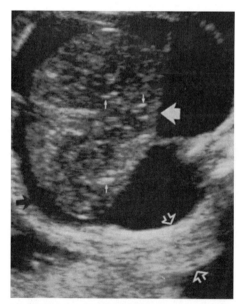

Figure 41-14—Viral calcification. The liver (large arrow) contains multiple tiny calcifications (small arrows). The fetus is also hydropic as shown by the presence of ascites (black arrow) and skin thickening (open arrows). At autopsy, it was determined that the fetus was infected with cytomegalovirus (CMV). (Reprinted with permission from Sohaey R, Woodward P, Zwiebel WJ: Fetal gastrointestinal anomalies. Semin Ultrasound CT MRI 17:51-65, 1996.)

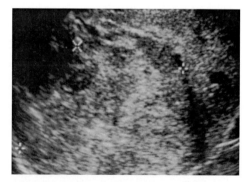

Figure 41-16—Hepatoblastoma. A large, heterogeneous, solid liver lesion (calipers) appeared in an 8-week interval. Hepatoblastomas are rarely detected in utero but should be suspected if a growing, solid liver mass is seen. (Reprinted with permission from Sohaey R, Woodward P, Zwiebel WJ: Fetal gastrointestinal anomalies. Semin Ultrasound CT MRI 17:51-65, 1996.)

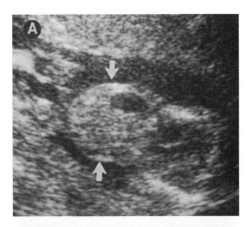

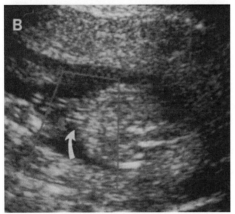

Figure 41-17—Omphalocele. (A) Transverse image of the fetal abdomen demonstrates a large abdominal wall defect. The liver and stomach are extracorporeal (arrows). **(B)** The umbilical cord inserts at the apex of the omphalocele (curved arrow). (Reprinted with permission from Sohaey R, Woodward P, Zwiebel WJ: Fetal gastrointestinal anomalies. Semin Ultrasound CT MRI 17:51-65, 1996.)

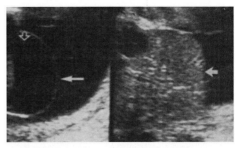

Figure 41-18—Omphalocele. Transverse images of a large, liver containing omphalocele (small arrow at right). The omphalocele membrane (long arrow) and ascites (open arrow) are clearly seen. (Reprinted with permission from Sohaey R, Woodward P, Zwiebel WJ: Fetal gastrointestinal anomalies. Semin Ultrasound CT MRI 17:51-65, 1996.)

omphalocele and gastroschisis; uncommon defects include the pentalogy of Cantrell, the limb–body wall complex, and the body stalk anomaly.

OMPHALOCELE

Herniation of bowel or liver into the base of the umbilical cord results in an omphalocele, which occurs in 1 in 4000 live births.[28, 49] Liver-containing omphaloceles are most common and are thought to be caused by failure of the lateral body folds to close. Bowel-containing omphaloceles probably result from failure of physiologically herniated bowel to return to the abdomen.[1, 50] Omphaloceles that contain only bowel are rare.

Ultrasound Findings

The liver-containing omphalocele tends to be a large, central defect easily seen with ultrasound

(Fig. 41–17). The umbilical cord insertion site is usually at the apex of the defect, but it can be eccentric.[22] An omphalocele membrane is almost always present and is composed of two layers, the inner peritoneal membrane and the outer amnion. (The amnion also covers the umbilical cord.) Ascites commonly is seen within the omphalocele sac and helps delineate the membranes (Fig 41–18).[22]

First-trimester diagnoses of liver-containing omphaloceles have been reported,[51, 52] and we have correctly diagnosed two 10-week omphaloceles at our institution (Fig. 41–19). The sonographic features of normal physiologic bowel herniation (see Fig. 41–3) into the umbilical cord have been discussed earlier. Whereas bowel herniation is normal in the first trimester, liver herniation is not normal. Liver-containing omphaloceles are larger, more homogeneous, and less echogenic than normal physiologic bowel herniation.[51, 52] If there is any doubt as to whether first-

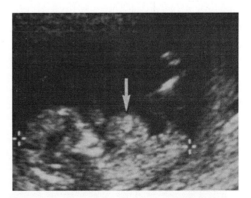

Figure 41-19—First-trimester omphalocele. Sagittal image of a 10-week embryo (calipers) shows extracorporeal liver (arrow). Follow-up sonography confirmed the diagnosis of an omphalocele. (Reprinted with permission from Sohaey R, Woodward P, Zwiebel WJ: Fetal gastrointestinal anomalies. Semin Ultrasound CT MRI 17:51-65, 1996.)

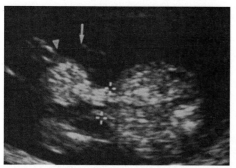

Figure 41-20—Bowel containing omphalocele.
The umbilical cord inserts (arrowhead) upon an
omphalocele that contains only bowel. The omphalocele
membrane is seen (arrow), helping to differentiate the
omphalocele from an umbilical hernia. (Reprinted with
permission from Sohaey R, Woodward P, Zwiebel WJ: Fetal
gastrointestinal anomalies. Semin Ultrasound CT MRI
17:51-65, 1996.)

trimester herniation into the cord is normal or
pathologic, the sonographer should re-image the
fetus after 14 weeks' menstrual age.[13] Abdominal
wall defects containing only bowel should never
be diagnosed earlier than 14 weeks.

As noted previously, it is rare for an omphalocele to contain only bowel (Fig. 41–20). Such
wall defects are commonly misdiagnosed as gastroschisis or are overlooked because they are
smaller than liver-containing omphaloceles.[53]
Differentiating between a bowel-only omphalocele and a small umbilical hernia also may be
difficult. An umbilical hernia should be covered
by skin and subcutaneous fat, whereas the omphalocele is covered only by the omphalocele
membrane.[53]

Prognosis and Associated Anomalies

The prognosis for the fetus with an omphalocele depends on the presence and severity of

associated anomalies. Ninety percent of fetuses
survive if an omphalocele is the sole anomaly,
but survival is only 20% to 30% if one or more
malformations are seen in addition to the omphalocele.[54, 55] Unfortunately, approximately two
thirds of fetuses with omphalocele have associated malformations. These include other gastrointestinal tract anomalies as well as anomalies of
the heart, genitourinary tract, and central nervous system.[28]

Chromosome abnormalities also are more
common in fetuses with omphalocele, occurring
in one third to one half of cases. The most
frequently associated chromosome defects are
trisomy 13 and 18.[22, 53, 56] Nyberg and colleagues[53]
showed a correlation between omphalocele contents and chromosome abnormalities. In their
series, the absence of liver in the sac strongly
correlated with an abnormal karyotype. All eight
of their fetuses with bowel-only omphalocele had
chromosome anomalies, while only 2 of 18 fetuses (11%) with liver-containing omphalocele
had an abnormal karyotype.[53]

GASTROSCHISIS

A gastroschisis results from a small, *paraum*-
bilical abdominal wall defect. The weakness in
the abdominal wall at this site may be secondary
to the normal involution of the right umbilical
vein,[50] or it may be due to ischemic damage from
disruption of the omphalomesenteric artery.[57]
Gastroschisis occurs in 1 in 4000 live births, a
rate similar to that for omphalocele.[28]

Ultrasound Findings

A gastroschisis defect may be more difficult to
visualize than an omphalocele defect. The defect
occurs to the *right* of the cord insertion and
usually is less than 2 cm in size (Fig. 41–21). No

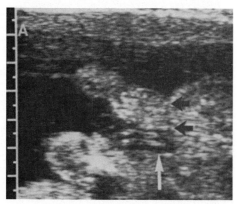
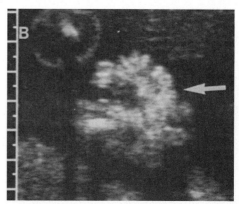

Figure 41-21—Gastroschisis. (A) A right-sided, paraumbilical abdominal wall defect is seen (black arrows). The
umbilical cord inserts normally (white arrow). **(B)** The extracorporeal bowel (arrow) is not confined by a membrane and is
seen free-floating in the amniotic fluid. (Reprinted with permission from Sohaey R, Woodward P, Zwiebel WJ: Fetal
gastrointestinal anomalies. Semin Ultrasound CT MRI 17:51-65, 1996.)

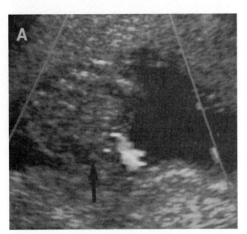
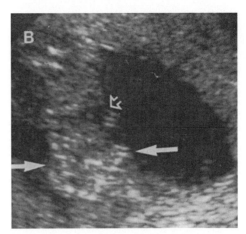

Figure 41-22—Gastroschisis: Pitfall. (A) The right paraumbilical region is obliterated because the fetus is positioned along the posterior uterine wall (arrow). This image is not an adequate cord insertion view. **(B)** Seconds later, the fetus moves away from the uterine wall and extracorporeal bowel is seen (solid arrows). The umbilical cord insertion is at the normal site (open arrow). (Reprinted with permission from Sohaey R, Woodward P, Zwiebel WJ: Fetal gastrointestinal anomalies. Semin Ultrasound CT MRI 17:51-65, 1996.)

membrane is present, and the herniated bowel is free-floating within the amniotic fluid.[10, 22] An adequate cord insertion view is crucial for the correct diagnosis of a gastroschisis. If only one margin of the cord is seen, a gastroschisis can be missed (Fig. 41–22). False-positive and false-negative diagnoses of abdominal wall defects have been reported. In these cases, either the umbilical cord was confused with extruded bowel or vice versa. Color Doppler examination should prevent such errors.[49]

In gastroschisis, extruded bowel is exposed to the amniotic fluid, since the bowel is not contained within a membrane. The bowel wall often is thickened, probably from exposure to fetal urine within the fluid, or perhaps from exposure to meconium, which may be present in small amounts.[34, 35, 58] Chemical irritation of extruded bowel may lead to bowel dilatation (Fig. 41–23)

and perforation.[22] Intra-abdominal bowel dilatation also can occur, secondary to obstruction, which is a particular problem in fetuses with small gastroschisis defects (Figs. 41–24 and 41–25). Fetuses with gastroschisis are at a higher than normal risk for intrauterine growth retardation and should be followed closely.

Prognosis

Gastroschisis, unlike omphalocele, tends to be an isolated anomaly. Non-bowel anomalies and chromosome abnormalities are not significantly increased in fetuses with gastroschisis,[22] and we do not routinely recommend amniocentesis at our institution for cases of gastroschisis.

Gastroschisis is associated, however, with other bowel-related anomalies such as bowel malrota-

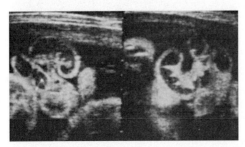

Figure 41-23—Gastroschisis complication. The extruded bowel is dilated, and bowel wall thickening is present (compare with the bowel in Figure 21*B*), most likely from chemical irritation by amniotic fluid contents. (Reprinted with permission from Sohaey R, Woodward P, Zwiebel WJ: Fetal gastrointestinal anomalies. Semin Ultrasound CT MRI 17:51-65, 1996.)

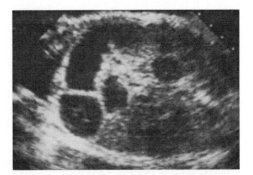

Figure 41-24—Gastroschisis complication. Coronal image of the fetal abdomen shows multiple dilated loops of intra-abdominal bowel in a fetus with a "tight" gastroschisis defect. (Reprinted with permission from Sohaey R, Woodward P, Zwiebel WJ: Fetal gastrointestinal anomalies. Semin Ultrasound CT MRI 17:51-65, 1996.)

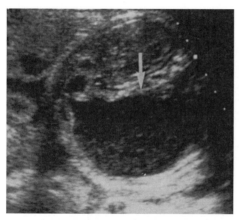

Figure 41-25—Gastroschisis complication. The stomach is obstructed and dilated (arrow) in this fetus with a gastroschisis in which the entire small bowel was extracorporeal. (Reprinted with permission from Sohaey R, Woodward P, Zwiebel WJ: Fetal gastrointestinal anomalies. Semin Ultrasound CT MRI 17:51-65, 1996.)

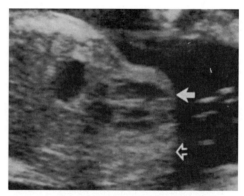

Figure 41-26—Pentalogy of Cantrell. The body wall defect involves the lower chest. The heart (solid arrow) and liver (open arrow) are in the omphalocele cavity. (Reprinted with permission from Sohaey R, Woodward P, Zwiebel WJ: Fetal gastrointestinal anomalies. Semin Ultrasound CT MRI 17:51-65, 1996.)

tion or nonrotation. The blood vessels supplying bowel may become torsed or compressed as they exit or return through the tight abdominal wall defect, resulting in bowel atresia and stenosis.[22]

The prognosis for gastroschisis is quite good. Mortality is less than 10% when fetuses deliver at a tertiary care center. Neonatal demise occurs from premature delivery, sepsis, and bowel ischemia.[54] The combined ultrasound findings of small bowel dilatation and mural wall thickening are tentatively associated with more severe intestinal damage.[59] At our institution, however, early delivery of fetuses with these findings is considered only if lung maturity has been established.

PENTALOGY OF CANTRELL

Pentalogy of Cantrell is a rare abdominal wall defect that involves the lower chest and upper abdomen. It is probably caused by failure of the lateral body folds to fuse in the thoracic region, with variable inferior extension of the fusion defect.[28] The pentalogy consists of omphalocele, ectopia cordis, intrinsic cardiac defects, diaphragmatic hernia, and a pericardial defect. The diagnosis should be suspected when an omphalocele seems unusually large and involves the cardiac apex (Fig. 41–26). Pentalogy of Cantrell is fatal and is associated with trisomies.[60]

LIMB–BODY WALL COMPLEX

Limb–body wall complex (LBWC) is characterized by multiple body defects such as ventral wall anomaly, craniofacial defects, limb amputations, and spinal dysraphism. Internal anomalies

are present in 95% of affected fetuses.[22, 61] The etiology for this severe anomaly complex is not known, but some believe it represents a severe form of amniotic band syndrome.[62] Others believe LBWC can be explained by early vascular disruption affecting many structures.[63] Sonography reveals a bizarre, large, eccentric thoracoabdominal wall defect that does not fit neatly into the gastroschisis or omphalocele categories. The defect is frequently left sided.[62] The combination of scoliosis and a bizarre abdominal wall defect should suggest the diagnosis of LBWC (Fig. 41–27). The condition is fatal.[22]

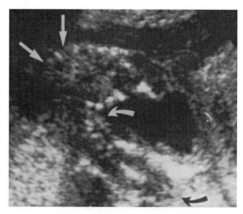

Figure 41-27—Limb-body wall complex. Coronal imaging of the fetus reveals an acute angle scoliosis (curved white arrow) and an atypical left lateral thoracoabdominal wall defect (straight white arrows). (For orientation purposes, the pelvis is marked with the curved black arrow. The fetal cranium is not visualized at this scan plane.) (Reprinted with permission from Sohaey R, Woodward P, Zwiebel WJ: Fetal gastrointestinal anomalies. Semin Ultrasound CT MRI 17:51-65, 1996.)

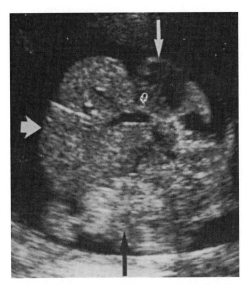

Figure 41-28—Body stalk anomaly. A fetal body is not recognizable. Instead, viscera, such as liver (short arrow), heart (long arrow), and bowel (black arrow), come in direct contact with amniotic fluid and placenta. There is complete evisceration. (Reprinted with permission from Sohaey R, Woodward P, Zwiebel WJ: Fetal gastrointestinal anomalies. Semin Ultrasound CT MRI 17:51-65, 1996.)

BODY STALK ANOMALY

The most severe abdominal wall defect is the body stalk anomaly, representing complete failure of formation of the body stalk. This rare anomaly presents as complete evisceration, and ultrasound reveals fetal viscera in contact with the placenta, without a recognizable body shape[58, 64] (Fig. 41–28).

REFERENCES

1. Moore KL: The digestive system: Esophagus, stomach, intestines, and major digestive glands. *In* Moore KL, Persaud TVN (eds): The Developing Human: Clinically Oriented Embryology. 5th ed. Philadelphia, WB Saunders, 1993.
2. Leopold G: Antepartum obstetrical guidelines. J Ultrasound Med 5:241, 1986.
3. Nelson N, Filly RA, Goldstein RB, et al: The AIUM/ACR antepartum obstetrical sonographic guidelines: Expectations for detection of anomalies. J Ultrasound Med 4:189, 1993.
4. Levine D, Callen PW, Goldstein RB, et al: Imaging the fetal abdomen: How efficacious are the AIUM/ACR guidelines? J Ultrasound Med 14:335–341, 1995.
5. Hadlock FP, Harrist RB, Carpenter RJ, et al: Sonographic estimation of fetal weight: The value of femur length in addition to head and abdomen measurements. Radiology 150:533–540, 1984.
6. Campbell S, Wilkin D: Ultrasonic measurement of fetal abdominal circumference in the estimation of fetal weight. Br J Obstet Gynaecol 82:689–697, 1975.
7. Chinn DH, Filly RA, Callen PW: Ultrasonic

8. Millener PB, Anderson NG, Chisholm RJ: Prognostic significance of nonvisualization of the fetal stomach by sonography. AJR Am J Roentgenol 160:827–830, 1993.
9. Goldstein I, Reede EA, Yarkoni S, et al: Growth of the fetal stomach in normal pregnancy. Obstet Gynecol 70:641–644, 1987.
10. Pretorius DH, Gosink BB, Clautice-Engle T, et al: Sonographic evaluation of the fetal stomach: Significance of nonvisualization. AJR Am J Roentgenol 151:987–989, 1988.
11. Zador IE, Bottoms SF, Tse GM, et al: Nomograms for ultrasound visualization of fetal organs. J Ultrasound Med 7:197–201, 1988.
12. Pareulekar SG: Sonography of normal fetal bowel. J Ultrasound Med 10:211–220, 1991.
13. Cyr DR, Mack LA, Schoenecker SA, et al: Bowel migration in the normal fetus: US detection. Radiology 161:119–121, 1986.
14. Nyberg DA, Dubinsky T, Resta RG, et al: Echogenic fetal bowel during the second trimester: Clinical importance. Radiology 188:527–531, 1993.
15. Karcnik TJ, Rubenstein JB, Swayne LC: The fetal presacral pseudomass: A normal sonographic variant. J Ultrasound Med 10:579–581, 1991.
16. Hogge WA, Hogge JS, Boehm CD, et al: Increased echogenicity in the fetal abdomen: Use of DNA analysis to establish a diagnosis of cystic fibrosis. J Ultrasound Med 12:451–454, 1993.
17. Dicke JM, Crane JP: Sonographically detected hyperechoic fetal bowel: Significance and implications for pregnancy management. Obstet Gynecol 80:778, 1992.
18. Louhimo I, Lindahl H: Esophageal atresia: Primary results of 500 consecutively treated patients. J Pediatr Surg 18:217–229, 1983.
19. Pretorius DH, Drose JA, Dennis MA, et al: Tracheo-esophageal fistula in utero. J Ultrasound Med 6:509–513, 1987.
20. Comstock CH: The antenatal diagnosis of diaphragmatic anomalies. J Ultrasound Med 5:391–396, 1986.
21. Bundy AL, Saltzman DH, Emerson D, et al: Sonographic features associated with cleft palate. J Clin Ultrasound 14:486–489, 1986.
22. Emanuel PG, Garcia GI, Angtuaco TL: Prenatal detection of anterior abdominal wall defects with US. RadioGraphics 15:517–530, 1995.
23. Sharony R, Sinow R, Asch M, et al: Prenatal ultrasound diagnosis of gastric outlet obstruction due to a pyloric web. Prenat Diagn 15:56–59, 1995.
24. Petrikovsky BM: First trimester diagnosis of duodenal atresia. Am J Obste Gynecol 171:569–570, 1994.
25. Nelson LH, Clark CE, Fishburne JI, et al: Value of serial sonography in the in utero detection of duodenal atresia. Obstet Gynecol 59:657, 1982.
26. Grosfeld JL, Rescorla FJ: Duodenal atresia and stenosis: Reassessment of treatment and outcome based on antenatal diagnosis, pathologic variance, and long-term follow up. World J Surg 17:301–309, 1993.
27. Boychuk RB, Lyons EA, Goodhard TK: Duodenal atresia diagnosed by ultrasound. Radiology 127:500, 1978.
28. Nyberg DA, Mack LA: Abdominal wall defects. *In* Nyberg DA, Mahony BS, Pretorius DH (eds): Diagnostic Ultrasound of Fetal Anomalies: Text and Atlas. St. Louis, CV Mosby, 1990, pp 395–432.

29. Touloukian RJ: Intestinal atresia. Clin Perinatol 5:3–18, 1978.
30. Goldstein RB, Filly RA: Diagnosis of meconium ileus in utero. J Ultrasound Med 6:663, 1987.
31. Boles ET Jr: Imperforate anus. Clin Perinatol 5:149–161, 1978.
32. Harris RD, Nyberg DA, Mack LA, et al: Anorectal atresia: Prenatal sonographic diagnosis. AJR Am J Roentgenol 149:395–400, 1987.
33. Hall JW, Tank ES, Lapides J: Urogenital anomalies and complications associated with imperforate anus. J Urol 103:810–814, 1970.
34. Kizilcan F, Karnak I, Tanyel FC, et al: In utero defecation of the nondistressed fetus: A roentgen study in the goat. J Pediatr Surg 29:1487–1490, 1994.
35. Fenton AN, Steer CM: Fetal distress. Am J Obstet Gynecol 83:354, 1962.
36. Mandell J, Lillehei CW, Greene M, et al: The prenatal diagnosis of imperforate anus with rectourinary fistula: Dilated fetal colon with enterolithiasis. J Pediatr Surg 27:82–84, 1992.
37. Grant T, Newman M, Gould R, et al: Intraluminal colonic calcifications associated with anorectal atresia: Prenatal sonographic detection. J Ultrasound Med 9:411–413, 1990.
38. Foster MA, Nyberg DA, Mahony BS, et al: Meconium peritonitis: Prenatal sonographic findings and their clinical significance. Radiology 165:661–665, 1987.
39. Chalubinski K, Deutinger J, Bernaschek G: Meconium peritonitis: Extrusion of meconium and different sonographical appearances in relation to the stage of the disease. Prenat Diagn 12:631–636, 1992.
40. Forouhar F: Meconium peritonitis: Pathology, evolution, and diagnosis. Am J Clin Pathol 78:208–213, 1982.
41. Park RW, Grand RJ: Gastrointestinal manifestations of cystic fibrosis: A review. Gastroenterology 81:1143–1161, 1981.
42. Finkel LI, Slovis TL: Meconium peritonitis, intraperitoneal calcifications, and cystic fibrosis. Pediatr Radiol 12:92–93, 1982.
43. McGahan JP, Hanson F: Meconium peritonitis with accompanying pseudocyst: Prenatal sonographic diagnosis. Radiology 148:125–126, 1983.
44. Suchet IB, Labatte MF, Dyck CS, et al: Fetal cholelithiasis: A case report and review of the literature. J Clin Ultrasound 21:198–202, 1993.
45. Brown DL, Teele RI, Doubilet PM, et al: Echogenic material in the fetal gallbladder: Sonographic and clinical observations. Radiology 182:73–76, 1992.
46. Schackelford GD, Kirks DR: Neonatal hepatic calcification secondary to transplacental infection. Radiology 122:753–757, 1977.
47. Berman B, Lim HW: Concurrent cutaneous and hepatic hemangioma in infancy: Report of a case and review of the literature. J Dermatol Surg Oncol 4:869–873, 1978.
48. Zelop C, Benacerraf BR: The causes and natural history of fetal ascites. Prenat Diagn 14:941–946, 1994.
49. Lindfors KK, McGahan JP, Walter JP: Fetal omphalocele and gastroschisis: Pitfalls in sonographic diagnosis. AJR Am J Roentgenol 147:797–800, 1986.
50. DeVries PA: The pathogenesis of gastroschisis and omphalocele. J Pediatr Surg 15:245, 1980.
51. Brown DL, Emerson DS, Shulman LP, et al: Sonographic diagnosis of omphalocele during 10th week of gestation. AJR Am J Roentgenol 153: 825–826, 1989.
52. Curtis JA, Watson L: Sonographic diagnosis of omphalocele in the first trimester of fetal gestation. J Ultrasound Med 7:97–100, 1988.
53. Nyberg DA, Fitzsimmons J, Mack LA, et al: Chromosomal abnormalities in fetuses with omphalocele: Significance of omphalocele contents. J Ultrasound Med 8:299–308, 1989.
54. Mayer T, Black R, Matlak ME, et al: Gastroschisis and omphalocele. Ann Surg 192:783–787, 1980.
55. Bair JH, Russ PD, Pretorius DH, et al: Fetal omphalocele and gastroschisis: A review of 24 cases. AJR Am J Roentgenol 147:1047–1051, 1986.
56. Gilbert WM, Nicolaider KH: Fetal omphalocele: Associated malformations and chromosomal defects. Obstet Gynecol 70:633–635, 1987.
57. Hoyme HE, Higginbottom MC, Jones KL: The vascular pathogenesis of gastroschisis: Intrauterine interruption of the omphalomesenteric artery. J Pediatr 98:228–231, 1981.
58. Kluck P, Tibboel D, Van Der Kamp AWM, et al: The effect of fetal urine on the development of the bowel in gastroschisis. J Pediatr Surg 18:47–50, 1983.
59. Bond SJ, Harrison MR, Filly RA, et al: Severity of intestinal damage in gastroschisis: Correlation with prenatal sonographic findings. J Pediatr Surg 23:520–525, 1988.
60. Ghidini A, Sitori M, Romero R, et al: Prenatal diagnosis of pentalogy of Cantrell. J Ultrasound Med 7:567–572, 1988.
61. Van Allen MI, Curry C, Gallagher L: Limb–body wall complex. I. Pathogenesis. Am J Med Genet 28:529–548, 1987.
62. Moerman P, Fryns JP, Vandenberghe K, et al: Constrictive amniotic bands, amniotic adhesions, and limb–body wall complex: Discrete disruption sequences with pathologic overlap. Am J Med Genet 42:470–479, 1992.
63. Hartwig NG, Vermeij-Keers C, De Vries HE, et al: Limb–body wall malformation: An embryologic etiology? Hum Pathol 20:1071–1077, 1989.
64. Potter EL, Craig JM: Pathology of the Fetus and Infant. Chicago, Year Book Medical Publishers, 1975, pp 388–392.

Chapter 42

The Fetal Genitourinary System

Roya Sohaey

Fetal genitourinary (GU) tract anomalies are common, accounting for 14 to 57% of all fetal malformations detected by prenatal ultrasound.[1, 2] Fetal GU anomalies range in severity from fatal disorders, such as renal agenesis, to cosmetic problems such as mild hypospadias. The goal of this chapter is to focus on the major GU anomalies that are seen in fetal life, with emphasis on renal agenesis, congenital hydronephrosis, and cystic disease of the kidneys. We will also review selected nonurinary tract anomalies, such as retroperitoneal masses and disorders of the fetal ovaries and testicles. Every attempt will be made to avoid repeating material included previously in Chapters 16 to 23.

EMBRYOLOGY

Before proceeding to GU anomalies per se, it is necessary to review certain aspects of GU embryology. This information, as presented in Chapter 16, is required for understanding anomalies that affect the fetal kidneys, ureters, bladder, and genital system. Table 42–1 reviews the basic embryologic sequences necessary for normal formation of the kidneys, ureters, and bladder. The formation of the genitourinary tract is complex, and many structures that are important in embryonic life, such as the pronephros, regress and do not produce crucial structures in the definitive (fetal) urinary tract.

The key feature of urinary tract development is the formation of a ureteral bud (metanephric diverticulum) from the caudal aspects of the primitive mesonephros. This ureteric bud must grow dorsal and cephalad to unite with the metanephric blastema (a mass of mesodermal cells) in order for the kidney to develop properly. If the ureteric bud fails to develop or does not meet the metanephric blastema, then induction of renal development fails and no kidney forms. This is the pathophysiology of renal agenesis. The ureteric bud divides and induces the metanephric blastema to form multiple calyces and lobes. The outlines of the lobes are visible on the surface of the kidneys throughout much of fetal life; therefore, the normal fetal kidney is a rather lumpy organ, compared with its smooth adult configuration. Fetal lobation sometimes persists into adulthood as a normal variant (see Chapter 17).[3]

Early in their development, the fetal kidneys are located in the pelvis. Through a process of differential growth, the kidneys eventually "rise" to their ultimate position in the flanks. As this transition occurs, arterial connections are sequentially established and obliterated until the permanent renal arteries (arising from the aorta) are established. If lower arterial connections do not degenerate, the kidney may be supplied by multiple renal arteries. If for some reason a kidney does not rise appropriately, or a permanent arterial connection is established more caudally than expected, then a pelvic ectopic kidney may occur. Another anomaly of renal position may occur if the two masses of metanephric blastema that form the kidneys fuse. In such cases, the kidneys are united in some sense, and they also may be ectopic. This union may result in a horseshoe kidney (central union, kidneys both in the flank area, albeit lower than expected), or crossed fused ectopy (kidneys fused and located on one side of the abdomen or pelvis).[3]

It should be noted that adrenal gland embryology is unrelated to GU tract embryology. The adrenal gland forms in the flank from neuroectoderm and mesoderm components.[3] Because the fetal adrenal glands are quite large, they can mimic the appearance of kidneys. In cases of renal agenesis, the adrenal glands may easily be mistaken for fetal kidneys.[4]

Table 42-1. Basic Embryology of the Genitourinary Tract

Primitive Structure	Final Structure in the Adult
Pronephros	Degenerates
Mesonephros (wolffian and müllerian)	Male: Efferent ductules of the testes, epididymis, vas deferens, seminal vesicle, ejaculatory duct
	Female: Fallopian tubes, uterus, upper vagina
Mesonephric diverticulum (ureteral bud)	Ureter, renal pelvis, calyces, collecting tubules
Metanephric blastema (needs ureteral bud induction)	Nephrons, renal connective tissue
Cloaca and allantois	Bladder and urethra

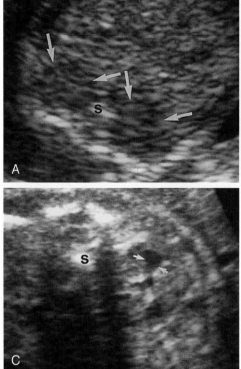

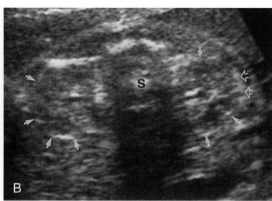

Figure 42-1—Normal Fetal Kidneys. (A) Early in the second trimester, normal kidneys are difficult to see. Transverse view through the fetal flank shows that the kidneys (arrows) are diffusely hypoechoic. **(B)** Later in the second trimester, the kidneys are more obvious (arrows). Note the echogenic rim surrounding the kidneys, representing Gerota's fascia (open arrows). **(C)** Corticomedullary differentiation can be seen in utero. The renal pyramid is hypoechoic (arrows) and should not be confused with a dilated calyx. S, spine.

NORMAL ULTRASOUND FINDINGS

It is recommended* that images of the fetal kidneys and bladder be obtained during every second and third trimester obstetric ultrasound examination, but normal fetal kidneys may be difficult to visualize early in the second trimester.

The normal appearance of the fetal kidneys is illustrated in Figure 42–1. The kidneys are mildly hypoechoic structures seen in the fetal flank area; they are round in cross-section and ovoid in longitudinal sections. Anatomic detail is limited in kidney views obtained in the early second trimester, but detail increases later in pregnancy, with the cortex, medulla, renal sinus, and Gerota's fascia becoming apparent.[4, 5]

Standard fetal renal measurements have been reported, but the experienced sonographer usually can easily detect abnormalities in renal size. As a rule of thumb, on a transverse image through the kidneys, the ratio of renal circumference (of one kidney) to abdominal circumference remains constant at 0.27 to 0.30 throughout the second and third trimesters (Fig. 42–2).[6] In other words, the cross-sectional renal circumference should not exceed approximately one third of the abdominal circumference. Renal length may be more difficult to assess subjectively (Fig. 42–3), and if renal size abnormalities are suspected, renal length should be compared with standard tables (Table 42–2).[7]

The adrenal glands can be visualized superior to the kidneys. They are hypoechoic and can mimic the kidneys early in the second trimester. Later in the second trimester, they develop a distinctive layered, or "ice cream sandwich," ap-

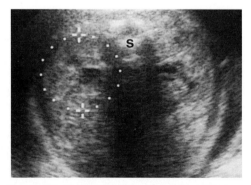

Figure 42-2—Renal Circumference. Axial view through the fetal flank shows measurement of the renal circumference (calipers). The renal circumference (of one kidney) should be 0.27 to 0.30 of the abdominal circumference. These kidneys were normal in size. S, spine.

---

*The American Institute of Ultrasound in Medicine (AIUM), The American College of Obstetrics and Gynecology (ACOG), and The American College of Radiology (ACR).

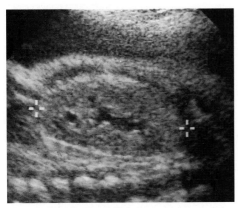

Figure 42-3—Renal Length. Longitudinal view of the kidney demonstrates the proper way to measure the maximum renal length (calipers). See Table 42–2 for expected renal lengths for various gestational ages.

Table 42-2. Mean Renal Lengths for Various Gestational Ages

Gestational Age (weeks)	Mean Length (cm)	SD	95% Cl	n
18	2.2	0.3	1.6–2.8	14
19	2.3	0.4	1.5–3.1	23
20	2.6	0.4	1.8–3.4	22
21	2.7	0.3	2.1–3.2	20
22	2.7	0.3	2.0–3.4	18
23	3.0	0.4	2.2–3.7	13
24	3.1	0.6	1.9–4.4	13
25	3.3	0.4	2.5–4.2	9
26	3.4	0.4	2.4–4.4	9
27	3.5	0.4	2.7–4.4	15
28	3.4	0.4	2.6–4.2	19
29	3.6	0.7	2.3–4.8	12
30	3.8	0.4	2.9–4.6	24
31	3.7	0.5	2.8–4.6	23
32	4.1	0.5	3.1–5.1	23
33	4.0	0.3	3.3–4.7	28
34	4.2	0.4	3.3–5.0	36
35	4.2	0.5	3.2–5.2	17
36	4.2	0.4	3.3–5.0	36
37	4.2	0.4	3.3–5.1	40
38	4.4	0.6	3.2–5.6	32
39	4.2	0.3	3.5–4.8	17
40	4.3	0.5	3.2–5.3	10
41	4.5	0.3	3.9–5.1	4

From Cohen HL, Cooper J, Eisenberg P, et al: Normal length of fetal kidneys: Sonographic study in 397 obstetric patients. AJR Am J Roentgenol 157:545–548, 1991. Used with permission.

pearance (Fig. 42–4). The layered appearance results because the adrenal cortex is hypoechoic relative to the adrenal medulla.[8]

The urinary bladder should be seen as a fluid-filled structure in the pelvis after 14 weeks menstrual age (Fig. 42–5).[9] When a normal-appearing urinary bladder is identified in the early second trimester, less concern for renal agenesis is felt when the kidneys cannot be visualized. The bladder, of course, fills gradually and empties periodically but rarely completely empties. Since the fetus normally fills and empties its bladder every 20 to 30 minutes,[10, 11] the sonographer may need to extend an examination to 60 to 90 minutes before diagnosing its absence.[4]

At this point, the reader should recall (from Chapter 35) that the fetal kidneys start to produce amniotic fluid at 9 weeks and are the main source of amniotic fluid after 16 weeks. Severe bilateral fetal renal abnormalities are associated with profound oligohydramnios from the midsecond trimester onward, but amniotic fluid volume may be normal or only mildly decreased early in pregnancy when renal production of amniotic fluid is less important.

GENDER DETERMINATION AND ANOMALIES

As will be seen subsequently, the determination of fetal gender is an essential diagnostic component of a number of genitourinary anoma-

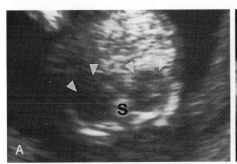
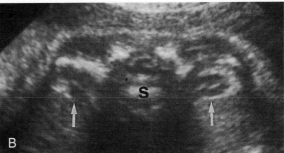

Figure 42-4—Normal Fetal Adrenal Glands. (A) Early in the second trimester, adrenal glands (arrowheads) are large and hypoechoic and can mimic fetal kidneys. **(B)** Later in pregnancy, adrenal glands have a layered "ice cream sandwich" appearance (arrows). The echogenic inside layer is the medulla, and the outer hypoechoic area is the adrenal cortex. The gland is surrounded by an outer echogenic rim, Gerota's fascia. S, spine.

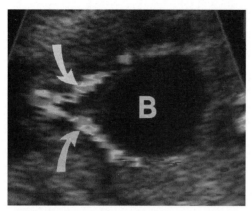

Figure 42-5—Urinary Bladder. The fluid-filled urinary bladder (B) is almost always seen after 13 to 14 weeks. The umbilical arteries (curved arrows) flank the urinary bladder.

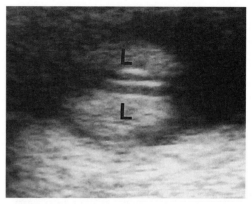

Figure 42-7—Female Fetus. Axial image through the perineum shows the labia majora (L).

lies. It is important, therefore to review this subject. Ultrasound is an accurate indicator of fetal gender. After 24 weeks, gender determination is possible with 92 to 99% confidence in more than 90% of fetuses.[12–14] Earlier (between 16 and 20 weeks), fetal genitalia can be successfully visualized 84% of the time.[15] The parents often want to know the gender of a fetus, and it has been shown that this and other information provided by fetal sonography increases bonding between the parents and their offspring.[12] Sonographic findings associated with the male gender include visualization of the testicles within a scrotum as well as the penis (Fig. 42–6). The testicle descends into the scrotum between 26 and 32 weeks' gestation,[12] and prominent female labia may be mistaken for the scrotum earlier in gestation. In females, the labia majora and minora can be visualized, as well as the clitoris (Fig. 42–7).

Clitoromegaly, which occurs normally in early gestation, may mimic a penis.[3, 16] Because of these and other pitfalls, it is wise to tell the parents that gender determination is not 100% accurate, especially in early pregnancy. Tell them, for instance, that they should not paint the baby's room blue just yet. When the fetal gender cannot be determined because the external genitalia have an ambiguous appearance, adrenal or endocrine abnormalities should be considered.[17]

The most common anomaly associated with the female gender is an ovarian cyst. This subject is discussed at the end of this chapter. Scrotal abnormalities that can be diagnosed in utero include hydrocele, testicular torsion,[18] and inguinal hernia (Fig. 42–8). A small hydrocele (fluid surrounding the testicle) is a common finding in utero and is normal. A large hydrocele is abnormal, however, and implies fluid-filled cysts along the path of the processus vaginalis.[3] Large hydroceles also may accompany hydrops. Testicular

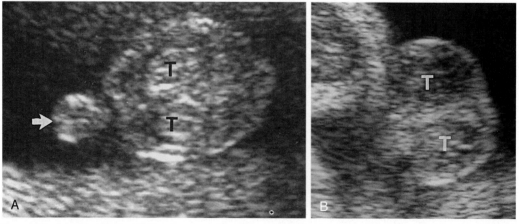

Figure 42-6—Male Fetus. **(A)** The diagnosis of gender can be made with a great deal of confidence in this case since a penis (arrow) is seen, as well as testicles (T), within the scrotum. **(B)** Coronal view through the scrotum confirms the presence of testicles (T) within the scrotum.

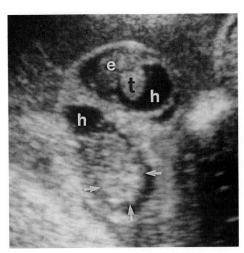

Figure 42-8—Inguinal Hernia. Prenatal assessment of the scrotum shows bilateral hydroceles (h). In addition, increased mass effect and echogenicity associated with the left scrotum (arrows) raised suspicion for bowel within the scrotal sac. After delivery, a reducible inguinal hernia was diagnosed. T, testicle; e, epididymis.

torsion may present as an asymmetric, heterogeneous testicle associated with a hydrocele. The in utero diagnosis of this condition is exceedingly rare and is associated with poor prospects for testicular salvage.[18, 19] Hypospadias occurs in 1/250 live births, and in utero ultrasound findings of hypospadias have been described recently.[20] This condition is characterized by a blunt-ending glans penis,[20] which produces an ultrasound appearance resembling a "circumcised" penis (Fig. 42–9). Abnormal penile curvature (chordae) may also be seen.[20]

RENAL AGENESIS

In the course of renal embryology, if the ureteric bud does not meet the metanephric blastema or the metanephric blastema simply does not form, renal agenesis may occur.[3] The incidence of bilateral renal agenesis is 1 in 3000 to 10,000 births, and it is a uniformly fatal anomaly.[21-23] Ultrasound identification of this condition early in the second trimester may be difficult, since the fetal kidneys normally are hard to see at that stage of gestation, and amniotic fluid volume may be relatively normal for reasons stated earlier (Fig. 42–10). However, the fetal bladder is seen in almost every normal fetus after 14 weeks,[9] and its nonvisualization should alert the sonographer to the possibility of renal agenesis.

Definitive ultrasound findings in renal agenesis are absence of the fetal kidneys and bladder.[4] Secondary findings that are helpful include se-

vere oligohydramnios after 16 weeks and nonvisualization of the renal arteries on color Doppler examination[24] (Fig. 42–10). In cases of severe oligohydramnios, the acoustic "window" provided by amniotic fluid is lost, and the visualization of fetal structure is limited proportionately. It may be very difficult to examine the fetal kidneys, therefore, at a time when clear visualization is most important. We have found that transvaginal imaging of the kidneys can be helpful in cases of oligohydramnios if the fetus is in a transverse lie or breech presentation. Rarely, instillation of sterile saline may be needed to better visualize fetal anatomy.[4] Magnetic resonance imaging also may be used to document the presence or absence of kidneys in cases of severe oligohydramnios.[25]

Renal agenesis in most cases is an isolated developmental defect. Associated cardiovascular anomalies, however, have been reported in 14% of cases.[23] Other anomalies accompanying renal agenesis are principally the secondary effects of severe oligohydramnios, including the well known Potter's syndrome.[4, 23] The latter includes pulmonary hypoplasia, limb deformities (abnormal positioning of the hands and feet, club feet, hip dislocation, bowed legs), and abnormal facies (low-set ears, redundant skin, parrot-beak nose, micrognathia, prominent inner canthus of the eyes). Potter initially ascribed these abnormalities to renal agenesis; however, the features of Potter's syndrome can be seen in any fetus suffering from severe oligohydramnios, regardless of the cause.[26] Recurrence risk for renal agenesis is 2 to 5%,[4, 27] and some cases demonstrate X-linked, autosomal recessive, or autosomal dominant inheritance patterns.[28, 29] We routinely suggest genetic counseling for all families in whom a fetus with renal agenesis has been identified.

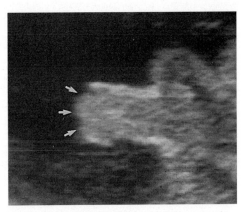

Figure 42-9—Hypospadias. The glans penis has a blunt, "circumcised" appearance (arrows). Normally, the glans penis has a more tapering shape. Postnatal evaluation showed a mild hypospadias.

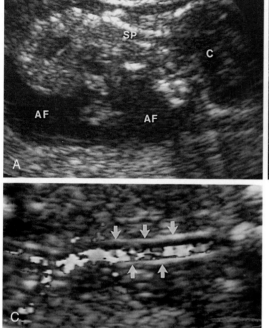

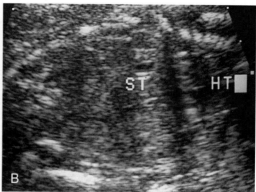

Figure 42-10—Renal Agenesis. (A) Ultrasound examination at 14 weeks demonstrates the presence of amniotic fluid (AF), albeit decreased. No bladder was visualized at this time. (Fetus is spine up in this sagittal view.) C, fetal cranium; SP, spine. **(B)** At 19 weeks, no amniotic fluid is present and the uterus is filled with fetal parts. (Fetal body seen in coronal view.) ST, stomach; HT, heart. **(C)** Color Doppler examination of the abdominal aorta and iliac arteries shows absence of renal arteries. Note the continuous echogenic lines representing the lateral and medial walls of the aorta (arrows), where the renal arteries should originate. In addition, the fetal kidneys and bladder were not seen.

The fatal consequences of bilateral renal agenesis notwithstanding, it should be noted that most cases of renal agenesis are unilateral and are identified incidentally during prenatal sonography or postnatal life.[4] A single, normal kidney more than meets the eliminatory needs of the organism throughout life. Amniotic fluid volume tends to be normal in cases of unilateral renal agenesis; therefore, Potter's syndrome is not an issue. Fetuses with unilateral renal agenesis should be examined closely in utero, however, to identify contralateral renal abnormalities. Müllerian duplication anomalies, as defined in Chapter 28, are particularly associated with unilateral renal agenesis; therefore, in a female fetus, postnatal evaluation of the uterus is important to

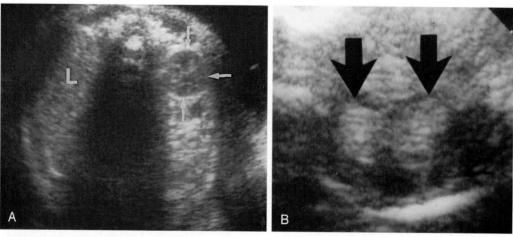

Figure 42-11—Unilateral Renal Agenesis. (A) During routine fetal ultrasound examination, the sonographer noted the presence of only one kidney (arrows). The right flank is filled with the posterior segment of the right lobe of the liver (L). **(B)** Postnatal examination confirmed the presence of only one kidney. Since the neonate was female, ultrasound of the pelvis was also performed. Transverse view through the neonatal uterus shows two endometrial cavities (black arrows). Müllerian anomalies, such as uterine duplication anomalies, are commonly associated with renal agenesis. (Reprinted with permission from Woodward PJ, Sohaey R, Wagnen BJ: Congenital uterine malformations. Curr Probl Diagn Radiol 24:177–197, 1995.)

identify bicornuate uterus or other müllerian anomalies[30, 31] (Fig. 42–11).

CONGENITAL HYDRONEPHROSIS

A dilated renal pelvis is the most common renal abnormality seen prenatally, and it is one of the most problematic from a diagnostic perspective. The renal pelvis is visualized in a large percentage of fetuses during prenatal ultrasound examination, and it is the difficult task of the ultrasound practitioner to determine whether the renal pelvis is normal in size or dilated. The renal pelvis should be measured anteroposteriorly on a transverse view of the fetal renal hilum (Fig. 42–12).

Many investigators have studied fetal renal pelviectasis (pelvic dilatation) and have followed fetuses with pelviectasis into childhood to determine whether renal damage occurs.[32–34] From these studies, suggestions have been made concerning the need for surgical correction of congenital hydronephrosis, and in this respect, the data from Corteville and associates (Table 42–3)[33] are particularly useful as a measure of the amount of dilatation that is significant at different gestational ages. Other investigators[34] have shown that pelvic dilatation is clinically significant and potentially requires surgical correction if the AP diameter (of the pelvis) measures greater than 5 mm between 15 and 20 weeks, greater than 8 mm between 20 and 30 weeks, and greater than 10 mm after 30 weeks. Calyceal dilatation accompanying pelvic dilatation is an important finding that implies clinically significant hydronephrosis. Finally, any degree of dilatation is considered significant if accompanied by cystic changes in the renal parenchyma.[35] At our institution, fetuses that are felt to have significant renal pelviectasis are followed serially with ultrasound at 4-week intervals to assess for progression and to evaluate the amniotic fluid volume. Serial examinations are important to determine whether the initial findings are persistent. Pro-

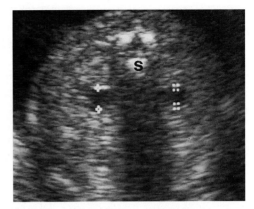

Figure 42-12—Mild Renal Pelviectasis. Transverse view through the fetal kidneys shows mild renal pelvis dilatation. Calipers measure the anteroposterior diameter of the renal pelvis. In this case, the dilatation resolved in utero. S, spine.

gressive hydronephrosis is associated with a more unfavorable outcome.[32–34]

Unilateral renal obstruction is not treated in utero. Attempts at urinary tract decompression for bilateral obstruction are discussed later. At birth, however, most fetuses with unilateral renal obstruction are stable, and immediate imaging of the kidneys is discouraged. Since most neonates are dehydrated and renal function is not optimal in the neonate, early imaging may underestimate the amount of obstruction present.[36] Instead, postnatal ultrasound should be performed at the end of the first week of life. If the renal pelvis continues to measure greater than 10 mm, we refer our patients to a pediatric urologist.

Although significant congenital hydronephrosis may result from vesicoureteral reflux, the usual cause is urinary tract obstruction. The most common site of obstruction is the ureteropelvic junction, followed by the ureterovesical junction.[37] Ureteral duplication anomalies cause obstruction of the renal upper pole calyces, often associated with an ectopic ureterocele at the bladder end of the ureter that drains the upper pole.[38] This subject is presented in more detail

Table 42-3. Thresholds for Counseling: Anteroposterior Pelvic Diameter

Anteroposterior Pelvic Diameter (mm)	CH (%) 14–23 wk	S/C (%) 14–23 wk	CH (%) 24–32 wk	S/C (%) 24–32 wk	CH (%) 33–42 wk	S/C (%) 33–42 wk
<3	0	0	0	0	0	0
4–6	41	19	38	13	0	0
7–9	53	40	33	6	67	50
>10	82	73	86	72	82	59

CH, Congenital hydronephrosis confirmed postnatally; S/C, postnatal surgery and/or evidence of renal compromise.
From Corteville JE, Gray DL, Crane JP: Congenital hydronephrosis: Correlation of fetal ultrasonographic findings with infant outcome. Am J Obstet Gynecol 165:384–388, 1991. Used with permission.

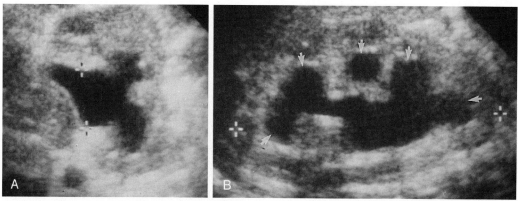

Figure 42-13—Ureteropelvic Junction (UPJ) Obstruction. (A) Axial view of the right kidney shows renal pelvis dilatation (calipers measure the anteroposterior diameter of the renal pelvis). (B) Longitudinal view of the kidney confirms the presence of pelviectasis as well as calyceal dilatation (arrows). Since a dilated ureter was not seen, the most likely point of obstruction is the UPJ (confirmed postnatally).

in Chapter 17. With duplication anomalies, the lower pole of the affected kidney may be affected by vesicoureteral reflux, which may be demonstrated postnatally. Reflux is probably impossible to visualize in utero, however. Bladder outlet obstruction also may cause significant hydronephrosis in utero, as discussed later.

The morphology of renal obstruction often helps identify the etiology. For instance, if the renal pelvis and calyces are visibly dilated but a dilated ureter is not seen, then the obstruction most likely is at the ureteropelvic junction (Fig. 42–13). Alternatively, a dilated ureter seen to the level of a normal-appearing bladder implies ureterovesical obstruction[39, 40] (Fig. 42–14). Vesicoureteral reflux also can cause generalized ureteral dilatation and should be a diagnosis of exclusion. When hydronephrosis affects only the upper pole of the kidney, a ureteral duplication anomaly should be anticipated, and an ectopic ureterocele may be seen in the bladder (Fig. 42–15).

Before leaving the subject of the morphology of urinary tract dilatation, it is worth noting that as a ureter dilates it also elongates.[41] The elongated ureter folds upon itself accordion-style, and for this reason a massively dilated ureter often appears as a series of cysts on ultrasound sections. The talented sonographer, however, can "connect the cysts" and demonstrate the tubular nature of the dilated ureter (Fig. 42–14).

Bladder outlet obstruction is often an obvious ultrasound diagnosis since the markedly enlarged, thick-walled bladder is readily seen. A variable degree of hydronephrosis is usually also seen.[4, 42] Bladder outlet obstruction occurs most commonly in male fetuses who are subject to the development of posterior urethral (not ureteral) valves.[42, 43] The largest bladders seen in utero are caused by posterior urethral valves, and these bladders often fill the abdominal cavity. The proximal urethra is usually dilated as well, giving the bladder a pear or keyhole shape[4] (Fig. 42–16). Renal findings vary in fetuses with posterior

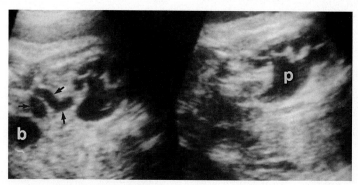

Figure 42-14—Ureterovesical Junction (UVJ) Obstruction. Long axis views of the fetal abdomen and pelvis show a markedly dilated renal pelvis (p), calyces, and a serpiginous dilated ureter (arrows) leading to a normal-appearing bladder (b). The level of obstruction is the UVJ (confirmed postnatally).

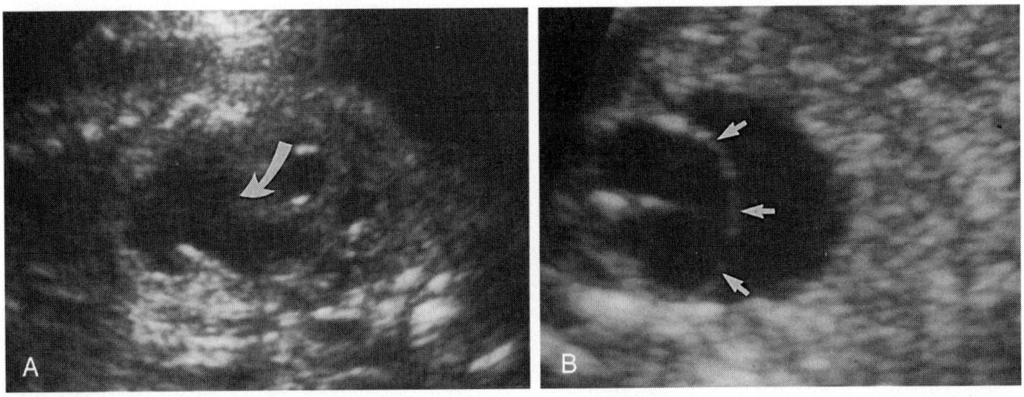

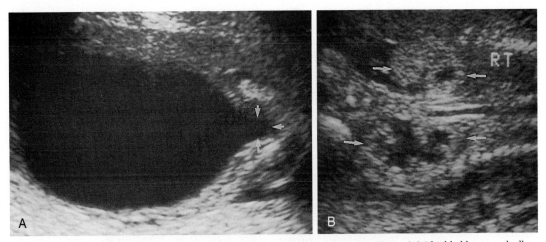

Figure 42-15—Duplicated Kidney with Ureteral Obstruction. (A) The upper pole collecting system is markedly dilated (curved arrow) while the lower pole collecting system is only mildly dilated. **(B)** In addition, a cystic "balloon-like" structure was seen in the bladder (arrows). This represents an ectopic ureterocele associated with the ureter that is draining the upper pole of the kidney. The ureter associated with the lower renal moiety often refluxes, leading to some dilatation of this collecting system as well.

urethral valves. In some cases, the kidneys are markedly hydronephrotic but otherwise normal in appearance. At the opposite extreme, the kidneys are small and echogenic, secondary to obstruction-induced cystic dysplasia.[44] Complete bilateral urinary tract obstruction occurring in utero is fatal in postnatal life, and in some cases intervention in utero is attempted. Bladder drainage with urinary electrolyte analysis (for prognostic purposes), and placement of vesicoamniotic shunts (when renal function seems reasonable) have been attempted with variable success. Further details can be found in references 45 through 48.

Partial posterior urethral valves, with mild or moderate urinary tract dilatation, carry a good prognosis if the amniotic fluid volume is suffi-cient to support respiratory development. The posterior urethral valves can usually be removed easily during the postnatal period. Rarely, bladder outlet obstruction is due to urethral strictures or agenesis,[4] and this diagnosis should be considered in the female fetus with a markedly distended bladder.

Peritoneal fluid seen in association with urinary tract obstruction most likely represents urinary ascites (Fig. 42–17). Furthermore, isolated ascites, seen in the *absence* of fetal hydrops, is most likely urinary in origin.[49] When ascites and urinary tract anomalies occur concomitantly, however, it should not be assumed that ascites is caused by the urinary tract disorder until hydrops is excluded. A careful search should be made for other findings associated with fetal hydrops.

Figure 42-16—Bladder Outlet Obstruction from Posterior Urethral Valves. (A) The bladder is markedly distended and fills the abdomen. The dilated proximal urethra (arrows) is seen and gives the bladder a "keyhole" or "pear-shaped" appearance. **(B)** Coronal image through the kidneys (arrows) shows that the left kidney is hydronephrotic while the right is small. Both kidneys are echogenic because of cystic dysplasia from long-standing obstruction.

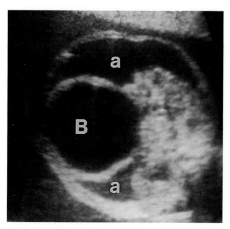

Figure 42-17—Urinary Ascites. The urinary bladder is distended (B) and urinary ascites is present (a). No other findings to suggest hydrops were seen. This fetus had posterior urethral valves at autopsy. Bladder decompression into the peritoneal space had occurred.

Since hydrops is not associated, per se, with urinary tract anomalies, the presence of hydrops implies other serious disorders.

RENAL CYSTIC DYSPLASIA

Cystic changes involving the renal parenchyma can occur secondary to genetic conditions or urinary tract obstruction, or in association with chromosome abnormalities and syndromes.[4, 50] Basically, if the kidney is damaged in any way, it responds by forming cysts. There are three major cystic renal disorders with which ultrasound practitioners should be familiar, as these conditions are seen fairly commonly during fetal life.

These are recessive polycystic kidney disease, multicystic dysplasia, and cystic dysplasia related to obstruction. In most cases, fetal cystic disorders can be diagnosed with precision on the basis of ultrasound findings.

AUTOSOMAL RECESSIVE POLYCYSTIC KIDNEY DISEASE

Autosomal recessive polycystic kidney disease (RPKD) is a genetic disorder that affects 1 of 40,000 neonates.[51] Since 1 in 112 of the population carries the gene for polycystic kidney disease, this anomaly is not rare, and obstetric ultrasound practitioners are likely to encounter fetuses affected by this condition.[50–52] Although the prognosis is somewhat variable for RPKD, the outlook generally is not good, and the identification of RPKD in fetal life portends severe involvement and a poor to grim prognosis, especially in the presence of oligohydramnios.[53]

The ultrasound findings in RPKD are characteristic. Both fetal kidneys tend to be markedly enlarged and highly echogenic[4] (Fig. 42–18). Corticomedullary differentiation, normally seen in the third trimester, is absent since both the cortex and medulla are affected.[54] The increase in renal echogenicity results from tubular ectasia, which is the hallmark of this disease. The ectatic tubules run perpendicular to the renal capsule[54] and produce innumerable interfaces that the ultrasound beam encounters as it traverses the kidneys. These interfaces, in turn, generate homogeneously increased echogenicity.[4] The ectatic or "cystic" tubules are too small for sonographic

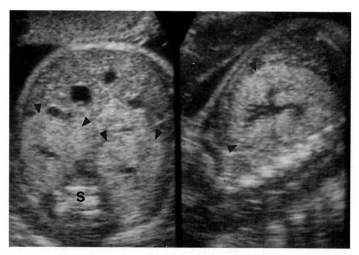

Figure 42-18—Autosomal Recessive Polycystic Kidney Disease. The kidneys (arrowheads) are enlarged and diffusely echogenic. Corticomedullary differentiation has been lost. This disease causes tubular ectasia, resulting in many ultrasound interfaces, thus causing the echogenic (not "cystic" per se) appearance seen with ultrasound. S, spine.

resolution, but rare larger cysts (called macro-cysts) may be present that can be resolved. The macrocysts seldom exceed 1 cm in size, in dis-tinction to other cystic conditions discussed later. Ultrasound findings for RPKD are usually, but not always, present by 24 weeks. Rarely, RPKD is inapparent until later in fetal life. Therefore, a normal ultrasound in a fetus "at risk" for RPKD does not always rule out its presence; serial ex-aminations into the third trimester may be neces-sary.[4] The amount of amniotic fluid varies in proportion to renal function, but some degree of oligohydramnios (usually progressive and severe) is the rule.[55, 56]

Fetuses with RPKD are not at an increased risk for associated malformations. In neonates, however, macrocysts may be visualized in the pancreas, liver, or other organs. Renal function varies in cases of RPKD, as discussed further in Chapter 21.

Autosomal dominant polycystic kidney disease (DPKD) is a common inherited cystic renal dis-order, which typically affects adults. Rarely, how-ever, DPKD is detected in fetal life and can mimic the appearance of RPKD. The principal ultrasound findings are echogenic, enlarged kid-neys[57] that rarely contain macrocysts. Differentia-tion between these conditions is accomplished with a family history, and with images of the parents' kidneys.

MULTICYSTIC DYSPLASIA

Multicystic dysplastic kidney (MCDK) is char-acterized by multiple cysts of varying sizes that do not communicate and are usually associated with renal impairment.[54] The pathophysiology of

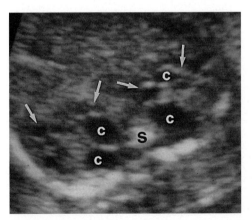

Figure 42-19—Bilateral Multicystic Dysplastic Kidneys (MCDK). Axial view through the fetal flank shows two kidneys (arrows) that are normal in size but their parenchyma is replaced by cysts (c). No amniotic fluid is present, reflecting the fact that most MCDK do not function. S, spine.

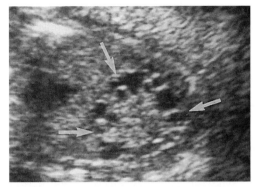

Figure 42-20—Multicystic Dysplastic Kidney (MCDK) and Renal Agenesis. The affected kidney (arrows) has multiple cysts of variable sizes throughout its periphery. The other kidney was absent.

MCDK is unclear, but two theories have been proposed. The first ascribes the dysplastic devel-opment to disorganization of renal structures be-cause of embryologic abnormalities.[4, 58, 59] The second relates the cystic changes in the renal parenchyma to urinary tract obstruction oc-curring early in fetal life.[42, 54, 60] Regardless of etiology, a kidney involved with MCDK is usually rendered useless. In the majority of cases, multicystic dysplasia is a unilateral renal abnor-mality that is incidentally noted on prenatal ultra-sound examination. In approximately 40% of cases, however, multicystic dysplasia is associated with a contralateral renal abnormality such as renal agenesis, congenital hydronephrosis, or multicystic dysplasia affecting both kidneys (20%).[4] If both kidneys are abnormal, resulting in severe renal impairment, the condition can be fatal.

The sonographic findings in MCDK are *mac-rocystic* changes in the affected kidney. Multiple cysts of varying sizes replace the renal paren-chyma (Figs. 42–19 and 42–20), and the kid-ney(s) may be so large that it fills the abdominal cavity. The principal differential consideration is severe hydronephrosis. It usually is possible to distinguish between these conditions by showing that the cysts do not communicate with a central pelvis. Additional differential considerations in-clude autosomal dominant polycystic kidney dis-ease (very rare in utero) and cystic dysplasia resulting from chronic renal obstruction. Primary multicystic dysplasia cannot be differentiated from cystic dysplasia related to obstruction unless ultrasound examinations initially demonstrate hy-dronephrosis, followed later by multicystic dys-plasia.

The natural history of an MCDK is gradual decrease of cyst size with possible ultimate disap-pearance of the kidney.[61, 62] In utero, the cysts may initially increase in size, and this finding should not dissuade the sonographer from making the correct diagnosis.[62] Further discussion of this matter is found in Chapter 21.

CYSTIC DYSPLASIA DUE TO OBSTRUCTION

Renal parenchymal cystic changes often occur in response to severe, long-standing renal obstruction.[42, 54] The cysts may be macroscopic or microscopic.[4, 44] In some cases, macroscopic cysts are seen to surround a dilated collecting system, whereas in other cases macroscopic parenchymal cysts develop in a previously obstructed kidney (Fig. 42–21). Microscopic cysts, on the other hand, may produce a small, echogenic kidney (Fig. 42–16). The occurrence of macroscopic or microscopic cysts in the presence of hydronephrosis is proof that hydronephrosis is clinically significant and has resulted in cystic dysplastic changes within the renal parenchyma. This gross manifestation of dysplasia is evidence that renal damage is extensive.[42, 44]

CONDITIONS ASSOCIATED WITH CYSTIC DISORDERS

Cystic disorders of the kidneys are associated with multiple syndromes and inheritable conditions, as summarized in Table 42–4.[4] The three most important associated entities are the VACTERL syndrome, the Meckel-Gruber syndrome, and trisomy 13.

The VACTERL syndrome is an acronym for multiple mesodermal anomalies that occur together: Vertebral anomalies, Anorectal atresia, Cardiovascular abnormalities, Tracheal Esopha-

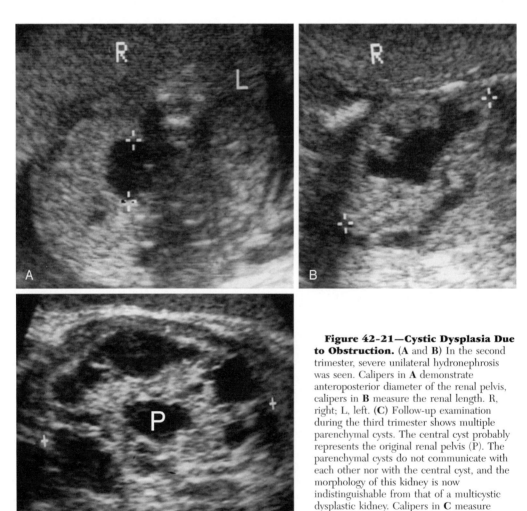

Figure 42-21—Cystic Dysplasia Due to Obstruction. (A and B) In the second trimester, severe unilateral hydronephrosis was seen. Calipers in **A** demonstrate anteroposterior diameter of the renal pelvis, calipers in **B** measure the renal length. R, right; L, left. **(C)** Follow-up examination during the third trimester shows multiple parenchymal cysts. The central cyst probably represents the original renal pelvis (P). The parenchymal cysts do not communicate with each other nor with the central cyst, and the morphology of this kidney is now indistinguishable from that of a multicystic dysplastic kidney. Calipers in **C** measure renal length.

Table 42-4. Cystic Renal Disease: Common Associations

Syndromes	VACTERL (50% with renal cysts)
	Meckel-Gruber (95% with renal cysts)
	Prune belly syndrome
	Asphyxiating thoracic dystrophy (Jeune's)
	Cerebrohepatorenal syndrome (Zellweger's)
Chromosome abnormalities	Trisomy 13 (33% with renal cysts)
	Trisomy 18 (10% with renal cysts)

geal fistula, *R*enal disorders, and *L*imb anomalies.[4, 63] If any one of these anomalies is identified in utero, the others should be sought. Vertebral anomalies seen in this syndrome range in severity from hemivertebrae to caudal regression.[64] Anal atresia and tracheoesophageal fistula may be difficult to diagnose in utero, as noted in previous chapters. Cardiac anomalies, when present, are nonspecific and may be complex.[4, 64] VACTERL renal anomalies tend to be cystic.[4] Limb anomalies range from radial ray anomalies to sirenomelia (fused lower extremities).[63, 64] The prognosis is usually poor for fetuses with the VACTERL association, but the recurrence risk for future pregnancies, fortunately, is low.

The Meckel-Gruber syndrome is most frequently characterized by a sloping forehead, posterior meningoencephalocele, polydactyly, and polycystic kidneys.[65-67] The condition is fatal in the perinatal period. A diagnosis of Meckel-Gruber syndrome should always be considered in a fetus with cystic dysplasia of the kidneys and encephalocele (Fig. 42–22). Since the Meckel-Gruber syndrome is an autosomal recessive trait, recurrence risk can be as high as 25%. Therefore, it is important for ultrasound practitioners to suggest this diagnosis in appropriate cases.

The final important association of cystic renal dysplasia is with chromosome abnormalities, and particularly with trisomy 13.[4] In most fetuses with trisomy-associated cystic renal disease, additional abnormalities are identified, including intrauterine growth retardation and craniofacial anomalies.[68] Because of the association with karyotype abnormalities, we recommend chromosome analysis in all pregnancies with unexplained renal cystic dysplasia.

NON–URINARY TRACT CYSTIC MASSES

The discussion of cystic renal masses is an apt springboard from which to consider other conditions that may present as a cystic abdominal or pelvic mass. Clearly, the urinary tract is the most common cause of such a mass in the fetus, but other diagnostic possibilities should always be considered. In the third trimester, the most common non–urinary tract and non–gastrointestinal tract cyst is a benign ovarian cyst.[4] Therefore, it is important to determine fetal gender if a cyst is identified in the fetal abdomen and the kidneys appear normal. Ovarian cysts result from maternal hormonal influence upon fetal ovaries causing the formation of functional cysts.[69-71] The sonographic appearance of the cyst depends on whether or not it is a complicated cyst.[4, 69] The uncomplicated ovarian cyst is usually unilocular, thin walled, and anechoic, but it may have a few internal septations. Cysts complicated by hemorrhage or torsion appear complex or solid. The cysts are often large enough to "rise" out of the pelvis and be located within the fetal abdomen.[4, 69] Following delivery, the maternal hormonal influence is discontinued, and most uncomplicated cysts resolve spontaneously (Fig. 42–23).[4] Fetuses with large cysts (greater than 10 cm) and complicated cysts usually need surgical

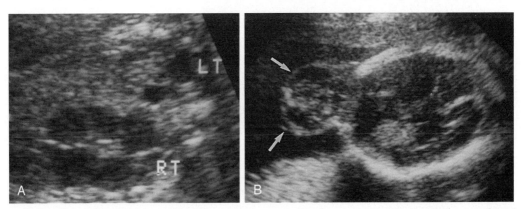

Figure 42-22—Meckel-Gruber Syndrome. (**A**) Bilateral cystic kidneys are present. RT, right kidney; LT, left kidney. (**B**) In addition, axial view through the fetal cranium reveals an occipital encephalocele (arrows demonstrate the extracranial brain tissue).

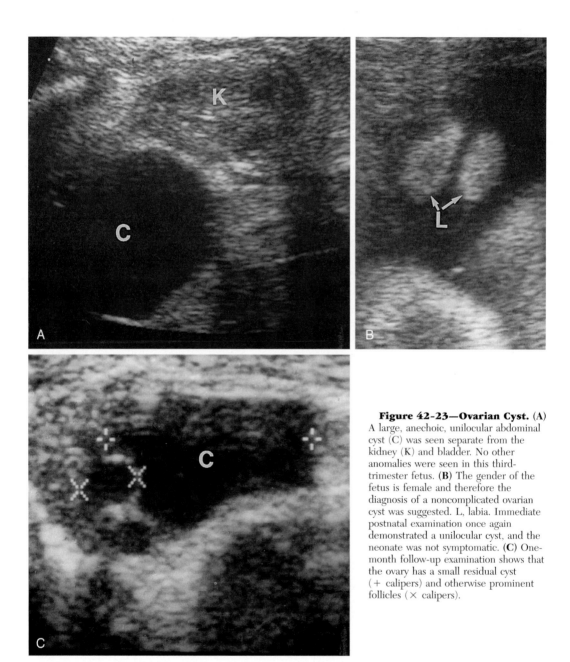

Figure 42-23—Ovarian Cyst. (A) A large, anechoic, unilocular abdominal cyst (C) was seen separate from the kidney (K) and bladder. No other anomalies were seen in this third-trimester fetus. **(B)** The gender of the fetus is female and therefore the diagnosis of a noncomplicated ovarian cyst was suggested. L, labia. Immediate postnatal examination once again demonstrated a unilocular cyst, and the neonate was not symptomatic. **(C)** One-month follow-up examination shows that the ovary has a small residual cyst (+ calipers) and otherwise prominent follicles (× calipers).

resection.[69] Salvaging ovaries that have torsed in utero is difficult.

Other causes for peritoneal cysts include mesenteric cysts, gastrointestinal duplication cysts, pseudocysts, and a persistent urachus. Mesenteric cysts are epithelialized congenital cysts that arise, as the name implies, from the mesentery.[72] With ultrasound, these cysts are indistinguishable from duplication cysts, which arise from the stomach or small bowel, and both mesenteric and duplication cysts are indistinguishable from ovarian cysts. Pseudocysts result from in utero bowel perforation, as noted in Chapter 41. These may be distinguished from the aforementioned cysts since they are more likely to be thick walled and calcified, contain internal echoes, and be often associated with bowel obstruction.[73] A urachal cyst characteristically lies in the midline anterior abdominal wall, between the bladder and umbilical cord attachments.[74] This location may be quite difficult to appreciate in the fetus, however. Urachal cysts are discussed briefly and illustrated in Chapter 23. The final consideration in the differential diagnosis of a cystic mass is the rare occurrence of an anterior meningocele or cystic intrapelvic sacrococcygeal teratoma.

RETROPERITONEAL MASSES

Solid retroperitoneal masses are exceedingly rare in the fetus and for that reason they will be considered only briefly. If a solid lesion appears to involve the fetal kidney, then in utero diagnosis of mesoblastic nephroma or, rarely, nephroblastomatosis should be considered.[75-77] These lesions, which are discussed further in Chapter 20, can grow rapidly in utero, leading to hydrops fetalis. Suprarenal masses seen in utero most commonly represent infradiaphragmatic pulmonary sequestration, adrenal hemorrhage, or neuroblastoma (discussed further in Chapters 24 and 39). Distinguishing features among these three diagnoses include (1) identification of a feeding vessel from the aorta to a pulmonary sequestration; (2) increase in size of a neuroblastoma, with subsequent development of hydrops fetalis; and (3) visualization of the typical sonographic evolution of a blood clot in cases of adrenal hemorrhage.[4]

REFERENCES

1. Quinlan RW, Cruz AC, Huddelston JF: Sonographic detection of fetal urinary tract anomalies. Obstet Gynecol 67:558–565, 1986.
2. Helin I, Persson P: Prenatal diagnosis of urinary tract abnormalities by ultrasound. Pediatrics 78:879–883, 1986.
3. Moore KL: The urogenital system. *In* Moore KL (ed): The Developing Human: Clinically Oriented Embryology. 4th ed. Philadelphia, WB Saunders, 1988, pp 246–255.
4. Grannum PA: The genitourinary tract. *In* Nyberg DA, Mahony BS, Pretorius DH (eds): Diagnostic Ultrasound of Fetal Anomalies: Text and Atlas. St. Louis, CV Mosby, 1990, pp 433–491.
5. Bowie JD, Rosenberg ER, Andreotti MD, et al: The changing sonographic appearance of fetal kidneys during pregnancy. J Ultrasound Med 2:505–507, 1983.
6. Grannum PA, Brachen M, Silverman R, et al: Assessment of fetal kidney size in normal gestation by comparison of ratio of kidney circumference to abdominal circumference. Am J Obstet Gynecol 136:249–254, 1980.
7. Cohen HL, Cooper J, Eisenberg P, et al: Normal length of fetal kidneys: Sonographic study in 397 obstetric patients. AJR Am J Roentgenol 157:545–548, 1991.
8. Oppenheimer DA, Carroll BA, Yousem S: Sonography of the normal neonatal adrenal gland. Radiology 146:157–160, 1983.
9. Clautice-Engle T, Pretorius DH, Budorick NE: Significance of nonvisualization of the fetal urinary bladder. J Ultrasound Med 10:615–618, 1991.
10. Campbell S, Wladimiroff JW, Dewhurst CJ: The antenatal measurement of fetal urine production. Br J Obstet Gynaecol 80:680–686, 1973.
11. Wladimiroff JW, Campbell S: Fetal urine production rates in normal and complicated pregnancy. Lancet 1:151–154, 1974.
12. Birnholz JB: Determination of fetal sex. N Engl J Med 309:942–944, 1983.
13. Elejalde BR, de Elejalde MM, Heitman T: Visualization of the fetal genitalia by ultrasonography: A review of the literature and analysis of its accuracy and ethical implications. J Ultrasound Med 4:633–639, 1985.
14. Benacerraf BR, Saltzman DH, Mandell J: Sonographic diagnosis of abnormal fetal genitalia. J Ultrasound Med 8:613–617, 1989.
15. Reece EA, Winn HN, Wan M, et al: Can ultrasonography replace amniocentesis in fetal gender determination during the early second trimester? Am J Obstet Gynecol 156:579–581, 1987.
16. Emerson DS, Felker RE, Brown DL: The sagittal sign: An early second-trimester sonographic indicator of fetal gender. J Ultrasound Med 8:293–297, 1989.
17. Cooper C, Mahony BS, Bowie JD, et al: Prenatal ultrasound diagnosis of ambiguous genitalia. J Ultrasound Med 4:433–436, 1985.
18. Gross BR, Cohen HL, Schlessel JS: Prenatal diagnosis of bilateral testicular torsion: Beware of torsions simulating hydroceles. J Ultrasound Med 12:479–481, 1993.
19. Rosenberg J, Zimmerman M: Case report: Intrauterine testicular torsion. J Med Soc NJ 81:320–321, 1984.
20. Sides D, Goldstein RB, Baskin LB, et al: Prenatal diagnosis of hypospadias. J Ultrasound Med 15:741–746, 1996.
21. Carter CO, Evans K: Birth frequency of bilateral renal agenesis. J Med Genet 18:158, 1981.
22. Potter EL: Bilateral absence of ureters and kidneys: A report of 50 cases. Obstet Gynecol 25:3–12, 1965.
23. Wilson RD, Baird PA: Renal agenesis in British Columbia. Am J Med Genet 21:153–169, 1985.
24. DeVore GR: The value of color Doppler sonography

in the diagnosis of renal agenesis. J Ultrasound Med 14:443–449, 1995.

25. Benson RC, Colletti PM, Platt LD, et al: MR imaging of fetal anomalies. AJR Am J Roentgenol 156:1205–1207, 1991.

26. Roodhooft AM, Birnholz JC, Holmes LB: Familial nature of congenital absence and severe dysplasia of both kidneys. N Engl J Med 310:1341–1345, 1984.

27. Schmidt W, Kubli F: Early diagnosis of severe congenital malformations by ultrasonography. J Perinat Med 10:233–241, 1982.

28. McPherson E, Carey J, Kramer A, et al: Dominantly inherited renal aplasia. Am J Med Genet 26:863–872, 1987.

29. Romero R, Cullen M, Grannum P, et al: Antenatal diagnosis of renal anomalies with ultrasound. III: Bilateral renal agenesis. Am J Obstet Gynecol 151:38–43, 1985.

30. Winkle CA: Diagnosis and treatment of uterine pathology. *In* Carr BC, Blackwell RE (eds): Textbook of Reproductive Medicine. East Norwalk, CT, Appleton & Lange, 1993, pp 481–504.

31. Banner EA: The ectopic kidney in obstetrics and gynecology. Surg Gynecol Obstet 121:32–36, 1965.

32. Anderson N, Clautice-Engle T, Allan R, et al: Detection of obstructive uropathy in the fetus: Predictive value of sonographic measurements of renal pelvic diameter at various gestational ages. AJR Am J Roentgenol 164:719–723, 1995.

33. Corteville JE, Gray DL, Crane JP: Congenital hydronephrosis: Correlation of fetal ultrasonographic findings with infant outcome. Am J Obstet Gynecol 165:384–388, 1991.

34. Mandell J, Blyth BR, Peters CA, et al: Structural genitourinary defects detected in utero. Radiology 178:193–196, 1991.

35. Blane CE, Barr M, DiPietro MA, et al: Renal obstructive dysplasia: Ultrasound diagnosis and therapeutic implications. Pediatr Radiol 21:274–277, 1991.

36. Laing FC, Burke VD, Wing VW, et al: Postpartum evaluation of fetal hydronephrosis: Optimal timing for follow-up sonography. Radiology 152:423–424, 1984.

37. Brown T, Mandell J, Lebowitz RL: Neonatal hydronephrosis in the era of sonography. AJR Am J Roentgenol 148:959–963, 1987.

38. Jeffrey RB, Laing FC, Wing VW, et al: Sonography of the fetal duplex kidney. Radiology 153:123–124, 1984.

39. Cohen HL, Haller JO: Diagnostic sonography of the fetal genitourinary tract. Urol Radiol 9:88–98, 1987.

40. Maizels M, Reisman ME, Flom LS, et al: Grading nephroureteral dilatation detected in the first year of life: Correlation with obstruction. J Urol 148:609–614, 1992.

41. Montana MA, Cyr DR, Lenke RR, et al: Sonographic detection of fetal ureteral obstruction. AJR Am J Roentgenol 145:595–596, 1985.

42. Glazer GM, Filly RA, Callen PW: The varied sonographic appearance of the urinary tract in the fetus and newborn with urethral obstruction. Radiology 144:563–568, 1982.

43. Doraiswamy NV, Al Badr MSK: Posterior urethral valves in siblings. Br J Urol 55:448–449, 1983.

44. Mahony BS, Filly RA, Callen PW: Fetal renal dysplasia: Sonographic evaluation. Radiology 152:143–146, 1984.

45. Glick PL, Harrison MR, Golbus MS, et al: Management of the fetus with congenital hydronephrosis. II. Prognostic criteria and selection of treatment. J Pediatr Surg 20:376–381, 1985.

46. Cobodny AH: Antenatal diagnosis and management of urinary abnormalities. Pediatr Clin North Am 34:1365–1371, 1987.

47. Adzick NS, Flake AW, Harrison MR: Recent advances in prenatal diagnosis and treatment. Pediatr Clin North Am 32:1103–1106, 1985.

48. Drugan A, Zador IE, Bathia RK, et al: First-trimester diagnosis and early in utero treatment of obstructive uropathy. Acta Obstet Gynecol Scand 68:645–649, 1989.

49. Zelop C, Benacerraf BR: The causes and natural history of fetal ascites. Prenat Diagn 14:941–946, 1994.

50. Reuss A, Wladimiroff JW, Niermeyer MF: Sonographic, clinical, and genetic aspects of prenatal diagnosis of cystic kidney disease. Ultrasound Med Biol 17:687–694, 1991.

51. Zerres K, Volpel MC, Weiss H: Cystic kidneys: Genetics, pathology, anatomy, and prenatal diagnosis. Hum Genet 68:104–135, 1984.

52. Kaplan BS, Kaplan P, De Chadareian JP, et al: Variable expression of autosomal recessive polycystic kidney disease and congenital hepatic fibrosis within a family. Am J Med Genet 29:639–647, 1988.

53. Bosniak MA, Ambos MA: Polycystic kidney disease. Semin Roentgenol 10:133–143, 1975.

54. Fong KW, Rahmani MR, Rose TH, et al: Fetal renal cystic disease: Sonographic-pathologic correlation. AJR Am J Roentgenol 146:767–773, 1986.

55. Luthy DA, Hirsch JH: Infantile polycystic kidney disease: Observations from attempts at prenatal diagnosis. Am J Med Genet 20:505–517, 1985.

56. Mahony BS, Callen PW, Filly RA, et al: Progression of infantile polycystic kidney disease in early pregnancy. J Ultrasound Med 3:277–279, 1984.

57. Journel H, Guyot C, Barc RM, et al: Unexpected ultrasonographic prenatal diagnosis of autosomal dominant polycystic kidney disease. Prenatal Diag 9:663–671, 1989.

58. Diard F, LeDosseur P, Cadier L, et al: Multicystic dysplasia in the upper component of the complete duplex kidney. Pediatr Radiol 14:310–313, 1984.

59. Newman LB, McAllister WH, Kissane J: Segmental renal dysplasia associated with ectopic ureteroceles in childhood. Urology 3:23–26, 1974.

60. Beck AD: The effect of intrauterine urinary obstruction upon the development of the fetal kidney. J Urol 105:784–789, 1971.

61. Pedicelli G, Jequier S, Bowen A, et al: Multicystic dysplastic kidneys: Spontaneous regression demonstrated with US. Radiology 161:23–26, 1986.

62. Hashimoto BE, Filly RA, Callen PW: Multicystic dysplastic kidney in utero: Changing appearance on US. Radiology 159:107–109, 1986.

63. Mahony BS: The extremities. *In* Nyberg DA, Mahony BS, Pretorius DH (eds): Diagnostic Ultrasound of Fetal Anomalies: Text and Atlas. St. Louis, CV Mosby, 1990, pp 492–562.

64. Temtamy SA, Miller JD: Extending the scope of the VATER association: Definition of the VATER syndrome. J Pediatr 85:345–349, 1974.

65. Fraser FC, Lytwyn A: Spectrum of anomalies in the Meckel syndrome, or: "Maybe there is a malformation syndrome with at least one constant anomaly." Am J Med Genet 97:67–73, 1981.

66. Mecke S, Passarge E: Encephalocele, polycystic kidneys, and polydactyly as an autosomal recessive

trait simulating certain other disorders: The Meckel syndrome. Ann Genet 14:97–103, 1971.

67. Salonen R: The Meckel syndrome: Clinicopathological findings in 67 patients. Am J Med Genet 18:671–689, 1984.

68. Benacerraf BR, Miller WA, Frigoletto FD Jr: Sonographic detection of fetuses with trisomy 13 and 18: Accuracy and limitations. Am J Obstet Gynecol 158:404–409, 1988.

69. Nussbaum AR, Sanders RC, Hartmann DS, et al: Neonatal ovarian cysts: Sonographic-pathologic correlation. Radiology 168:817–821, 1988.

70. DeSa DJ: Follicular ovarian cysts in stillbirths and neonates. Arch Dis Child 50:45–50, 1975.

71. Carlson DH, Griscom NT: Ovarian cysts in the newborn. AJR Am J Roentgenol 116:664–672, 1972.

72. Vanek VW, Phillips AK: Retroperitoneal, mesenteric, and omental cysts. Arch Surg 119:838–842, 1984.

73. McGahan JP, Hanson F: Meconium peritonitis with accompanying pseudocyst: Prenatal sonographic diagnosis. Radiology 148:125–126, 1983.

74. Sepulveda W, Bower S, Dhillon HK, et al: Prenatal diagnosis of congenital patent urachus and allantoic cyst: The value of color flow imaging. J Ultrasound Med 14:47–51, 1995.

75. Ehman RI, Nicholson SF, Machin GA: Prenatal sonographic detection of congenital mesoblastic nephroma in a monozygotic twin pregnancy. J Ultrasound Med 2:555–557, 1983.

76. Geirrson RT, Ricketts NEM, Taylor DJ, et al: Prenatal appearance of a mesoblastic nephroma associated with polyhydramnios. J Clin Ultrasound 13:488–490, 1985.

77. Ambrosino MM, Hernanz-Schulman M, Horii SC, et al: Prenatal diagnosis of nephroblastomatosis in two siblings. J Ultrasound Med 9:49–51, 1990.

Chapter 43

Fetal Musculoskeletal Diagnosis

Roya Sohaey

The majority of malformations affecting the fetal musculoskeletal system are classified as skeletal dysplasias. Since over 200 skeletal dysplasias have been described,[1, 2] an in-depth evaluation of all fetal skeletal abnormalities is beyond the scope of this book. The goal of this chapter is to discuss the common, severe dysplasias that result in short-limbed dwarfism. Prenatal ultrasound identification of these more severe dysplasias is usually possible. We also briefly discuss some focal skeletal abnormalities and arthrogrypotic conditions (fetal movement abnormalities). First, however, we introduce a practical approach to skeletal abnormalities.

While published guidelines[3, 4] do not require visualization of all the extremities during a routine obstetric ultrasound examination (see Chapter 33), we feel that the sonographer should note the presence of four extremities and normal fetal movement during all second- and third-trimester examinations. Fortunately, the femur length (a measurement obtained routinely) is an excellent predictor of serious skeletal dysplasias;[5, 6] however, other extremity abnormalities may be noted incidentally during the examination. Figure 43–1 suggests an approach for the sonographer or physician who incidentally sees an extremity abnormality. The reader should be aware that skeletal abnormalities can be among the most difficult to diagnose, and referral centers should be consulted for complex cases.

SHORT-LIMBED DWARFISM

Skeletal dysplasias occur in approximately 0.024% to 0.076% of births, and unfortunately most are lethal disorders. Lethal skeletal dysplasias account for 51% of all skeletal dysplasias.[1, 2, 7–9] Fetuses with skeletal dysplasia are commonly referred to as short-limbed dwarfs. The sonographer may be asked to evaluate a fetus at risk for skeletal dysplasia because of a family history for the disorder, but more commonly a skeletal dysplasia is diagnosed unexpectedly, based on abnormalities seen during an ultrasound examination performed for some other reason.[8]

Short-limbed dwarfism is detectable during ultrasound scanning because the femur is usually the most severely affected long bone; the femur

length should always be measured after the first trimester (Fig. 43–2). In other words, the most sensitive measurement for detecting skeletal dysplasia is the routinely obtained femur length.[5, 6] Measuring all the long bones is not necessary on a routine basis and does not increase the sensitivity for detecting a generalized skeletal dysplasia.[5] After a short femur has been detected, however, measuring all the extremities will confirm generalized involvement and may help in the differential diagnosis of a skeletal dysplasia.[8, 10–12] Table 43–1 lists the expected long bone lengths at varying gestational ages and is provided as a reference.[11]

Since not all bones are equally affected when bone shortening occurs, certain "patterns" of dwarfism have been described.[8, 12, 13] The three bone-shortening patterns described are rhizomelia, mesomelia, and acromelia. With rhizomelia, the most proximal bone in the extremity (i.e., humerus or femur) is the shortest. With mesomelia, the middle segment of an extremity (i.e., radius, ulna, tibia, fibula) is the shortest, whereas the acromelia pattern results in severe shortening of distal segments (hands and feet). Overall bone shortening is called micromelia. Although the pattern of bone shortening may help in differentiating among skeletal dysplasias, more often the pattern is not as important as the severity of micromelia. All too often, fetal micromelia is quite severe and associated with a grave prognosis.

We will discuss the four most common short-limbed disorders: osteogenesis imperfecta, thanatophoric dysplasia, achondroplasia, and achondrogenesis.[7, 8, 12] Some less common skeletal dysplasias will be referred to as we consider these four common disorders, mostly in reference to differential diagnosis. The identification of a severe skeletal dysplasia allows for family counseling, pregnancy management decisions, and the ability to direct appropriate postnatal diagnostic evaluation.[8]

OSTEOGENESIS IMPERFECTA

Osteogenesis imperfecta (OI) is a disorder of Type I collagen that results in abnormally short and fragile bones. Manifestations of OI are not

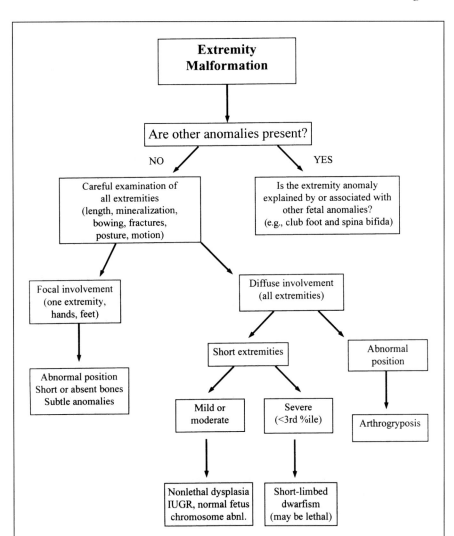

Figure 43-1—An Algorithmic Approach for Extremity Malformations. IUGR = intrauterine growth retardation.

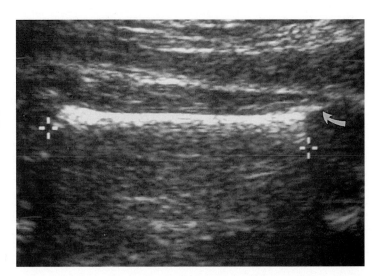

Figure 43-2—Femur Length. The longest measurement of the femur that is closest to the transducer should be used (calipers). Only the diaphysis should be measured; the specular echo distal to the diaphysis (arrow) should not be included in the measurement.

Table 43-1. Normal Bone Lengths and Biparietal Diameters at Various Menstrual Ages

Menstrual Age (Wk)	Biparietal Diameter	Femur	Tibia	Fibula	Humerus	Radius	Ulna
13	2.3 (0.3)	1.1 (0.2)	0.9 (0.2)	0.8 (0.2)	1.0 (0.2)	0.6 (0.2)	0.8 (0.3)
14	2.7 (0.3)	1.3 (0.2)	1.0 (0.2)	0.9 (0.3)	1.2 (0.2)	0.8 (0.2)	1.0 (0.2)
15	3.0 (0.1)	1.5 (0.2)	1.3 (0.2)	1.2 (0.2)	1.4 (0.2)	1.1 (0.1)	1.2 (0.1)
16	3.3 (0.2)	1.9 (0.3)	1.6 (0.3)	1.5 (0.3)	1.7 (0.2)	1.4 (0.3)	1.6 (0.3)
17	3.7 (0.3)	2.2 (0.3)	1.8 (0.3)	1.7 (0.2)	2.0 (0.4)	1.5 (0.3)	1.7 (0.3)
18	4.2 (0.5)	2.5 (0.3)	2.2 (0.3)	2.1 (0.3)	2.3 (0.3)	1.9 (0.2)	2.2 (0.3)
19	4.4 (0.4)	2.8 (0.3)	2.5 (0.3)	2.3 (0.3)	2.6 (0.3)	2.1 (0.3)	2.4 (0.3)
20	4.7 (0.4)	3.1 (0.3)	2.7 (0.2)	2.6 (0.2)	2.9 (0.3)	2.4 (0.2)	2.7 (0.3)
21	5.0 (0.5)	3.5 (0.4)	3.0 (0.4)	2.9 (0.4)	3.2 (0.4)	2.7 (0.4)	3.0 (0.4)
22	5.5 (0.5)	3.6 (0.3)	3.2 (0.3)	3.1 (0.3)	3.3 (0.3)	2.8 (0.5)	3.1 (0.3)
23	5.8 (0.5)	4.0 (0.4)	3.6 (0.2)	3.4 (0.2)	3.7 (0.3)	3.1 (0.4)	3.5 (0.2)
24	6.1 (0.5)	4.2 (0.3)	3.7 (0.3)	3.6 (0.3)	3.8 (0.4)	3.3 (0.4)	3.6 (0.4)
25	6.4 (0.5)	4.6 (0.3)	4.0 (0.3)	3.9 (0.4)	4.2 (0.4)	3.5 (0.3)	3.9 (0.4)
26	6.8 (0.5)	4.8 (0.4)	4.2 (0.3)	4.0 (0.3)	4.3 (0.3)	3.6 (0.4)	4.0 (0.3)
27	7.0 (0.5)	4.9 (0.3)	4.4 (0.3)	4.2 (0.3)	4.5 (0.2)	3.7 (0.3)	4.1 (0.2)
28	7.3 (0.5)	5.3 (0.5)	4.5 (0.4)	4.4 (0.3)	4.7 (0.4)	3.9 (0.4)	4.4 (0.5)
29	7.6 (0.5)	5.3 (0.5)	4.6 (0.3)	4.5 (0.3)	4.8 (0.4)	4.0 (0.5)	4.5 (0.4)
30	7.7 (0.6)	5.6 (0.3)	4.8 (0.5)	4.7 (0.3)	5.0 (0.5)	4.1 (0.6)	4.7 (0.3)
31	8.2 (0.7)	6.0 (0.6)	5.1 (0.3)	4.9 (0.5)	5.3 (0.4)	4.2 (0.3)	4.9 (0.4)
32	8.5 (0.6)	6.1 (0.6)	5.2 (0.4)	5.1 (0.4)	5.4 (0.4)	4.4 (0.6)	5.0 (0.6)
33	8.6 (0.4)	6.4 (0.5)	5.4 (0.5)	5.3 (0.3)	5.6 (0.5)	4.5 (0.5)	5.2 (0.3)
34	8.9 (0.5)	6.6 (0.6)	5.7 (0.5)	5.5 (0.4)	5.8 (0.5)	4.7 (0.5)	5.4 (0.5)
35	8.9 (0.7)	6.7 (0.6)	5.8 (0.4)	5.6 (0.4)	5.9 (0.6)	4.8 (0.6)	5.4 (0.4)
36	9.1 (0.7)	7.0 (0.7)	6.0 (0.6)	5.6 (0.5)	6.0 (0.6)	4.9 (0.5)	5.5 (0.3)
37	9.3 (0.9)	7.2 (0.4)	6.1 (0.4)	6.0 (0.4)	6.1 (0.4)	5.1 (0.3)	5.6 (0.4)
38	9.5 (0.6)	7.4 (0.6)	6.2 (0.3)	6.0 (0.4)	6.4 (0.3)	5.1 (0.5)	5.8 (0.6)
39	9.5 (0.6)	7.6 (0.8)	6.4 (0.7)	6.1 (0.6)	6.5 (0.6)	5.3 (0.5)	6.0 (0.6)
40	9.9 (0.8)	7.7 (0.4)	6.5 (0.3)	6.2 (0.1)	6.6 (0.4)	5.3 (0.3)	6.0 (0.5)
41	9.7 (0.6)	7.7 (0.4)	6.6 (0.4)	6.3 (0.5)	6.6 (0.4)	5.6 (0.4)	6.3 (0.5)
42	10.0 (0.5)	7.8 (0.7)	6.8 (0.5)	6.7 (0.7)	6.8 (0.7)	5.7 (0.5)	6.5 (0.5)

Mean values (cm); value of 2 SD in parentheses.

From Merz E, Kim-Kern MS, Pehl S: Ultrasonic measurements of fetal limb bones in the second and third trimesters. J Clin Ultrasound 15:175–183, 1987. Reprinted by permission of John Wiley & Sons, Inc.

only skeletal but also include ligaments, teeth, the ears, the sclera, and the skin. The clinical features of OI include multiple long bone fractures, short limbs, deafness, and abnormal dentition. OI occurs in 1 in 20,000 to 30,000 births. Inheritance patterns may be autosomal recessive or dominant, but new mutations account for most cases.[14–16]

Four types of OI, based on clinical and radiologic features, have been described by Sillence and coworkers.[14, 15] OI Type II, the lethal form, is identified most commonly in utero. Types I, III, and IV may not be identified during prenatal ultrasound examination, or they may be difficult to differentiate from other causes of short-limbed dwarfism.[8, 16] For our purposes, we will describe the characteristic sonographic findings of Type II osteogenesis imperfecta.

OI may be detected during routine ultrasound examination, or a patient may be referred for ultrasound examination because of a family history for the disorder. In OI Type II, the findings are usually severe and are seen by the early second trimester. A normal ultrasound examination after 17 weeks in a fetus at risk for OI basically excludes this lethal condition.[17] The sonographic findings of multiple fractures and severe shortening of the long bones in the early second trimester suggests lethal OI Type II. Additional features include polyhydramnios, platyspondyly (short, flattened vertebral bodies), hypoechogenic skeleton (particularly the skull), and rib fractures.[17] Other dysplasias may demonstrate bone fractures; however, in OI, fractures are the *predominant* finding, and the majority of fetuses have numerous visible fractures (Fig. 43–3). The lower extremities are affected more than upper extremities.[16] A "wrinkled" appearance of bone is characteristic; this represents a multitude of fractures along the cortical surface.[17] Bone angulation is also often seen with OI; however, bowing of bone can also be seen with other dysplasias. If the bowing involves only the femur and tibia, then the diagnosis of campomelic dysplasia should be considered. Campomelic dysplasia is rare but characterized by the triad of (1) sharp, bowing angulation of the femur and tibia; (2) hypoplastic fibula; and (3) hypoplastic scapula.[12, 17, 18]

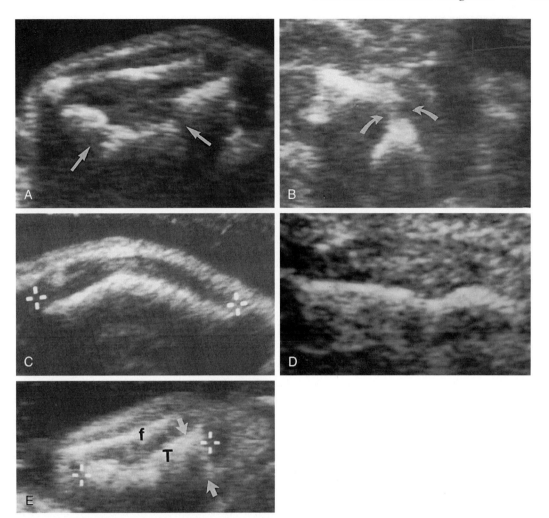

Figure 43-3—Osteogenesis Imperfecta Type II: Long Bone Findings (multiple cases). (A) Multiple fractures in a single bone. The tibia contains two discrete fractures (arrows) and the midshaft is displaced. **(B)** Angulated short bone. An acute angulation of the femur has occurred at a fracture site (arrows). Note that the femur is markedly short. **(C)** Bowing. The femur (calipers) is bowed but fractures are not seen. **(D)** Wrinkled bone. In this case, discrete fractures are not seen, but the cortical surface of the bone is undulating and irregular, implying the presence of multiple fractures. **(E)** Thickened bone. The tibia (T) is markedly thickened (arrows), presumably from callus formation and poor mineralization. Poorly mineralized bone appears "thickened" because the sound beam is not attenuated normally and both the near and far margins of the bone are seen. f, Fibula.

Bone demineralization is a classic radiographic finding in OI, but, unfortunately, fetal bone mineralization is difficult to assess with ultrasound. Studies have shown that ultrasound detects only severe bone demineralization.[16, 17] The fetal calvarium is the best structure to evaluate for bone mineralization (Fig. 43–4). If the sonographer can see the fetal brain "too well," then calvarial ossification may be abnormal. Another feature that suggests bone demineralization is "thick"-appearing long bones (Fig. 43–3). The normally mineralized bone attenuates the sound beam, and as a result the distal bone margin is not seen. Sound penetrates demineralized bone, however, allowing for visualization of the distal margin of

the bone. The bone appears thick because both the near and far surfaces are seen.[10] Bone thickening also occurs from callus formation, in response to multiple fractures.[12, 16, 17] Calluses from multiple fractures gives the ribs a beaded appearance (Fig. 43–5).[17]

In summary, the diagnosis of lethal OI Type II should be considered in the short-limbed dwarf with multiple limb fractures that may be accompanied by bone bowing, demineralization, and thickening. Nonlethal OI may present with congenital bowing and normal mineralization. The principal differential consideration is campomelic dysplasia, which is an autosomal recessive skeletal disorder.[19] Congenital hypophosphatasia

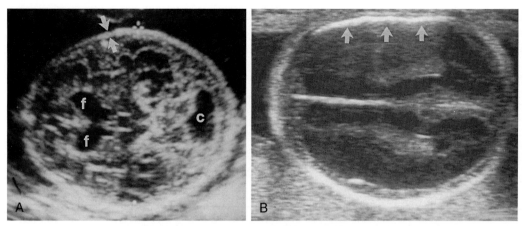

Figure 43-4—Osteogenesis Imperfecta Type II: Poor Mineralization. A poorly ossified calvarium is seen in two different fetuses with OI. **(A)** The thin calvarium (arrows) results in excellent visualization of the fetal brain. f, Frontal horns, c, cisterna magna. **(B)** The calvarium in this fetus with OI is thin and soft. Mild transducer pressure deforms the skull (arrows show flattening of the near field skull).

is another fatal autosomal recessive disease that results in short limbs and severe bone demineralization and, therefore, can mimic OI in utero. However, the reported prenatal cases of this rare congenital disorder have not been characterized by multiple fractures.[17]

If further prenatal diagnosis of OI is necessary, invasive tests such as chorionic villus sampling, DNA linkage, or biochemical studies are now available.[16] The management of OI in the perinatal period depends on the severity and type of disease. The optimal mode of delivery for nonlethal forms of OI is unclear. Cesarean section has been recommended in the past, but several case

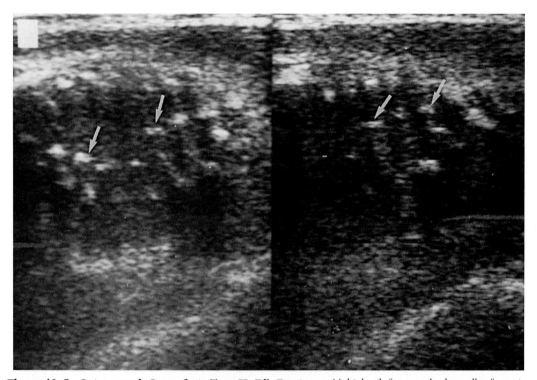

Figure 43-5—Osteogenesis Imperfecta Type II: Rib Fractures. Multiple rib fractures lead to callus formation. The resultant sonographic appearance is of multiple echogenic foci in the ribs, giving the ribs a "beaded" appearance. (Arrows point to some of the fractures.) (Reprinted with permission from Sohaey R, Zwiebel WJ: The fetal thorax: Noncardiac chest anomalies. Semin Ultrasound CT MRI 17:34–50, 1996.)

reports have shown that vaginal delivery in infants with nonlethal OI does not result in an increased number of bone fractures.[20, 21]

THANATOPHORIC DYSPLASIA

Probably the most common lethal skeletal dysplasia, thanatophoric dysplasia derives its name from the Greek, meaning "death bearing."[7, 22] Thanatophoric dysplasia (TD) has a sporadic incidence and therefore most cases are detected incidentally during ultrasound examination or at birth.[13, 23] Two types of TD have been described, but these probably represent variability, not heterogeneity, of the disorder. The hallmark of both types is generalized, severe bone shortening.

Characteristic ultrasound features of thanatophoric dysplasia include marked extremity shortening and the cloverleaf skull deformity[12] (Fig. 43–6). Fetuses with thanatophoric dysplasia have marked shortening of all the long bones; however, the proximal long bones may be more affected than more distal segments (rhizomelic pattern). The cloverleaf skull deformity occurs from premature closure of calvarial sutures (craniosynostosis). A large calvarium with a trilobed appearance and concomitant hydrocephalus is typically seen.[12, 24, 25]

While the visualization of a cloverleaf skull and short limbs should lead the sonographer to the specific diagnosis of TD, only 14% of fetuses with this condition have a cloverleaf skull.[10] Rarely, a cloverleaf skull can also be seen with homozygous achondroplasia.[26, 27] To differentiate between these two lethal disorders, simply look at the parents of the fetus. In the case of homozygous achondroplasia, one or usually both the parents have heterozygous achondroplasia.[27, 28] Other sonographic findings in TD include flat vertebral bodies (Fig. 43–7), a narrow spinal canal, bowed limbs, and soft tissue (skin) redundancy.[12] The spine findings may be difficult to see with ultrasound and may require x-ray confirmation.[9] Approximately 50% of TD cases present with polyhydramnios.[23]

As the name implies, TD is lethal. Other extremely rare, lethal short-limbed dysplasias may mimic TD, and postnatal radiography and histologic evaluation are often required to make the diagnosis with confidence. These other rare dysplasias are also lethal; therefore, the rule that severe bone shortening (severe micromelia) carries a poor prognosis is applicable, even if the final diagnosis is unknown.

ACHONDROPLASIA

Achondroplasia is a disorder of endochondral bone formation that has an autosomal dominant mode of inheritance. Either heterozygous or homozygous forms can occur. Heterozygous achondroplasia occurs in 1 per 26,000 births,[29] and the great majority of these cases (80%) are due to spontaneous mutation.[13] People with heterozygous achondroplasia have normal mental and sexual development.[13, 29, 30] Physical features of heterozygous achondroplasia include moderate rhizomelic features (femora and humeri shortening greater than that of other long bones); a large head with frontal bossing (prominent forehead), a depressed nasal bridge; short, "trident" hands; and excessive lumbar lordosis.[13]

Homozygous achondroplasia is a lethal genetic disorder. The most common cause of death is respiratory difficulty secondary to a small thorax.[31, 32] A fetus carries a 0.002% risk for homozygous achondroplasia if one of the parents has heterozygous achondroplasia. This risk exists because of the possible occurrence of a spontaneous mutation of the unaffected gene from the

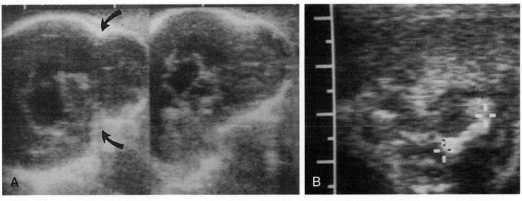

Figure 43-6—Thanatophoric Dwarf. (A) The fetal calvarium is abnormally shaped. Craniosynostosis (early suture closure), seen here involving the coronal sutures (arrows), leads to a clover leaf–shaped skull. **(B)** The extremities are markedly short. Femur length is only 10 mm in this late second trimester fetus.

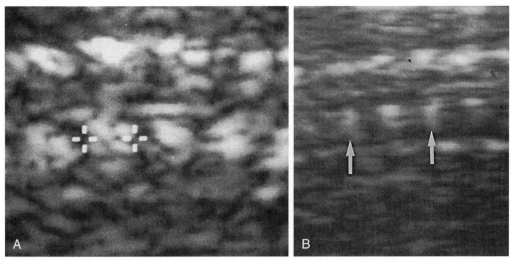

Figure 43-7—Thanatophoric Dwarf: Platyspondyly (Flat Vertebral Bodies). (A) Normal. This image shows measurement of a normal vertebral body in the craniocaudal dimension. **(B)** In this fetus with thanatophoric dwarfism, the vertebral bodies are flat (arrows) and the intervertebral space seems excessively large (compare with **A**).

nonachondroplastic parent. Marriage between people with heterozygous achondroplasia is not uncommon, however, and fetuses from these unions carry a 25% risk of homozygous achondroplasia. Therefore, the distinction among heterozygous achondroplasia, homozygous achondroplasia, and an unaffected fetus is often important. Sonographic findings permit differentiation among these three diagnoses.[31]

Heterozygous achondroplasia shows progressive proximal long bone shortening on sequential ultrasound studies, with normal mineralization and absence of fractures (Fig. 43–8). The chest size is normal throughout gestation, but the biparietal diameter (BPD) and head circumference tend to be larger than expected for gestational age, and typically are above the 97th percentile at birth.[8, 31, 33] Other sonographic findings with heterozygous achondroplasia include frontal bossing on profile images of the fetal head, trident hands, and flat, nonflared iliac bones. Patel and Filly[31] studied fetuses at risk for heterozygous achondroplasia (fetuses from unions between people with heterozygous achondroplasia) and showed that affected fetuses begin to demonstrate femoral lengths below the 3rd percentile between 18 and 26 weeks' menstrual age, compared with the BPD. Others have shown that by 27 weeks' gestational age, the femur length is always less than the 5th percentile.[8] Therefore, it is difficult to exclude the diagnosis of heterozygous achondroplasia until late in the second trimester or early in the third trimester. On the other hand, fetuses with normal interval femur length growth during the second trimester and femur lengths greater than 3.4 cm at 26 weeks'

BPD age are unlikely to be affected by the achondroplasia gene.[31]

Sonographic findings for homozygous achondroplasia are similar to those of heterozygous achondroplasia, but they are much more severe.[31–33] In some cases, the features of homozygous achondroplasia resemble those of thanatophoric dysplasia.[28, 31] Patel and Filly's study[31] of fetuses at 25% risk for homozygous achondroplasia (fetuses in which both parents have achondroplasia) shows that affected fetuses had femoral lengths below the third percentile standard compared with the BPD at 17 weeks. Also, these fetuses demonstrated severe progressive femoral length shortening at 20 to 23 weeks' BPD age.[31] As mentioned previously, differentiation between homozygous achondroplasia and thanatophoric dwarfism can usually be made simply by looking at the parents of the affected fetus. With achondroplasia, one or both of the parents will have heterozygous achondroplasia.

In most cases of in utero evaluation for achondroplasia, the parents are at risk for carrying a fetus with this disorder, and the sonographer is asked to rule in or rule out the diagnosis. Serial ultrasonic examinations are recommended. A reasonable approach is to begin these studies at the 14th week of gestation with subsequent examinations at 17, 20, 23, and 27 weeks.[18, 31] Normal interval growth by 27 weeks should help confirm a normal (unaffected) fetus. A fetus affected with early, severe bone shortening (less than the third percentile by 14 to 17 weeks) is at risk for homozygous achondroplasia, whereas progressive bone shortening suggests heterozygous achondroplasia.[31]

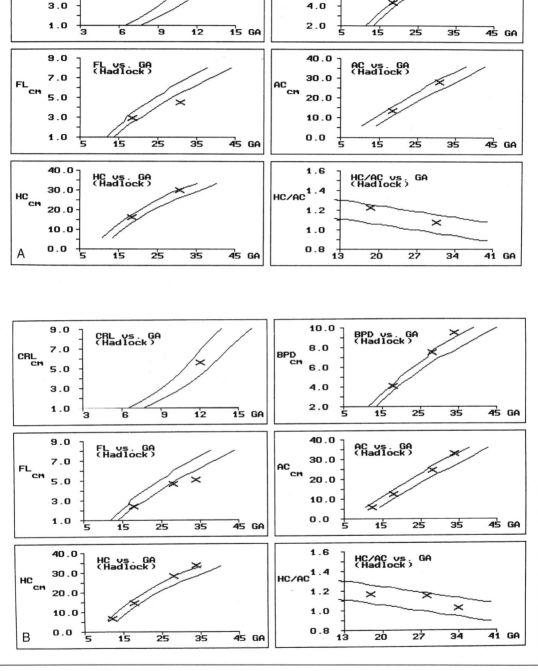

Figure 43-8—Heterozygous Achondroplasia Growth Pattern. (**A** and **B**) Prenatal ultrasound growth curves of two fetuses with heterozygous achondroplasia (representing two different pregnancies from one mother with heterozygous achondroplasia). Both fetal growth curves show progressive femur length shortening (FL$_{cm}$) with advancing gestational age. The femur length is within normal limits at 17 weeks but progressively "falls" from the curve. The femurs measure less than the 5th percentile (bottom line of growth curve) by 27 weeks. Note that the head measurements are greater than expected, a finding typical for neonates with heterozygous achondroplasia. CRL = crown rump length; GA = gestational age; BPD = biparietal diameter; FL = femur length; AC = abdominal circumference; HC = head circumference.

ACHONDROGENESIS

Achondrogenesis is an autosomal recessive condition that represents another type of lethal dwarfism. Because cartilage growth is disorganized, skeletal growth is absent or severely retarded.[34] The shortest bone lengths of all fetuses with skeletal dysplasia occur with achondrogenesis.[7] Most cases of achondrogenesis do not carry a positive family history and probably occur as mutations. Radiologic findings include poorly ossified or nonossified spine and calvaria; flared, fractured ribs; poorly ossified pelvis; absent sacrum; and absent pubis.[8]

Ultrasound examination in achondrogenesis reveals severe micromelia early in gestation (by 19 weeks). Most cases also show poor vertebral body ossification and variable calvarial hypomineralization. Additional findings include a narrow thorax, deformed extremity bones (fractures and bowing), polyhydramnios, and hydrops. Achondroplasia can mimic thanatophoric dysplasia or other lethal dysplasias with severe micromelia.[12]

DIFFERENTIATING BETWEEN THE LETHAL DYSPLASIAS

In summary, most lethal dysplasias are identifiable by prenatal ultrasound examination. The femur length should be measured routinely in all second- and third-trimester fetuses. A fetus with a markedly short femur (less than the 95th percentile) is at an increased risk for a significant skeletal dysplasia. Most of these fetuses have markedly short femurs in the second trimester (femur length 5 mm or more below the second standard deviation).[6] The four most common dysplasias include osteogenesis imperfecta, thanatophoric dysplasia, achondroplasia, and achondrogenesis. Table 43–2 reviews the characteristic sonographic finding for each diagnosis. Sometimes it is difficult to differentiate among these four causes of short-limbed dwarfism; however, the sonologist can take solace in the fact that it is usually *not* difficult to differentiate between a lethal short-limbed dysplasia and one of the many nonlethal short-limbed syndromes.

FOCAL LIMB ABNORMALITIES

Focal musculoskeletal anomalies either may be part of a generalized fetal disease process or may represent an isolated finding. If isolated, they often carry an excellent prognosis. On the other hand, the association of a focal limb abnormality with other structural defects often signals the presence of a fetal syndrome or chromosome abnormality. The detection of associated structural defects can often lead the sonologist to a more accurate diagnosis. Although I cannot discuss all focal limb abnormalities, I have chosen some relatively common anomalies that the sonographer may encounter.

Table 43-2. Characteristic Sonographic Findings in Common Lethal Skeletal Dysplasias

Skeletal Dysplasia	Characteristic Sonographic Findings
Osteogenesis imperfecta (Type II)	Micromelia by 17 weeks
	Long bones: bowing, fractures, callus
	Ribs: beaded
	Poor mineralization: thin skull, thick bones
Thanatophoric dysplasia	Severe micromelia (rhizomelia pattern)
	Cloverleaf skull (in minority of cases)
	Flat vertebral bodies
	Redundant skin
Homozygous achondroplasia	Micromelia by 17 weeks
	May resemble thanatophoric dysplasia
	Parent with heterozygous achondroplasia
Achondrogenesis	Most severe micromelia
	Poor or absent mineralization of long bones, calvarium, and spine

Clubfoot

With an incidence of 3 per 1000 live births, congenital clubfoot (talipes) is a common birth defect detectable in utero.[35] A variety of abnormal foot positions can be seen with clubfoot; however, the majority exhibit talipes equinovarus.[36] With this deformity, the sole of the foot is turned inward (varus) and the foot is adducted and flexed at the midtarsal joints (giving a "hoof-like," or equine, appearance).[12, 36]

Ultrasound shows a foot that is deviated medially, with respect to the lower leg. The following is a good rule of thumb to keep in mind in visualizing the lower extremities: a coronal plane through the lower leg should show the foot in short axis (Fig. 43–9). If a long axis of the foot is seen while the coronal plane of the tibia and fibula is also seen, an abnormal foot position may be present (Fig. 43–10).[12, 37, 38] Depending on the amount of plantar flexion in clubfoot, the foot may also be foreshortened. Fetal foot length is usually the same as the femur length,[39] and the foot length can easily be determined in the second and third trimester (Fig. 43–9). Care must be taken not to overdiagnose clubfoot, since

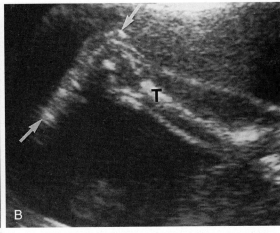

Figure 43-9—Normal Lower Extremity Foot Orientation. (A) With normal shin/foot orientation, a coronal plane through the tibia (T) and fibula (f) ends with the foot (arrows) in short axis. (Imagine that the toes are pointing at you.) (B) Sagittal plane through the tibia (T) ends with the foot in long axis. (Imagine the foot in profile.) (C) Foot length measurements (calipers) can be performed either on the sagittal (profile) or the plantar (sole) image of the foot. T = toes; H = heel.

sometimes a fetus simply holds the foot in a position suspicious for clubfoot.[37, 38] To avoid this, the sonographer should view the foot position for several minutes and watch the leg as it moves away from the uterine wall. Sometimes transducer "prodding" of the fetus is necessary to

move the legs.[37] If the fetal foot cannot straighten, the diagnosis of clubfoot should be made.

In the majority of cases, clubfoot is seen in concert with other structural abnormalities.[12, 37, 38] Congenital clubfoot may be associated with neural tube anomalies, skeletal dysplasia, musculoskeletal anomalies, oligohydramnios, and chromosome anomalies (i.e., trisomy 18, trisomy 13).[12, 37, 38] Any cause of decreased fetal movement (akinesia) can lead to clubfoot. Since 23% of fetuses with clubfoot have an abnormal karyotype, chromosome analysis should be considered.[37] However, the fetus with isolated clubfoot carries a much lower risk for aneuploidy, and in several large studies of fetuses with chromosome abnormalities, in all cases other structural abnormalities were visualized during the prenatal scan.[37, 38, 40, 41]

Fetal Hand Abnormalities (Polydactyly, Clinodactyly, Overlapping Digits) (Fig. 43–11)

Polydactyly (extra fingers) is usually detected in the fetus with other anomalies. Polydactyly inheritance may be autosomal dominant (as an isolated finding),[36] and the sonographer may be asked, therefore, to look for polydactyly when

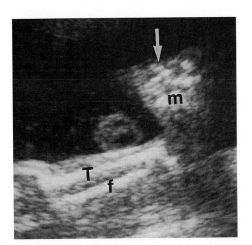

Figure 43-10—Club Foot. Coronal plane through the tibia (T) and fibula (f) shows the long axis of the medially deviated foot (arrow). The long axis of the metatarsal bones (m) is seen in the same plane as the coronal plane of the tibia and fibula (compare with Figure 43–9). The fetus maintained this abnormal foot position throughout the examination and was born with bilateral club feet.

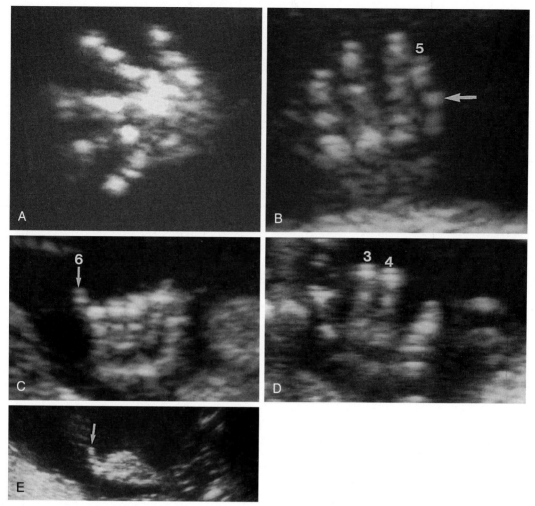

Figure 43-11—Fetal Hand Anomalies. (A) Normal extended fetal hand. **(B)** Clinodactyly. Hypoplasia of the middle phalanx (arrow) of the fifth finger (5) results in medial deviation of the tip of the finger. This fetus had trisomy 21. **(C)** Polydactyly. Fingers 1–5 are flexed; a sixth finger is extended (6). We were looking for polydactyly in this fetus because an older sibling had polydactyly (inheritance can be autosomal dominant). **(D)** Syndactyly. The third (3) and fourth (4) fingers remained together throughout the examination and the neonate had soft tissue syndactyly at birth. **(E)** Clenched hand. This fetus with multiple anomalies had clenched hands and overlapping fingers. The index finger (arrow) overlaps the other fingers. Chromosome analysis revealed trisomy 18.

there is a family history of this disorder. Either way, ultrasound is effective for detecting supernumerary digits, but care must be taken because false-positive diagnoses of polydactyly have been reported.[12] Polydactyly can be associated with chromosome abnormalities (e.g., trisomy 13) and skeletal dysplasias (e.g., short-rib polydactyly syndrome, chondroectodermal dysplasia).[12] The recognition of polydactyly in conjunction with more severe anomalies can help narrow the differential diagnosis. Isolated polydactyly carries an excellent prognosis and usually does not warrant amniocentesis.

Clinodactyly refers to hypoplasia of the middle phalanx of the fifth digit, which results in medial deviation of the tip of the finger.[42] Over 30 syn-

dromes are associated with clinodactyly,[13] but this finding also occurs in the normal population (12% of Japanese school children and 1% of Americans have clinodactyly).[42] An association between clinodactyly and trisomy 21 has been described[43]; however, this association is not strong enough to warrant amniocentesis for isolated clinodactyly. Other findings associated with trisomy 21 are discussed in Chapter 45; when these anomalies are seen in association with clinodactyly, amniocentesis may be warranted.[43]

A fetus will normally hold its hand in a neutral, mildly flexed position but will occasionally extend and flex its fingers fully. A consistently clenched hand or overlapping digits is not a normal hand position, and observance of it should lead the sonographer to search carefully for other anomalies. A clenched hand with overlapping fingers (usually the index finger overlapping the middle finger) is seen most often in fetuses with trisomy 18.[44] As with the other hand anomalies discussed in this section, a clenched hand and overlapping fingers are usually seen in conjunction with other more obvious anomalies.

Amniotic Band Syndrome

A relatively common cause for focal extremity abnormalities is the amniotic band syndrome. Occurring in 1 of every 1200 births, amniotic band syndrome results in asymmetric (or focal) limb and body wall abnormalities.[45–47] The pathogenesis is thought to be in utero rupture of the amnion leading to entanglement of fetal tissue by the amnion. The chorionic side of the amnion restricts fetal motion and causes edema and amputation of fetal parts. The extremities are usually affected, but deformities can involve any part of the fetus. Ultrasound findings are variable and include visualization of the amniotic bands, absence of fetal parts, and skin edema (Fig. 43–12). In severe cases, the fetal trunk or head may be involved, and bizarre facial, cranial, or abdominal wall defects can be seen. The prognosis depends on the body parts involved. Amniotic band syndrome is usually sporadic and not associated with chromosome abnormalities.

IMPAIRED FETAL MOVEMENT

As part of the routine real time ultrasound evaluation of the fetus, the sonographer develops an eye for normal fetal movement (see Chapter 35) and positioning. Abnormal fetal movement or lack of fetal movement is an important diagnosis and can be a serious finding. Arthrogryposis is a term applied to a large group of conditions that result from lack of fetal movement.[48, 49] Abnormalities of the brain, spinal cord, peripheral nerves, muscles, or connective tissue can result in lack of movement.[48, 49] The resultant effect of these conditions is joint contractures, abnormal hand and foot positioning, and other neuromuscular defects. Ultrasound findings include limitation of motion, contractures, clubfeet, and overlapping fingers (Fig. 43–13).[48] Since limb growth is altered by restriction of motion, most fetuses demonstrate some degree of limb shortening and underossification,[49] but usually not to the same

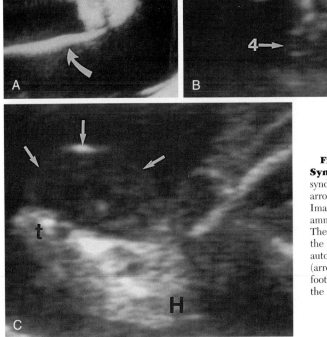

Figure 43-12—Amniotic Band Syndrome. Two fetuses with amniotic band syndrome. In **A,** the amnion is seen (curved arrow) detached and entrapping a fetal limb. **(B)** Image through the foot of another fetus with amniotic band syndrome shows toe amputations. The first (1) and the fourth (4) toes are seen but the others are absent. H = heel. (Proved at autopsy.) **(C)** In addition, soft tissue swelling (arrows) is seen along the dorsum of the other foot. t = Toes; H = heel. The amnion restricts the limb, causing edema and amputations.

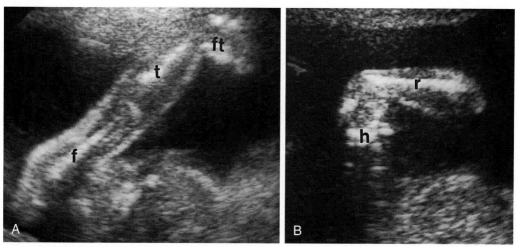

Figure 43-13—Arthrogryposis. This fetus did not move much during the examination. **(A)** Sagittal view through the fetal body and legs shows that the legs are hyperextended. F = femur; t = tibia; ft = foot. **(B)** Both hands (h) were held tightly flexed, in relation to the forearm. r = Radius. Fetus was diagnosed with Pena Shokeir syndrome after birth.

degree as fetuses with lethal skeletal dysplasias. A small chest and pulmonary hypoplasia may be present if the muscles of the chest wall are affected. Polyhydramnios may be present if swallowing is impaired.[48] Since trisomy 18 is the most common syndrome associated with arthrogryposis,[50] we routinely suggest chromosome analysis when this diagnosis is suspected.

REFERENCES

1. Camera G, Mastroiacovo P: Birth prevalence of skeletal dysplasias in the Italian multicentric monitoring system for birth defects. *In* Papadatos CJ, Bartsocas CS (eds): Skeletal Dysplasias. New York, Alan R. Liss, 1982, pp 441–449.
2. Oriole IM, Castilla EE, Barbosa JG: Birth prevalence rates of skeletal dysplasias. J Med Genet 23:328–332, 1986.
3. American Institute of Ultrasound in Medicine: 1994 Guidelines for Performance of the Antepartum Obstetrical Examination. From AIUM Executive Office, 14750 Sweitzer Lane, Suite 100, Laurel, MD 20707-5906.
4. American College of Radiology: ACR Standard for Antepartum Obstetrical Ultrasound, 1995. From American College of Radiology, 1891 Preston White Drive, Reston, VI 22091.
5. Heffe FN, Prescott GH, Watson PT: Utility of a screening examination of the fetal extremities during obstetrical sonography. J Ultrasound Med 5:639–645, 1986.
6. Kurtz AB, Needleman L, Wapner RJ, et al: Usefulness of a short femur in the utero detection of skeletal dysplasias. Radiology 177:197–200, 1990.
7. Goncalves L, Jeanty P: Fetal biometry of skeletal dysplasias: A multicentric study. J Ultrasound Med 13:977–985, 1994.
8. Spirt BA, Oliphant M, Gottlieb RH, et al: Prenatal sonographic evaluation of short-limbed dwarfism: An algorithmic approach. RadioGraphics 10:217–236, 1990.
9. Pretorius DH, Rumack CM, Manco-Johnson ML, et

10. al: Specific skeletal dysplasias in utero: Sonographic diagnosis. Radiology 159:237–242, 1986.
10. Bowerman RA: Anomalies of the fetal skeleton: Sonographic findings. AJR Am J Roentgenol 164:973–979, 1995.
11. Merz E, Kim-Kern MS, Pehl S: Ultrasonic measurements of fetal limb bones in the second and third trimesters. J Clin Ultrasound 15:175–183, 1987.
12. Mahony BS: The Extremities. *In* Nyberg DA, Mahony BS, Pretorius DH (eds): Diagnostic Ultrasound of Fetal Anomalies: Text and Atlas. St Louis, CV Mosby, 1990, pp 492–562.
13. Taybi H: Radiology of Syndromes and Metabolic Disorders. 2nd ed. Chicago, Year Book Medical Publishers, 1983.
14. Sillence DO, Senn A, Danks DM: Genetic heterogeneity in osteogenesis imperfecta. J Med Genet 16:101–116, 1979.
15. Sillence DO, Barlow KK, Garber AP, et al: Osteogenesis imperfecta type II: Delineation of phenotype with respect to genetic heterogeneity. Am J Med Genet 17:407–423, 1984.
16. Bulas DI, Stern HJ, Rosenbaum KN, et al: Variable prenatal appearance of osteogenesis imperfecta. J Ultrasound Med 13:419–427, 1994.
17. Munoz C, Filly RA, Golbus MS: Osteogenesis imperfecta type II: Prenatal sonographic diagnosis. Radiology 174:181–185, 1990.
18. Byers PH, Tsipouras P, Bonadio JF, et al: Prenatal lethal osteogenesis imperfecta (OI type II): A biochemically heterogeneous disorder usually due to new mutations in the genes for type I collagen. Am J Med Genet 42:237–248, 1988.
19. Houston CS, Opitz JM, Spranger JW, et al: The campomelic syndrome: Review. Am J Med Genet 15:3–28, 1983.
20. Carlson JW, Harlass FE: Management of osteogenesis imperfecta in pregnancy. J Reprod Med 38:228–232, 1993.
21. Kuller J, Bellantoni J, Dorst J, et al: Obstetric management of a fetus with nonlethal osteogenesis imperfecta. Obstet Gynecol 72:477–479, 1988.
22. Maroteaux P, Lamy M, Robert JM: Le nasisme thanatophore. Presse Med 75:2519–2524, 1967.

23. Isaacson G, Blakemore KJ, Chervenak FA: Thanatophoric dysplasia with cloverleaf skull. Am J Dis Child 137:396–398, 1983.

24. Elejalde BR, de Elejalde MM: Thanatophoric dysplasia: Fetal manifestations and prenatal diagnosis. Am J Med Genet 22:669–683, 1985.

25. Stamm ER, Pretorius DH, Rumack CM, et al: Kleeblattschadel anomaly: In utero sonographic appearance. J Ultrasound Med 6:319–324, 1987.

26. Brahmam S, Jenna R, Wittenauer HJ: Sonographic in utero appearance of Kleeblattschadel syndrome. J Clin Ultrasound 7:481–484, 1979.

27. Mahony BS, Filly RA, Callen PW, et al: Thanatophoric dwarfism with the cloverleaf skull: A specific antenatal sonographic diagnosis. J Ultrasound Med 4:151–154, 1985.

28. Langer LO, Spranger JW, Greinacher I, et al: Thanatophoric dwarfism: A condition confused with achondroplasia in the neonate, with brief comments on achondrogenesis and homozygous achondroplasia. Radiology 92:285–303, 1969.

29. Oberklaid F, Danks DM, Jensen F, et al: Achondroplasia and hypochondroplasia. J Med Genet 16:140–146, 1979.

30. Krane SM, Schiller AL: Hyperostosis, neoplasms, and other disorders of bone and cartilage. *In* Petersdorf RG, Adams RD, Braunwald E, et al (eds): Harrison's Principles of Internal Medicine. 10th ed. New York, McGraw-Hill, 1983, pp 1963–1972.

31. Patel MD, Filly RA: Homozygous achondroplasia: US distinction between homozygous, heterozygous, and unaffected fetuses in the second trimester. Radiology 196:541–545, 1995.

32. Aterman K, Welch JP, Taylor PG: Presumed homozygous achondroplasia: A review and report of a further case. Pathol Res Pract 178:27–39, 1983.

33. Horton WA, Rotter JI, Kaitila I, et al: Growth curves in achondroplasia. Birth Defects 13:101–107, 1977.

34. Saldino RM: Lethal short-limbed dwarfism: Achondrogenesis and thanatophoric dwarfism. AJR Am J Raentgenol 112:185–197, 1971.

35. Cowell HR, Wein BK: Genetic aspects of clubfoot. J Bone Joint Surg 62:1381–1384, 1980.

36. Moore KL: The articular and skeletal systems. *In* Moore KL (ed): The Developing Human: Clinically Oriented Embryology. 2nd ed. Philadelphia, WB Saunders, 1977, pp 301–314.

37. Benacerraf BR: Antenatal sonographic diagnosis of congenital clubfoot: A possible indication for amniocentesis. J Clin Ultrasound 14:703–706, 1986.

38. Hashimoto BE, Filly RA, Callen PW: Sonographic diagnosis of clubfoot in utero. J Ultrasound Med 5:81–83, 1986.

39. Campbell J, Henderson A, Campbell S: The fetal femur/foot length ratio: A new parameter to assess dysplastic limb reduction. Obstet Gynecol 72:181–184, 1988.

40. Benacerraf BR, Frigoletto FD: Prenatal ultrasound diagnosis of clubfoot. Radiology 155:211–213, 1985.

41. Jeanty P, Romero R, d'Alton M, et al: In utero sonographic detection of hand and foot deformities. J Ultrasound Med 4:595–601, 1985.

42. Tetamy S, McKusick V: Brachydactyly as an isolated malformation. *In* Bergsma D (ed): The Genetics of Hand Malformations. New York, Alan R. Liss, 1978, pp 187–225.

43. Benacerraf BR, Osathanondh R, Frigoletto FD: Sonographic demonstration of hypoplasia of the middle phalanx of the fifth digit: A finding associated with Down syndrome. Am J Obstet Gynecol 159:181–183, 1988.

44. Benacerraf BR, Miller WA, Frigoletto FD: Sonographic detection of fetuses with trisomies 13 and 18: Accuracy and limitations. Am J Obstet Gynecol 158:404–409, 1988.

45. Kalousek DK, Bamforth S: Amnion rupture sequence in previable fetuses. Am J Med Genet 31:63–73, 1988.

46. Lockwood C, Ghidini A, Romero R: Amniotic band syndrome in monozygotic twins: Prenatal diagnosis and pathogenesis. Obstet Gynecol 71:1012–1016, 1988.

47. Mahony BS, Filly RA, Callen PW, et al: The amniotic band syndrome: Antenatal diagnosis and potential pitfalls. Am J Obstet Gynecol 152:63–68, 1985.

48. Robinson YJ, Rouse GA, De Lange M: Sonographic evaluation of arthrogrypotic conditions. J Diagnostic Medical Sonography 10:18–22, 1994.

49. Hall JG: Analysis of Pena Shokeir phenotype. Am J Med Genet 25:99–117, 1986.

50. Hecht F, Hecht BK: Chromosome 18, trisomy 18. *In* Buyse ML (ed): Birth Defects Encyclopedia. Dover, DE, Center for Birth Defects Information, 1990, pp 385–386.

Chapter 44

The Placenta, Umbilical Cord, and Membranes

Roya Sohaey

Nonfetal structures, such as the placenta, umbilical cord, and membranes, are often ignored by sonographers and physicians alike. However, knowledge of the development and ultrasound features of these structures is crucial for fetal assessment. The placenta is arguably the most important organ of pregnancy. As the "warehouse" for the pregnancy, the placenta provides the fetus with oxygen and nutrition. Placental pathology can be seen with ultrasound, often prior to affecting the fetus. In this chapter, I review normal placental morphology and location, as well as common placental disorders such as abnormalities of placental size and location, and placental hemorrhage.

The placenta is gaining prominence; be aware that placental assessment is required in current obstetric guidelines.[1, 2] Although routine visualization of the umbilical cord is not required by published obstetric guidelines, abnormalities involving the umbilical cord are often seen incidentally and may carry important implications for the outcome of a pregnancy. This chapter, therefore, also reviews some common umbilical cord findings such as nuchal cord positioning, the significance of a two-vessel cord, and umbilical cord mass lesions. Membranes seen within an amniotic cavity can suggest a variety of diagnoses that I also discuss here. Multiple gestation is a special situation in pregnancy with a gamut of diagnostic dilemmas and fetal problems. Much of this material is outside the scope of this text, but I include the sonographic tools available to distinguish among the different types of multiple gestations. These tools include evaluation of the separating membrane and placentas in twinning.

Basically, this chapter concentrates on the "disposable" parts of a pregnancy — parts that seem unimportant once a healthy baby is born yet are essential in the formation of that baby.

PLACENTA

The Normal Placenta

The embryology of the placenta is briefly discussed in Chapter 36 and should be reviewed at this time. Basically, the placenta is derived from both maternal decidua basalis (decidual reaction of the endometrium in response to pregnancy) and fetal chorionic villi (formed from the fetal trophoblasts). The fetal chorionic villi initially uniformly surround the gestational sac. Subsequently, the part of the villi that lies in contact with the maternal decidua basalis proliferates, and the remaining portion involutes. This results in visible thickening of part of the decidua and villi, representing the chorionic frondosum seen by ultrasound (Fig. 44–1).[3, 4]

The placenta grows throughout pregnancy, but this growth is most rapid during the first half of pregnancy. At term, the placenta measures 15 to 20 cm in diameter and weighs 400 to 600 gm (approximately 1 pound).[5–8] The placenta is a disc-like structure with two surfaces. The fetal surface is lined by amnion, and beneath the amnion is the chorion, subchorionic fibrin, and branches of the umbilical arteries and veins. The maternal surface, also called the basilar plate, is in direct contact with the maternal endometrium.

Placental findings seen with ultrasound in the first trimester are reviewed in Chapter 36 and will not be repeated here. In the second trimes-

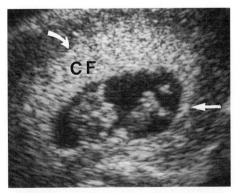

Figure 44-1—The Chorionic Frondosum. Focal thickening of the chorionic villi leads to formation of the chorionic frondosum (CF), site of the future placenta. Notice that the margin of the chorionic frondosum and the nonplacental chorionic villi have regressed (straight arrow). The curved arrow delineates the placental-myometrial junction.

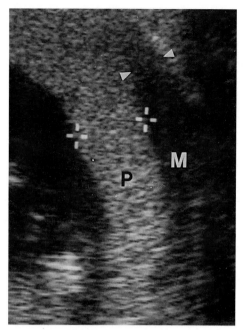

Figure 44-2—Second Trimester Placenta. The normal second trimester placenta (P) is of uniform thickness (calipers) and homogeneously echogenic. A normal hypoechoic myometrial zone should be seen throughout pregnancy (M, arrowheads).

ter, the normal placenta is homogeneously echogenic and of uniform thickness (Fig. 44–2). After 25 weeks, cystic, calcific, and hypoechoic areas are often seen in the normal placenta.[5, 7] These foci become more numerous as the placenta matures. The placenta is normally located in the fundus or body of the uterus, and it should not cover the internal os of the cervix.

Placental Size

The true size or volume of the placenta is very difficult to measure with ultrasound. However, the sonographer can estimate placental size by measuring placental thickness (distance between the placenta/myometrium interface and the placenta/amnion interface) (Fig. 44–2). The placenta grows approximately 1 mm per week of gestation.[6, 7] Therefore, the 10-week placenta measures approximately 1 cm, and the term placenta measures approximately 3 cm. A placenta measuring greater than 4.5 cm, at any time, is considered too thick.[5] Unfortunately, these measurements are not absolute by any means, and placental thickness is also related to the amount of placenta attached to the uterus.[5] In other words, if the placenta attaches to a relatively small area of endometrium, it may appear excessively thick; alternatively, a thin placenta may be seen if a large area of uterus is providing the "anchor" for the placenta.

Overall, assessment of placental size tends to be subjective, but the experienced sonographer usually will notice the excessively thick or excessively thin placenta. Excessively large placentas have been found to be associated with maternal diabetes, maternal or fetal anemia, chronic intrauterine infection, and hydrops fetalis (Fig. 44–3). Unusually small placentas are rarer and hard to detect but can be seen in pregnancies complicated with maternal hypertension, preeclampsia, polyhydramnios, and fetal intrauterine growth retardation (from any cause, including chromosome abnormalities such as trisomy 18 and trisomy 13).[5, 7, 9]

Placental Morphology: Hypoechoic, Cystic, and Calcified Structures

The placenta, like all organs, ages. As it matures, the placenta loses its homogeneous echogenicity, and cystic, calcific, and hypoechoic foci

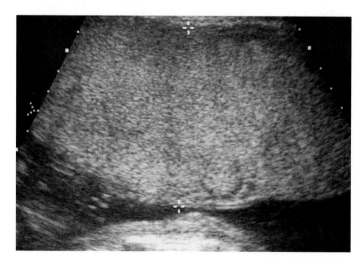

Figure 44-3—Placentomegaly. The placenta is excessively large and thick (calipers measured a thickness of 8 cm) in this pregnancy complicated with nonimmune hydrops fetalis.

are frequently seen. Small hypoechoic or cystic lesions are usually of no clinical significance and are commonly seen after 25 weeks' menstrual age (Fig. 44–4).[5, 7, 9] The sonographer should be concerned about these lesions under the following circumstances: (1) if they are seen prior to 20 to 25 weeks' menstrual age; (2) if they are numerous (greater than the three or four foci); and (3) if they are large (greater than 3 cm).[7]

Hypoechoic and cystic placental lesions usually represent intervillous thrombus (IVT), subchorionic fibrin, decidual septal cysts, placental "lakes," or areas of placental infarction.[5, 7, 9] Pathologically, an intervillous thrombus (IVT) is a small (usually less than 3 cm) focus of coagulated blood in the intervillous space. Leakage of fetal blood cells into the placenta results in a coagulation cascade by maternal blood; thus, the major component of the thrombus is maternal blood, not fetal blood.[8] Pathologically, IVT is seen in 20% to 50% of full-term pregnancies.[8] Although IVT is a normal finding, it also can be associated with elevated maternal serum alpha-fetoprotein (AFP) levels, toxemia, and hydrops fetalis.[10, 11] Decidual septal cysts form within the placenta as decidual cells degenerate. They may be anechoic or hypoechoic and are seen in 10% to 20% of placentas at term in normal pregnancies.[8] Placental "lakes" are usually located near the fetal surface of the placenta and are hypoechoic lesions in which slow-flowing blood is seen (Fig. 44–5). They represent blood flow within large intervillous spaces.[8, 9] Placental lakes decompress at delivery; although they tend to be larger than the other placental lesions discussed, the pathologist usually sees only small areas of fibrin deposition

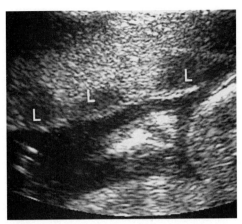

Figure 44-5—Placental Lakes. Unlike the hypoechoic structures seen in Figure 44–4, these hypoechoic foci (L) are larger, are located at the fetal surface of the placenta, and blood flow is seen within them.

upon examining the placenta.[8] Ultrasound cannot precisely differentiate among many of the hypoechoic and cystic lesions seen; however, seeing numerous placental "holes" may be significant, reflecting placental insufficiency. Basically, extensive intraplacental lesions may cause villus compression, which can lead to placental compromise.[11]

Most focal placental abnormalities are of no clinical significance, but placental infarction can be life-threatening to the fetus. Small, localized placental infarctions are common, tend to occur at placental margins, and are usually not clinically significant. Centrally located and large placental infarctions are associated with pregnancy-induced hypertension, intrauterine growth retardation, and fetal death.[7, 12] They are most commonly associated with placental abruption.[7, 12] Unfortunately, most infarctions are not seen with ultrasound, although some reports of hyperechoic and hypoechoic foci representing placental infarctions have been published.[13, 14] Color Doppler and power Doppler techniques may improve the sensitivity of ultrasound for detecting placental infarction by showing areas of decreased perfusion more clearly.[7]

Placental calcifications occur normally as the placenta ages. In the 1970s, and 1980s, investigators tried with much effort to correlate the amount and distribution of placental calcifications with fetal lung maturity. They had hoped for a noninvasive way of determining fetal lung maturity. Grannum and colleagues[15] proposed a placenta "grading" system. By this system, a grade 0 placenta is homogeneous and without calcification; a grade 1 placenta contains a small number of diffusely scattered calcifications; a grade 2 placenta has basilar plate (junction of

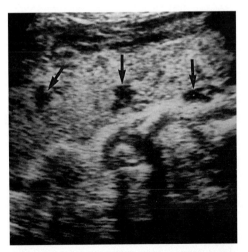

Figure 44-4—Hypoechoic Placental Structures. Most likely representing intervillous thrombi or decidual septal cysts, multiple hypoechoic foci (arrows) were seen in this third trimester placenta. A normal pregnancy ensued.

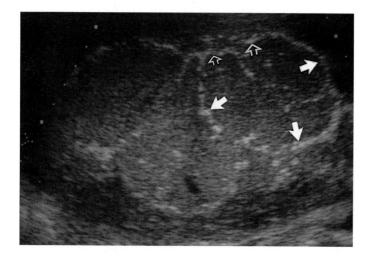

Figure 44-6—Grade 3 Placenta. Extensive placental calcification is seen. Basilar calcification (open arrows) as well as compartmental or "cotyledon" distribution of calcifications (arrows) makes this a grade 3 placenta.

placenta and uterus) calcifications; and a grade 3 placenta (Fig. 44–6) has calcified compartments (also known as cotyledons). Grade 0 placentas are typically seen in the first trimester; grade 1 placentas are normally seen between 14 and 34 weeks, and grade 2 placentas are seen after 30 weeks. However, only 30% of term placentas reach grade 3 status, and the grade 3 distribution of calcifications is rarely seen prior to 36 weeks.[16] Unfortunately, this grading system did not correlate well with fetal lung maturity, but investigators have found that grade 3 placentas seen earlier than expected are associated with fetal growth retardation, maternal hypertension, and oligohydramnios.[16–18]

Placental Tumors

Rarely, focal placental abnormalities represent true placental tumors. Placental tumors are categorized as nontrophoblastic, trophoblastic, and metastatic. Nontrophoblastic tumors are benign and include chorioangiomas (also known as hemangiomas) and teratomas. The incidence of chorioangiomas may be as high as 1% as seen in pathologic material.[8] When seen by ultrasound,[5, 7, 19–22] chorioangiomas measure 1 to 5 cm in diameter and are located on the fetal side of the placenta. They are usually hypoechoic, rounded, noncalcified, and located near the umbilical cord insertion site (Fig. 44–7). Differential diagnostic considerations include placental abruption and other causes for placental mass lesions (discussed previously). Since chorioangiomas often contain mild to moderate blood flow, as seen with spectral and color Doppler imaging, differentiation from other lesions is usually possible. Larger chorioangiomas (greater than 5 cm) are more frequently associated with complications such as hydrops fetalis, polyhydramnios, elevated mater-

nal serum AFP levels, thrombocytopenia, low birth weight, and fetal anemia. Complications occur more commonly if the chorioangioma is located near the umbilical cord insertion site or if multiple tumors are present.

Teratomas are rare tumors that have been detected prenatally.[7, 23] Unlike chorioangiomas, teratomas are more likely to contain calcification (40%). Teratomas may represent an abnormal form of twinning.

Trophoblastic tumors, also known as gestational trophoblastic neoplasia, are discussed in detail in Chapter 36 and will not be discussed here. The classic sonographic appearance is of a cystic mass that fills the uterus (Fig. 44–8). Metastatic tumors are exceedingly rare and represent metastasis from either primary maternal

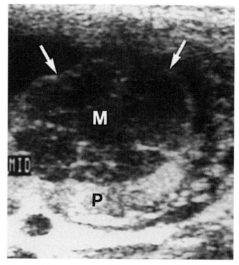

Figure 44-7—Placental Chorioangioma. A large hypoechoic mass (M, arrows) is located on the fetal side of the placenta (P) and proved to be a chorioangioma after delivery.

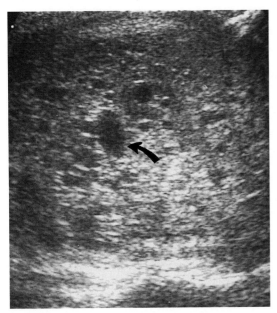

Figure 44-8—Gestational Trophoblastic Neoplasia. The uterus is filled with a complex cystic mass (curved arrow points to the largest cyst) representing trophoblastic disease. In this case, a complete molar pregnancy was diagnosed.

tumors (such as breast, bronchus, melanoma, and medulloblastoma) or primary fetal tumors (such as neuroblastoma and leukemia).[24, 25]

Placental Abruption

Premature separation of the placenta from the uterus results in hemorrhage and is defined as a placental abruption. Placental abruption is implicated in 16% to 25% of perinatal deaths.[26, 27] The signs and symptoms of placental abruption are nonspecific and include painless vaginal bleeding (often severe), preterm labor, disseminated intravascular coagulation (DIC), and fetal distress or death. Placental abruption is seen in approximately 0.5% to 1.3% of gestations.[26–28] Risk factors associated with abruption include multiple gestations, chorioamnionitis, prolonged rupture of membranes, maternal smoking, and hypertension (both essential and pregnancy-induced).[28] A spectrum of ultrasound findings associated with abruption has been described.[29, 30]

The sonographic appearance of a placental hemorrhage depends on the location and age of the hemorrhage. Blood changes its appearance with time. An acute hemorrhage is hyperechoic or isoechoic to the placenta; within the first week, the blood clot becomes hypoechoic and by 2 to 3 weeks becomes anechoic (Fig. 44–9). Nyberg and colleagues[30] describe three easy to identify anatomic locations for placental hemorrhage: periplacental (also called marginal or subchorionic hemorrhage), preplacental, and retroplacental. The great majority of abruptions are periplacental, and ultrasound may show the detached placental edge as well as the accompanying hematoma (Fig. 44–10). These abruptions are caused by a marginal separation of the placenta and tend to carry a good prognosis. Retroplacental abruption occur in 16% of pregnancies complicated with placental abruption.[30] They are caused by bleeding from a retroplacental vessel and carry a worse prognosis than periplacental abruptions.[29, 30] Since acute hemorrhage may be isoechoic to the placenta, a retroplacental hemorrhage may initially appear as an abnormally thickened placenta. Preplacental hematomas are rare (4% of abruptions).[30] The hematoma is located between the placenta and its covering mem-

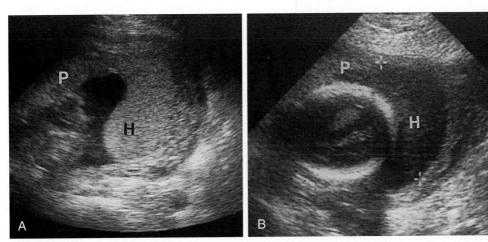

Figure 44-9—Placental Abruption. (**A**) In the acute setting, a periplacental hemorrhage (H) is isoechoic with the placenta (P). (**B**) A few hours later, the hematoma (H) has become more hypoechoic, compared with the placenta (P).

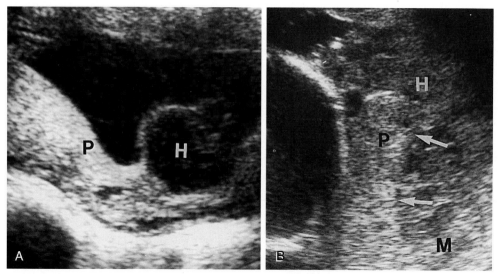

Figure 44-10—Periplacental (Marginal) Abruption (2 cases). (**A**) A small marginal hematoma (H) is seen adjacent to the placenta (P). Only the most inferior portion of the placenta has detached, and the hemorrhage is old (the hematoma is almost anechoic). (**B**) A larger, more acute marginal abruption is present. A large amount of placenta (P) has detached (arrows) and the hematoma (H) is more echogenic than is seen in (A). (M represents the myometrium). Both pregnancies were complicated with maternal hemorrhage, but the fetuses were normal.

branes (Fig. 44–11). Fetal hypoxemia and demise can occur if the umbilical cord insertion site is compressed by the hemorrhage.[8, 29, 31]

Fetal mortality from placental abruption is related to the amount of placental detachment. Greater than 50% detachment results in 75% mortality.[29] In many instances, a woman with bleeding will have a normal ultrasound examination, and in these cases an abruption has probably occurred but is not seen. Placental abruptions

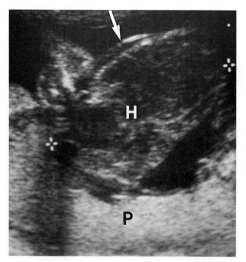

Figure 44-11—Preplacental Hemorrhage. A hematoma (H) has accumulated between the fetal surface of the placenta (P) and the placental membranes (arrow). This type of placental hemorrhage is rare and can mimic a placental tumor (see Figure 44–7).

that are "sonographically silent" may carry a better prognosis than those that are not.[30]

In summary, careful ultrasound evaluation of the placenta is crucial in any pregnant woman with vaginal bleeding. If a hematoma is not apparent, a placental abruption may still be present; however, the prognosis for the pregnancy is more favorable.[30] When a hematoma is seen, the sonographer should try to identify the location of the abruption (periplacental, retroplacental, or preplacental). Also, the sonographer should try to identify the size of the hematoma and amount of placenta detached, and estimate its approximate age. Serial ultrasound examinations may be indicated to assess the evolution of the hematoma and to prove thereby that a focal collection of blood is a hematoma and not a placental mass. Fetal mortality is associated with the extent of placental detachment (greater than 50% detachment), the volume of hematoma (greater than 60 cc), and the location of the hematoma (retroplacental is worse).[29, 30]

Placenta Previa and Other Placental Implantation Abnormalities

Normally, the placenta is located in the fundus or body of the uterus. Placenta previa is defined as a low-lying placenta that covers a portion or all of the internal cervical os.[3, 5, 7, 9] This condition occurs in 0.3% to 1% of pregnancies and is more common in multiparous women, women with previous cesarean sections, older women, and smokers.[3, 32, 33] These associations may be explained. Multiple pregnancies cause irreversible damage to uterine decidua, leading to low placental implantation in the uterus.[7] Women who smoke have placental hypertrophy (thought to be induced by carbon monoxide hypoxemia), and the resultant larger placenta is more likely to cover the internal os.[3, 33] Cesarean section scarring of the lower uterine segment may result in failure of the lower uterine segment to grow during pregnancy and therefore normal placental "migration" is stunted.[32]

It is interesting that the placenta that appears low-lying in the second trimester may "move away" or "migrate" as pregnancy advances. The reason for this is at least twofold. With advancing gestation, the lower uterine segment preferentially elongates, carrying the placenta toward the fundus and away from the cervical os.[5] Trophotropism is an alternative mechanism by which placentas may "migrate."[34] Since the lower uterine segment is an area of relatively poor blood flow, the placenta that implants there may atrophy, and the portion implanted at the more vascular rich fundus or corporeal region proliferates. This gives the impression that the placenta has "moved away" from the internal os. Regardless of the mechanism, it is important for the sonographer and physician to understand that placenta previa seen in the second trimester does not mean that a placenta previa will be present at birth.

Once again, we stress the importance of seeing both the placenta and the internal cervical os in order to diagnose or exclude placenta previa. In the majority of patients, transabdominal scanning (using a partially filled bladder as an acoustic window) is adequate to evaluate the cervix and the position of the placenta fully. However, on occasion, visualization is hampered by fetal parts, focal myometrial contraction, or an overly distended bladder. An overly distended maternal bladder causes approximation of the anterior and posterior portions of the lower uterine segment and can mimic a previa (Fig. 44–12). Overall, transabdominal technique alone has been shown to carry a 6% false-positive rate for the diagnosis of placenta previa.[35] Translabial ultrasound technique (also known as transperineal technique) is an easy, quick, and painless way to image the internal os of the cervix and should be attempted when abdominal imaging is suboptimal.[5, 36, 37] A schematic of this method is provided in Figure 44–13.

In our department, we do not hesitate to use this technique whenever better imaging of the cervix is needed. We have yet to have a patient refuse or complain about a translabial ultrasound examination. The patient is told that a noninvasive ultrasound examination of her cervix needs to be performed, and the technique is explained to her. She is then asked to empty her bladder completely. Her hips are elevated by a pillow or rolled towel. We simply ask her then to drop her knees apart as we do not feel that the lithotomy position is required. A 3.5- or 2.5-megahertz sector transducer is covered (either by a marketed transducer cover, cellophane wrap, or condom), and sterile gel is placed on the outside of the covering. The transducer is gently placed slightly above the introitus, below the symphysis pubis, between the labia majora. A sagittal plane is acquired and shows the collapsed vaginal walls (essentially being used as an acoustic window), the bladder anteriorly (to the right of the screen

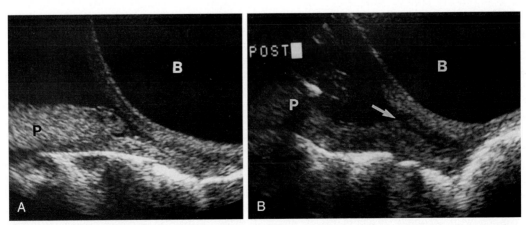

Figure 44-12—Pseudo Placenta Previa. (**A**) The maternal bladder (B) is overly distended, causing the anterior and posterior uterine walls to oppose. The placenta (P) seems to cover the cervical os. (The image is taken in a sagittal plane using the bladder as an acoustic window.) (**B**) The patient was asked to empty her bladder partially; the resultant image (taken in the same plane as [A]) shows that the internal cervical os (arrow) is clear of placental tissue (P).

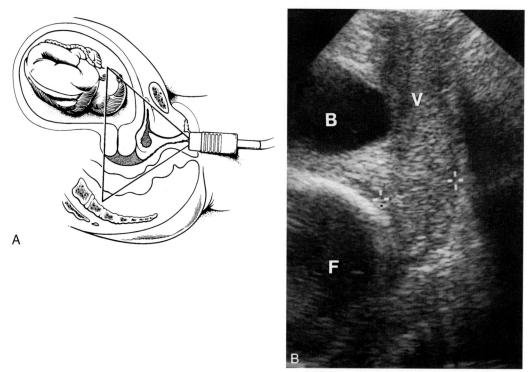

Figure 44-13—Translabial Technique. (**A**) Schematic of the translabial technique (please see text for details regarding performing this examination). (Reprinted with permission from Bowie JD: The placenta. *In* Rifkin MD (ed): Radiologic Society of America 1991 Ultrasound Omnibus. Oak Brook, IL, RSNA Publications, 1991, pp 159–170.) (**B**) Translabial ultrasound image performed in the sagittal plane (standard plane for this technique) shows the vagina (V) as a longitudinal structure (used as an acoustical window). The bladder (B) is to the left of the vagina and the vagina ends at the cervix (calipers). The fetal head (F) is against the internal cervical os (left caliper).

in real time), and the cervix (Fig. 44–13). The cervix is usually at an angle to the collapsed vagina. The entire internal cervical os is visualized by "sweeping" the beam in the sagittal and coronal plane. Translabial imaging allows for excellent visualization of the cervix during the latter second and third trimesters. The endovaginal probe can provide similar visualization of the cervix,[38] but in our experience translabial imaging almost always answers the question of the presence or absence of placenta previa, particularly in the third trimester. However, during the first trimester and earlier in the second trimester, transvaginal imaging of the cervix is preferred.

Different types of placenta previa may occur. A complete placenta previa completely covers the internal cervical os. Complete placenta previas are usually easily identified with ultrasound (Fig. 44–14). Rarely, a complete placenta previa can resolve with time,[37] but these previas tend to be asymmetric complete previas in which only an edge of the placenta completely covers the os. Women with complete placenta previa are watched carefully in the late third trimester and delivered by cesarean section prior to the onset of labor.

Presenting as a greater diagnostic and management challenge is the placenta that lies close to but does not completely cover the internal os. This type of previa is often referred to as a marginal, partial, or incomplete placenta previa (Fig. 44–15).[5, 9] Translabial ultrasound may be necessary to identify these previas accurately. Also, with this technique the os-placenta distance can be measured and may help determine the prognosis for the pregnancy.[37] A recent study of 40 women with suspected placenta previa showed that an os-placenta distance measurement of greater than 2 cm is associated with a high likelihood for safe vaginal delivery. Alternatively, only 1 of 11 patients with an os-placenta distance of less than 1 cm was able to deliver vaginally.[37] Obviously, the clinical presentation is very important in determining management, but sonographic findings may help predict outcome.

Vasa previa and marginal sinus previa are two special conditions to stress so that they are not confused with each other. Both are "vessel previas." With vasa previa, umbilical cord vessels overlie (or are very near to) the internal os of the cervix.[5, 7, 9] Vasa previa occurs if there is a velamentous insertion of the cord (instead of

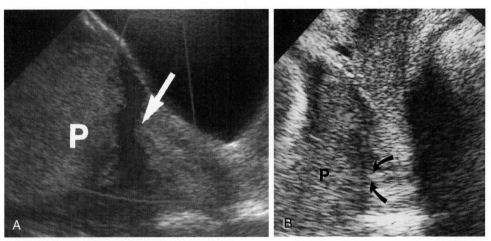

Figure 44-14—Complete Placenta Previa (2 different cases). (**A**) Sagittal transabdominal view of the lower uterine segment shows the placenta (P) completely covering the internal cervical os (arrow). (**B**) Translabial technique was used in another case better to visualize a suspected case of placenta previa. The internal os (arrows) is seen well and is covered by the placenta (P).

the umbilical cord originating from the expected location on the fetal surface of the placenta, it originates at the placental margin or even at a distance from the placenta) (Fig. 44–16) and the placenta is low lying. Alternatively, umbilical vessels supplying an accessory lobe of the placenta (also known as a succenturiate lobe) may cross the internal os. A vasa previa bleeds fetal blood, and fetal exsanguination can occur.[7] Routine ultrasound examinations carry a low sensitivity for detecting vasa previa, but case reports have been published.[39, 40] Marginal sinus previa is much more common than vasa previa and represents a variant of marginal placenta previa. With marginal sinus previa, placental vessels (at the edge of a low-lying placenta) lie near the internal os and cause bleeding (Fig. 44–17). The bleeding is usually maternal blood. The cord origin is normal, and umbilical vessels are not involved in the previa. Determining where the

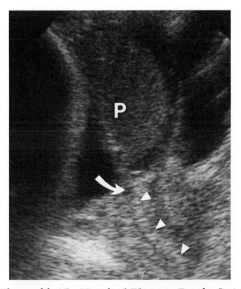

Figure 44-15—Marginal Placenta Previa. Sagittal transabdominal view of the lower uterine segment shows that inferior placental edge ends at the cervical internal os (curved arrow). The cervical canal is seen well (arrowheads). Notice that the hypoechoic myometrial zone between the placenta (P) and the bladder is well maintained, making placenta accreta unlikely. This previa did not resolve with time.

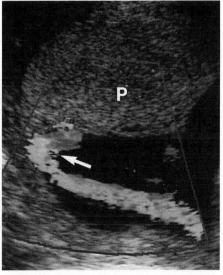

Figure 44-16—Velamentous Cord Insertion. Longitudinal image of the placenta (P) shows that the umbilical cord originates from the placental margin (arrow) and not from the fetal surface of the placenta (as would be expected).

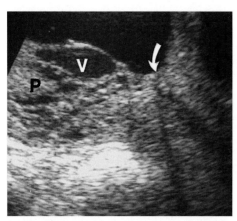

Figure 44-17—Marginal Sinus Previa. Although the placenta (P) ends 3 to 4 cm from the internal cervical os (curved arrow), a large placental vein (V) lies close to the internal os. Marginal sinus previa is a variant of marginal placenta previa, and this patient was symptomatic.

placental cord origin is located helps differentiate between vasa previa and marginal sinus previa.

Placenta Accreta

An important disorder of placental implantation is placenta accreta. Normally, the endometrial decidua provides a barrier to myometrial invasion by placental trophoblasts.[32, 41] If there is deficient development or scarring of the decidua, the placenta may attach too well and invade beyond the boundary of the endometrial decidua. Three types of accreta have been described:[3, 5, 7–9, 41] placenta accreta is defined as

villi penetrating the underlying decidua but not invading the myometrium; placenta increta demonstrates invasion of the myometrium; and placenta percreta represents villi that invade the uterine serosa and can extend into adjacent organs such as the urinary bladder or bowel. Clinical sequelae vary and include retained placenta after delivery and hemorrhage, often necessitating emergency hysterectomy or angiographic embolization. Placenta accreta is rare in an otherwise normal pregnancy;[8] however, the incidence in patients with placenta previa is 10%.[32] This is probably due to the relatively poor local blood supply of the lower uterine segment endometrium, disposing this segment to deficient decidualization. If placenta previa and a history of previous cesarean section are present, the risk for placenta accreta is approximately 25%. With additional prior cesarean section surgeries and the presence of a placenta previa, the incidence increases to as much as 67% if four prior cesarean sections have been performed.[32] The uterine scarring from cesarean section and the presence of a low-lying placenta set up the lower uterine segment for invasion.

Prospective sonographic diagnosis of placenta accreta is possible. Finberg and colleagues[41] describe three ultrasound findings for placenta accreta; this guide was used in a high-risk group to identify 18 patients with placenta accreta correctly and rule out placenta accreta in 16. The criteria (used in the third trimester) included (1) thinning (less than 1 mm) or absence of the hypoechoic myometrial zone. This zone lies between the placenta and the echodense boundary

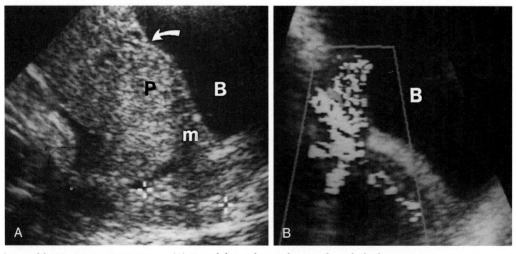

Figure 44-18—Placenta Percreta. (**A**) Transabdominal sagittal image through the lower uterine segment in a patient with multiple previous cesarean section surgeries. A placenta previa is present as demonstrated by placental (P) covering of the internal cervical os (calipers delineate the cervical canal). The normal hypoechoic myometrial zone (m) is focally disrupted (curved arrow). (**B**) Color Doppler imaging at the area of percreta shows placental vessels invading the urinary bladder (B).

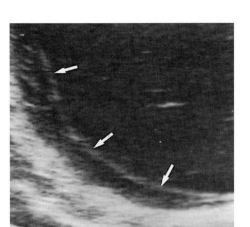

Figure 44-19—Chorioamniotic Separation. A peripheral uterine membrane is seen (arrows) separate from the fetus and the placenta. This patient had an amniocentesis earlier in her pregnancy, and the membrane represents separation of the amniotic membrane from the chorion. It is not associated with any adverse outcome for the pregnancy.

representing the uterine serosa and the posterior bladder wall; (2) thinning, irregularity, or focal disruption of the hyperechoic uterine serosa/bladder wall boundary; (3) the presence of a focal masslike extension of placental tissue beyond the uterine serosa (Fig. 44–18). Basically, a hypoechoic subplacental zone is usually seen in pregnancy and represents a myometrium/venous structure normally free of placental invasion (see Fig. 44–2).[41, 42] With placenta accreta, this zone is obliterated. However, the sonographer should be cautioned that false-negative cases occur, particularly in the low-risk patient.

Placental Membranes

Intrauterine septations and membranes are commonly seen and include chorioamniotic separation (usually after amniocentesis), amniotic

bands, uterine synechiae and membranes associated with multiple gestations.[9] As discussed in Chapter 36, the chorion and amnion may not fuse until 17 weeks' gestational age.[4] Once fused, chorioamniotic separation can occur as a result of amniocentesis. Chorioamniotic separation is a "benign" finding that should not be confused with amniotic band syndrome, which results from rupture of the amnion (discussed in detail in Chapter 43). Also, old periplacental hemorrhage becomes anechoic and can mimic chorioamniotic separation. On ultrasound examination, a peripheral membrane is seen separate from the fetus (the fetus is not entangled within the membrane as seen with amniotic band syndrome) and not necessarily adjacent to the placenta (as would be expected with periplacental hemorrhage) (Fig. 44–19).

Intrauterine synechiae are endometrial scars that are visualized in the gravid uterus as they are stretched taut with uterine growth. They appear to be intra-amniotic but are actually endometrial and are covered by a layer of amnion and chorion.[9] Synechiae are thick (usually thicker than other membranes seen in pregnancy) and broad-based (Fig. 44–20). Most patients have a previous history of uterine curettage. Placental margins occasionally implant upon the base of a synechiae. The fetus moves freely around the synechiae. They are usually incidental findings; however, an association between intrauterine synechiae and abnormal fetal presentation (breech or transverse) has been suggested.[9]

Membranes Associated with Twinning

Multiple gestations occur in approximately 1% of births but account for up to 13% of neonatal deaths.[43] Twins represent the most common form of multiple gestations. These high-risk pregnan-

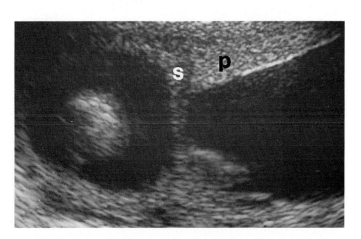

Figure 44-20—Uterine Synechia. Transverse image of the uterine fundus shows a thick, broad-based membrane(s). Notice that the placenta (p) implants upon the base of the synechia. This patient had a history of several uterine curettage procedures.

cies deserve special attention by the sonographer. Twins are at an increased risk for congenital abnormalities, preterm delivery, and intrauterine growth restriction. The first trimester is the best time to evaluate the chorionicity and amnionicity of twinning. Chorionicity and amnionicity are presented in schematic form in Figure 44–21.

One third of twin gestations arise from a single fertilized ovum and are called monozygotic twins ("identical twins" to lay people). Two thirds of twins come from separate fertilized ova and are known as dizygotic twins ("fraternal twins").[4, 24, 44] The number of amniotic and chorionic membranes in a twin gestation depends *both* on the zygocity and the time of separation of the fertilized ovum (in the case of monozygotic twinning). Dizygotic twins are always dichorionic and diamniotic. In other words, they have separate placental sites and four layers in their separating membrane (two amnion layers and two chorion layers). As a pregnancy advances, the two placental sites can approximate each other and resemble a single placenta, but vascular connections

between the placentas are not present. Monozygotic twins have any combination of membrane choices.[4, 24, 44] They are most commonly monochorionic, diamniotic (60%), but they can be dichorionic, diamniotic (30%), or rarely they are monochorionic, monoamniotic (10%). The chorionicity and amnionicity of monozygotic twinning depends on when the fertilized ovum separated.

Monochorionic, diamniotic twins share a single placental mass, and a very thin membrane (two layers of amnion) separates the twins. Placental vascular connections can occur between the fetuses, which can lead to twin-twin transfusion.[45-47] In this scenario, one twin (the "pump" twin) transfuses blood to the other twin (the "recipient" twin). The pump twin may subsequently suffer from intrauterine growth retardation and oligohydramnios. The oligohydramnios is sometimes so severe that the twin is "trapped" by its membrane along the sidewall of the uterus (Fig. 44–22). The recipient twin suffers from polyhydramnios and hydrops fetalis. The prognosis for both twins is usually poor. The sonogra-

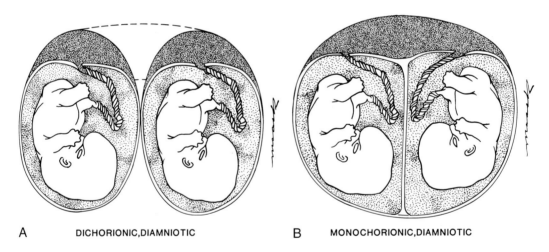

A   DICHORIONIC, DIAMNIOTIC

B   MONOCHORIONIC, DIAMNIOTIC

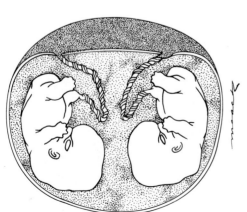

C   MONOCHORIONIC, MONOAMNIOTIC

Figure 44-21—Membranes Associated with Twinning. (**A**) *Dichorionic, diamniotic twins.* Each twin is invested within its own chorion and amnion, and therefore the separating membrane contains four layers. Two separate placentas are present, but they may appear fused (dotted lines) as they approximate each other. (**B**) *Monochorionic, diamniotic twins.* Each twin is invested with its own amnion, but they share the chorionic membrane and therefore the separating membrane contains only two layers. The twins also share a placenta. (**C**) *Monochorionic, monoamniotic twins.* A single chorion and amnion invests both twins, therefore no separating membrane is present. The twins share a placenta. (Reprinted with permission from Sohaey R, Woodward PJ: The spectrum of first trimester ultrasound findings. Curr Probl Diagn Radiol 25:55–75, 1996.)

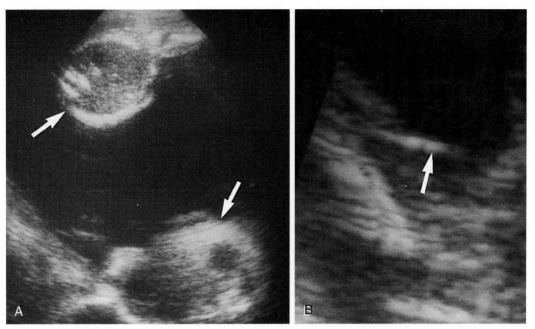

Figure 44-22—Twin-twin Transfusion. (**A**) Transverse image through the uterus shows two fetuses (arrows). The smaller twin is "stuck" against the anterior uterine wall (severe oligohydramnios is present), while the larger twin lies gravity-dependent along the posterior uterus (severe polyhydramnios is present). (**B**) By carefully searching along the peripheral margins of the smaller "stuck" twin, the sonographer was able to see a very thin membrane (arrow).

pher who notices fluid or growth discrepancies between twins should be highly suspicious of this diagnosis. Monochorionic, monoamniotic twins carry a poor prognosis. In this rare type of twinning, no separating membrane is present and the fetuses are at risk for cord entanglement. Mortality in this group is reported as high as 50%.[44]

All twin gestations, with the exception of the rare monochorionic monoamniotic twinning, contain a separating membrane between the fetuses. The first trimester is the best time to evaluate this membrane and therefore determine amnionicity and chorionicity. The membrane of dichorionic, diamniotic twinning is composed of four layers and is therefore thick (Fig. 44–23).

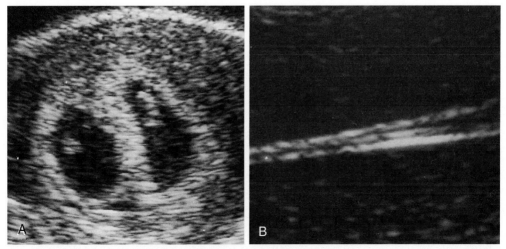

Figure 44-23—Dichorionic, Diamniotic Twins. (**A**) In the first trimester, the membrane separating the twins is thick, and it is easy to determine chorionicity and amnionicity. (**B**) During the third trimester, high-resolution imaging of the membrane using a high-frequency transducer may be necessary to show more than two layers (in this case we could resolve only three) between dichorionic, diamniotic twins.

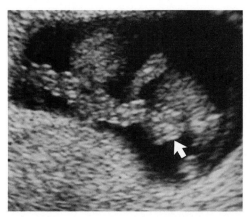

Figure 44-24—First-Trimester Umbilical Cord. By 10 weeks, the umbilical cord is coiled and seen well. A focal echogenic bulge at the base of the cord (arrow) represents normal physiologic bowel herniation and should not be confused with a cord mass or abdominal wall defect.

The membrane of a monochorionic, diamniotic gestation is composed of two layers and is therefore thin. The visualization of two separate placentas helps correctly diagnose dichorionic, diamniotic twinning; however, separate placentas often lie adjacent to each other and may appear as a single placental mass. By the third trimester, all membranes appear thin and it is much more difficult to determine the type of twinning that has occurred. High-resolution, high-frequency evaluation of the membrane may help delineate the number of layers within it (Fig. 44–23).

Umbilical Cord

The umbilical cord is easily seen with ultrasound and therefore abnormalities of the umbilical cord are often incidentally noted by the sonographer. As discussed in Chapters 36 and 41, the first-trimester umbilical cord is also easily seen. Between 7 and 12 menstrual weeks, normal bowel herniation can be seen at the base of the cord and should not be mistaken for an abdominal wall defect (Fig. 44–24).[4] The normal umbilical cord contains two arteries and one vein. As reviewed in Chapter 35, the umbilical arteries initially arise from the aorta and become branches of the internal iliac arteries. The umbilical arteries carry deoxygenated blood to the placenta and the umbilical vein carries oxygenated blood to the fetus. The cord matrix is composed of Wharton jelly. The umbilical cord grows until the end of the second trimester and attains an average diameter of 1.7 cm and a length of 50 to 60 cm by term.[48] Spiraling of the umbilical cord is variable (0 to 40 twists) and occurs by 9 weeks.[49]

The Two-Vessel Umbilical Cord

A single umbilical artery is seen in 0.2% to 1% of pregnancies,[9, 50] and this results in a two-vessel umbilical cord (Fig. 44–25). Atrophy or atresia of a previously formed umbilical artery is hypothesized as the cause for two-vessel umbilical cords.[4, 9, 50] Two-vessel umbilical cords are associated with chromosome abnormalities and fetal malformations. Anomalies associated with a two-vessel cord have been reported in every organ system and also with trisomy 18, trisomy 13, Turner syndrome, and triploidy.[9, 50, 51] Therefore, the prenatal detection of a single umbilical artery should alert the sonographer to look carefully at the rest of the fetus. Nyberg and associates[50] have shown that prenatal ultrasound reliably

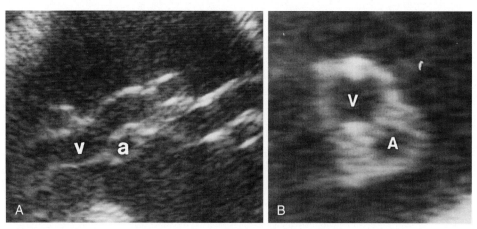

Figure 44-25—Two-Vessel Umbilical Cord. Longitudinal (**A**) and transverse (**B**) views of the umbilical cord show a two-vessel cord (a, umbilical artery; v, umbilical vein). No other fetal anomalies were seen.

detects concurrent fetal abnormalities when a two-vessel cord is seen. We do not routinely recommend amniocentesis in cases of isolated two-vessel umbilical cord.

Nuchal Cord

In approximately 25% of pregnancies, the umbilical cord encircles the fetal neck (nuchal cord).[52] The majority of nuchal cords are a single loop, but multiple loops can occur.[9, 52] An association between nuchal cord and excessive umbilical cord length, small fetuses, and polyhydramnios has been reported. The fetus with a nuchal cord may be at risk for fetal distress.[53, 54] However, asymptomatic nuchal cords are most common, and it is difficult for the sonographer and physician to determine which nuchal cords are significant and which are incidental findings.

Studies have shown that the presence of two or more tight nuchal loops are more likely to be associated with fetal distress.[9, 55] Indentation of the fetal skin by a "tight" cord can be seen

prenatally (Fig. 44–26).[55] Causes for false-positive diagnoses include seeing a cord that is simply draped behind the neck as well as in front of the neck but does not encircle the neck. Color Doppler imaging often facilitates the diagnosis. We routinely look for nuchal cord in fetuses with abnormal nonstress tests (NST) or when the patient complains of decreased fetal movement.

Cord Prolapse and Presentation

The umbilical cord should not precede the fetus through the birth canal. If the cord is the presenting part and the endocervical canal opens, the umbilical cord can prolapse (Fig. 44–27) and be compressed. Cord presentation and prolapse are associated with a high perinatal mortality.[56] Prenatal diagnosis of cord presentation in a term fetus may lead to immediate delivery by cesarean section. Preterm infants are usually managed expectantly with serial ultrasound examinations, and sometimes the mother is placed on bed rest

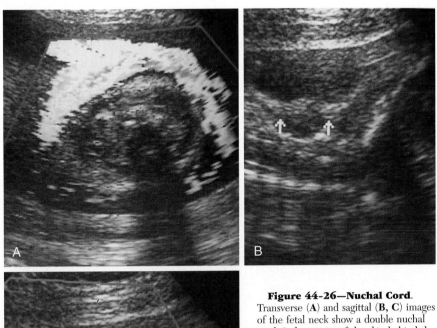

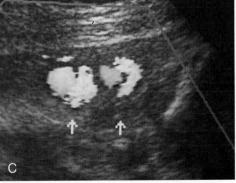

Figure 44-26—Nuchal Cord. Transverse (**A**) and sagittal (**B, C**) images of the fetal neck show a double nuchal cord. Indentations of the skin behind the neck (arrows in B and C) imply that the nuchal cord is "tight." This fetus also had an abnormal nonstress test and was delivered shortly after the ultrasound examination. (Notice that the color Doppler helps confirm the skin indentations are from the umbilical cord.)

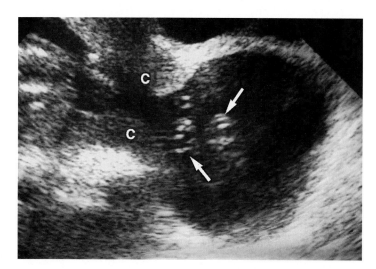

Figure 44-27—Cervical Incompetence with Umbilical Cord Prolapse. Sagittal transabdominal view of the lower uterine segment in a second-trimester pregnancy shows that the cervix has dilated prematurely (c). Fetal membranes, amniotic fluid, and the umbilical cord (arrows) have prolapsed into the vagina.

in the Trendelenburg position. Since current obstetric guidelines require the visualization of the cervix and internal os in every second and third-trimester case, cord presentation or prolapse should be diagnosable.

Umbilical Cord Mass Lesions

Umbilical cord cysts and tumors are rare (Fig. 44–28).[57] Umbilical cord cysts tend to occur near the fetal end of the cord and can be central or eccentrically positioned relative to the umbilical vessels.[58–60] They originate from omphalomesenteric or allantoic duct remnants. These same embryologic tissues give rise to portions of the body wall, gastrointestinal system, and genitourinary system. It is therefore understandable that um-

bilical cord cysts have been found to be associated with fetal anomalies.[57] Therefore, sonographic detection of an umbilical cord cyst should prompt a careful search for associated anomalies. First-trimester cysts are more common and are of less clinical significance.[61]

True tumors of the umbilical cord are even rarer than umbilical cord cysts.[57, 62–64] The majority are hemangiomas and tend to occur near the placental end of the cord. They are variable in size and appearance (solid or multicystic). Hemangiomas can cause fetal demise, fetal hydrops, umbilical cord hemorrhage, and premature delivery.[62, 63] Umbilical cord teratomas are rare. They may resemble hemangiomas but are more likely to contain calcification or bone.[64] Umbilical cord hematomas rarely occur

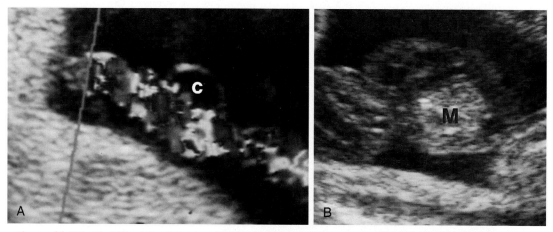

Figure 44-28—Umbilical Cord Cyst and Hemangioma (2 different cases). (**A**) A thin-walled anechoic mass represents an incidental umbilical cord cyst (c) seen in the first trimester. (**B**) This solid echogenic umbilical cord mass (M) is a hemangioma (diagnosed histologically after a normal full-term delivery).

without prior manipulation of the cord—i.e., ultrasound-guided cord puncture performed for the purpose of sampling fetal blood.

REFERENCES

1. American Institute of Ultrasound in Medicine: 1994 guidelines for performance of the antepartum obstetrical ultrasound examination. A.I.U.M. Executive Office, 14750 Sweitzer Lane, Suite 100, Laurel, MD 20707–5906.
2. American College of Radiology: ACR standard for antepartum obstetrical ultrasound, 1995. ACR, 1891 Preston White Drive, Reston, VA 22091.
3. Harris RD, Barth RA: Sonography of the gravid uterus and placenta: Current concepts. AJR Am J Roentgenol 160:455–465, 1993.
4. Moore KL: The fetal membranes and placenta. *In* Moore KL: The Developing Human: Clinically Oriented Embryology. 4th ed. Philadelphia, WB Saunders, 1988, pp 96–122.
5. Bowie JD: The placenta. *In* Rifkin MD (ed): Radiologic Society of North America 1991 Ultrasound Syllabus. Oak Brook, IL, RSNA Publications, 1991, pp 159–170.
6. Hoddick WK, Mahony BS, Callen PW, et al: Placental thickness. J Ultrasound Med 4:479–482, 1985.
7. Harris RD, Cho C, Wells WA: Sonography of the placenta with emphasis of pathological correlation. Semin Ultrasound CT MRI 17:66–88, 1996.
8. Fox H: Pathology of the placenta. *In* Bennington JL (ed): Major Problems in Pathology. Philadelphia, WB Saunders, 1978, pp 1–37.
9. Nyberg DA, Finberg HJ: The placenta, placental membranes, and umbilical cord. *In* Nyberg DA, Mahony BS, Pretorius DH (eds): Diagnostic Ultrasound of Fetal Anomalies: Text and Atlas. St Louis, CV Mosby, 1990, pp 623–675.
10. Kelly RB, Nyberg DA, Mack LA, et al: Sonography of placental abnormalities and oligohydramnios in women with elevated alpha-fetoprotein levels: Comparison with control subjects. AJR Am J Roentgenol 153:815–819, 1989.
11. Fleischer AC, Kurtz AB, Wapner AJ, et al: Elevated alpha-fetoprotein and a normal fetal sonogram: Association with placental abnormalities. AJR Am J Roentgenol 150:881–883, 1988.
12. Naeye RL: Placental infarction leading to fetal or neonatal death: A prospective study. Obstet Gynecol 50:583–588, 1977.
13. Jauniaux E, Campbell S: Antenatal diagnosis of placental infarcts by ultrasonography. J Clin Ultrasound 19:58–61, 1991.
14. Levine AB, Frieden FJ, Stein JL, et al: Prenatal sonographic diagnosis of placental infarction in association with elevated maternal serum alpha-fetoprotein. J Ultrasound Med 12:169–171, 1993.
15. Grannum RA, Berkowitz RL, Hobbins JC: The ultrasonic changes in the maturing placenta and their relationship to fetal pulmonic maturity. Am J Obstet Gynecol 133:915–922, 1979.
16. Petrucha RA, Platt LD: Relationship of placental grade to gestational age. Am J Obstet Gynecol 144:733–737, 1982.
17. Hopper KD, Komppa GH, Williams BP, et al: A reevaluation of placental grading and its clinical significance. J Ultrasound Med 3:261–266, 1984.
18. Kazzi GM, Gross UL, Solol RJ, et al: Detection of intrauterine growth retardation: A new use of sonographic placental grading. Am J Obstet Gynecol 145:733–737, 1983.
19. Laing ST, Woo JSK, Wong VCW: Chorioangioma of the placenta: An ultrasonic study. Br J Obstet Gynaecol 89:480–482, 1982.
20. Spirt BA, Gordon L, Cohan WN, et al: Antenatal diagnosis of chorioangioma of the placenta. AJR Am J Roentgenol 135:1273–1275, 1980.
21. Willard DA, Moeschler JB: Placental chorioangioma: A rare cause of elevated amniotic fluid alpha-fetoprotein. J Ultrasound Med 5:221–222, 1986.
22. O'Malley BP, Toi A, deSa DJ, et al: Ultrasound appearances of placental chorioangioma. Radiology 138:159–160, 1981.
23. Williams VL, Williams RA: Placental teratoma: Prenatal ultrasonographic diagnosis. J Ultrasound Med 13:587–589, 1994.
24. Fox H: Non-trophoblastic tumors of the placenta. *In* Fox H (ed): Obstetrical and Gynecological Pathology. 3rd ed. Edinburgh, Churchill Livingstone, 1987, pp 1030–1044.
25. Pollack RN, Pollak M, Rochon L: Pregnancy complicated by medulloblastoma with metastases to the placenta. Obstet Gynecol 81:858–859, 1993.
26. Douglas RG, Buchman MI, MacDonald PF: Premature separation of the normally implanted placenta. J Obstet Gynaecol Br Emp 62:710–736, 1955.
27. Knab DR: Abruptio placentae: An assessment of the time and method of delivery. Obstet Gynecol 52:625–629, 1978.
28. Saftlas AF, Olson DR, Atrash HK, et al: National trends in the incidence of abruptio placentae: 1979–1987. Obstet Gynecol 78:1081–1086, 1991.
29. Nyberg DA, Mack LA, Benedetti TJ, et al: Placental abruption and placental hemorrhage: Correlation of sonographic findings with fetal outcome. Radiology 164:357–361, 1987.
30. Nyberg DA, Cyr DR, Mack LA, et al: Sonographic spectrum of placental abruption. AJR Am J Roentgenol 148:161–164, 1987.
31. Spirt BA, Kagan EH, Rozanski RM: Abruptio placentae: Sonographic and pathologic correlation. AJR Am J Roentgenol 133:877–881, 1979.
32. Clark SL, Koonings PP, Phelan JP: Placenta previa/accreta and prior cesarean section. Obstet Gynecol 66:89–92, 1985.
33. Williams MA, Mittendorf R, Lieberman E, et al: Cigarette smoking during pregnancy in relation to placenta previa. Am J Obstet Gynecol 165:28–32, 1991.
34. Finberg HJ: The placenta and trophotropism: Recent observations on placenta previa and placenta abruption. Advances in Sonography: Syllabus of the 4th Annual Meeting of Society of Radiologists in Ultrasound, Chicago, 1995, pp 82–84.
35. Laing FC: Placenta previa: Avoiding false-positive diagnosis. J Clin Ultrasound 9:109–111, 1981.
36. Hertzberg BS, Bowie JD, Carroll BA, et al: Diagnosis of placenta previa during the third trimester: Role of transperineal sonography. AJR Am J Roentgenol 159:83–87, 1992.
37. Dawson WB, Dumas MD, Romano WM, et al: Translabial ultrasonography and placenta previa: Does measurement of the os-placenta distance predict outcome?. J Ultrasound Med 15:441–446, 1996.
38. Timor-Tritsch IE, Monteagudo A: Diagnosis of placenta previa by transvaginal sonography. Ann Med 25:279–283, 1993.
39. Nelson LH, Melone PJ, King M: Diagnosis of vasa

previa with transvaginal and color flow Doppler ultrasound. Obstet Gynecol 76:506–509, 1990.

40. Hsieh FJ, Chen HF, Ko TM, et al: Antenatal diagnosis of vasa previa by color flow mapping. J Ultrasound Med 10:397–399, 1991.

41. Finberg HJ, Williams JW: Placenta accreta: Prospective sonographic diagnosis in patients with placenta previa and prior cesarean section. J Ultrasound Med 11:333–343, 1992.

42. Callen P, Filly R: The placental subplacental complex: A specific indicator of placental position on ultrasound. J Clin Ultrasound 8:21–26, 1980.

43. Crane JP: Sonographic evaluation of multiple pregnancy. Semin Ultrasound CT MRI 5:144–156, 1984.

44. Benirschke K, Kim CK: Multiple pregnancy. Parts I, II. N Engl J Med 288:1276–1284, 1329–1336, 1973.

45. Mack LA, Patten R, Cyr DR, et al: Disparity of amniotic fluid volume in twin pregnancies: The problem of the stuck twin. Radiology 169:209, 1988.

46. Pretorius DH, Manchester D, Barkin S, et al: Doppler ultrasound of twin transfusion syndrome. J Ultrasound Med 7:117–124, 1988.

47. Rausen A, Seki M, Strauss L: Twin transfusion syndrome: A review of 19 cases studied at one institution. J Pediatr 66: 613–628, 1965.

48. Weissman A, Jakobi P, Bronshtein M, et al: Sonographic measurements of the umbilical cord and vessels during normal pregnancies. J Ultrasound Med 13:11–14, 1994.

49. Lacro RV, Jones KL, Benirschke K: The umbilical cord twist: Origin, direction, and relevance. Am J Obstet Gynecol 157:833–838, 1987.

50. Nyberg DA, Mahony BS, Luthy D, Kapur R: Single umbilical artery: Prenatal detection of concurrent anomalies. J Ultrasound Med 10:247–253, 1991.

51. Byrne J, Blanc WA: Malformations and chromosome anomalies in spontaneously aborted fetuses with single umbilical artery. Am J Obstet Gynecol 151:340–342, 1985.

52. Miser WF: Outcome of infants born with nuchal cords. J Fam Pract 34:441–444, 1992.

53. Spellacy WN, Gravem H, Fisch RO: The umbilical cord complications of true knots, nuchal coils, and cord around the body. Am J Obstet Gynecol 94:1136–1140, 1966.

54. Stembera ZK, Horska S: The influence of coiling of the umbilical cord around the neck of the fetus on its gas metabolism and acid-base balance. Biol Neonate 20:214, 1972.

55. Finberg HJ: Umbilical cord and amniotic membranes. *In* McGahan JP, Porto M (eds): Obstetrical Ultrasound: A Systematic Approach. Philadelphia, JB Lippincott, 1994, pp 104–133.

56. Hales ED, Westney LS: Sonography of occult cord prolapse. J Clin Ultrasound 12:283–285, 1984.

57. Dudiak CM, Salomon CG, Posniak HV, et al: Sonography of the umbilical cord. RadioGraphics 15:1035–1050, 1995.

58. Heifetz SA, Rueda-Pedraza E: Omphalomesenteric duct cysts of the umbilical cord. Am J Pediatr Pathol 1:325–335, 1983.

59. Sachs L, Fourcroy JL, Wenzel DJ, et al: Prenatal detection of umbilical cord allantoic cyst. Radiology 145:445–446, 1982.

60. Frazier HA, Guerriere JP, Thomas RL, et al: The detection of a patent urachus and allantoic cyst of the umbilical cord on prenatal ultrasonography. J Ultrasound Med 11:117–120, 1992.

61. Skibo LK, Lyons EA, Levi CS: First-trimester umbilical cord cysts. Radiology 182:719–722, 1992.

62. Resta RG, Luthy DA, Mahony BS: Umbilical cord hemangioma associated with extremely high alpha-fetoprotein levels. Obstet Gynecol 72:488–491, 1988.

63. Seifer DB, Ferguson JE, Behrens CM, et al: Non-immune hydrops fetalis in association with hemangioma of the umbilical cord. Obstet Gynecol 66:283–286, 1985.

64. Smith D, Majmudar B: Teratoma of the umbilical cord. Hum Pathol 16:190–193, 1985.

Chapter 45
Glossary of Common Anomalies and Syndromes

Roya Sohaey

In this brief chapter, I list anomalies that are known to be associated with certain drugs, syndromes, and chromosome abnormalities. The goal of these lists is to help the sonographer anticipate what he or she might see when asked to examine a fetus at risk for anomalies. For example, a patient may have had a previous fetus with Meckel-Gruber syndrome and is now pregnant again and coming for an ultrasound examination.

It is beyond the scope of this book to discuss all known syndromes, so I tried to choose the ones that are most common. Teratogens are also briefly discussed since a patient may inadvertently become pregnant while taking a known teratogen and the sonographer may be asked to evaluate the fetus. Finally, common anomalies that may occur with trisomy 21, trisomy 18, trisomy 13, and Turner syndrome are also listed.

PROVEN TERATOGENS[1]

Captopril—Small fetal head (hypocalvarium)

Carbamazepine—Neural tube defects, cardiac anomalies

Coumarin derivatives—Spontaneous abortion, intrauterine growth retardation (IUGR), open and closed neural tube defects, cardiac anomalies, scoliosis, limb hypoplasia, cleft palate

Ethanol (alcohol)—IUGR, microcephaly, microphthalmia, micrognathia, hypoplastic maxilla, cardiac anomalies, genitourinary anomalies, radioulnar synostosis, Klippel-Feil anomaly (described below), diaphragmatic hernia

Lithium—Cardiac anomalies, neural tube defects

Paramethadione—Spontaneous abortion, IUGR, cardiac anomalies

Phenytoin—Microcephaly, hypertelorism, cleft lip/palate, distal finger hypoplasia, short neck

Retinoic acid (vitamin A)—Hydrocephalus, neural tube defects, microphthalmia, microcephaly, cardiac defects, limb abnormalities, cleft palate

Sodium iodide—Ablation of fetal thyroid gland

Valproic acid—Neural tube defects, cardiac anomalies, microcephaly, hypertelorism, protruding eyes, micrognathia, hydrocephalus, cleft lip/palate, limb reduction, scoliosis, renal hypoplasia, duodenal atresia, hand deformity

COMMON SYNDROMES[2]

Apert syndrome—Coronal craniosynostosis, acrocephaly, beaked nose, hypertelorism, hydrocephalus, syndactyly. Autosomal dominant inheritance

Beckwith-Wiedemann syndrome—Macroglossia, visceromegaly (usually kidneys involved), omphalocele, hemihypertrophy, Wilms tumor, hypoglycemia at birth. Autosomal dominant inheritance

CHARGE association—*C*olobomatous malformation (eye anomaly), *h*eart defect, *a*tresia of the choanae, *r*etarded growth, *g*enital anomaly, and *e*ar anomaly. Sporadic incidence

Crouzon syndrome—Brachycephaly, prominent forehead, proptosis, midface hypoplasia, beaked nose, short upper lip. Autosomal dominant inheritance

de Lange syndrome—Cardiac malformation, dysplastic kidneys, cleft palate, genital anomalies, microcephaly, IUGR. Autosomal dominant inheritance

Fryns syndrome—Diaphragmatic hernia, central nervous system anomalies, renal cysts, distal limb anomalies, facial anomalies. Autosomal recessive inheritance

Holt-Oram syndrome—Upper extremity anomalies (usually radial defects), cardiac malformations. Autosomal dominant

Jeune syndrome (asphyxiating thoracic dysplasia)—Skeletal dysplasia with mild to moderate rhizomelic long bone shortening and small thorax, polydactyly, renal dysplasia. Autosomal recessive inheritance

Klippel-Feil deformity—Short neck, cervical vertebrae fusion, cervical myelomeningocele, iniencephaly. Sporadic inheritance pattern

Meckel-Gruber syndrome—Occipital encephalocele, cystic kidneys, polydactyly, microcephaly, cleft palate. Autosomal recessive inheritance

Megacystis-microcolon-hypoperistalsis syndrome—Bladder dilatation, hydronephrosis, microcolon, dilated duodenum. Autosomal recessive inheritance (usually female)

Noonan syndrome—Cystic hygroma, IUGR, cardiac anomalies. May be autosomal dominant inheritance. Phenotypically, resemble Turner syndrome

Pierre-Robin syndrome—Micrognathia, cleft palate, abnormal eyes. Sporadic inheritance pattern

Robert syndrome—Severe micromelia (may have absent limbs), cardiac anomalies, facial cleft, genitourinary anomalies. Autosomal recessive inheritance

Short-rib polydactyly syndrome—Micromelia, small chest from short ribs, renal cystic dysplasia, polydactyly. Autosomal recessive inheritance

Tuberous sclerosis—intracranial calcifications, cardiac rhabdomyoma, renal angiomyolipoma, renal cysts. Autosomal dominant inheritance

COMMON CHROMOSOME ABNORMALITIES[3-5]

Trisomy 21 (Down Syndrome)

Often normal on ultrasound examination

Major anomalies:
    Cardiovascular malformations (especially endocardial cushion defect)
    Duodenal atresia
    Cystic hygroma
    Hydrocephalus

Minor findings (second-trimester markers seen between 14 and 21 weeks' menstrual age):
    Nuchal fold thickening (>6 mm)
    Mild femoral and humeral bone shortening
    Mild fetal renal pelviectasis
    Hyperechoic bowel
    Intracardiac echogenic focus
    Fifth finger clinodactyly
    Sandal gap foot deformity

Trisomy 18

Rarely a normal ultrasound examination

Major anomalies:
    Early and symmetric intrauterine growth retardation (IUGR)
    Cardiac defects in 90%
    Microcephaly
    Central nervous system anomalies
    Gastrointestinal system anomalies
    Genitourinary tract anomalies

Minor anomalies (rarely isolated):
    Clenched hand with overlapping fingers
    Choroid plexus cysts
    Dolichocephaly
    Micrognathia
    Two-vessel umbilical cord
    Rockerbottom feet

Trisomy 13

Rarely a normal ultrasound examination

Major anomalies:
    Holoprosencephaly
    Cardiovascular anomalies
    Renal cystic dysplasia
    Omphalocele
    Hypotelorism or cyclopia
    Midline or bilateral cleft lip/palate

Minor anomalies (rarely isolated):
    Polydactyly
    Rockerbottom feet
    Two-vessel umbilical cord
    Low-set ears

Turner Syndrome (45X)

May have a normal ultrasound examination

Major anomalies:
    Cystic hygroma
    Hydrops fetalis
    Cardiovascular malformation (particularly coarctation of the aorta)
    Renal agenesis

Minor anomalies:
    Nuchal thickening
    Horseshoe kidneys
    Short stature

REFERENCES

1. Briggs GG, Freeman RK, Yaffe SJ: Drugs in Pregnancy and Lactation. Baltimore, Williams & Wilkins, 1990.
2. Nyberg DA: Appendix B. *In* Nyberg DA, Mahony BS, Pretorius DH (eds): Diagnostic Ultrasound of Fetal Anomalies: Text and Atlas. St. Louis, CV Mosby, 1990, pp 750–757.
3. Nyberg DA, Crane JP: Chromosome abnormalities. *In* Nyberg DA, Mahony BS, Pretorius DH (eds): Diagnostic Ultrasound of Fetal Anomalies: Text and Atlas. St. Louis, CV, Mosby, 1990, pp 676–724.
4. Benacerraf BR, Nadel A, Bromley B: Identification of second-trimester fetuses with autosomal trisomy by use of a sonographic scoring index. Radiology 193: 135–140, 1994.
5. Benacerraf BR: Use of sonographic markers to determine the risk for Down syndrome in second-trimester fetuses. Radiology 201:619–620, 1996.

Section 9
Superficial Structures

A variety of anatomic structures can, of course, be called "superficial." With respect to ultrasound diagnosis, however, "superficial structures" usually refer to the thyroid and parathyroid glands, the breast, and the scrotum. In this section of the text, we review the essential aspects of ultrasound examination of these organs.

Ultrasound continues to be the principal method for imaging the scrotum, and it is used widely for breast examination. The use of ultrasound for thyroid and parathyroid evaluation has decreased in recent years, as noted in the chapter that follows. Nonetheless, it is necessary for ultrasound practitioners to be familiar with the examination of these glands.

Chapter 46

The Thyroid and Parathyroid

William J. Zwiebel

THYROID ANATOMY

The thyroid gland[1, 2] consists of two lobes lying to the right and left of the trachea at the base of the neck, as illustrated in Figure 46–1. Each lobe is broad inferiorly and tapers superiorly. The size of the thyroid gland varies with age and body size, but in adults each lobe does not usually exceed 4 cm in length: 2 cm anteroposterior (AP) and 2 cm transverse. The lobes are connected by a band of thyroid tissue, called the isthmus, that passes anterior to the trachea.

Embryologically, the thyroid is derived from the fourth brachial pouch and "descends" from the base of the tongue to the base of the neck. The thyroglossal duct remnant, located in the midline of the neck, marks the route of descent of the thyroid, and thyroglossal duct cysts may occur in this location. Excessive "descent" may cause the lower pole of the thyroid to lie within the superior mediastinum, or it may cause ectopic thyroid tissue to lie wholly within the mediastinum.

The thyroid gland is closely associated with the carotid arteries, the internal jugular veins, the sternomastoid muscles, the longus colli muscles, and the esophagus, as shown in Figure 46–2. The esophagus commonly lies posterior to the left thyroid lobe and may be mistaken for thyroid or parathyroid pathology (Fig. 46–3).

Ultrasound examination shows that the thyroid is homogeneous in texture and relatively echogenic compared with the nearby sternomastoid muscle (Fig. 46–3). One can judge whether the echogenicity of a patient's thyroid is normal by comparing the patient's thyroid with the examiner's thyroid (assuming that the examiner has a normal gland). A large, longitudinally oriented vein, called the inferior thyroid vein, often is visible on images of the inferior poles of the thyroid. The inferior thyroid artery may be visualized in the same location.

PARATHYROID ANATOMY

Most individuals have four parathyroid glands, two located posterior to the lower lobes of the thyroid and two posterior to the upper lobes (see Figure 46–1). Thirteen percent of normal individuals have more than four glands: furthermore, parathyroid gland location is somewhat variable.[3–5] The two upper glands may be positioned anywhere from the upper thyroid pole to the thyroid isthmus. In a small percentage of individuals the superior gland may lie cephalad to the upper thyroid pole, posteromedial to the esophagus, or near the *inferior* thyroid artery. The inferior parathyroids also may be ectopic. These glands originate in the neck of the embryo and migrate with the thymus gland. They usually end up behind, or just inferior to, the lower thyroid poles, but about 13% descend into the superior mediastinum, and a small number fail to descend completely. The latter end up posterior to the upper or midportion of the thyroid gland rather than behind the lower pole. What all this amounts to is that enlarged parathyroid glands may not be found sonographically at the expected location. To make matters worse, a parathyroid gland may occasionally be embedded in the posterior aspect of the thyroid, mimicking a thyroid nodule. Normal parathyroid glands do not exceed 5 mm in any dimension and are rarely visualized with ultrasound because of their small size and because they typically are isoechoic with the thyroid tissue.

SONOGRAPHIC TECHNIQUE

Adequate visualization of the thyroid and parathyroid glands is predicated on hyperextending

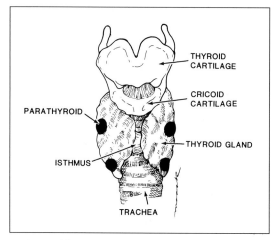

Figure 46-1—Location of the thyroid and parathyroid glands. The parathyroid glands are posterior to the thyroid glands.

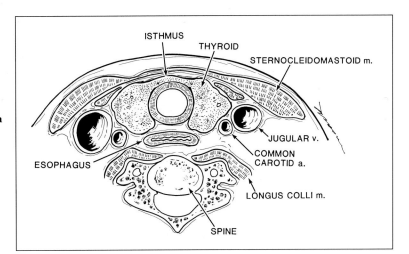

Figure 46-2—Cross-section of the thyroid gland and surrounding structures.

the patient's neck, which raises these glands from behind the sternum to a sonographically visible location. Neck hyperextension is accomplished by having the patient lie in a supine position with a pillow or other suitable bolus behind the shoulders. The glands then are scanned longitudinally and transversely with a high-frequency linear array transducer (7.5 or 10 MHz).

FOCAL THYROID MASSES

Thyroid pathology is outlined in Table 46–1. Before proceeding, please review this classification, as this material is not repeated in the text. Focal thyroid masses, or "nodules," are of three principal varieties: benign adenomas, cysts, and carcinomas. Adenomas, as discussed later, are extremely common, accounting for about 85% of palpable thyroid masses.[6] Some adenomas are

Table 46-1. Classification of Thyroid Pathology

Focal Masses
   Adenoma
   Carcinoma
      Papillary
      Follicular
      Anaplastic
   Cystic adenoma or carcinoma
   Lymphoma
   Asymmetric goiter
Diffuse Disorders
   Graves disease (also called toxic goiter)
   Multinodular goiter°
   Simple or nontoxic goiter°
   Endemic goiter°
   Hashimoto thyroiditis
   Subacute thyroiditis
   Reidel thyroiditis

°These disorders are related morphologically.
Compiled from information in Larsen PR, Ingbar SH: The thyroid gland. *In* Wilson JD, Foster DW (eds): Williams' Textbook of Endocrinology. 8th ed. Philadelphia, WB Saunders, 1992, pp 357–487.

hyperfunctioning and may even be functionally autonomous. These hyperfunctioning adenomas cause hyperparathyroidism and suppress the rest of the thyroid gland. Other adenomas function at about the same level as the normal thyroid or function less than normal thyroid.

Some investigators differentiate between adenomas and adenomatous nodules, from the perspective that adenomas are true neoplasms arising de novo from the thyroid, whereas adenomatous nodules are hyperplastic and represent overgrowth of normal follicular tissue. It is implied, for instance, that a solitary hyperfunctioning adenoma is a neoplasm, whereas multiple nodules present in diffuse nodular goiter (discussed later) are hyperplastic. Larsen and Ingbar, in their extensive treatise on thyroid disease,[1] discourage such differentiation because adenomas and so-called adenomatous nodules cannot be differentiated histologically. We will follow their example and use the term "adenoma" throughout this chapter, rather than adenomatous nodule.

Virtually all thyroid cysts are in fact adenomas that have undergone cystic degeneration; thus, these cysts often have a thick wall and often contain solid elements. Unfortunately, carcinomas also can exhibit cystic degeneration and are indistinguishable from benign cysts.

Thyroid cancers come in three principal varieties: papillary, follicular, and anaplastic. Fortunately, 50% to 70% of thyroid cancers are papillary, which is the most benign variety, and 10% to 15% are follicular, which is slightly more malignant but generally is curable. About 10% of thyroid cancers are anaplastic, and these are fast growing, widely metastasizing tumors to which the patient usually succumbs within months of diagnosis. Table 46–2 classifies thyroid cancers and describes the salient features of each variety.[1]

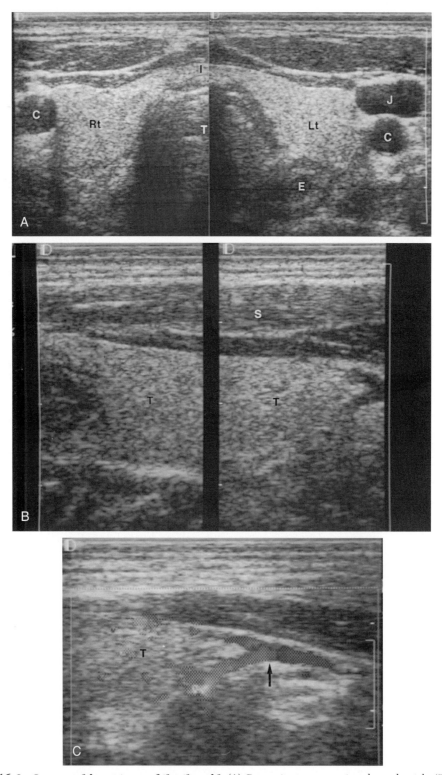

Figure 46-3—Sonographic anatomy of the thyroid. (A) Composite transverse view shows the right (Rt) and left (Lt) thyroid lobes, the thyroid isthmus (I), the trachea (T), the left jugular vein (J), the right and left common carotid arteries (C), and the esophagus (E). (B) Composite longitudinal view of the thyroid (T). Left, upper pole; right, lower pole. S, sternomastoid muscle. (C) Longitudinal view of the inferior thyroid pole (T), showing the inferior thyroid vein (arrow).

Table 46-2. Thyroid Cancer

Follicular Epithelium Origin

Papillary carcinoma	50%–70% of thyroid cancer; younger age (half before age 40 yr); 2–3 times more common in women than men. Least deadly; 6.5% death rate from tumor in 25-year follow-up
Follicular carcinoma	10%–15% of thyroid cancer; usually over 40 yr of age; 2–3 times more common in women than men. Slightly more deadly than papillary, with greater tendency for vascular invasion and hematogenous metastasis; 10-year survival, 44%–86%
Hürthle cell carcinoma	Variant of follicular carcinoma in which so-called Hürthle cells predominate
Anaplastic carcinoma	About 10% of thyroid cancer. Older age group (usually over 50 yr); slight female predominance. Highly malignant, with rapid local growth as well as diffuse and early metastasis. Not sensitive to radio-iodine therapy. Death usually within months

Perifollicular Origin

Medullary cancer	1%–2% of thyroid cancer; occurs past 40 yr of age; slight female predominance. More malignant than follicular carcinoma but not as deadly as anaplastic carcinoma. May be hormonally active, producing a variety of hormones, including calcitonin and ACTH. Component of multiple endocrine adenomatosis (MEN) syndrome
Lymphoma	Lymphoma of the thyroid is rare and most commonly associated with Hashimoto thyroiditis

Compiled from information in Larsen PR, Ingbar SH: The thyroid gland. *In* Wilson JD, Foster DW: Williams' Textbook of Endocrinology. 8th ed. Philadelphia, WB Saunders, 1992, pp 357–487.

"Sea" of Nodules, Few Cancers

Focal thyroid masses, or nodules as they often are called, are extremely common.[2, 6–16] Ultrasound studies have demonstrated one or more thyroid nodules in about 40% of asymptomatic adults who have no history of thyroid disease. A large autopsy-based study showed a similar prevalence (49%) of asymptomatic nodules and also demonstrated that nodule prevalence increases with age. *Palpable* thyroid nodules are much less common than the occult nodules detected in autopsy or ultrasound studies. The prevalence of *palpable* thyroid nodules in adults is 7% to 21%.

The clinical challenge with respect to thyroid nodules is to identify a few carcinomas residing in a "sea" of benign nodules, for although thyroid nodules are very common, thyroid cancer is relatively uncommon. The annual detection rate for thyroid cancer in the United States is 4/1000 adults, which is relatively low.[9] The incidence of thyroid cancer is greater in patients subjected to thyroid irradiation in childhood, but even in these individuals, two thirds of palpable nodules are benign, and those that are malignant are usually well-differentiated papillary or follicular lesions.

Ultrasound Features of Nodules

The introduction of high-resolution ultrasound in the early 1980s was greeted with great enthusiasm, as a potential means for differentiating between benign and malignant thyroid nodules. Unfortunately, as time passed and comprehensive studies were conducted, it became apparent that ultrasound could not reliably separate benign and malignant thyroid nodules. In spite of this failing, ultrasound practitioners should be aware of the features that *suggest* either benignity or malignancy. Most benign nodules either are isoechoic or hypoechoic, relative to normal thyroid. Malignant nodules also are hypoechoic, so this feature is not helpful in differentiating between benign and malignant lesions. Findings that suggest benignity (Table 46–3; Fig. 46–4) include the following:[17–19]

- Clearly defined margins are comforting, as malignant nodules tend to be invasive and poorly marginated.
- A thin, echolucent halo surrounding the *entire* lesion is particularly suggestive of benignity, as

Table 46-3. Ultrasound Features of Thyroid Nodules Suggesting Benignity or Malignancy

Benign
Clearly defined margins
Thin, complete halo
Solid, hyperechoic
Cystic
Peripheral eggshell calcification
Malignant
Poorly defined margins
Hypoechoic
Punctate bright reflections
Cervical adenopathy

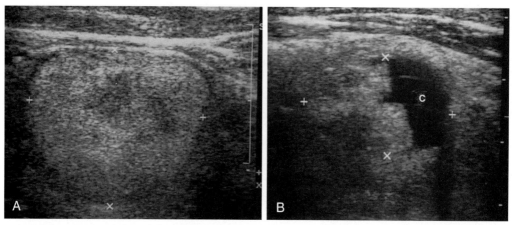

Figure 46-4—Benign appearance of thyroid masses. (A) A well-defined nodule (cursors) is surrounded by a thin, hypoechoic "halo." Slight central heterogeneity is probably due to necrosis. (B) Partial cystic degeneration (C) is evident in this benign nodule (cursors).

a halo is present in only 4% of malignant nodules.

- Cystic degeneration, with variable debris and solid elements, is a common feature in benign nodules; unfortunately, cystic degeneration also is present in 26% of malignant nodules.
- Increased echogenicity (relative to normal thyroid) in a completely solid nodule is virtual proof of benignity, since thyroid cancers are invariably hypoechoic. Unfortunately, increased echogenicity is rare.
- Peripheral eggshell calcification also is highly suggestive of benignity but is only rarely seen.

Ultrasound features that suggest malignancy (Table 46–3) are poorly defined and irregular margins; diffuse, punctate, bright internal reflections (especially in papillary carcinoma); and cervical lymphadenopathy associated with a thyroid mass (discussed later). Of particular concern is a hypoechoic nodule that is poorly marginated, as shown in Figure 46–5. Such a lesion is likely to be thyroid cancer, particularly if the nodule is associated with cervical lymphadenopathy.[17–19]

Color and spectral-Doppler sonography have been evaluated but found not useful for determining whether a thyroid nodule is benign or malignant. Vascularity appears more related to the size of the nodule and the state of thyroid activity than to anything else.[2]

Cervical Lymph Nodes

Ultrasound findings are helpful for differentiating among normal, inflamed, and neoplastic cervical lymph nodes.[2] Normal nodes are hypoechoic and ovoid, with a long axis that is distinctly larger than the short axis. Inflamed nodes are

enlarged but retain the normal relationship of length to thickness. Neoplastic nodes are characterized by increased thickness; i.e., they are rounder than normal. If the transverse diameter is more than half of the length of the node, then neoplasia is likely.

The Role of Ultrasound

As noted earlier, the attractiveness of ultrasound for assessment of focal thyroid disease has dimmed because of inability to distinguish benign from malignant lesions. The attractiveness of ultrasound also has dimmed because most palpable nodules now are investigated directly with percutaneous needle aspiration, performed without image assistance. The reader might wonder, therefore, why we have included the thyroid in this text. We included the thyroid because ultrasound still is used occasionally for assessment of this organ, and therefore ultrasound practitioners should be familiar with this subject. The indications for thyroid ultrasound are the following.[2, 20–23]

1. Ultrasound is a convenient way to determine that a cervical mass arises from the thyroid, rather than from an adjacent structure such as a lymph node.
2. Patients with thyroiditis or multinodular goiter sometimes present with asymmetric gland enlargement mimicking a discrete nodule. Ultrasound can document that the gland is diffusely abnormal and direct the clinical evaluation appropriately.
3. Ultrasound is very helpful for directing fine-needle aspiration biopsy when nonguided biopsy has failed to produce diagnostic material

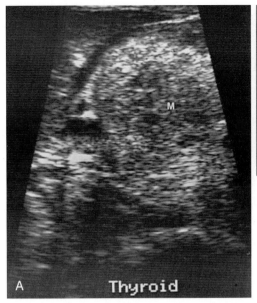

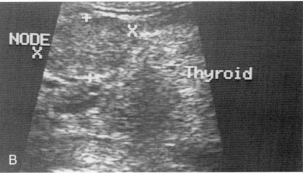

Figure 46-5—Thyroid carcinoma (papillary). (A) An ill-defined, hypoechoic, lobulated mass (M) is visible in the right thyroid lobe on this transverse image. **(B)** An enlarged lymph node (cursors) is seen adjacent to the thyroid.

(i.e., when only blood or necrotic debris is obtained). In these instances, the aspiration needle can be directed into solid elements of the nodule, as outlined in Table 46–4.

4. Ultrasound can be used to guide fine-needle aspiration of nonpalpable nodules that are "cold" scintigraphically.

5. Ultrasound can be used to detect recurrent

Table 46-4. Recommended Technique for Needle Aspiration of Thyroid Nodules, Parathyroid Adenomas, or Cervical Lymph Nodes°

Transducer	7- to 10-MHz linear array
Needle	Standard 26-gauge 1.5-inch hypodermic needle (cutting needle can be used but is hard to get through the skin)
Antisepsis	Scrub transducer face with surgical antiseptic solution used to cleanse patient's skin. Apply transducer directly to skin *without* a plastic or rubber sheath, which degrades the image.
Orientation	Position yourself, the patient, and the ultrasound machine such that (1) you can look directly at the image monitor, and (2) the orientation of the image matches the orientation of the patient. I often place the patient between the ultrasound machine and myself, so that I am looking across the patient to the monitor.
Stabilization	The trick of ultrasound guidance is to hold the transducer (and image) very still. To this end, the operator should sit on a chair or stool in a comfortable position and rest the forearm of the limb holding the transducer on the examining table or on the patient's chest, to stabilize the transducer during needle insertion.
Technique	a. Localize the target (nodule, lymph node, etc.) and plan your "attack" before you scrub.
	b. Choose the needle insertion site and mark it prior to antiseptic scrub.
	c. Scrub the patient's neck and the transducer and anesthetize the insertion site (use ultrasound guidance to ensure adequate anesthesia all the way to the target).
	d. Localize the nodule and insert the needle *in line with the image plane*.
Aspiration	a. Use a 10-cc syringe with intervening tubing.
	b. Have someone else apply suction to the syringe, if needed.
	c. Move needle brusquely up and down through the lesion under ultrasound guidance.
	d. The goal is to get a few drops of material in the needle hub.
	e. If aspiration produces too much material or blood, remove syringe and move the needle through the lesion *without aspiration*. Capillary action will be enough to acquire material.
	f. Put a drop of aspirate on each of two slides and smear each. Flush residual material into nonbacteriostatic saline (*not formalin*).
	g. Obtain about three samples (or more if you do not believe you have attained adequate material).
Color Doppler	Color Doppler may be used to identify large cervical or thyroid vessels, but it tends to frighten the examiner since the thyroid is extremely vascular.

°As recommended by Carl Reading, MD, and the Mayo Clinic (Hopkins CR, Reading CC: Thyroid and parathyroid imaging. Semin Ultrasound CT MRI 16:279–295, 1995), and endorsed by me.

tumor in the neck after thyroidectomy for thyroid cancer. Ultrasound generally is not needed in patients with well-differentiated follicular or papillary thyroid cancer, as these tumors take up iodine and can be identified scintigraphically. Ultrasound is useful, however, for detecting recurrent tumor that does not take up iodine.

6. Ultrasound can be used to direct palliation of tumor recurrences with percutaneous injection of 100% ethyl alcohol.

7. Ultrasound can be used similarly for alcohol ablation of autonomous functioning thyroid nodules in hyperthyroid patients. The subject of alcohol ablation of thyroid nodules is out of the scope of this chapter. For technical details, the reader is referred to references 2 and 21 through 23.

The Role of Scintigraphy

Scintigraphy with iodine-123 (^{123}I) has been the mainstay of thyroid imaging, but the role of this modality also has been questioned in recent years.[8, 24] "Hot" nodules that take up ^{123}I in excess of the surrounding thyroid have a low probability of malignancy, estimated at 1% to 4%.[2] Warm nodules, having uptake about the same as that of the surrounding thyroid, are usually adenomas but have about a 10% chance of being malignant.[3] Cold nodules have about a 10% to 25% chance of malignancy and require aspiration biopsy; nevertheless, the great majority of cold nodules are benign. Recent clinical practice has tended to skip scintigraphy and proceed directly to percutaneous biopsy of palpable thyroid nodules in euthyroid patients.

DIFFUSE THYROID DISEASE

In most cases, diffuse thyroid disease presents with goiter, or thyroid enlargement, and in most instances it is obvious that thyroid enlargement is diffuse on physical examination. The exception to this rule occurs when thyroid enlargement is asymmetric, mimicking a focal mass. The main causes of diffuse thyroid enlargement (see Table 46–1) are multinodular goiter, Graves disease, and Hashimoto thyroiditis, and ultrasound practitioners should be particularly cognizant of these conditions, which are emphasized in this chapter. Subacute thyroiditis and Reidel struma are uncommon diffuse thyroid disorders that are mentioned briefly.

Multinodular Goiter

Multinodular goiter is a chronic, slowly developing disorder characterized by the formation of multiple adenomas within the thyroid gland. Since this condition develops slowly over time, it usually is inapparent until the middle years or late in life. Initially, multinodular goiter is euthyroid, and many cases are diagnosed incidentally on physical examination. There is a tendency, however, for hyperthyroidism to develop as a late manifestation, and some cases, therefore, are diagnosed because of thyrotoxic manifestations.

The ultrasound findings in multinodular goiter are true to the name; the gland is diffusely en-

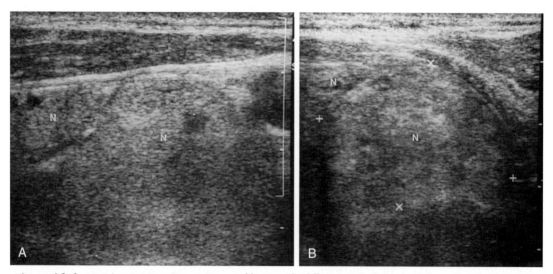

Figure 46-6—Multinodular goiter. A 54 year old man with "fullness" in the left side of the neck. **(A)** A longitudinal view of the right lobe shows two nodules (N). **(B)** A transverse view of the left lobe shows two more nodules (N). On realtime examination, nodules of various sizes were seen throughout the gland, which was grossly enlarged. Cursors, thyroid margins.

larged and studded with numerous discrete nodules (Fig. 46–6) that are iso- or hypoechoic with respect to normal thyroid tissue. The surface of the gland may be distorted by the nodules. The more the gland is scrutinized, the more nodules become apparent. Some nodules may have a surrounding halo, and others may show cystic changes.

Simple or Nontoxic Goiter

The term "simple or nontoxic goiter" refers to diffuse thyroid enlargement without other abnormalities and without hyperthyroidism. The most common example is endemic goiter, which occurs in areas where iodine is deficient in the food supply, but nontoxic goiter may have other causes or may be idiopathic. The enlarged gland initially is homogeneous, which differentiates this condition from multinodular goiter, but there is a tendency for adenomas to form over time, ulti-

mately leading to a multinodular appearance, as described above.

Diffuse Toxic Goiter

Graves disease, or diffuse toxic goiter, refers to generalized thyroid enlargement associated with thyrotoxicosis that usually is severe. Associated eye findings may be present, including proptosis and dysfunction of extraocular muscles. Graves disease is quite different from simple or multinodular goiter. This is a complex autoimmune disease, the etiology of which is not entirely understood.

Ultrasound in Graves disease (Fig. 46–7) reveals diffuse glandular enlargement and uniform decrease in thyroid echogenicity. The surface of the gland may be lobulated, but discrete nodules are absent. These features are consistent with histologic findings principally consisting of diffuse inflammation. A massive increase in vascularity is typical in Graves disease and results in a

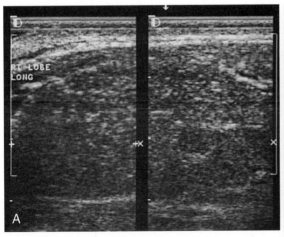

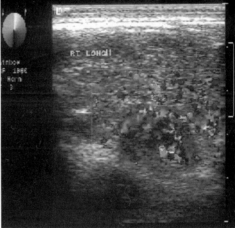

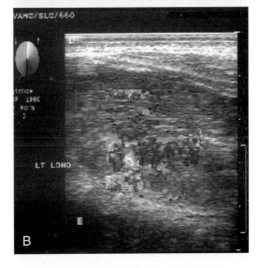

Figure 46-7—Graves disease. (A) A composite longitudinal view shows an enlarged (5 cm long), hypoechoic, and slightly heterogeneous gland. **(B)** Color Doppler images of the right (top) and left (lower) lobes show a massive increase in blood flow, known as the thyroid inferno. See Color Figure 46–7B following page 532.

color Doppler appearance called the "thyroid inferno."[25]

Hashimoto Thyroiditis

Hashimoto thyroiditis is more properly called chronic lymphocytic thyroiditis. This is a fairly common autoimmune disorder, typically seen in young or middle-aged women, that is characterized histologically by lymphomatous infiltration, fibrosis, and the formation of lymphoid follicles. The gland is diffusely enlarged but painless, and the condition often is asymptomatic and diagnosed only because of neck swelling.

Hashimoto disease is characterized sonographically by multiple hypoechoic areas (lymphoid tissue) separated by echogenic, thickened fibrous strands. The result is a bizarre sonographic appearance, without any detectable normal parenchyma. Discrete thyroid nodules and adjacent lymphadenopathy may be detected occasionally. In its end stage, Hashimoto thyroiditis results in diffuse thyroid scarring manifested as a small, ill-defined, heterogeneous gland.

Subacute Thyroiditis

Subacute thyroiditis is an uncommon manifestation of viral infection of the thyroid. The condition often presents following a typical viral infection (flu or upper respiratory), with severe thyroid pain and slight-to-moderate goiter. Sonography shows a hypoechoic, diffusely enlarged gland (Fig. 46–8).

Reidel Thyroiditis

This rare condition is characterized by extensive fibrosis of the thyroid and adjacent structures. Fibrosis develops insidiously, and the heralding signs are compression of structures adjacent to the thyroid, including the trachea, the esophagus, or the recurrent laryngeal nerve. Reidel thyroiditis produces a heterogeneous sonographic appearance, with a poorly defined gland, like the late stages of Hashimoto thyroiditis.

PARATHYROID PATHOLOGY

Practically speaking, the only parathyroid condition of concern to sonologists is adenoma formation, as parathyroid carcinoma is a rare condition.[2] A parathyroid adenoma may occur as a primary disorder in otherwise healthy individuals, and in such cases the clinical manifestations are termed "primary hyperparathyroidism." Parathyroid adenomas also may develop secondary to chronic renal failure, in which case the term "secondary hyperparathyroidism" is used. In either case, the clinical result is elevated serum parathyroid hormone, calcium, and phosphate levels, which are associated with increased osteoclastic activity in bone. Primary hyperparathyroidism almost always is caused by a single parathyroid adenoma. Secondary hyperparathyroidism typically results from hyperplasia of all the glands, but a large adenoma may develop in one or more glands.

Ultrasound Findings

About 70% to 80% of parathyroid adenomas can be detected sonographically by searching carefully for a mass located in the vicinity of the thyroid gland.[5, 26, 27] The great majority of parathyroid adenomas are well defined, hypoechoic, and uniform in texture (Fig. 46–9) and are elongated in the cephalocaudal plane. The hypoechoic appearance is caused by the uniform cellularity of these tumors, without echo-generating interfaces. On occasion, a parathyroid adenoma may be isoechoic or hyperechoic relative to the thyroid, or it may contain internal cystic

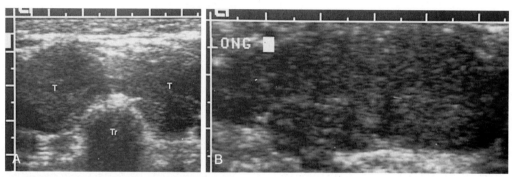

Figure 46-8—Hashimoto thyroiditis. (A) A transverse scan shows massive thyroid (T) enlargement in comparison to the size of the trachea (Tr) (compare with normal proportions shown in Fig. 46–3). Note that the gland is strikingly hypoechoic. **(B)** Longitudinal view of the right thyroid lobe showing generalized hypoechogenicity and minimal heterogeneity.

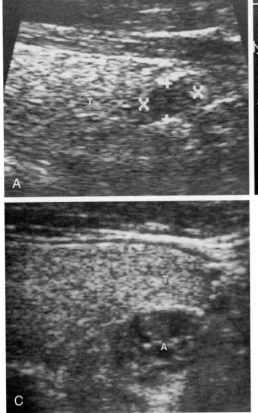

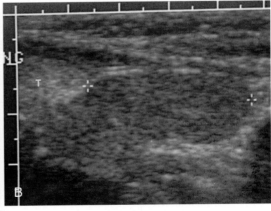

Figure 46-9—Parathyroid adenoma. (A) Longitudinal view of a typical 1-cm parathyroid adenoma (cursors) posterior to the lower pole of the thyroid (T). **(B)** Longitudinal view of a typical 3-cm parathyroid adenoma (cursors) located inferior to the lower thyroid (T) pole. **(C)** Longitudinal view of a slightly echogenic and heterogeneous parathyroid adenoma (A) adjacent to the lower thyroid (T) pole.

spaces. Peripheral vascularity often is visible on color Doppler examination, and this feature helps differentiate between parathyroid adenomas and cervical lymph nodes, which have central vascularity.

Parathyroid adenomas usually are located posterior to the thyroid gland and are near the great vessels of the neck. They may appear imbedded in the thyroid gland, in which case differentiation from a thyroid nodule is difficult. This differentiation is aided in some cases by an echogenic band separating the parathyroid adenoma from the adjacent thyroid. Most parathyroid adenomas are 8 to 15 mm in maximum dimension, but they may be as large as 5 cm in size.[2] Adenomas arising in the upper parathyroid glands usually are located behind the midlevel of the thyroid, whereas lower-gland adenomas are typically located behind or below the lower thyroid poles. Adenomas arising in the lower glands may lie beneath the sternum and in such cases can be seen only with hyperextension of the neck or with swallowing, which transiently elevates the thyroid. If an adenoma is not identified initially, have the patient sip water through a straw and watch for a parathyroid adenoma to appear from beneath the sternum.

As noted at the beginning of this chapter, a small number of parathyroid glands may be located anywhere from the base of the tongue to the level of the thymus. Adenomas in these glands are difficult or impossible to detect with ultrasound, but they may be localized with scintigraphy, magnetic resonance imaging, or computed tomography.

The Role of Ultrasound

In medical centers with experienced parathyroid surgeons, preoperative localization of parathyroid adenomas is not necessary, as morbidity is rare with parathyroidectomy in experienced hands.[2] It may be argued, however, that preoperative localization permits selective surgery on only one side of the neck in patients with primary hyperthyroidism. The role of preoperative localization is limited in secondary hyperthyroidism. Subtotal parathyroidectomy is required in patients with secondary hyperthyroidism, and in these individuals all four glands must be exposed surgically, even if ultrasound shows a large, "dominant" adenoma.

Perhaps the greatest advantage of parathyroid ultrasound occurs in patients with postoperative recurrence of hyperparathyroidism. In this setting, ultrasound can identify 60% to 80% of residual adenomas.[3, 28, 29] Ultrasound is inexpensive and convenient and probably should be used before more expensive imaging procedures. If an adenoma is not identified sonographically in a postoperative patient, then scintigraphy with ^{99m}Tc sestamibi, computed tomography, or magnetic resonance imaging may be used to identify potentially ectopic glands.[2] With this approach, the reoperative success rate is as high as 90%.[3, 28]

A final application of ultrasound for parathyroid adenoma is to guide percutaneous needle insertion for alcohol ablation of the adenoma.[2] As of this writing, alcohol ablation has been successful in obliterating postoperative adenoma recurrences, and this method may have application as a primary mode of therapy. For further details, see references 30 through 33.

REFERENCES

1. Larsen PR, Ingbar SH: The thyroid gland. *In* Wilson JD, Foster DW: Williams' Textbook of Endocrinology. 8th ed. Philadelphia, WB Saunders, 1992, pp 357–487.
2. Hopkins CR, Reading CC: Thyroid and parathyroid imaging. Semin Ultrasound CT MRI 16:279–295, 1995.
3. Price DC: Radioisotopic evaluation of the thyroid and the parathyroids. Radiol Clin North Am 31:991–1015, 1993.
4. Freitas JE, Freitas AS: Thyroid and parathyroid imaging. Semin Nucl Med 24:234–245, 1994.
5. Gooding GA: Sonography of the thyroid and parathyroid. Radiol Clin North Am 31:967–989, 1993.
6. Mills LC: Management of the thyroid nodule. Hahnemann Journal of Medicine, Hahnemann University, Philadelphia, Fall 1978, pp 8–9.
7. Ezzat S, Sarti DA, Cain DR, et al: Thyroid incidentalomas; Prevalence by palpation and ultrasonography. Arch Intern Med 154:1838–1840, 1994.
8. Mazzaferri EL: Thyroid cancer in thyroid nodules: Finding a needle in the haystack. Am J Med 93:359–362, 1992.
9. Gharib H: Final-needle aspiration biopsy of thyroid nodules: Advantages, limitations, and effect. Mayo Clin Proc 69:44–49, 1994.
10. Gharib H, Goellner JR: Fine-needle aspiration biopsy of the thyroid: An appraisal. Ann Intern Med 118:282–289, 1993.
11. Horlocker TT, Hay JE, James EM, et al: Prevalence of incidental nodular thyroid disease detected during high-resolution parathyroid ultrasonography. *In* Medeiros-Neto G, Gaotam E (eds): Frontiers in Thyroidology. Vol 2. New York, Plenum, 1986, pp 1309–1312.
12. Funari M, Campos Z, Gooding AW: MRI and ultrasound detection of asymptomatic thyroid nodules in hyperparathyroidism. J Comput Assist Tomogr 16:615–619, 1992.
13. Brander A, Viikinkoski P, Nickels J, et al: Thyroid gland: Ultrasound screening in middle-aged women with no previous thyroid disease. Radiology 173:507–510, 1989.
14. Bruneton J, Balu-Maestro C, Marcy P, et al: Very high frequency (13 MHz) ultrasonographic examination of the normal neck: Detection of normal lymph nodes and thyroid nodules. J Ultrasound Med 13:87–90, 1994.
15. Akerstrom G, Malmaeus J, Bergstrom R: Surgical anatomy of the human parathyroid glands. Surgery 95:14–21, 1984.
16. Goepfert H, Calender DL: Differentiated thyroid cancer: Papillary and follicular carcinomas. Am J Otolaryngol 15:167–179, 1994.
17. Solbiati L, Volterrani L, Rizzatto G, et al: The thyroid gland with low uptake lesions: Evaluation by ultrasound. Radiology 155:187–191, 1985.
18. Schober O, Muller ST, Schwarzrock R: Zur Bedeutung der Sonographie bei Schilddrusenerkrankungen. *In* Schmidt HAE, Adam WE (eds): Imaging of Metabolism and Organ Function. New York, Schattauer, 1984, pp 752–756.
19. Schwarzrock R, Muller ST, Schober O, Hundeshagen H: Bedeutung der Sonographie für die Diagnose der Schilddrusenmalignome. Akt Endokr Stoffwf:107–120, 1983.
20. Simeone JF, Daniels GH, Hall DA, et al: Sonography in the follow-up of 100 patients with thyroid carcinoma. AJR Am J Roentgenol 148:45–49, 1987.
21. Boland GW, Lee MJ, Mueller PR, et al: Efficacy of sonographically guided biopsy of thyroid masses and cervical lymph nodes. AJR Am J Roentgenol 161:1053–1056, 1993.
22. Livraghi T, Paracchi A, Ferrari C, et al: Treatment of autonomous thyroid nodules with percutaneous ethanol injection: 4-year experience. Radiology 190:529–533, 1994.
23. Goletti O, Monzani F, Lenziardi M, et al: Cold thyroid nodules: A new application of percutaneous ethanol injection treatment. J Clin Ultrasound 22:175–178, 1994.
24. Oommen R, Walter NM, Tulasi NR: Scintigraphic diagnosis of thyroid cancer. Acta Radiol 35:222–225, 1994.
25. Ralls PW, Mayekawa DC, Lee KP, et al: Color-flow Doppler sonography in Graves disease: "Thyroid inferno." AJR Am J Roentgenol 150:780–784, 1988.
26. Reading CC: Thyroid, parathyroid, and cervical nodes. *In* Rifkin MD (ed): Syllabus: Special Course—Ultrasound. Oak Brook, IL, RSNA, 1991, pp 363–377.
27. Wolf RJ, Cronan JJ, Monchik JM: Color Doppler sonography: An adjunctive technique in assessment of parathyroid adenomas. J Ultrasound Med 13:303–308, 1994.
28. Grant CS, van Heerden JA, Charboneau JW, et al: Clinical management of persistent and/or recurrent primary hyperparathyroidism. World J Surg 10:555–565, 1986.
29. Higgins CB: Role of magnetic resonance imaging in hyperparathyroidism. Radiol Clin North Am 31:1017–1028, 1993.
30. Karstrup S, Hegedus L, Holm HH: Ultrasonically guided chemical parathyroidectomy in patients with primary hyperparathyroidism: A follow-up study. Clin Endocrinol 38:523–530, 1993.
31. Solbiati L, Giangrande A, DePra L, et al: Percutaneous ethanol injection of parathyroid tumors under US guidance: Treatment for secondary hyperparathyroidism. Radiology 155:607–610, 1985.

32. Karstrup S, Transbol I, Holm HH, et al: Ultrasound-guided chemical parathyroidectomy in patients with primary hyperparathyroidism: A prospective study. Br J Radiol 62:1037–1042, 1989.

33. Kitaoka M, Fukagawa M, Ogata E, et al: Reduction of functioning parathyroid cell mass by ethanol injection in chronic dialysis patients. Kidney Int 46:1110–1117, 1994.

Chapter 47

Assessment of Breast Lesions

William J. Zwiebel

One of the first medical applications of ultrasound was for the detection of breast lesions, as reported by Wild and Neil in 1951.[1] In this and subsequent work, it was recognized that ultrasound can differentiate between breast cysts and solid masses, and this capability continues to be the most valued contribution of ultrasound to breast lesion diagnosis. During the early 1980s, considerable experimental work was done on ultrasound examination of the entire breast, using water path scanners (Fig. 47–1). It was hoped that this application would increase the detection rate for cancers in radiographically dense breasts. This hope faded with time, however, as it became apparent that both the false-positive and false-negative rates for ultrasound diagnosis were excessive.[2, 3] As a result, ultrasound breast screening has been abandoned, and ultrasound now is used strictly for assessment of mass lesions detected with mammography or physical examination. This restriction does not diminish the value of breast ultrasound, which is evident in the fact that virtually all radiology departments offering mammography also offer adjunctive breast ultrasound.

ANATOMY

The anatomy of the breast is illustrated in Figures 47–1 and 47–2. Note in these figures the presence of Cooper ligaments, which are strongly echogenic and easily seen with ultrasound. Cooper ligaments divide the breast tissue into irregular segments that sometimes resemble mass lesions; furthermore, Cooper ligaments sometimes mimic the appearance of breast cancer (discussed later), for they are highly attenuating and may cast acoustic shadows. Pseudotumors caused by Cooper ligaments probably accounted for most of the false-positive examinations in the days of ultrasound breast "screening."

A second noteworthy feature of breast anatomy is the echogenicity of fat and glandular tissue. Breast fat is markedly hypoechoic, whereas glandular tissue is medium in echogenicity (Fig. 47–1). The hypoechoic appearance of breast fat contrasts sharply with that of intra-abdominal fat, which typically is quite echogenic. The cause of this variance in fat echogenicity has not been evaluated in detail.

Additional important aspects of breast anatomy are illustrated in Figures 47–1 and 47–2, and the reader should review these details before proceeding with the text.

Localization of Breast Lesions

Ultrasound practitioners should be familiar with the customary methods for describing the location of breast lesions. The first method refers to the quadrant in which the lesion is located (upper inner, upper outer, lower inner, and lower outer). The second localizing method is to envision each breast as a clock (while facing the patient), with the nipple at the center. Lesions are described by their location on the face of the imaginary clock. For example, a lesion in the upper outer quadrant of the left breast would be located at 1 or 2 o'clock, and a lesion in the upper outer quadrant of the right breast would be located at 9 or 10 o'clock. A lesion directly above the nipple in either breast would be at 12 o'clock, and so on.

Regardless of the method used for describing the location of a breast lesion, it is essential to ensure that the lesion examined sonographically is in fact the same lesion seen mammographically or palpated by the referring clinician.[4] Of particular concern is the scenario in which a benign cyst visualized with ultrasound is mistaken for a nearby carcinoma, which is visible mammographically but not sonographically. To this end, it is good policy to examine a patient's mammograms immediately before performing breast sonography. Scrutinize the location of the lesion as well as its size and appearance. Be sure that all these features are concordant between the mammographic and sonographic findings. If in doubt, mark the location of the lesion with a metallic skin marker and obtain repeat mammographic views.[4] Alternatively, for breast cysts, the lesion may be drained percutaneously, followed by a repeat mammogram to ensure that it has "disappeared" from view.

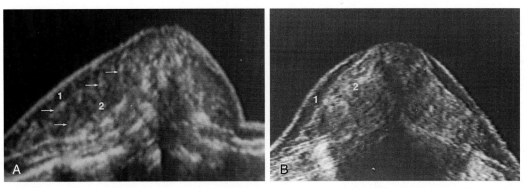

Figure 47-1—Ultrasound breast anatomy (water path scan). Longitudinal (**A**) and transverse (**B**) views illustrate the sonographic anatomy of the breast. The subcutaneous fat (1) is hypoechoic compared with the glandular parenchyma (2). Cooper ligaments (arrows) are seen as curvilinear structures in (**A**). The patient shown in (**A**) is 48 years old; the patient shown in (**B**) is 32 years old. Note that the glandular tissue in (**A**) is less echogenic than that in (**B**) due to fat replacement associated with aging.

ULTRASOUND NONVISUALIZATION

A discrete breast lesion detected by palpation or mammography that cannot be identified with ultrasound should be considered malignant until proved otherwise. One should not assume that a breast mass is benign or nonexistent simply because it cannot be detected with ultrasound, because the ultrasound false-negative rate for palpable lesions is as high as 45% in some studies.[3] It can be argued that these studies were performed with inferior equipment by today's standards,[5] but it is clear, nonetheless, that ultrasound does not detect a substantial number of breast cancers.[3, 4, 6]

ULTRASOUND TECHNIQUE

The patient is examined in the supine position, with the side of the chest to be examined elevated with a triangular sponge or other bolus. Elevating the chest distributes the breast tissue medially, providing a more uniform thickness of tissue and stabilizing the breast somewhat. Without elevation of the chest, the breast tends to fall toward the axilla and is more difficult to examine. A linear array transducer with an output frequency of 7.5 to 10 MHz (or higher) is used. In my institution, the ultrasound examination is focused on the specific area of interest, and unaffected areas of the breast are not examined. This practice eliminates problems with false-positive studies (discussed previously).

APPLICATIONS

The following are widely accepted applications of breast ultrasound:[2–4, 6, 7]

Cyst/Solid Mass Differentiation. The most common and perhaps the most valuable use of ultrasound is to differentiate between cysts and solid lesions detected mammographically. Ultrasound should be used to *prove* that a lesion *thought* to be a cyst is in fact a cyst. There is no point in using ultrasound for a lesion that is thought to be a cancer mammographically as such a lesion must be biopsied regardless of the ultrasound findings. Classic ultrasound cyst features (cited below) prove benignity, and no

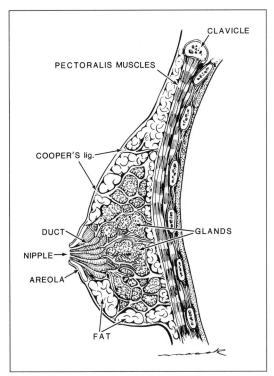

Figure 47-2—Breast anatomy. Note that Cooper ligaments segment the breast parenchyma into irregular chambers.

further follow-up is needed. Ultrasound is said to be 96% to 100% accurate for differentiating between cysts and solid masses in the breast.[3, 7]

Palpable Mass Not Seen Mammographically. When a palpable mass cannot be identified mammographically, ultrasound may be used to determine whether the mass is cystic or solid. As noted, a cystic appearance ensures benignity, but nonvisualization with ultrasound does *not* ensure that the lesion is benign.

Palpable Mass in a Young Woman. In women less than 30 years of age, it is very likely that a palpable breast lesion is benign, and the use of mammography is undesirable due to concerns of increased sensitivity of breast tissue to the carcinogenic effects of irradiation. Ultrasound is used to determine whether a palpable lesion is a cyst, and hence benign, or is solid. If the lesion is solid, then a single-view mammogram may be obtained to look for microcalcifications. The ultrasound and mammographic features then are scrutinized with respect to potential benignity or malignancy.[3, 5] This information, coupled with clinical factors, is used to determine whether the mass can be followed or should be biopsied.

Assessment of the Infected Breast. Ultrasound is an effective means for determining whether a frank abscess, requiring drainage, is present in an infected breast. Breast infection (mastitis) usually occurs in lactating women and causes exquisite pain that may preclude effective physical diagnosis of an abscess.

Guidance for Invasive Procedures. Ultrasound can be used to guide aspiration or core biopsy of mammographically identified lesions and masses that are palpable but not visualized with mammography. Ultrasound also can be used to place localization wires or other appliances for open biopsy of nonpalpable masses.

NON-APPLICATIONS

The use of ultrasound as a screening measure for breast cancer is strongly discouraged for three reasons.[2, 3, 6] First, the false-positive and false-negative rates are excessive. As noted previously, up to 45% of palpable breast masses cannot be identified with ultrasound;[3] furthermore, in one study 25% of nondetected masses were carcinomas.[6] Second, microcalcifications that represent the earliest detectable stages of carcinoma development cannot be seen with ultrasound. Finally, ultrasound screening potentially can reveal large numbers of benign lesions, leading to unnecessary biopsy.[2]

The use of ultrasound for evaluating asymmetric densities seen with mammography also is strongly discouraged.[3] The clinical utility of this application has not been proved, and there is great concern with respect to potential false-negative ultrasound studies.

The use of ultrasound to differentiate between benign and malignant solid masses is gaining popularity, but this application of ultrasound is not universally accepted practice as of this editing. One notable study[5] reported good results for sonographic differentiation of benign and malignant solid lesions, but it is not fully accepted that ultrasound features can make this differentiation reliably. It is common practice to biopsy virtually all breast lesions that are solid on ultrasound examination, but this practice may change within a short time after publication of this work. The reader is advised, therefore, to consult current literature with respect to this issue.[2, 3, 6, 8]

Finally, ultrasound has not been found to have a useful role for assessment of augmented breasts, contrary to some reports that state otherwise.[3]

ULTRASOUND FEATURES OF COMMON BREAST LESIONS

Cysts

Breast cysts occur most frequently between the ages of 35 and 50 years and are the most common palpable breast masses.[9] Ultrasound can detect cysts as small as 2 mm. The classic cyst features that confirm benignity (Fig. 47–3) are the following: (1) an imperceptible wall, (2) a smooth inner surface, (3) anechoic contents, and (4) a strong backwall (far wall) echo or enhanced through-transmission of ultrasound.[2, 3, 9] When these features are evident, a breast cyst can be regarded as benign with 96% to 100% accuracy, and no further evaluation or follow-up is needed. It is *not* necessary to aspirate or biopsy cysts with a benign appearance.

Unfortunately, all breast cysts do not exhibit classic benign features. Some cysts are slightly septate, and others have diffuse or dependent internal echoes. Internal echoes may be spurious artifacts that can be removed by adjusting instrument settings. In other cases, however, echoes are bonafide reflections from debris within the cyst fluid, which may include blood and milk of calcium. In up to 25% of benign cysts, enhanced through-transmission cannot be demonstrated.[9] Finally, some cysts may have thick (and possibly irregular) walls or may contain mural soft tissue nodules, and these cysts are particularly worrisome.

So, what should the sonologist do when an atypical breast cyst is encountered? Unfortu-

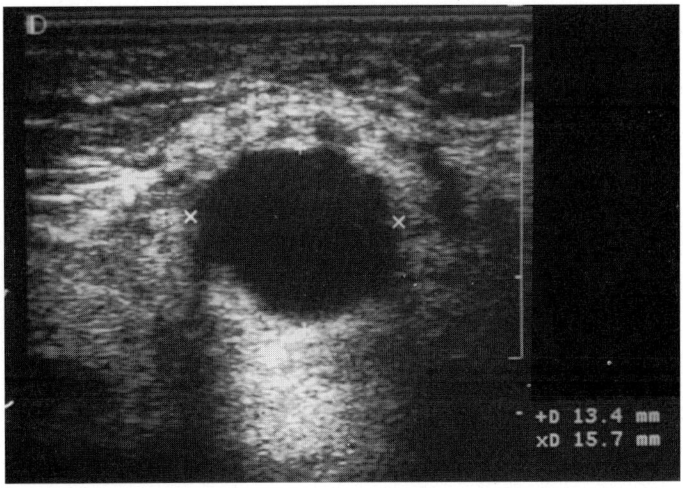

Figure 47-3—Breast cyst.
Ultrasound confirms classic cyst features in a nonpalpable breast mass detected by mammography. The cyst is anechoic, is smoothly marginated, and shows enhanced through-transmission of ultrasound.

nately, there is no clear answer. If echoes disappear with "tuning" of the ultrasound instrument, the operator may be convinced that the lesion meets criteria for benignity. If the cyst is slightly septate, or if the cyst contains dependent debris or debris that moves with agitation, then it appears reasonable to follow the lesion if all other features suggest benignity.[2] If the cyst wall is thick or a mural nodule is suggested, then biopsy is recommended, because such a lesion either may be a carcinoma arising in a cyst or a carcinoma with cystic degeneration.[2] *Cyst aspiration with cytologic analysis does not appear helpful for differentiating benign and malignant cysts.* In one series, cytology was negative in 38% of malignant breast cysts.[10] Pneumocystography may help determine whether a cyst is benign or malignant. In this procedure, the cyst is aspirated percutaneously and filled with air for subsequent mammographic assessment.[10] If the inner surface is smooth or minimally septate, the cyst very probably is benign. If the inner surface is irregular or a mural nodule is present, then the cyst should be biopsied.

Solid Masses

As stated previously, the biopsy of solid breast masses generally is recommended as of this editing, but ultrasound may be used increasingly in the future to ascertain whether a solid lesion has benign characteristics and is amenable to conservative follow-up (without biopsy).[2, 3, 5, 6, 9] Ultrasound practitioners, therefore, should recognize features that suggest benignity or malignancy (Table 47–1). Benign solid masses[2, 3, 5] (Fig. 47–4) tend to be well defined, smoothly marginated, and iso- or hypoechoic relative to glandular tissue. An oval shape is common, with the long

axis of the ovoid *parallel* to the skin. Some benign lesions may be *gently* lobulated or may have a thin, echogenic "pseudocapsule." Intense hyperechogenicity strongly suggests benignity but is an uncommon finding.

Malignant lesions (breast cancers) typically look quite different from benign masses. They are poorly defined and hypoechoic, and because they are markedly attenuating they cast distal acoustic shadows (Fig. 47–5). Additional features suggesting malignancy are branching or spiculated borders, angular margins, calcification, "tethering" of surrounding structures, and thickening or puckering of the overlying skin. Elongated malignant masses typically are oriented with the long axis of the lesion perpendicular to the skin (in contradistinction to a benign lesion). This orientation apparently results from the predilection of cancers to grow along the course of ducts.

Table 47-1. Benign Versus Malignant Appearance of Breast Masses

Benign
    Classic cyst appearance
    Hyperechoic (very likely benign)
    Iso- or hypoechoic, but nonshadowing
    Clearly defined margins
    Smooth or gently lobulated
    Round or ovoid
    Long axis parallel to skin (if ovoid)
    No malignant features
    Long axis of lesion perpendicular to skin
Malignant
    Cyst with a mural nodule
    Hypoechoic
    Distal acoustic shadow
    Poorly defined margins
    Angular, irregular, spiculated, or highly lobular
    Tethering of surrounding structures
    Thickening or puckering of overlying skin

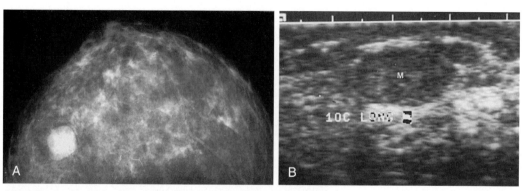

Figure 47-4—Benign solid mass (fibroadenoma). (A) A craniocaudad mammogram shows a well-defined mass located laterally in the left breast. **(B)** Ultrasound shows a homogeneous, well-defined, hypoechoic mass (M) in a corresponding location (1 o'clock [labeled 1 OC]). The size and shape of the mass agreed with the mammographic appearance. Note that the long axis of this benign mass is parallel to the skin.

Pseudomasses

As noted, Cooper ligaments may surround segments of breast parenchyma in such a way as to create a masslike appearance. Such errors can be avoided by examining a lesion in multiple projections and thinking three-dimensionally. If a rounded lesion becomes strikingly triangular as the image plane changes, then an anatomic pseudomass is likely.

Abscesses

Breast abscesses[3, 4] have a variety of appearances. They may be irregular or hypoechoic or contain echogenic debris. Uncomplicated mastitis produces increased parenchymal echogenicity in the affected area, possibly associated with skin thickening. In some cases, multiple small abscesses may be present that are not amenable to drainage. The goal of ultrasound is to differentiate between mastitis that can be treated with antibiotics and an abscess that requires incision and drainage. It is not likely that a breast abscess

large enough to require drainage will be overlooked with ultrasound, but it is possible to mistake a cyst for an abscess.

INTERVENTIONAL PROCEDURES

Ultrasound is an excellent medium for guiding percutaneous biopsy of breast lesions.[3, 6] There are two major forms of biopsy: needle aspiration and core biopsy with an automated cutting needle. The technique recommended for ultrasound-guided breast biopsy is virtually the same as that described for thyroid biopsy in Chapter 46, and the reader is referred to that chapter for further details. Three points specific to breast biopsy should be noted, however. First, 4 to 6 core samples (Fig. 47–6) of solid masses should be obtained (in different parts of the mass) to reduce the possibility of sampling error. Second, the needle should be oriented more or less parallel to the chest wall to avoid inadvertent puncture of the lung and resultant pneumothorax. Finally, direct pressure should be applied to the

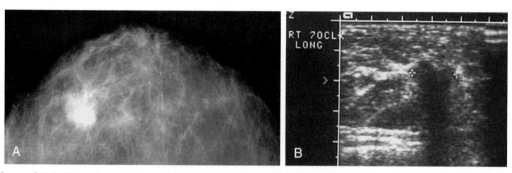

Figure 47-5—Breast cancer (nonpalpable, infiltrating ductal adenocarcinoma). (A) A craniocaudad mammogram of the right breast shows a mass with potentially malignant features, but a cyst could not be excluded on this or other views. **(B)** Ultrasound identified an ill-defined, slightly irregular mass (cursors) that was hypoechoic, yet strongly attenuating. The size and location (7 o'clock) of the mass corresponded precisely with mammographic findings.

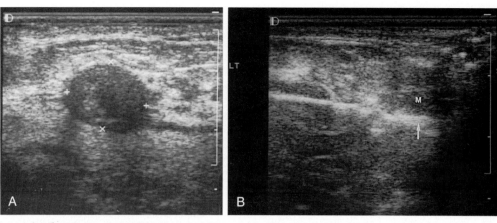

Figure 47-6—Ultrasound-guided breast biopsy of benign mass (focal fat necrosis). (A) Ultrasound demonstrates a well-defined, hypoechoic, but slightly heterogeneous mass (cursors; maximum dimension, 14 mm). This represented a nonpalpable, incidental finding *not* seen mammographically but near a cyst that *was* visible on the mammogram. **(B)** Image obtained during core biopsy shows the needle (arrows) within the mass (M).

biopsy site at the end of the procedure to prevent the formation of a large hematoma. (Ecchymosis and slight tenderness are expected sequelae of breast biopsy.)

REFERENCES

1. Wild LL, Neil D: The use of high frequency ultrasonic waves for detecting changes of texture in the living tissue. Lancet 1:655–657, 1951.
2. Bassett LW, Kimme-Smith C: Breast sonography. AJR Am J Roentgenol 156:449–455, 1991.
3. Jackson VP: The role of US in breast imaging. Radiology 177:305–311, 1990.
4. Venta LA, Dudiak CM, Salomon CG, Flisak ME: Sonographic evaluation of the breast. RadioGraphics 14:29–50, 1994.
5. Stavros AT, Thickman D, Rapp CL, et al: Solid breast nodules: Use of sonography to distinguish between benign and malignant lesions. Radiology 196:123–134, 1995.
6. Gordon PB, Goldenberg SL, Chan NHL: Solid breast lesions: Diagnosis with US-guided fine-needle aspiration biopsy. Radiology 189:573–580, 1993.
7. Reynolds HE, Jackson VP: The role of ultrasound in breast imaging. Appl Radiol 19:55–59, 1991.
8. Jackson VP: Management of solid breast nodules: What is the role of sonography? Radiology 196:14–15, 1995.
9. Ikeda DM, Adler DD, Helvie MA: Breast ultrasound. Appl Radiol 17:19–24, 1991.
10. Tabar L, Pentek Z, Dean PB: The diagnostic and therapeutic value of breast cyst puncture. Radiology 141:659–663, 1981.

Chapter 48

The Scrotum

William J. Zwiebel

ANATOMY

The scrotum is divided into two compartments by a fibrous septum called the median raphe. Each compartment contains a testicle, epididymis, and spermatic cord. The anatomy of the scrotum[1-9] is outlined in Figures 48–1 through 48–4. Please review these figures now as they contain essential information that is not repeated in the text.

From an ultrasound perspective, each testis is homogeneous and medium in echogenicity (Fig. 48–5). The outer border is smooth and well defined. The tunica albuginea, which covers the testis and epididymis and lines the scrotal sac, usually is not resolved but may be seen occasionally as a fine echogenic border surrounding the testis. In adults, each testis measures 3 to 5 cm in length and 2 to 3 cm in diameter.[2, 4] Age-related standards for testicular size in children are available in pediatric textbooks. The testes are relatively hypoechoic before the age of puberty and achieve adult echogenicity thereafter.[5]

The mediastinum testis is seen regularly as a strongly echogenic, longitudinally oriented band running along the posterior aspect of the testis (Fig. 48–5C). On transverse section, the mediastinum may appear solid or may be seen to split into two layers at the surface of the testis. A

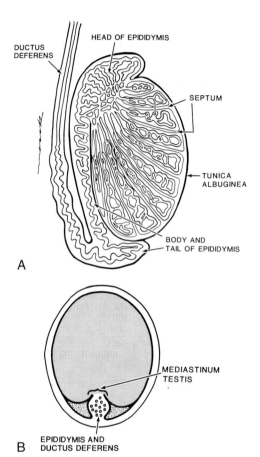

Figure 48-2—Scrotal anatomy. (A) The testis is divided into chambers by fibrous septa (not visible with ultrasound). Myriad seminiferous tubules converge on the epididymis as shown. The epididymis is divided for descriptive purposes into the head (located superiorly), the body, and the tail (located inferiorly). The ductus deferens parallels the epididymis but cannot be identified as a discrete structure on ultrasound images. **(B)** The tunica albuginea lines the scrotal sac, envelops the testis and epididymis, and forms the mediastinum, which contains the body of the epididymis and the ductus deferens. The arrangement is analogous to the chest, in which the pleura lines the chest cavity, envelops the lungs, and encloses the mediastinum.

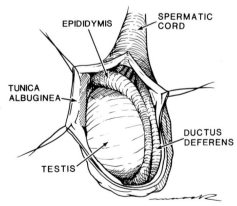

Figure 48-1—Scrotal anatomy. Each testis and epididymis is suspended in a sac formed by the tunica albuginea and the wall of the scrotum (not shown). The tunica albuginea lines the sac and covers the testis, epididymis, and ductus deferens.

prominent hypoechoic band occasionally is seen traversing the testis obliquely, from the mediastinum to the opposite surface. This band is caused by a prominent artery and vein (called the transmediastinal vessels), as is readily apparent with color Doppler.[8, 9]

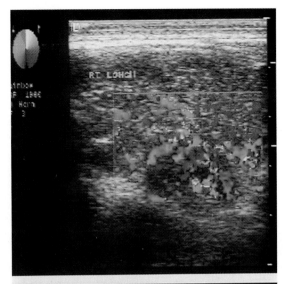

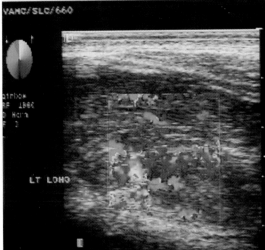

Figure 46-7B—Graves Disease. Color Doppler images of the right (top) and left (lower) lobes show a massive increase in blood flow, known as the thyroid inferno.

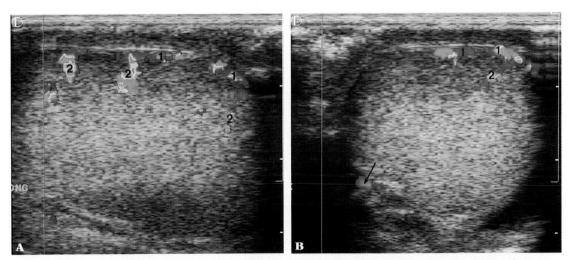

Figure 48-6—Normal Testicular Vessels. (A) Longitudinal and **(B)** transverse images show capsular (1) and centripetal (2) arteries. Flow is visible in the spermatic artery (arrow) within the mediastinum testis.

PLATE VII

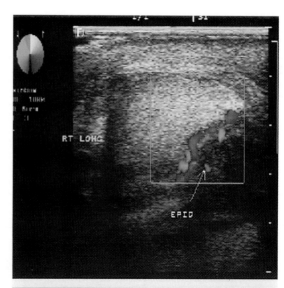

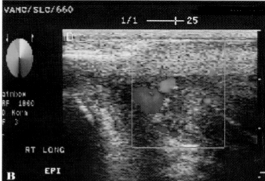

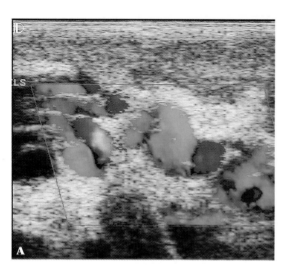

Figure 48-12A—Varicocele. Color Doppler image shows huge serpiginous vessels along the spermatic cord.

Figure 48-14B—Epididymitis. Color flow images show luxuriant flow in the body (upper) and head (lower) of the epididymis.

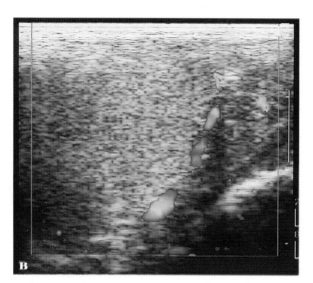

Figure 48-16B—Testicular Torsion. The unaffected testis shows abundant flow that is detected easily.

PLATE VIII

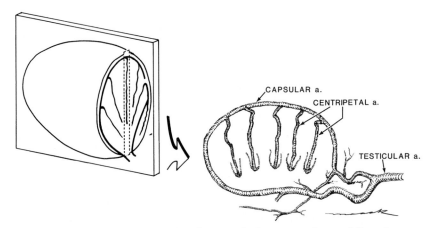

Figure 48-3—Vascular anatomy of the testis. The testicular (or spermatic) artery follows the course of the epididymal body through the mediastinum testis and gives off "capsular" branches that circle *around* the periphery of the testis, beneath the tunica albuginea. The capsular arteries give off centripetal arteries that course through the testis toward the mediastinum and then loop back for a short distance as the recurrent rami. The venous drainage (not shown) parallels the arterial distribution.

The arterial supply and venous drainage of the scrotal contents[6-9] are illustrated in Figures 48–3 and 48–4. Blood vessels are readily seen in and about the testis with color Doppler sonography (Fig. 48–6). The capsular and centripetal arteries are seen most easily, and recurrent rami (branches) are seen occasionally. Flow in the centripetal vessels is from the capsular arteries to the mediastinum. Veins also may be seen within the testis, but it should be noted that the recurrent arterial rami flow in the same direction as the veins and differentiation between these vessels can be made only with spectral Doppler.

Arterial flow in the testis and epididymis characteristically exhibits low-resistance features, including continuous flow in diastole (Fig. 48–6*B*).

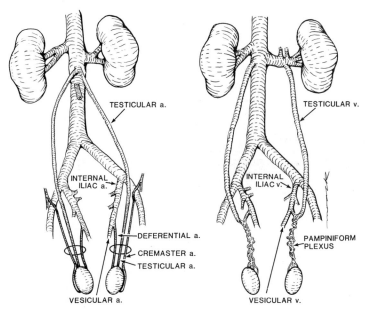

Figure 48-4—Arterial supply and venous drainage of the scrotal contents. Each testicular artery arises from the aorta and extends directly to the testicle and epididymis, following the course of the spermatic cord and the body of the epididymis. The arterial supply to scrotal structures other than the testis and epididymis is via the cremasteric and deferential branches, which originate from the internal iliac arteries, as shown. The principal arterial supply to the testis and epididymis is via the testicular artery, but anastomotic channels exist among all the scrotal arteries, permitting collateral flow. The venous drainage of each testis and epididymis is via a network of tiny veins called the pampiniform plexus. This network gradually coalesces to form two or three veins that follow the spermatic cord and unite as the spermatic vein. On the left, the spermatic vein drains into the ipsilateral renal vein, and on the right, the spermatic vein drains into the inferior vena cava.

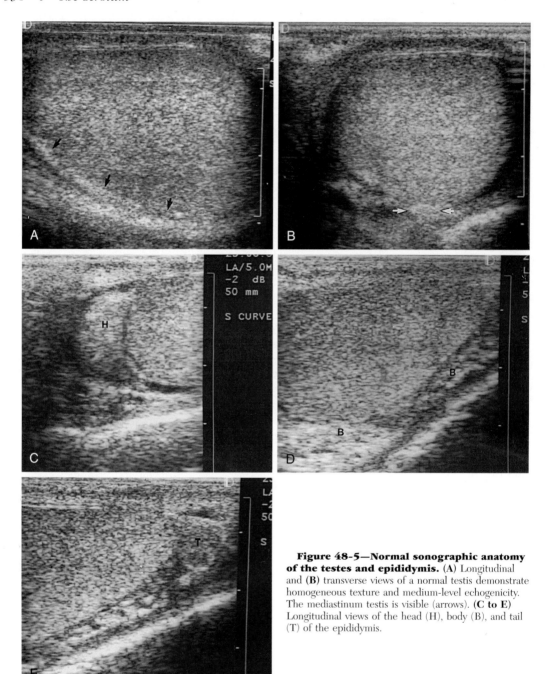

Figure 48-5—Normal sonographic anatomy of the testes and epididymis. (A) Longitudinal and **(B)** transverse views of a normal testis demonstrate homogeneous texture and medium-level echogenicity. The mediastinum testis is visible (arrows). **(C to E)** Longitudinal views of the head (H), body (B), and tail (T) of the epididymis.

In contrast, the flow pattern in extragonadal vessels has high-resistance features. It is important not to mistake extragonadal flow signals for testicular flow. Peak systolic velocity in testicular arteries ranges from 4 to 19 cm per sec (mean, 9.7 cm per sec); end-diastolic velocity from 1.6 to 6.9 cm per sec (mean, 3.6 cm per sec); and the resistivity index ranges from 0.48 to 0.75 (mean, 0.62).[6] These values may be of use occasionally, but in most clinical situations, spectral

Doppler features of testicular flow are assessed qualitatively rather than quantitatively.

SONOGRAPHIC TECHNIQUE

A linear array transducer with a frequency output of 7 to 10 MHz is used to examine the testes. Several scanning approaches may be used. One method is to place towels between the patient's legs to support the scrotum. Another

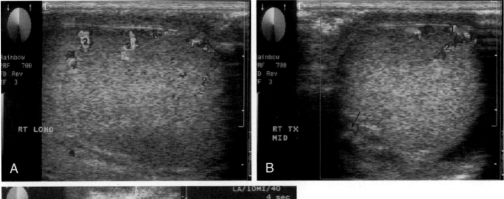

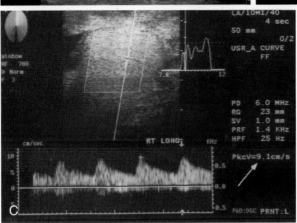

Figure 48-6—Normal testicular vessels. (A) Longitudinal and **(B)** transverse images show capsular (1) and centripetal (2) arteries. Flow is visible in the spermatic artery (arrow) within the mediastinum testis. See Color Figure 48–6*A* and *B* following page 532. **(C)** Normal low-resistance Doppler features of testicular and epididymal flow are shown (arrow; peak systolic velocity is 9.1 cm/sec).

method is to use one hand to hold the scrotum and the other hand to maneuver the transducer. While this method provides optimal control of the movable scrotal contents, it requires the presence of a second individual to operate the ultrasound controls.

The first step in scanning the scrotum is to get oriented. The examiner then obtains a set of scans oriented longitudinal and transverse to the axis of each testis and epididymis. A composite transverse view showing both testes is useful for comparing testicular size. Pathologic findings are portrayed in whatever image plane best documents the abnormality, but longitudinal and transverse views should be used whenever possible as an aid to orientation.

Color Doppler examination must be conducted with the instrument set to detect low-velocity flow (i.e., low pulse repetition frequency). Relatively high-gain settings typically are needed to detect the weak flow signals produced by small testicular vessels.

ULTRASOUND OBJECTIVES

Many ultrasound examinations are performed because a mass is palpated in the scrotum. The principal objective here is to determine the loca-tion of the palpable abnormality, as well as its gross anatomic features. Mass location is important since epididymal masses almost invariably are benign, whereas testicular masses may be malignant. Anatomic features are equally important, since testicular cysts are benign, but solid testicular lesions may be malignant. The simple ability of ultrasound to confirm precisely the location and nature of scrotal pathology is of great clinical utility.

Scrotal swelling is another common indication for scrotal ultrasound. The objective here is to determine whether the scrotal contents are normal or contain pathology accounting for the swollen state. For example, scrotal swelling often is due to hydrocele (the accumulation of fluid in the scrotal sac). A hydrocele may be idiopathic or may be caused by pathology such as a testicular neoplasm. Scrotal swelling also may be caused by large epididymal cysts that are identified readily with ultrasound. Swelling often precludes adequate assessment of the scrotal contents by palpation.

Scrotal pain, often associated with swelling, is another frequent indication for ultrasound. Likely causes are infection (epididymitis or orchitis); a tumor which has bled, producing a painful hematoma; a spontaneous epididymal hematoma;

or testicular torsion. Ultrasound can help with identification of all these conditions.

The final common indication for scrotal ultrasound is trauma. Penetrating injuries must be explored surgically, but closed contusion and crush injuries are treated conservatively, if possible. In many cases, pain and swelling preclude adequate physical examination of the traumatized scrotum, and ultrasound is the only alternative for assessing the condition of the scrotal contents. Of greatest concern is to determine that the testicle is intact and perfused. Testicular fracture or devitalization is an indication for surgical exploration.

TESTICULAR CYSTS

Benign cysts of the testis[2-4] are idiopathic and are common. The incidence of benign cysts increases with patient age, and such cysts are identified in 8% of adults examined sonographically. In most cases a single cyst is present, and it is uncommon to encounter more than three benign cysts in a given individual. Most cysts are 1 cm or less in size, but cysts up to several centimeters in diameter occur occasionally.

Testicular cysts may be divided into two varieties: those located on the surface and those located deeper within the parenchyma. Surface cysts are called tunica cysts, since they are thought to arise in the tunica albuginea. These cysts may be palpable, leading to ultrasound investigation. Deeper cysts are thought to be caused by dilatation of the sperm-collecting tubules, called the rete testes. These are not palpable and occasionally may be seen in association with epididymal cysts.

The most important point about testicular cysts from an ultrasound perspective is to differentiate between these benign lesions and other cystic pathology, including abscesses, hematomas, and cystic neoplasms. Testicular cysts (Fig. 48–7)

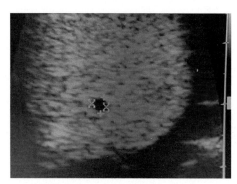

Figure 48-7—Testicular cyst. A testicular cyst (cursors) of less than 3 mm is visible.

may be considered benign if they exhibit the following features: (1) anechoic contents; (2) sharply defined, exquisitely thin, or invisible walls; (3) bright backwall or enhanced through-transmission of ultrasound; and (4) no solid elements. Cysts meeting these criteria may be regarded as inconsequential and require no follow-up.

TESTICULAR TUMORS

Testicular neoplasms are classified and described in Table 48–1.[2, 4, 10] Please review this table to obtain an overview of testicular tumors. Testicular neoplasms occur most frequently between the ages of 25 and 35 years and usually are malignant. The prognosis generally is excellent, however, and 5-year survival is 90% overall with timely use of surgery and radiation or chemotherapy.[10] Testicular tumors usually present in two ways: as a palpable but otherwise asymptomatic mass, or with sudden pain and swelling due to hemorrhage. In some cases the latter presentation follows minor trauma, whereas in others hemorrhage occurs spontaneously. A small number of patients present with signs and symptoms resulting from metastases.

Both lymphatic and hematogenous metastasis may occur with testicular neoplasms. Lymphatic nodal metastasis from the left testis tends to occur at the junction of the left renal vein and inferior vena cava (IVC). Lymphatic nodal metastasis from the right testis is apt to occur along the right lateral surface of the IVC, in the area from the renal vein distally. These locations correspond to the IVC insertion sites of the renal veins. Hematogenous metastasis is usually to the lungs.

The sonographic presentation of testicular neoplasms[2, 10] is nonspecific (Fig. 48–8). They usually are well-defined, hypoechoic lesions with varying degrees of heterogeneity due to hemorrhage, liquefaction necrosis, and calcification. When a mass suggestive of a testicular neoplasm is found, the abdomen should be scanned for evidence of metastasis, with particular attention to the para-aortocaval region (Fig. 48–9).

Whereas ultrasound is almost 100% sensitive in detecting testicular neoplasms and can separate intratesticular and extratesticular pathology with about 98% accuracy,[2] ultrasound cannot differentiate among histologic types of tumors, nor can it differentiate between malignant and benign lesions. These deficiencies notwithstanding, certain features suggest one tumor or another, and these are worth mentioning.[2, 10]

- Seminomas usually are homogeneous, fine grained, and well defined.

Table 48-1. Classification of Testicular Neoplasms

Seminoma	Most common (40%–50% primary testicular cancer). Least aggressive testicular cancer and exquisitely radiosensitive. Tend to occur in older age group
Mixed germ cell tumor	Accounts for 40% of primary testicular neoplasms. Mixture of different germ cell types. Teratocarcinoma/teratoma/embryonal cell carcinoma is most common and is an aggressive tumor
Embryonal cell carcinoma	Most aggressive primary germ cell tumor, as indicated by tunica invasion, testicular contour irregularity, and areas of hemorrhage or necrosis
Teratoma	Benign version of teratoma more common in children; most adult teratomas are malignant, but of low grade.[10] Origin from all three germ cell layers. May contain dermal elements, bone, etc., similar to ovarian teratomas
Choriocarcinoma	Rare but highly malignant. Metastasis often is presenting feature. Hemorrhage and necrosis common
Stromal tumor	Stromal tumors are uncommon but may present with feminizing effects or precocious puberty in children. Leydig cell tumor is the most common member of this class
Lymphoproliferative tumor	Acute leukemia, chronic leukemia, and non-Hodgkin lymphoma commonly involve the testes, especially in children
Metastases	Metastases from aggressive non-lymphoid tumors are uncommon

- Multifocal masses suggest seminoma, lymphoproliferative tumors, or metastases. Seminoma is multifocal within a single testis. Bilateral testicular involvement most commonly occurs with lymphoproliferative tumors (discussed later) and rarely with metastasis of other tumors *to* the testes.

- Extension beyond the tunica albuginea and into contiguous structures suggests a highly aggressive tumor such as embryonal cell carcinoma, choriocarcinoma, or mixed germ cell tumor.

- Teratoma and teratocarcinoma are analogous to their ovarian relatives in that they may contain material from all three germ layers. They commonly are cystic, calcified, and heterogeneous. A teratoma may present as a cyst with a thick, echogenic wall.[10]

Occult Testicular Tumors

As many as 15% of testicular neoplasms present with metastases in the *absence* of a palpable testicular mass.[2] In addition, precocious puberty in boys occasionally may be caused by a testicular neoplasm that cannot be palpated. Ultrasound is an extremely valuable means for locating the primary tumor in both of these cases. On rare occasions, testicular tumor metastasis is diagnosed but testicular ultrasound is negative, or only a small calcified scar is found. These occurrences are attributed to spontaneous regression or "burn-out" of the primary tumor.

Secondary Testicular Tumors

Lymphoproliferative malignancies are the most common secondary tumors of the testes. Acute leukemia involves the testes in 64% of cases, chronic leukemia in 24%, and non-Hodgkin lymphoma in 18.6%.[10] The detection of occult leukemic rests in the testes is of particular importance, as such rests may persist in children even though the bone marrow is free of tumor following treatment. Lymphoproliferative neoplasms usually present with diffuse hypoechogenicity and slight heterogeneity (Fig. 48–10).[2, 10]

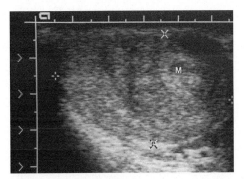

Figure 48-8—Testicular neoplasm. A longitudinal view of the affected testis shows a 1-cm mass (M) surrounded by a hematoma. Patient was a 26 year old man with swelling and pain after minimal trauma. Mixed germ cell tumor.

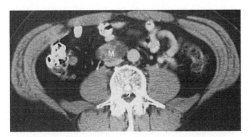

Figure 48-9—Paracaval metastasis (right testicular seminoma). Contrast-enhanced CT scan shows a heterogeneous mass (M) anterior to the inferior vena cava and about 4 cm below the right renal vein (not shown).

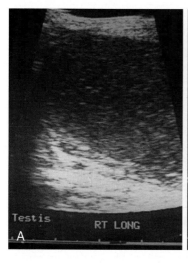
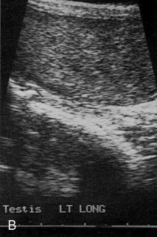

Figure 48-10—Non-Hodgkin lymphoma. (A) The right testicle is enlarged and diffusely hypoechoic due to lymphomatous infiltration. **(B)** The left testicle is normal. Note difference in size and echogenicity.

Involvement usually is *bilateral*, and the testes may be normal in size or enlarged. A second presentation consists of multiple focal hypoechoic areas. Metastasis to the testicles from non-lymphoproliferative tumors is uncommon and may be from a wide variety of sources. The tumor of origin usually is highly malignant.

Testicular Tumor Mimics

As noted earlier, the sonographic appearance of testicular masses is nonspecific, and it is useful, on occasion, to remind the referring practitioner of this fact. Lesions that can mimic the appearance of neoplasms include abscesses, inflamed areas (without frank abscess formation), contusions, hematomas, and infarcts.[1, 2, 10] Two neoplasm mimics are of particular note:

1. Small crescentic lucencies representing focal inflammation may occur in the periphery of the testis adjacent to the epididymis in patients with acute epididymitis.[2]
2. Infarcts can produce hypoechoic lesions. These are peripheral, wedge-shaped (not round), devoid of mass effect, and nonpalpable (soft). They may occur following infection, torsion, or trauma.[1, 2] Tumors, in contrast, are round, hard, and palpable and often have mass effect.

TESTICULAR CALCIFICATION

Two varieties of calcification occur in the testes: macrocalcifications of several millimeters in diameter or punctate microcalcifications.[2, 4] The larger variety are thought to be tumors that have regressed spontaneously, or dystrophic calcification from infarction or infection. The punctate

variety are idiopathic and of no known clinical significance. One or two punctate calcifications are seen occasionally as incidental findings; 10 to 12 are seen rarely; and on very rare occasions innumerable punctate calcifications are found in otherwise normal testes.

UNDESCENDED TESTIS

The incidence of undescended testis is 4% in neonates and less than 1% in adults; nonetheless, failure of testicular migration from the abdominal cavity through the inguinal canal and into the scrotum is significant.[2, 4] The undescended testis is subject to atrophy, infarction, and a 50-fold increase in testicular cancer risk (compared with a fully descended testis). Nondescended testes are bilateral in 10% of cases.

If a testicle fails to descend by 1 year of age, then surgery is recommended to place the testis in the scrotum and thereby prevent the aforementioned complications. About 80% of undescended testes are palpable. The main value of ultrasound is in localizing those that are nonpalpable, and the success rate in this endeavor is high (80% to 97%).[2, 4] The search for an undescended testis should begin at the scrotum and proceed upward through the inguinal canal and then into the pelvis. Most undescended testes are located in the inguinal canal and below the inguinal ring, accounting for the high rate for ultrasound detection. An ovoid, hypoechoic soft tissue mass should be sought. If the testis has remained undescended for a long period, it may be atrophic and much smaller than expected for the patient's age.

A second role for ultrasound is surveillance for tumor development in undescended testes in older individuals who have not been treated surgically. Such surveillance should continue until age 35 years, after which the risk of cancer decreases.[2] If the patient has both an undescended and a descended testis, both should be examined as there is increased risk for tumor development in the descended testis, as well as in the undescended testis.

EPIDIDYMAL MASSES

Whereas testicular masses are often malignant, epididymal masses almost invariably are benign, and most are cysts.[2, 4, 10] One or more epididymal cysts may be found in about 40% of adult men examined sonographically.[2] Most are located in the epididymal head, but they may occur anywhere in the epididymis. In some cases they are palpable; in other cases they are found incidentally. They may be single, multiple, unilateral, or bilateral. Some may be clustered and multilocular. Extensive epididymal cyst formation may mimic the appearance of a loculated hydrocele, as discussed later. Most epididymal cysts are 2 to 3 mm in diameter, but larger cysts are common, and some may be several centimeters in size. They usually are anechoic on ultrasound and have invisible walls, as seen in Figure 48–11. The etiology of epididymal cysts is not entirely clear. Some may represent spermatoceles, which are encapsulated collections of sperm. It is said that epididymal cysts containing diffuse or dependent echoes probably are spermatoceles, but this hypothesis has not been proved.

Tumors of the epididymis are exceedingly rare,[2, 4, 10] and besides cysts, the only common lesions of the epididymis are inflammatory masses and hematomas. Inflammatory masses are discussed later in this chapter. Hematomas of the epididymis or cord usually occur in the context of trauma but may occur spontaneously or in association with vigorous exercise. An epididymal hematoma usually presents as a hard, palpable (and possibly tender) mass that may mimic a testicular neoplasm. Alternatively, scrotal pain from the hematoma may mimic testicular torsion. On ultrasound examination, a hematoma has a hypoechoic or heterogeneous appearance and clearly is extratesticular. In some cases, the hematoma may have multiple locules of differing echogenicity. A varicocele (discussed next) is a common associated finding, suggesting that rupture of a varix may be the cause in some cases.

VARICOCELE

Another common cause of epididymal mass is a varicocele, or dilatation of the "pampiniform plexus" of veins that drain the testis and epididymis.[2–4] These veins normally are quite small but for unknown reasons dilate in some individuals, forming a tangle of large veins that accompanies the spermatic cord and may extend along the course of the epididymis. In some cases, dilated veins may even extend into the substance of the testis. Varicoceles are more common on the left side of the scrotum than the right, and this predilection may relate in some undefined way to the insertion of the left spermatic vein into the left renal vein. The right renal vein generally drains into the inferior vena cava. In some individuals, a varicocele contributes to low sperm count and infertility. Persistent elevation of testicular temperature, due to hyperemia, is the postulated cause, but the exact cause is unknown.

In most instances, varicocele is a clinical diagnosis, as the tangle of veins is easily palpated and feels like a "bunch of worms." Ultrasound is required when the nature of the palpable mass is unclear, and it also is helpful in some infertile men in whom the presence or absence of varicocele cannot be determined by palpation. In any case, varicocele is diagnosed with color Doppler ultrasound if a large number of veins of unusually large size are seen in the spermatic cord or epididymis (Fig. 48–12). Normal veins are 2 mm or less in size,[4] but this appears to be a somewhat arbitrary number, and the diagnosis of varicocele is based more on judgment than on individual vein size.[3] Straining or the Valsalva maneuver may be required to maximally distend the veins. Varicoceles frequently are incidental findings on ultrasound examination and should not be confused with other pathology.

HYDROCELE

The term "hydrocele" refers to the accumulation of an abnormal volume of fluid in the scro-

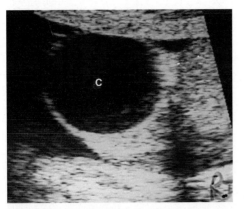

Figure 48-11—Epididymal cyst (C). The margins are smooth, and enhanced through-transmission of ultrasound is evident. Note dependent low-level echoes.

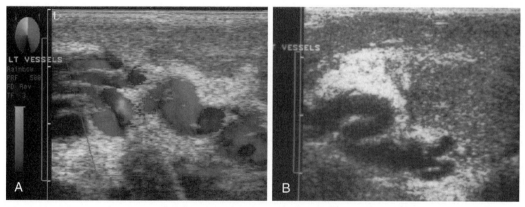

Figure 48-12—Varicocele. (A) Color Doppler image shows huge serpiginous vessels along the spermatic cord. See Color Figure 48–12A following page 532. **(B)** Black-and-white image of large vessels in the epididymis.

tum.[1-4] Hydrocele is the most common cause of scrotal swelling and is a normal finding in utero and in neonates. Hydroceles presenting in adults often are idiopathic, but they also can result from infection, tumor, torsion, infarction, or trauma. In an idiopathic or uncomplicated hydrocele, the fluid typically is anechoic, and the testicle appears to "swim" within a water bath (Fig. 48–13A).

So-called "complicated hydroceles" contain proteinaceous material, blood, or purulent debris. These may be highly loculated, and it may be hard to differentiate between a loculated hydrocele and multiple large epididymal cysts. The key point here is that a hydrocele substantially surrounds the testis whereas epididymal cysts tend to displace the testis. In addition to locula-

tion, complicated hydroceles may exhibit diffuse, fine-grained echogenicity or dependent echogenic debris. Infected hydroceles typically are attended by findings of epididymo-orchitis, as discussed next. Postsurgical hydroceles that contain a large amount of blood may have a bizarre, multilocular appearance, as seen in Figure 48–13B. On rare occasions, chronic hydroceles may exhibit moderate or high levels of echogenicity due to the presence of proteinaceous material or cholesterol crystals within the fluid.

INFECTION OF THE SCROTAL CONTENTS

Infection is the most common cause of acute scrotal pain and tenderness. In the great majority

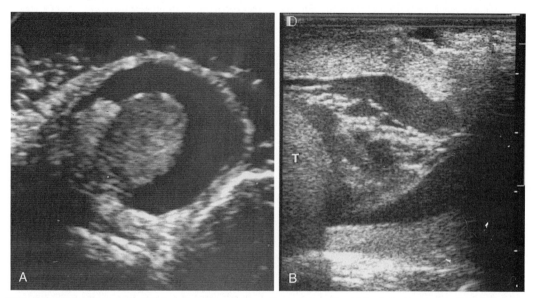

Figure 48-13—Hydrocele. (A) A water path scan shows the testicle and epididymis "swimming" in fluid. **(B)** A loculated, postsurgical hydrocele is present inferior to the testis (T).

of cases, the scrotal contents are infected[1, 3, 4, 7] by sexually transmitted organisms (principally *Neisseria gonorrhoeae* and *Chlamydia trachomatis*) that "ascend" through the genital tract. The tail of the epididymis is infected first and then the infection spreads throughout the epididymis (epididymitis). The infection may then extend to the testis (orchitis). Finally, the organism may spread to the scrotal cavity, generating an infected hydrocele.

Besides the usual sexually transmitted infections, the scrotal organs may be infected hematogenously by *Treponemas (T. pallidum)*; by fungi, including *Blastomyces, or, Coccidioides*; by *Mycobacterium tuberculosis;* and by the mumps virus. Hematogenous infections such as mumps may produce orchitis without epididymitis. Noninfectious epididymo-orchitis occurs rarely and is caused by reaction to medications such as the cardiac drug amiodarone.

Our discussion of the ultrasound manifestations of scrotal infection will be confined to the common sexually transmitted infections. Ultrasound is a useful method for confirming the diagnosis of epididymitis or orchitis and for excluding other pathology that may cause acute scrotal pain or swelling. The principal findings are enlargement and decreased echogenicity of the affected structures, accompanied by increased blood flow on color or spectral Doppler examination (Fig. 48–14).[1, 4, 7] In some cases, only the epididymis is involved, whereas in others, both the epididymis and testis may be infected. A small hydrocele usually is present, and in some cases the scrotal wall may be inflamed and thickened. If only one epididymis/testis is infected, marked differences in organ size and blood flow are evident from one side of the scrotum to the other. Finally, a focal, hypoechoic area of inflammation may be seen occasionally in the periphery of the testis, adjacent to an infected epididymis, and this may mimic a testicular tumor, as noted previously.

Most cases of epididymo-orchitis are treated successfully and resolve, but untreated or undertreated cases may present with finding of chronic epididymitis or abscesses. Chronic epididymitis is manifested as diffuse thickening and heterogeneity of the epididymis. Hydrocele usually is present as well, and this may be loculated or may contain echogenic material. Abscesses may occur in the epididymis or testis in patients with chronic infection. These appear as heterogeneous masses (Fig. 48–15) or as fluid collections

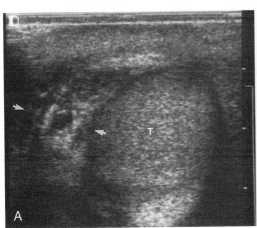
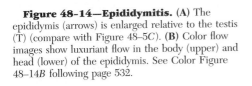
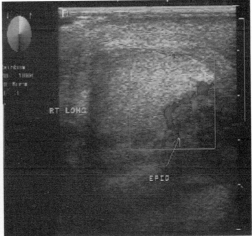
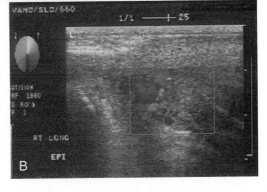

Figure 48-14—Epididymitis. (A) The epididymis (arrows) is enlarged relative to the testis (T) (compare with Figure 48–5C). **(B)** Color flow images show luxuriant flow in the body (upper) and head (lower) of the epididymis. See Color Figure 48–14B following page 532.

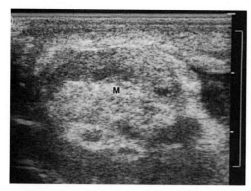

Figure 48-15—Chronic abscess. Patient is a 50 year old man with a tender mass above the right testis for 2 to 3 weeks. A 2- × 3-cm, heterogeneous mass (M) is visible in the epididymis. After the patient underwent an unsuccessful course of antibiotic therapy, surgery revealed a chronic abscess.

with irregular walls and perhaps with diffuse or dependent debris. If an abscess is confined to a testicle, it may easily be mistaken for a tumor with central hemorrhage or necrosis, unless the clinical history specifically suggests infection.

TESTICULAR TORSION

Torsion refers to twisting of the testis within the scrotal sac, such that the supply and drainage vessels are compressed and the blood supply to the testis is cut off.[1, 3, 4, 7, 11] Torsion results from abnormal mobility of the testis, due in turn to deficient or absent attachment of the mediastinum testis to the scrotal wall. Torsion usually occurs in children or young adults, and two peaks of incidence have been noted: the neonatal period and puberty. Although scintigraphy continues to be utilized for diagnosis of testicular torsion, Doppler ultrasound has become the predominant diagnostic method. Ultrasound is 86% to 100% sensitive and virtually 100% specific in the diagnosis of testicular torsion.[11]

The pathologic consequences of testicular torsion are divided into four phases, as outlined in Table 48–2.[4] Of greatest importance is the acute phase, which encompasses the first 6 hours after torsion has occurred.[1, 4, 7] If the testis is detorsed during this period, then viability may be restored.

During this phase, the testis is normal in size or enlarged and is hypoechoic (compared with the opposite testis) due to congestion. A small hydrocele may be present, and the scrotal wall may be swollen. The initial effect of testicular torsion is restriction of venous drainage, which is followed in turn by restriction of arterial flow. The testicle initially becomes engorged with blood as a result of venous occlusion, which is why it usually is swollen and hypoechoic on ultrasound examination. Doppler findings are key to the diagnosis of testicular torsion (Fig. 48–16).[1, 4, 7, 11] On color Doppler examination, blood flow is visibly diminished or absent in the torsed testis (as compared with the opposite testis). Spectral Doppler either shows absence of blood flow or damped, low-amplitude signals in the torsed testicle.

Two pitfalls are noteworthy with respect to testicular torsion diagnosis.[1, 4, 11] First, blood flow is cut off completely in the affected testis only with fairly marked levels of torsion. With torsion of 360 degrees or less, Doppler diagnosis is based on qualitative differences in arterial flow signals in the affected and unaffected testes. These differences may be subtle or even absent.[11] Second, a torsed testis may undergo spontaneous detorsion followed by a period of hyperemia. If the testis is examined during the hyperemic period, increased blood flow might be mistaken for orchitis.[4]

SCROTAL TRAUMA

As noted earlier, penetrating scrotal trauma generally requires surgical exploration and is not the subject of ultrasound examination. Ultrasound is extremely useful, however, in concussion or crush injuries of the scrotum that are difficult to evaluate clinically because of pain and scrotal swelling.

The primary role of ultrasound in scrotal trauma is to determine whether the testes are intact and whether nonviable tissue is present.[1, 7, 12] Improved salvage of traumatized testes can be achieved if testicular rupture is recognized early and treated surgically.[12] Blunt injuries of the scrotum may result in contusion, laceration, or complete fracture of a testicle. Contusion pro-

Table 48-2. Stages of Testicular Torsion

Acute	Initial 6 hours	Congestion; hypoechoic, possibly enlarged
Early subacute	1–4 days	Congestion, liquefactive necrosis; hypoechoic, enlarged, anechoic areas
Late subacute	5–10 days	Gradual decrease in findings
Chronic	> 10 days	Testis small and hypoechoic; epididymis enlarged and hyperechoic

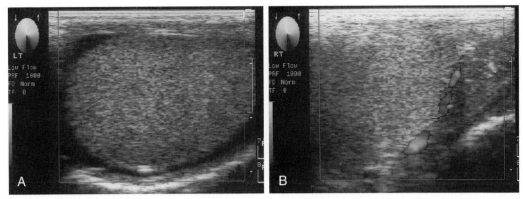

Figure 48-16—Testicular torsion. (**A**) No flow is evident in the affected testicle. A small hydrocele is present. (This testicle was slightly hypoechoic on realtime examination, but this cannot be appreciated here.) (**B**) The unaffected testis shows abundant flow that is detected easily. See Color Figure 48–16*B* following page 532.

duces testicular swelling as well as heterogeneous or hypoechoic areas caused by tissue damage and hemorrhage. With laceration, a break is visible internally and perhaps on the testicular surface. With fracture, two or more isolated portions of the testis are present. The blood supply may be compromised to one or more of the testicular fragments, and Doppler ultrasound is a convenient way to assess this possibility.

The epididymis also may be injured, and in such cases it may be swollen and heterogeneous due to hemorrhage. A large hematocele typically is present in trauma patients due to hemorrhage from the testis or other scrotal contents. An acute hematocele is homogeneous, and the fluid is echogenic to varying degrees. Subacute hematoceles are heterogeneous due to clot formation and the extrusion of serum from the clot. A chronic hematocele is represented as a loculated fluid collection, which in some cases may have a bizarre appearance.

REFERENCES

1. Tumeh SS, Benson CB, Richie JP: Acute diseases of the scrotum. Semin Ultrasound CT MRI 12:115–130, 1991.
2. Doherty FJ: Ultrasound of the nonacute scrotum. Semin Ultrasound CT MRI 12:113–156, 1991.
3. Watson LR, Abbitt PL, Woodard LL, Howard SS: Applied scrotal sonography. Appl Radiol 20/12:27–35, 1991.
4. Gerscovish EO: High-resolution ultrasonography in the diagnosis of scrotal pathology: I. Normal scrotum and benign disease. J Clin Ultrasound 21:355–373, 1992.
5. Hamm B, Fobbe F: Maturation of the testis: Ultrasound evaluation. Ultrasound Med Biol 21:143–147, 1995.
6. Middleton WD, Thorne DA, Melson GL: Color Doppler ultrasound of the normal testis. AJR Am J Roetgenol 152:293–297, 1989.
7. Horstman WJ, Middleton WD, Melson GL, Siegel BA: Color Doppler US of the scrotum. RadioGraphics 11:941–957, 1991.
8. Middleton WD, Bell MW: Analysis of intratesticular arterial anatomy with emphasis on transmediastinal arteries. Radiology 189:157–160, 1993.
9. Fakhry J, Khoury A, Barakat K: The hypoechoic band: A normal finding on testicular sonography. AJR, Am J Roentgenol 153:321–322, 1989.
10. Gerscovich EO: High resolution ultrasonography in the diagnosis of scrotal pathology: II. Tumors. J Clin Ultrasound 21:375–386, 1993.
11. Frush DP, Babcock DS, Lewis AG, et al: Comparison of color Doppler sonography and radionuclide imaging in different degrees of torsion in rabbit testes. Acad Radiol 2:945–951, 1995.
12. Lupetin AR, King W, Rich PJ, Lederman RB: The traumatized scrotum. Radiology 148:203–207, 1983.

Index

ISBN 0-7216-6947-6

90038

9 780721 669472